Encounters wit

CHILDREN

Pediatric Behavior and Development

Visit our website at **www.mosby.com**

Encounters with
CHILDREN

Pediatric Behavior and Development

SUZANNE D. DIXON, M.D., M.P.H.

Emeritus Professor of Pediatrics
University of California, San Diego, La Jolla, California;
Clinical Faculty, University of Washington, Seattle, Washington;
Great Falls Clinic, Great Falls, Montana;

MARTIN T. STEIN, M.D.

Professor of Pediatrics
Director, Developmental and Behavioral Pediatrics
University of California, San Diego
La Jolla, California

THIRD EDITION

Mosby

St. Louis Baltimore Boston Carlsbad Chicago Minneapolis New York Philadelphia Portland
London Milan Sydney Tokyo Toronto

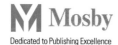
Dedicated to Publishing Excellence

Acquisitions Editor: Liz Fathman
Developmental Editor: Peggy Perel
Project Manager: Patricia Tannian
Production Editor: Gail Stobaugh
Design Manager: Gail Morey Hudson
Cover Design: Teresa Breckwoldt
Cover Illustration: Michelle E. Lambert

THIRD EDITION

Mosby, Inc.
A Harcourt Health Sciences Company
11830 Westline Industrial Drive
St. Louis, Missouri 63146

Printed in the United States of America

International Standard Book Number 0-323-00253-6

99 00 01 02 03 CL/QF 9 8 7 6 5 4 3 2 1

CONTRIBUTORS

SUZANNE D. DIXON, M.D., M.P.H.
Emeritus Professor of Pediatrics, University of California, San Diego, La Jolla, California;
Clinical Faculty, University of Washington, Seattle, Washington;
Behavioral and Developmental Pediatrics, Great Falls Clinic, Great Falls, Montana;
Medical Director and Editor, The Parenting Institute

MARIANNE E. FELICE, M.D.
Professor and Chair, Department of Pediatrics, University of Massachusetts Medical School;
Pediatrician-in-Chief, University of Massachusetts Memorial Children's Medical Center
Worcester, Massachusetts

LAWRENCE S. FRIEDMAN, M.D.
Associate Professor, Pediatrics and Medicine
Chief, Division of Primary Care Pediatrics and Adolescent Medicine
University of California, San Diego, La Jolla, California

MICHAEL J. HENNESSY, M.D.
Orthopedic Surgeon, Great Falls Clinic
Great Falls, Montana

SUSAN L. INSTONE, M.D., D.N.Sc., C.P.N.P.
Assistant Professor of Nursing, Hahn School of Nursing & Health Sciences
University of San Diego, San Diego, California

JENNIFER MAEHR, M.D.
Instructor of Pediatrics, University of Maryland at Baltimore
Baltimore, Maryland

NANCY MANN, M.D.
Pediatric Coordinator, Department of Family Medicine, Idaho State University
Pocatello, Idaho

PHILIP R. NADER, M.D.
Professor of Pediatrics, Chief, Division of Community Pediatrics, University of California, San Diego
La Jolla, California

MARTIN T. STEIN, M.D.
Professor of Pediatrics, Director, Developmental and Behavioral Pediatrics, University of California, San Diego
La Jolla, California

MARIA TROZZI, M.D.
Assistant Professor of Pediatrics, Boston University School of Medicine;
Director of the Good Grief Program, Boston Medical Center
Boston, Massachusetts

YVONNE VAUCHER, M.D., M.P.H.
Professor of Pediatrics, University of California, San Diego
La Jolla, California

ROBERT DAVID WELLS, Ph.D.
Associate Professor of Pediatrics, and Psychiatry, University of California, San Francisco
San Francisco, California

JOHN B. WELSH, M.D.*
Professor of Pediatrics, University of California, San Diego
La Jolla, California

*Deceased

FOREWORD TO THE FIRST EDITION

This is a wonderful, timely book. Written for primary care practitioners who care for children and their families, it will meet an increasing need in pediatric care. At a time when the Task Force of the American Academy of Pediatrics has recommended a knowledge of child development for all pediatricians, when the American Nursing Association has developed a career for graduate nurses in primary care (the Pediatric Nurse Practitioner), and at a time when the public is for more support and guidance in parenting roles, the Committee on Psychosocial Development of Children and Families of the Academy of Pediatrics has published a series of guidelines for primary care physicians to enhance their attention to child and family development on routine visits to their caregiver. These guidelines are a help, but they need just such a volume as this to enhance their meaning and their value. The "lists" of items to be identified at these routine visits will be of no value to either pediatrician or targeted family unless they form a bridge for communication between the physician and parents and child. If the questions are asked simply as questions, the parents will feel bombarded by a new set of demands to answer in a relatively meaningless fashion. The already-too-pathological model of looking for and identifying failures in the parent will be made into a longer list by developmental questions aimed at looking for failure in the child and in the parent. If, on the other hand, with this textbook as a backdrop, the primary caregiver can participate in the enormous richness of the child's and parent's development as his or her area to share with families, he or she will feel the excitement of the developing child and family. If he or she can understand and participate in the emotional and cognitive development of the child as well as in his* physical development, the caregiver will feel the rewards of a deepening relationship with the parents in his or her care, for the child's development is the language of the parent. If the caregiver demonstrates a real understanding and gives a sense of caring for these aspects of the child's development, every parent will feel supported and cared for. In these days, new parents are no longer backed up by extended families, by strong cultural belief systems, or by support systems which are meaningful in the area about which they care the most—becoming a successful parent. As women must go to work (and over half of mothers of young children are in the work force now), their need for backup, for information, and for guidance in their precious job of childrearing is even greater. It is a time when we, as caring physicians and PNPs, can play a vital role in advo-

---

*For simplicity's sake, I shall use the masculine pronoun for the child, the feminine for the parent.

cacy for the child and in enhancing the joy and assurance of the parenting role. Our opportunity to play a vital role in the family with attention to anticipatory guidance is out of proportion to the time and effort it will take from us. Each routine visit will become valued and valuable to us, as well as to parents. If we indeed transmit a sense of caring, of joining in each parent's job of parenting, we can establish rewarding roles for ourselves.

Having been in pediatric practice for 35 years now, I know that I personally would have "burned out" 25 years ago if I had not shared the child's development as a mutual goal with parents in my care. The quest for physical disease and for physical milestones is too sparse and unrewarding for most active minds at routine visits. They all too quickly become "routine." But the kind of shared knowledge and the kind of relationships with each family which this book will enhance at each visit can make the practice of primary care an act and a pleasure.

In Stein's chapter on interviewing, he displays the respect for children which underlies each subsequent chapter. He and Dixon give one a real sense of "how" to make and keep a working relationship with each set of parents at each visit. For it is within the context of relationships that a caregiver can be of any meaningful help to parents. Also, as the relationship deepens over time, the shared values deepen. I find that I no longer need to search for meaningful questions with the patients with whom I have developed a relationship. They bring me the important questions all too readily. Hence, each visit should be seen as an opportunity to strengthen and deepen the relationship between you and the parents. This is the reason why the child's development is such a critical ground for shared understanding.

Enhancing your relationship is also a reason for being sure that you hit "paydirt" in at least one area at each visit. You can recognize "paydirt," for the parent will lean forward, her face will become intense as her involvement with what you are saying becomes more and more obvious. I always try to be sure that I touch on one meaningful area for each parent and that I provide an opportunity for her (and him) to share the intensity of her own feelings as we approach such an area. With this concept of paydirt in mind, the concept of anticipatory guidance is a powerful one, because every parent will recognize her need for information and support you are offering as she approaches a new development phase in the child. If she can share her own feelings and anxiety with you as you share your development knowledge with her, you will be of real value to her.

Coincident with our capacity for conquering and preventing physical disease, we are becoming more sensitized to our capacity for the prevention of psychological disorders and for improving the quality of life for the children in our care. Prevention, intervention, and quality of life are becoming catchwords in pediatrics. Plasticity, the capacity of a developing organism to find pathways around a deficit or to recover from an insult, is a concept we can all utilize in pediatrics if we are aware of its forces and have a deeper understanding of its mechanisms in development. This book can provide such an understanding for pediatricians and for nurse practitioners.

The format of each chapter is economical and helpful. The theoretical base for the developmental processes which can be profitably addressed at each stage of development is excellent. The attention to deepening the relationship with parents and child is accompanied by specific questions which will help the practitioner. The section on what to observe, how to observe is followed by specific suggestions of how to share this with parents at each visit in infancy and toddlerhood. Sharing the developmental exam with parents is the most powerful way of achieving an effective working relationship to improve the child's outcome that I have found. I can then couch advice and anticipatory guidance without threat to our relationship or to the parent's feeling of competence because we have shared this mutually satisfying observation. I need this kind of communication at each visit. These chapters by Dixon, Stein, and Kaiser are rich in these values for all those involved in primary care.

Stein prepares us in the perinatal period for preventing the "vulnerable child syndrome." Dixon says "parents of premature infants are premature, too." Kaiser addresses the important issue of mothers dealing with sibling rivalry in the post partum period. Each chapter addresses the cognitive and social progress of the child and the appropriate parental responses, which one can elicit at each well baby visit. The meaning and use of stranger anxiety at 8 months, of magic and fantasies in the third and fourth years are beautiful essays and should be read by all who are interested in small children.

Putnam and Nader address the issues of the preschool and school-aged child in the same valuable format. Pediatric practitioners will not only better understand the developmental issues, but the practical questions and observations of each area which should be addressed are clear and helpful.

Marianne Felice outlines the issues of preadolescence and adolescence for practitioners in a sympathetic way which will allow us to respect the adolescent's turmoil and need for privacy, but which will also help us to enhance our relationship with him and to address his issues in a straightforward, helpful manner. I find that adolescents with whom I've grown up are extremely grateful for my continued deep involvement with them. Although they may guard themselves with me from time to time, they use me in crises—drugs, sex, and other acting out periods—and remember my caring relationship later by bringing their own children to me. I now have more grandchildren than children in my practice. A real reward for all these years!

The last two chapters are as helpful as any in the book. The chapter on which books to have available by Felice, Caffery and Kaiser is very good. The marvelous chapter on children's drawings—their meaning and their use in enhancing a pediatrician's relationship with his parents—is by John Welsh, a pediatrician practicing for 35 years. It is not only delightful but also insightful and wonderful in presenting a whole new system for communication for diagnostic work with children.

I wish I'd written this book, for it is sure to be a classic for pediatric practitioners. In their famous longitudinal study of the development of temperament, Thomas and colleagues found that the relationships of families with the observer pediatricians proved to be amazingly effective in alleviating potential psychological problems: 68% of the patients with mild or moderate symptoms improved markedly and 50% with real psychopathology improved with their team's preventive approach. I believe that pediatricians and pediatric nurse practitioners are in a unique position to provide the kind of relationship, insight, and therapeutic support which most parents will utilize to prevent disorders in their children. But pediatricians will need an understanding of normal development and of establishing supportive relationships in working with families to do that. This volume will go a long way toward providing that for primary caregivers.

T. Berry Brazelton, M.D.

Professor of Pediatrics
Harvard School of Medicine
Chief, Child Developmental Unit
Children's Hospital Medical Center
Boston, Massachusetts

BIBLIOGRAPHY

Brazelton TB: Anticipatory guidance. *Pediatr Clin North Am* 1975;22:553.

Brazelton TB: Developmental framework of infants and children: A future for pediatric responsibility. *J Pediatr* 1985;27:14

Brazelton TB: Developmental framework of infants as an opportunity for early intervention for pediatricians, in Green M (ed): *The Psychosocial Aspects of the Family*. Skillman, NJ, Johnson and Johnson Publishers, Lexington Books, pp 53-65.

Committee on Psychosocial Development of Children and Families. *Guidelines for Health Supervision*. Evanston, Ill, American Academy of Pediatrics, 1985.

Thomas A, Chess S, Brick HG: *Temperament and Behavior Disorders in Children*. New York, University Press, 1968.

PREFACE TO THE THIRD EDITION

The evolution of this book now spans more than two decades of dramatic changes in the training and practice of medicine. The original goal—to bring fundamental principles and strategies of child development into a clinically useful, easily digestible form for child health care clinicians—seems as robust and relevant as when we began. This remains our aim in the Third Edition. While being responsive to the new realities in child health care practice and in the lives of children and families, we think that our original basic perspectives are still the right ones today. This edition finds these perspectives enhanced by new research, a tightening of content, more case studies, and new formats that facilitate learning.

All chapters have been updated, including new material from research in child development and incorporating new perspectives and policies as in the following examples:

- A new conceptual framework that informs us on motor development is presented in the chapters on reach and walking.
- The "Back To Sleep" message, which has reduced the occurrence of sudden infant death syndrome, significantly changes our advice on infant sleep position and urges play in the prone position to keep motor development on track.
- New appreciation of the importance of breast feeding for early brain development and optimal health prompts a new emphasis for active promotion of nursing, along with an understanding of the psychological barriers that prevent women from successful nursing.

Every chapter has something new, but also retains what we can now see are enduring views. We were surprised to find that some ideas that seemed cutting edge at the first edition are now "classics" and are retained. Less perennial material has been pruned.

New realities in medical care required some changes for this edition. For example, because newborn stays are shorter and a lot of early infant care now occurs at home, in the office and by phone, a rearrangement of the chapters dealing with these issues was in order. For the office setting, we have tried to emphasize ways to do this work in an efficient, almost automatic way. This is of increasing importance in an ever-tightening, managed care marketplace. The chapters on practice organization, on interviewing, and on the use of drawings attempt to help the professional get back in control of the clinical encounter. This is in response to what we know to be the needs of clinicians as they experience rapid changes in the delivery of health care.

This edition also reflects societal changes that impact our work. Examples of this type of change include the shifts in the adolescent chapters that were prompted by the cultural and educational changes in the lives of young people. They are growing up faster in many ways. On the other end of the age spectrum, the growing proportion of multiple births and very low birth weight babies means that the issues in the care of the high-risk neonate have changed, and new sections have been added to the book to address them. The chapter on special families continues to evolve, reflecting societal changes in families and a growing awareness of what that means for kids. The Internet has invaded, expanded, and challenged all our lives; in response, we recommend specific principles on how to use that source of information in pediatric practice and provide suggestions on general parenting sites that we know to be good.

Some entirely new sections have been added for this edition. The chapter on loss is a strong addition because it gives developmental perspective on these ordinary and sometimes extraordinary occurrences, from the death of a pet or relative to school-based violence. The entire section on cross-cultural issues is new. Although a proper discussion of cultural and medical anthropology is beyond this volume, we have tried to integrate some principles from those disciplines that influence practice regularly. The importance of understanding the influence of temperament on behavior is given a stronger emphasis at all ages. Finally, the parent resource section has been entirely redone. The references are updated and annotated to be maximally tailored to specific users.

New formatting should make this volume even more accessible to the reader. Boxes and bullets help to emphasize key points, give quick summaries, and provide lists of clinical pearls. We have added many more case studies to introduce developmental and behavioral themes, to illustrate how these issues present in practice at various times in children and adolescents, and to suggest practical strategies on how to address issues. We have tried to divide equally the use of feminine and masculine pronouns throughout the text to reflect the diversity of clinicians, patients, and parents.

This edition should be even more fun to read, inspiring a practice that is even more fun to do. Our expanding knowledge of young people means that child development has never been more exciting than it is at the dawn of the 21st century; we hope that this book enriches child health care provider to the same level of excitement.

Suzanne D. Dixon, M.D.
Martin T. Stein, M.D.

PREFACE TO THE FIRST EDITION

The purpose of this volume is to suggest one explicit approach to the integration of child behavior evaluation and developmental assessment into the practice of pediatric primary care. With increasing frequency, pediatric caregivers seek out this integration as they attempt to meet the psychosocial as well as the physical needs of their patients (Reisinger and Bires, 1980). As much as 40% of a primary care practitioner's time may be spent in assessment and counseling in matters that pertain more to psychological growth than physical growth (Chamberlain, 1974). Parents' concerns, laid out in questions to their pediatric caregivers, are largely in psychosocial areas (McCune et al., 1984; Hickson et al., 1983). Indeed there is evidence that psychosocial factors may go unrecognized as a basis for many encounters or illnesses and may be the source of poor compliance and complicating factors in the most ordinary of pediatric encounters (Starfield et al., 1980). Many factors may be contributing to the recent and growing emphasis in pediatrics, i.e., a decrease in morbidity from infectious disease, improved perinatal conditions with resultant decrease in mortality, smaller families, a decrease in the extended family support structure, and a growing consciousness of the impact of psychological factors on the future of children (Yancy, 1975; Hickson et al., 1983). In addition, there has been an increase in pediatric care providers, so that now there are more pediatricians, pediatric nurse practitioners and physician's assistants who are involved in the direct care of children. Family medicine residencies now offer a greater exposure to the care of pediatric patients in the context of their families. Particular needs of children find more focus in these specialized settings and with practitioners specially trained in the care of children.

The specialty of pediatric medicine, in itself a young discipline, grew out of both a sociological and medical awareness of childhood as a distinct period of life. Prior to this century, children were viewed as miniature adults and adolescence was not recognized as a special period of life at all. An awareness of the extent and complexity of the differences in physiology of both sick and well children has emerged in the 20th century. The technology of medicine has been applied to the study of organ ontogeny, embryology, cell physiology, and the basis for physiologic growth regulations. Children form marvelous models for study of physiologic maturation. The study of psychological growth of children and its impact on their overall well-being has increased in the second half of this century and is beginning to show a significant effect on pediatric medicine.

In light of these changes, the significant gap in the attention to and remediation of behavioral problems in comparison with the attention received by somatic dysfunction is striking (Starfield and Borkowf, 1960). The disciplines of psychology, sociology, education, psycholinguistics, neuropsychology, anthropology, and child psychiatry are all adding new information to the data bank on normal and abnormal development. We know more today than ever about the development of the child (Elkind, 1981). In spite of the increasing degree of sophistication and specificity, this data base is not often seen as readily applicable to clinical settings. Scholarly journals from these social science disciplines are usually not read by clinicians, or if they are, the studies seem unintelligible, complex in design, and analysis, and are written in seemingly foreign tongues. Practical answers to the issues presented every day in clinical practice seem elusive. The clinician may feel himself like a rat in a maze looking for a way out when he attempts to enter the world of social sciences. This volume was developed in response to the need to infuse child development into pediatrics with a scholarly approach that is still practical and focused.

TRAINING IN BEHAVIOR AND DEVELOPMENT

There are many good reasons why the social and behavioral sciences may seem an alien territory for the clinician. Traditional training programs have offered little in formal education in the behavioral sciences (Dworkin et al., 1979). Newer programs, in line with recommendations of the Task Force for Pediatric Training (American Academy of Pediatrics, 1978) are beginning to have this input (Richmond, 1975). Most programs, however, still rely upon casual integration of behavior and development into training. Many institutions report that they lack trained personnel and a curriculum to do this in a more formal way. When this kind of integration is attempted in many pediatric programs, it is presented as "soft" (i.e., intuitive versus scientific) and as such is given little time or credibility. This may be a reaction to limitations in available professional expertise and to information found in the medical literature on psychosocial issues. This body of information is largely ignored in traditional training programs and the new material that is constantly under development in the professional social science world is not readily integrated into medical curricula.

The level of scholarly input in behavioral medical science has not kept up with that of the physical sciences. Written material that is presented for the clinician in a readable form is often "a pathological model"—an emphasis on delays in development or behaviors that indicate pathology (Brazelton, 1975). It is assumed that the disease model of physical illness can be utilized in a similar fashion when assessing child development and behavioral issues. Although surveillance for developmental disability remains an important part of pediatric practice, it is not what clinicians find most often among their daily concerns. In general, they must deal with a normal child growing up in her own style, at her own rate in a family interested in optimizing its children's lives, and not just avoiding psychoses or other major handicaps.

In the conceptualization and organization of this book, we have sought to remediate some of these gaps in professional child health training. We have developed an approach that is different than a disease surveillance model. This volume is designed to be used as part of formal child health training programs as well as a guide to "mid-career" clinicians who want to upgrade their knowledge and expertise in this area. Indeed, some of our most gratifying responses to this work have been from well-established physicians who are delighted with the new dimensions this material adds to their practices.

A SYNTHESIS

From the literature of pediatrics, psychiatry, anthropology, and psychology, salient and clinically relevant points in child development have been refocused in a form that we hope the clinician will find readable, digestible and easily integrated into clinical pediatric practice. It serves as an outline of child development for the clinician.

This work presents a model for considering one or more aspects of development at each health supervision encounter. We have attempted to integrate issues of both parent and family development into this model.

This is a how-to-do-it book—how to integrate the monitoring, supporting, and assessing of developmental processes into the usual course of pediatric care. It is the transposition of behavioral science into primary care settings. This transposition allows the clinician to vary his approach to well child care with each encounter. The child and the family have different agendas at different ages; so should the clinician. This changing agenda instills a freshness into the practice of pediatrics that in our experience adds to professionalism and enjoyment in primary care. Casey and Whitt (1980) and Hoekelman (1975) have shown this reordering of well child care to include changing developmental concerns does not result in a decline in the quality of surveillance of medical care. In addition, this approach may even be cost-effective in the delivery of comprehensive preventive medicine, the foundation of pediatrics. This clinical model of practice does not represent a deviation from the basic philosophy of pediatric care. Rather, it allows for the integration of behavioral issues and traditional pediatric care in a way that is practical, intellectually secure, and palatable to pediatric clinicians.

THE DEVELOPMENT OF THIS BOOK

We, the authors and contributors, are active pediatric caregivers, working in an urban primary care center of a university hospital and/or in private practice. We all participate in medical student, nurse practitioner, housestaff, and fellowship training in addition to maintaining our own practices. Clinical and basic research supplement our primary focus as clinicians. We have all struggled with the process and content of teaching behavioral pediatrics within primary care. We have participated in curriculum development and have experimented with many formats for presenting behavioral and developmental concepts and skills. Some of the material fits into lecture form; most is best presented in seminars through assigned readings and discussion of topics presented in an abbreviated form here. Some of the most effective but costly teaching occurs individually with students and residents as we discuss or examine a specific patient; we use the model presented in this book in that setting.

As teacher-clinicians in general pediatrics, the need for this book was identified by the pediatric housestaff. As clinicians we stretched our imaginations in order to discover ways to teach normative development at each well child encounter, identifying basic issues and moving away from the pathologic model. To spark enthusiasm for primary care issues in residents, whose minds wee preoccupied with intravenous orders and respirator settings, we soon realized that the *dynamic* changes in children from visit to visit had to be identified and placed in precise focus. Residents could not be allowed to slip into monotonous listing of developmental milestones, or they lost interest and enthusiasm. Each visit was seen as a unique challenge, and the residents requested that we write down the principles and focus of our teaching method. They did not want another textbook, but a practical how-to-do-it manual. With this handbook, we have attempted to meet that need.

The volume then is a practice manual, a curriculum component for clinicians at several stages in their own professional development, an outline of child development presented in a novel and clinically relevant way. This work grew out of pediatric primary care and we hope it adds excitement and vitality to that setting.

Suzanne D. Dixon, M.D.
Martin T. Stein, M.D.

REFERENCES

American Academy of Pediatrics: *The Future of Pediatric Education: The Task Force Report.* Evanston, Ill, American Academy of Pediatrics, 1978.

Brazelton TB: Anticipatory guidance. *Pediatr Clin North Am* 1975; 22:533-544.

Casey PH, Whitt JK: Effect of the pediatrician on the mother-infant relationship. *Pediatrics* 1980; 65:815-820.

Chamberlain RW: Management of preschool behavior problems. *Pediatr Clin North Am* 1974; 21:33-47.

Dworkin RH, Shonkoff JP, Leviton A, et al: training in developmental pediatrics: How practitioners perceive the gap. *Am J Dis Child* 1979; 133:709-712.

Elkind D: *The Hurried Child: Growing Up Too Soon.* Redding, Mass, Addison Wesley, 1981.

Hickson GB, Altemeier WA, O'Connor S: Concerns of mothers seeking care in private offices: Opportunities for expanding services. *Pediatrics* 1983; 72:619-624.

Hoekelman RA: What constitutes adequate well baby care? *Pediatrics* 1975; 55:313.

McCune Y, Richardson M, Powell J: Psychosocial health issues in pediatric practice: Parents' knowledge and concerns. *Pediatrics* 1980; 74:183-190

Reisinger KS, Bires JA: Anticipatory guidance in pediatric practice. *Pediatrics* 1980: 66:889-899

Richmond JB: An idea whose time has arrived. *Pediatr Clin North Am* 1975; 22:517-523.

Starfield B, Borkowf S: Physician's recognition of complaints made by parents about their children's health. Pediatrics 1960; 43:168

Starfield B, Gross E, Wood M, et al: Psychosocial and psychosomatic diagnosis in primary care of children. *Pediatrics* 1980; 66:159-167.

Yancy WS: Behavioral pediatrics and the practicing pediatrician. *Pediatr Clin North Am* 1975; 22:685-694.

ACKNOWLEDGMENTS

This book reflects the work of many people throughout nearly two decades of its evolution. Throughout it all we would like first and foremost to thank our own families for their unwavering support and patience. They continue to provide support, perspective, and continuing real-life experience. Thanks to Mike, Mary, Ryan, Colin, Neil, Josh, Ben, and Sarah. Without them we could not have pulled it all off.

We would also like to thank the generations of students, interns, residents, fellows, and colleagues who have given us new insights, valuable feedback, and continuing prompts for intellectual growth and development ourselves. Thank you for the questions asked, the observations brought forward, and the clinical dilemmas we have tried to solve together.

To the children and families whose lives we have shared in clinical care, thank you for the rich experience that we hope we have brought to the successive editions of this work. Each encounter is an opportunity for learning and growth.

Thanks to Mr. Bergman and his talented art students from the Charles M. Russell High School in Great Falls, Montana, who shared their outstanding work, a worthy tribute to their school's namesake.

The influence of mentors and teachers has become so ingrained now that we can hardly identify all the specifics that they have given us. The discipline of behavioral and developmental pediatrics has come of age during the evolution of this volume, and the pillars of that field inform this work. Some of those whose ideas influence this work most directly are Benjamin Spock, T. Berry Brazelton, Marshall Klaus, John Kennell, Julius Richmond, William Carey, and Morris Green. John Welsh continues to sit on our shoulders, inspiring this work and serving as a model of the best in pediatric care. We miss him.

Finally, we very much appreciate the outstanding clerical and editorial support provided by Andrea Cody. She has grown up with us in the evolution of this book, and we could not have done it without her.

Suzanne D. Dixon, M.D.
Martin T. Stein, M.D.

CONTENTS

Encounters with
CHILDREN

Pediatric Behavior and Development

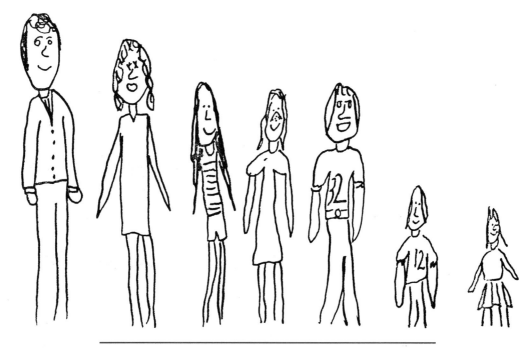

"Seeing the child in the context of the family." By Susan, age 11.

CHAPTER 1

PERSPECTIVES AND FORMAT: WHAT THIS BOOK IS ALL ABOUT

■ Suzanne D. Dixon
■ Martin T. Stein

Child development is a basic science of child health care; it is the backbone of pediatric medicine. The expected and healthy changes in the child are part of the appraisal of well-being that distinguishes pediatric medicine from adult health care. Without the knowledge of developmental change, we can't say that our health assessment of a child is complete. The imperative to monitor physical growth is coupled with the need to monitor psychological growth and well-being. This is the everyday work of pediatric care.

In spite of the importance of development and behavior to the work of child health care, specific training in the discipline of child development is often meager at the preprofessional level and during residency training in pediatrics and family medicine. Awareness is growing of the need to provide more content in this area in teaching and training. Most medical schools have an introductory course in human development that often is the first and only behavioral science course on normal human development given to students. At the residency level, pediatrics now has a mandate to provide at least one rotation on developmental and behavioral issues.[1] This may or may not include a specific curriculum in normal child development. The experience for residents is often dependent on the training, interest, and clinical practice of faculty mentors. A new guideline for residency training in developmental and behavioral pediatrics will focus the content of training on the normal child.[1] The input is usually also variable in family medicine and psychiatry. For those training in the allied health professions, most curricula have just a smattering of this material.

The irony of this situation is that these small infusions of information into the lives of the individuals who will care directly for children come at a time when we know much about the developmental processes and behavioral issues. Developmental psychology, the study of early human development and behavior, has exploded with information in the last half century. We know more than ever about the development of children and adolescents, and yet the translation of that information to child health care providers represents only a fraction of what is available. Part of the difficulty in bridging that gap is that information from developmental psychology remains unavailable—unavailable because it is written in big textbooks or in journals that are not on medical shelves or is presented at conferences that attract few health professionals. Psychologists seem to speak a different language and organize information in different ways, and the research applications of their work often seem far from clinical life. So the clinician stays relatively starved in this time of plenty.

BRAIN DEVELOPMENT

Recent discoveries in neuroscience also introduce an opportunity for clinicians to view early child development in new ways. The discoveries that link brain maturation with function bridge the fields of developmental neurology, child development, and pediatrics. The neurological underpinnings of predicted behavioral changes are being elucidated more and more each day. For example, the decrease in spontaneous smiling and crying at 2 to 3 months of age (see Chapter 8) is correlated with the emergence of cortical inhibition of brainstem circuits. The onset of fear of strangers between 7 and 10 months of age (see Chapter 11) has been correlated with an emerging ability to retrieve stored representations of the past and to compare past and present. These observations occur simultaneously and predictably with maturational changes in the prefrontal cortex, hippocampus, and the limbic systems.[2] Correlations of brain maturation and behavior gain greater significance to the clinician when these discoveries are understood in the context of ongoing brain development throughout childhood. The "hard wiring" of the brain at birth has about 100 billion neurons and 50 trillion synapses. In the first year of life the number of synapses increases twentyfold. As new synapses form, others drop out in a process called "pruning."[3] Those synaptic connections that are preserved are activated frequently in association with specific environmental stimulation. Less active synapses are lost. These discoveries in anatomical-behavioral interface in nonhuman primates support a belief long held among pediatricians that "within genetic restraints . . . the central nervous system displays tremendous plasticity, allowing itself to be critically shaped through its interactions with the environment."[4]

A convergence is growing of knowledge about the developing child from developmental psychology, neurosciences, sociology, and anthropology. As we enter the twenty-first century, we can look forward to a continuing interweaving of insights from these various disciplines to define the increasingly rich tapestry of the development of the child. The clinician should be ready to add these emerging understandings to a solid background in this area.

A GUIDE FOR LEARNING

This book was designed to remedy the present situation in part. Information from developmental psychology has been reviewed, digested, translated, and presented in a form and format that should be easy for the clinician to read. It is an introduction to the science of child development presented in a way that seems familiar to those in child health care. It serves as a guide to clinically applicable aspects of developmental psychology, a mini-course for those who wish to expand their fund of knowledge in this basic science. This information is integrated into the form that is most familiar to those who are in child health care. Material is presented in an abbreviated form to match the pacing and culture of clinical settings. Learners at several different levels will find this useful.

Medical Students

Students going through their basic science courses in human development may use this as a basic or supplemental book to learn about child and adolescent development. The cases will be of interest for small study groups, and the topical material may augment lectures or other readings. During the clinical years, medical students will find this of use in understanding their patients during core and elective rotations in pediatrics, family medicine, or psychiatry. In addition to looking at the developmental age chapters as they encounter children of those ages, students will discover that chapters such as interviewing (Chapter 3), understanding illness (Chapter 24), and the use of drawings (Chapter 25) seem particularly relevant to the medical student rotation.

Residents

The first edition of this book was created with residents in mind. Faced with teaching these busy people about development in an applied way, the authors, all academicians in busy university training programs, pulled together core material in a digestible form. We think this is still vital to pediatric training, particularly now when more is demanded in terms of mandated rotations and competency in behavioral and developmental pediatrics. We also think this work is of use for residents in family medicine, psychiatry, and combined med-ped programs. Seminar series, preclinic conferences (especially continuity clinics), and online use in clinic sessions are suggested venues. The age-linked chapters will be helpful in really learning from continuity patients, whereas the interviewing chapter (Chapter 3) seems a natural for the early internship orientation conference. Chronic illness and loss chapters (Chapters 24 and 26) fit well into inpatient rotations.

Fellows

Fellows in behavioral and developmental pediatrics, child neurology, and child psychiatry have used this text as part of the structured learning of normal child development and as a complement to their experiences with atypical development, behavioral problems, and serious pathology in behavioral medicine. A solid grounding in normal development prepares the learner at this level to distinguish and characterize deviations from the norm. These chapters form an outline, a beginning for a course of study at this level. Additional readings in selected areas are listed as references that will allow for more expanded learning. The chapters may also serve as teaching topics for fellows' presentations.

Established Clinicians

Many physicians, perhaps realizing the gap in their own training and recognizing the prominence of development and behavior in practice, will find this of value in updating their knowledge. Whether for recertification preparation or private study, this information should be of use. For this group, the conceptual framework and new ways to frame their clinical experiences seem to have been the most interesting. Private study groups and seminars for seasoned clinicians have taken the outline of this book as a model. The chapters on theories (Chapter 2), drawings (Chapter 25), and special families (Chapter 24) seem to draw the most attention from this group, although the age-linked chapters can add new life to health supervision visits.

Midlevel Professionals

Nurse practitioners and physician assistants have used this as a core and supplemental text for their child health training. Given that many of them will be doing health supervision visits in a primary care setting, this is certainly appropriate. For those already in the field we hope this will add dimension and understanding to their everyday work.

Allied Health Professionals

Therapists of several types, those in child life programs, and social work students and professionals have used this book in training for an understanding of the child and family. Although the format may not be completely aligned with how and when they see families, the topics are of importance to all of their work.

All the groups noted above have a lot to learn about child development (a term we prefer because it encompasses physical, as well as psychological, growth and is less discipline-specific than developmental psychology). And this book in no way can present it all. It is a distillation, a translation that the authors felt was the *most* relevant material for child health care providers. The hope is that this will be a start, a guide to new insights about children and their families.

This is not a comprehensive text; many good ones are available for the learner who wants more. The Coles' text and that by Laura Berk are examples.[5,6] We have had to leave many topics behind; we hope readers will be enticed to go back and pick up these dropped threads. Finally, this is a work that deals with normal child development, not developmental problems, behavioral concerns, or issues. Those are best understood by a clinician firmly grounded in normal processes, so this work forms a foundation for pursuing those other areas.[7-9]

GUIDE FOR PRACTICE

The science presented here is an applied one. The authors have taken the theoretical concepts or the experimentally derived observations and brought them into a clinical format. Salient processes, behavioral observations, and assessment suggestions are presented so that the clinician can not only learn, but also use this information. Clinical application of critical knowledge is the goal here. This task demands that the clinician have a clear understanding of the processes in question so that he or she can come to the daily clinical encounters with a vision of what to plan, observe, and ask. Toward that end, we have defined one or more prominent issues at each age on which to focus. We have made some arbitrary choices and know that a complete developmental appraisal is not a part of every chapter. In defense of this approach, we have appreciated through the years of practice and teaching that time is not sufficient to do everything at every visit. It is just not practical, given the time constraints under which most clinicians practice. Rushing through long lists of developmental questions and giving long lists of "anticipatory guidance" dictums are neither productive nor satisfying for the family or the clinician. The risk is obvious: you cover everything and nothing. You lose the chance to really get to know a child and family and the opportunity to address what really concerns them at that time. The parents' agenda for the visit may remain hidden, and they will leave dissatisfied. You are unlikely to build a relationship with a family, which, in the end, is your strongest therapeutic tool for intervention and support. If you don't have that, you are unlikely to be effective in getting the best for your patient. And ineffectiveness is the worst form of inefficiency.

Efficiency in developmental surveillance at each health supervision visit is a goal of this book.[10] We cannot add much more to the shrinking time that we have with patients in a primary care setting, so these moments have to be well thought out and productive. Most families want and look to the child health care provider to give them insight and guidance about their child's growth and development. This can be done if the visit has the following characteristics:

■ *Well planned* to highlight the child's abilities and anticipate the parents' questions and concerns
■ Uses parent and office staff input and *observation* in a systematic way
■ Builds a *relationship with the family* that allows for members to bring forward concerns about behavior and development
■ Grounded in an understanding of the *child as an individual*
■ Given context in terms of an understanding of the *environment* in which the child lives

This volume aims to provide the clinician with the tools to put these components in place. Then the wise clinician can set the stage. This means setting the agenda for the visit ahead of time through an anticipation of the issues that are likely to be most salient, important, and most available for assessment and review. The next step is setting the stage so that information and observations are gathered with efficacy and efficiency. The way that the office is set up (see Chapter 3), what toys are laid out for play, how weighing and measuring are used as data gathering points, and how and when play, questions, and comments are placed in sequence all contribute to an automatic developmental data gathering and to the convenience of a developmental perspective. Setting the stage is a vital first step. The clinician has to be ready, as well as the office.

The physician can establish an internal map of child development by understanding the sequence of, for example, language (Chapter 13) or motor development (Chapters 9 and 11) or the progression of how the child develops a self-concept (Chapter 15). Then comes the ability to quickly map onto that matrix every behavior or utterance of the child in that domain. If you know what you want to see (Does he grab for the stethoscope? How many parts of a person does he draw?) or hear (How is mom coping with temper tantrums? Is the child reading at school?), your time with a family from the moment that the visit begins can be more efficient. Focused questions and observations are the key. Families will feel that you understand them and their child if you bring this individualized appraisal to the visit. And because you have defined your territory of concern and issues of behavior and development, families will become more efficient purveyors of information at subsequent visits. They will do more and more of the work for you as you highlight the developmental processes and how these emerge and progress. The kids are guaranteed to show you what they are about if you catch them with tasks of interest at their level and give them the support they need to be free to perform. Developmental monitoring will then not be an add-on, but woven into the fiber of the whole visit with data emerging from all aspects of the encounter.

GETTING THE MOST OUT OF EACH VISIT

With the stage set for a developmental perspective, the clinician is then in a position to influence how a family sees a child and how members handle routine care and exceptional circumstances. Commenting on the child's behavior, demonstrating competencies of the child, or reflecting on the parents' stated or unstated concerns offers an intervention, however brief. Referral for services outside the office can be made thoughtfully. Advice about the management of feeding issues, sleep concerns, minor illness, and other daily matters becomes the matrix for gathering data and developing relationships rather than routine annoyances that prompt rote responses. A developmental rethinking of these opportunities gives perspective on these frequent concerns. They add energy to the appraisal rather than serving as an energy drain. Small problems become big opportunities.

For the clinician, this developmental perspective does not and should not mean doing more work, but working smarter during the time with families at each encounter. The tighter the time constraints are in primary care, the more important it is to carefully prioritize and orchestrate each visit. With the information and guidance provided here, the clinician should be able to move toward that goal.

Clinicians today often feel frustrated because they believe they don't have the time to really get into the concerns of a child and family. Increasingly, paperwork soaks up the day. Through a conscious reorganization of how visits go, the provider can address areas of concern, say something meaningful, and build on a relationship developed over time. A sense of control and accomplishment can be realized through this kind of approach. The relationship with families is our most powerful tool and our greatest personal reward.

This book, then, is a guide for learning and a guide for practice. It is meant to be useful for learning one of the vital basic sciences of pediatric health care and to be a guide for adding behavioral and developmental depth to the practice of pediatric medicine. The underlying tenets and the form and format of this book were designed to reach those goals.

BASIC TENETS

The following perspectives guide and inform this work:
■ *Most children are normal.* This book is based on the fact that most children are developmentally normal and that most children a pediatric clinician sees will have concerns that are broadly within the normal range. This means that the clinician will be monitoring and supporting normal developmental processes. However, even within the range of normal will be hurdles, problems, and concerns that should be addressed by the knowledgeable clinician. Some of these will be developmental variation,[11] some based on differences in

temperament in child and family,[12] and some based on stressors that are all too common for children and families. Most unusual behaviors are both explainable and adaptive if seen within the broader context of the individual child and family. Cross-cultural, socio-economic, geographical, and even political forces are active in shaping the boundaries of what is normal versus abnormal. The clinician must be well grounded in what is normal and what variation might be expected in order to support and advise families appropriately in all these circumstances. In addition, we believe we have the chance to support optimal development for each child through recognition of strengths within this normal range. We hope that the clinician will not see his or her job as merely being a marauder for pathology, fueled only by the identification of delays or problems, which are issues that will come up for a minority of patients. This kind of "negative model" is not what parents want, and it shortchanges what clinicians can do for kids and families.[13]

∎ *The processes of development have consistencies, but also variation.* Herein lies the richness of diversity. Developmental psychology provides us with the science to understand the sequences of progress and age ranges of expectations. These are important parameters in child health care. We hope that this book provides an understanding of these expectations. However, we hope that the clinician won't be satisfied with only looking at the numbers or the specific age of accomplishments. That perspective eliminates a lot of the fun and excitement of seeing children over time. The individual way that a given child realizes these gains and weaves these into his or her individual makeup and circumstances adds excitement to each child's course. We hope that this book inspires the clinician to look at and enjoy this variation, confident that the child's behavior falls within the range of expectations. A solid grounding in normal child development means that the clinician can then work with a family with confidence, knowing what calls for intervention and what calls for only explanation or support.

∎ *Most families want to do the best for their children and will make good choices if they have the right information and support.* No matter the circumstance or situation, parents around the globe want their children to do well, and they do their best with whatever resources they have to see that this happens. Those resources are often physical ones, but also include knowledge, their own life experiences, their definition of *well*, their family and community support systems, and their energy. If mistakes are made, they are usually grounded in poor information, reduced energy or resources, or failure to appreciate the child's perspective or abilities. The pediatric clinician can remedy the latter issue by presenting the child's issues. He or she may have to serve as the interpreter of the child's behavior, help identify needs, or mark the exhibited strengths. The clinician may also help to identify resources both internal and external to the family. With the assumed shared goal of what's best for the child, the clinician and family form an alliance toward that end.

This is very different than the hierarchical or dictatorial relationship that has been an historical medical model of care. The clinician can share information and the child's needs and perspectives (material presented in this volume), and the family can bring its own insights, goals, and situations that are important to the whole picture. Premature prescriptive advice and an emphasis on shortcomings generally aren't helpful and drain energy from rather than add it to a family system. Look for strengths and build on them.

As stated by Dr. Benjamin Spock in his half-century bestseller for parents, "Trust yourself. You know more than you think you do."[14] The clinician should start with that same sense of trust in the parents, at least at the basic level of caring and commitment.

■ *Gains in developmental competency in a child always start a cascade of changes in the child and his environment.* With each new skill the child's view of self and place in the world is altered. A new skill may mean that the care required changes. And this in turn results in alterations in how the child is viewed and understood by the family. For the clinician then, each developmental gain calls for a look at other areas of the child's functioning, the response in the family, and what has changed in terms of required supports. This means that the clinician must do the following:
1. Anticipate the change in the child
2. Identify and acknowledge the change
3. Anticipate the ripples that may accompany change

For example, when the child starts to be mobile, cognitive abilities around spatial relations and sense of self are changed because the child can move through space and literally change perspective. At the same time the child becomes energized to explore, demands more of a role in feeding himself or herself, and starts to become anxious with separations. Sleep issues predictably come up in this beginning of discipline and sleep management, and issues of safety change dramatically. In this circumstance, the clinician should note the big shift and help the family discover what should be done differently (see Chapter 13). This kind of integrated understanding of what development means and demands goes beyond the checklist mentality that often is presented as developmental monitoring in practice. For this reason, this book is presented thematically and tries to identify family developmental issues along with those of the child at each step.

■ *Interventions should be guided by strengths, not deficits.* The initial approach to understanding a situation or developing an intervention is to identify the strengths and capacities because in those are energy for change. Building on developmental strengths will enable the child and family to find detours around difficulties; beating on the family about deficits will not result in gains. This doesn't mean a Pollyannaish denial or glossing over of difficulties. It does mean that one understands the basic developmental processes clearly and can identify ways to get to the goal in spite of carefully characterized barriers. The primary care physician, seeing a child and family over time, should be in a good position to see the big picture and to bring the capabilities forward when a problem must be faced. These may be found in the child, the family, or the many levels of the environment. Pat answers, rote approaches, or prepackaged programs are unlikely to be successful unless they are responsive to individual differences.

■ *Children will readily display the cutting edge of their developmental competency.* Children readily practice emerging skills if given the correct prompt to show them off. Competencies are most often obvious to parents as well, although parents might not always know what they are seeing or where the skill comes from or is going toward. Developmental appraisal, then, is not hard if the clinician knows the focused questions to ask and how to observe behavior as it emerges in a supportive setting. Kids and parents do all the work; we just need to set the stage and watch and listen. Trainees often ask with wonder how we know that a child will do a certain task with blocks or that the elements of a typical child's drawing of a person add up to the child's correct age, as if it's a miracle. Maybe it is, but it's a miracle that can be easily anticipated if we know the sequence of development and what behavioral issues are likely to come up at a given age. Through a knowledge of child development, we should be efficient and even downright lazy as we get the kids and families to present most of the data we need. For this reason, it's not necessary to run the gamut of questions or tests at every session with the child who has followed a typical course. Focused observations and questions are at the core of "developmental surveillance,"[15,16] the proper professional role for the child health care provider. Deviance from expectations, however, presents the imperative to look at issues further.

THE BOOK SETUP

This book is laid out, in the main, in chapters that coincide with the recommended schedule of health supervision visits.[17] These are the "encounters" that provide the child health care provider with an opportunity to evaluate and support a child and family. For each of these visits, we have defined one or more closely related issues or themes that typically come to the fore at that time for the child and the family. These behavioral and developmental processes are explored in the chapter. The developmental foundations for issues are laid out, as well as the typical progression into later ages. For example, walking at 1 year gives us a chance to focus on motor development and movement. The precursors, processes, and progression of gross motor movement are all discussed in that chapter (Chapter 12), although we would not expect a 1-year-old to display the more advanced aspects of movement presented. We can then use that visit for special emphasis, giving the family some specialized information and giving ourselves a chance to really focus on one aspect of development. An expanded exploration of one issue in depth at each encounter and varied themes for each visit add interest, intellectual challenge, and saliency to the visit. Of course, other issues may present themselves at that time through questionnaires, historical issues, or in the interview. Concerns about motor development, for example, usually prominent at 1 year, may surface at another time. Cross-referencing will help the clinician be responsive to individual issues as they come up. However, over time, we will cover all the areas of development with a child and family and our areas of focus and concern will sensitize the family to the issues such that they will be more likely to bring specific observations and concerns forward.

  This approach is different than going through a checklist of everything at every visit. Parent questionnaires or lists (see Appendix for several suggestions) can be used if desired to catch concerns that may not come up in the discussion, although that seems unlikely. These should be completed before the visit, if used. The focus or agenda may have to change based on that information. A list of questions should not be asked by the clinician directly except in rare cases. A better use of professional time, in our view, is to really provide an in-depth approach to the cutting-edge issues at that time, addressing concerns that have saliency for the child and family. Seeing the child with a family and looking at the changes that are important for care are more interactive and targeted than going through a long litany that is unlikely to stick and certainly seems less satisfying than what we are proposing. Our approach should also give the clinician a sense of empowerment in setting the agenda for the visit, a feeling that is all too scarce in this age of child health care.

Case Presentations

Each chapter is illustrated by brief cases that serve several purposes. First, the opening vignette illustrates the chapter theme as it may present itself in clinical practice. By the end of the chapter, the reader should be able to comprehend the theme and have the skills to explore and manage the issue or case for themselves. Other cases within the chapter's text may illustrate the specific point discussed or highlight a clinical dilemma or management issue that a specific theme suggests. Adult learners, particularly clinicians, learn best from cases, so we hope these will solidify the concept presented in didactic form. The reader is encouraged to use his or her own clinical cases to reflect on developmental and behavioral themes.

Data Gathering

Observation, history taking, and assessment are the structure of primary health care, so most chapters finish with how to approach the issues or themes in these formats. Through the collection of these three types of data, we hope that the clinician can get all the information needed on the issue in a clear and efficient way. In many cases, models for specific questions and activities are suggested. In others, topics for discussion are suggested, to be explored with solid, age-appropriate interviewing techniques as presented in Chapter 3. Anticipatory guidance is the foundation for preventive health care for kids, so it's no surprise that this section addresses issues of behavior and development, using what we have learned about the processes of development to anticipate the next event and to help parents support their children. Guidance for the use of other professional and community resources is also found in these sections.

Issue Chapters

Some chapters develop issues that are not age linked, such as the chapters on office environment, on handling loss, and on the use of children's drawings. These chapters serve as background for the developmental and behavioral issues addressed at each age and concerns that go across childhood and adolescence. We hope that the reader will read them and go back to them as needed when issues or special concerns emerge. The chapter on developmental theory (Chapter 2) presents views on children from the several perspectives that shape our understanding of children. Reference to these theories will come up in the age-specific chapters as they apply to issues at that age. The chapter on drawings (Chapter 25) will help the reader to appreciate the drawings that are used throughout the book; reading it should make all the illustrations more meaningful.

Each of these chapters, as well as the age-specific ones, can be used as a seminar topic, the focus of a preclinic conference, or the subject of study group. The references at the end will be helpful to the reader who wishes to pursue the topic in greater depth. Seen as a whole they form a course in human development. The shuffle of topics was determined by the child health encounter, not the area of development or strictly age progression. This format should make it more familiar to the child health care provider.

A Word About the Drawings

Throughout this book, children's drawings are used to illustrate each chapter. As cute as these may be, they are not merely decorative. As an integral part of each chapter, they serve to highlight what we think are the key developmental issues presented in the chapter. They may illustrate the developmental process at that age, as in the school-age drawings of kids in their wider world. Or they may show how kids see an issue, as in the powerful drawings of divorce, death, and illness in the chapters devoted to those topics. Or they may reveal psychological processes that are important at particular ages but are unavailable for direct discussion, such as the "shooting kisses" drawing in the prenatal interview chapter or the dynamics seen in the other family drawings. The drawings by adolescents show the turbulence and complexity of that age far more clearly than we could ever explain. The stark frankness of the children's work calls themes out emphatically, adding punch to the ideas presented in the written word. Often we have heard from readers of previous editions that a particular drawing is long remembered, and the ideas it illustrated hang on that image. We hope that the drawings will continue to provide that rich memory prompt.

At even a more basic level, the use of drawings themselves illustrates a key tenet of this work—children themselves will tell us what they are up to and what they are about if we set the stage and then listen and look. They will do the work of demonstrating their own developmental progress if we lay out the opportunity. We can trust them to show us what they are working on, and our own work with them and their families follows from that. We can use the kids as forthright accomplices to reveal where they are and what they are thinking and feeling. In this book, their artwork tells a vital part of the story. Don't skip the drawings.

REFERENCES

1. Coury D et al: Curricular guidelines for residency training in developmental-behavioral pediatrics, *J Dev Behav Pediatr* 20(suppl S1-S38):2, 1999.
2. Herschkowitz N, Kagan J, Zilles K: Neurobiological bases of behavioral development in the first year, *Neuropediatrics* 28:296, 1997.
3. Shore R: *Rethinking the brain: new insights into early development*, New York, 1997, Families and Work Institute.
4. Wang P: Book review of Capute AJ, Accardo PJ: Developmental disabilities in infancy and childhood. In *Am J Ment Retard* 101(6):647, 1996.
5. Cole M, Cole SR: *The development of children*, ed 3, New York, 1996, WH Freeman and Co.
6. Berk L: *Infants, children and adolescents*, ed 3, Boston, 1999, Allyn and Bacon.
7. Levine MD, Carey WB, Crocker AC, editors: *Developmental-behavioral pediatrics*, ed 2, Philadelphia, 1992, WB Saunders.
8. Parker S, Zuckerman B: *Handbook of developmental and behavioral pediatrics*, Boston, 1995, Little, Brown.
9. Lewis M, editor: *Child and adolescent psychiatry*, Philadelphia, 1997, Williams & Wilkins.

10. Dworkin PH: British and American recommendations for developmental monitoring: the role of surveillance, *Pediatrics* 84:1000, 1989.
11. American Academy of Pediatrics: *Diagnostic and statistical manual for mental health disorders: pediatric and adolescent version (DSM-PC)*, Elk Grove Village, Ill, 1996, American Academy of Pediatrics.
12. Carey WB, McDevitt SC: *Coping with children's temperament*, New York, 1995, Basic Books.
13. Brazelton TB: *Touchpoints*, ed 7, New York, 1992, Addison-Wesley.
14. Spock B, Parker S: *Dr. Spock's baby and child care*, New York, 1998, Pocket Books.
15. Dworkin PH: Developmental screening: expecting the impossible? *Pediatrics* 83:619, 1989.
16. Dworkin PH: British and American recommendations for developmental monitoring: the role of surveillance, *Pediatrics* 84:1000, 1989.
17. American Academy of Pediatrics: *Guidelines for health supervision III*, Elk Grove Village, Ill, 1997, American Academy of Pediatrics.

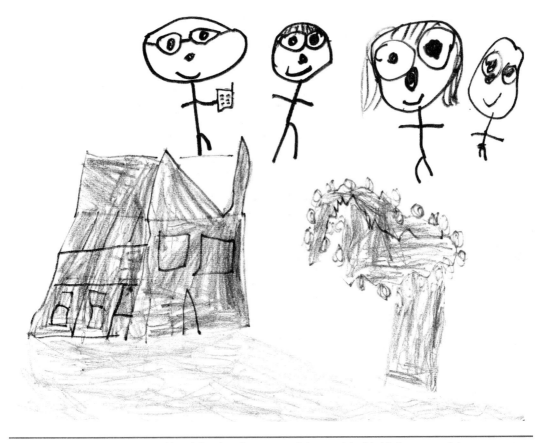

A 5-year-old boy shows himself with his family on top of the world with his house and the orange tree below.

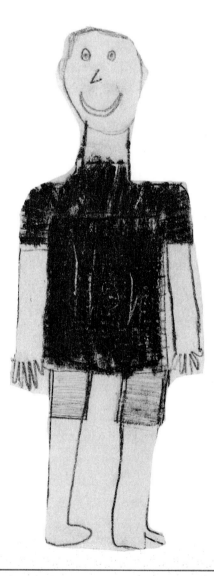

A self-portrait. By Neil Hennessy, age 8 (original in pencil and red and blue crayon).

THEORIES, CONCEPTS, AND CULTURAL DIMENSIONS OF DEVELOPMENT

■ Suzanne D. Dixon

The study of child development has flourished in the twentieth century with the application of increasingly sophisticated observational and experimental techniques in this field. We know more than we ever have about the processes of development in children.[1] Investigators focus, however, on different aspects of development and, even within shared areas, may not agree on the meaning of the behavior that they study. As stated by Cole and Cole,[2] no theory "gives unity to the entire body of relevant scientific knowledge of human development."

The infusion of this body of knowledge into clinical training and practice has lagged behind the explosion of information. Further, without an understanding of the theoretical framework(s) upon which new research is based, the clinician often has a hard time understanding, evaluating, and using these insights even if they are made available.[3] The purpose of this chapter is to provide a brief synopsis of the theoretical perspectives that guide our current understanding of development in children. These perspectives will then enable the clinician to gain insight into the processes of development that underlie every encounter. Because child development is a basic science behind pediatric practice, it behooves us to have at least a beginning knowledge of it, such as that provided here. I hope that this chapter prompts enough interest and excitement among clinicians that they want to learn more about this area of science and that texts of developmental psychology will join this volume on the shelf. Current ones, from which we have drawn throughout this book, include those by Berk[4] and by Cole and Cole,[2] but many are available. This chapter is a start and, I hope, an enticement to learn more about the science of child development.

My own experience with adding the study of the theories of child development to residency and fellowship training is that this body of knowledge enhances the expertise of trainees in clinical dealings with children. Students and residents are given an educated, broad view of the child rather than the mandate to memorize facts, milestones, and rigid standards. This background enriches their clinical experiences by adding intellectual depth. Theories and perspectives open eyes to behaviors that otherwise might have passed unheeded. Older staff physicians have requested many of these materials as well, sensing that some new understandings will enhance their considerable personal experience. It helps them add dimension to what they see and do every day and provides the intellectual background for their work. For all of us the theoretical perspectives guide and give meaning to what we see in clinical encounters.

Throughout this volume we have taken an eclectic approach to understanding child development, pulling some concepts and applications from several different theoretical models that seem to make sense in specific clinical settings or around specific clinical issues. As clinicians we can do that; we are not wedded to one perspective or another. And it's a good thing that we have the freedom to draw insights from varying schools because no single one of them explains the richness of even one of the many children we see. This chapter, then, prepares the reader for some insights brought forward in the chapters that follow.

Different periods of a child's development seem to fit one perspective better than other periods, and different areas of development are addressed by various theoretical models. The clinician can choose from these theoretical spotlights for guidance on a particular child with a particular concern. This flexible approach, however, demands a solid knowledge of these perspectives. I hope that this chapter provides some of that and sets the stage for the rest of the book.

MATURATIONAL THEORY-NORMATIVE APPROACH

The maturational theory-normative approach school regards development as the inevitable unfolding of events determined internally by the forces of genetics and the neuromaturational processes that the genes direct. This perspective, propagated in the first half of this century by Gesell, drew heavily from 18th and 19th century thinkers.[5-10] This perspective is the one most familiar to pediatricians because it runs parallel to our understanding of embryology, developmental physiology, and physical growth. It is also the perspective that underlies much of the traditional, often rudimentary material on child development that was presented in school and training. In this model, behavior depends entirely on neurological and physical maturation. The child is seen as an immature or incomplete organism, moving in predictable patterns of behavior during the course of continuous maturation. Gesell[6,7] and other proponents of this model[11,12] gave us extensive data on the normative course of development, providing the earliest and most enduring standards to expectations of typical development.[7,13,14] This approach allows easy clinical assessment and the systematic classification of children as delayed, deviant, or normal based on the timing of emergence of specific skills.[11] Most of the usual development tests are based on this foundation. Development is seen as continuous. The child's place in the continuum compared with that of his age-mates is the basis for a diagnostic formulation. The child's environment is seen as having an impact in a subordinate way; it may have detrimental impact and impede the developmental sequence.[7] Temperament and individual issues are acknowledged, but their role in determining development is seen as minimal.

Today we retain the norms of expected development in children that were built upon this perspective,[14] but no one now weighs in on the extreme view that nature alone determines development. The powerful role of the environment has been identified and is incorporated into more recent perspectives. Further, the discontinuities in developmental processes, abrupt shifts in competencies, and the new abilities that seem to appear without

BOX 2-1	KEY POINTS—MATURATIONAL THEORIES

Regular, universal sequence present in development.
Age norms for developmental milestones.
Development arises from internal factors, neuromaturational forces.
Psychological change linked to physical development.
Environment contributes in minor way.

antecedent are all at odds with orthodox maturational models (Box 2-1). Much of the complexity and variability in development is left unexplained by this model.

Some of the poor predictors in early assessment based on this scheme may be explained by the gaps in this theoretical model. For example, the outcome for the premature infant weighing more than 1500 g is much better predicted by his interaction with mother than by the pattern of early development (see Chapter 7). Further, affective and cognitive development are not adequately addressed in this model and are only tightly squeezed into its framework with ranges of norms that give general guidelines. The major contribution of maturational theory stems from the valuable norms it has provided for the systematic observation of development in children. We still need and use these today.

PSYCHOSEXUAL THEORY AND PSYCHOANALYTIC MODELS

Freud made a significant contribution to our understanding of personality development through his retrospective observations and thoughtful theoretical formulations.[15-18] He drew our attention to the consequences in later life of early childhood experience and the centrality of emotional life in shaping personality (Box 2-2). This model emphasizes the importance of the unconscious and conscious mental processes that allow children to develop a concept of themselves as individuals and of their place in society. This self-concept results from the interface of a particular child's inner needs (biological drives) with the demands of the external world around him (social expectations), which are viewed as conflicting.

BOX 2-2	KEY POINTS—PSYCHOSEXUAL THEORIES

Emotional life has powerful influence on behavior and development.
Unconscious processes shape behavior, concurrent and ongoing.
Interactions between parent and child influence personality, resiliency, adjustment, and behavior into adulthood.
Individual's life history is unique and worthy of study and understanding.

Each stage in life revolves around the resolution of a particular "psychosexual" conflict. These stages are as follows:

- *Oral phase* (infancy, 0 to 18 months), in which the act of feeding is central
- *Anal phase* (toddlerhood, 18 months to 3 years), emphasizing the pleasures and demands of elimination
- *Phallic stage* (3 years to 6 years), bringing the identification of a sexual self
- *Latency period* (school-age, 6 years to 11 years), characterized by an increase in control of sexual drives (i.e., bodily pleasures and aggressive tendencies)
- *Genital stage* (adolescence to adulthood), in which relationships with individuals outside the family grow and mature while the young person separates from his parents.

Successful resolution of specific inner conflicts at each stage leaves the child ready for a new level of emotional and social maturity. Disruptions or abnormalities at a specific stage (e.g., anal) are seen as the basis for psychic difficulty (e.g., obsessive behavior) that continues into adult life, resulting in conflicting difficulties (neuroses) or major psychological disturbances (psychoses).

Orthodox psychoanalytic theory was not based on direct observations of children, but on adult memories. It has not been submitted to experimental testing. This perspective has been described as having an inherent cultural, historical, and perhaps male bias.[19-21] The terms used in this theory are now a part of everyday life (e.g., ego, libido, Freudian slip, repression), but a widespread commitment to the original formulation of this perspective no longer exists. Specific reviews of this theory refute the existence of the oedipal phase particularly and the link between stage arrest and later problems. We must acknowledge the considerable contribution that Freud brought to the field of human development. Some of the enduring Freudian insights and principles are the following:

- Children do have an active mental life even before the emergence of speech.
- This mental life contributes to the child's adjustment both at that time and later in life.
- Unconscious wishes and thoughts influence both present and future behavior.
- The place of the child's interpersonal experience with loved ones, most often his parents, is central to his overall adjustment and later functioning as an individual.
- The ability to form relationships with others is determined in part by these primary interactions and the gradual process of separation and individuation. Families are vital to the healthy development of children.

These principles add insight into the development of self through the interactions with primary caregivers.

Following Freud, other important theoreticians emerged and provided additional insight. Margaret Mahler and colleagues taught that a child's mental and physical relationship with his mother gradually moves from one of total symbiosis (as in pregnancy) to independence through a series of stages in the first 3 years of life.[22] These predictable landmarks of emotional development allow for the child's increasingly solid sense of self as an individual, unique, and competent person.

Erik Erikson formulated a useful structure in which to understand the stages of emotional development throughout the life cycle. His **psychosocial theory** is shown in Table 2-1.[19,23] Each stage is characterized by negotiation of one central issue that is necessary for emotional advancement to the next stage. Erikson's schema is attractive because it applies themes that can encompass several areas of development. Variation in when these stage-

Stage	Age	Issue
TABLE 2-1 ■ Erikson's Stages of Development		
1	Birth-18 mo	Trust vs. mistrust
2	18 mo-3 yr	Autonomy vs. shame and doubt
3	3-6 yr	Initiative vs. guilt
4	6-11 yr	Industry vs. inferiority
5	Adolescence	Identity vs. role confusion
6	Young adulthood	Intimacy vs. isolation
7	Adulthood	Generativity vs. stagnation
8	Old age	Ego integrity vs. despair

locked tasks occur is based on forces of culture, family, individual differences, and the changing demands of society. Erikson's theory extends through adulthood, highlighting some of the generic issues confronting parents as part of their own development. These insights can contribute to our assessment of families as we provide support and sometimes intervention. Similar to most pediatric clinicians, Erikson believed that "the child can be trusted to obey the inner laws of development." Under this umbrella, child rearing becomes a child-response event rather than a prescriptive or adult-directed process. These Ericksonian broad themes can help us step back from specific issues or behaviors that are brought to our attention clinically. If we see what the child's "big job" is at that stage, we can often find a way out of a dilemma.

> *Kari, age 5, was always the object of her mother's annoyance. Everything in her room was a mess, and when she was given the order to clean it up, the task was overwhelming. She just left it and skipped out. Her mother asked advice about this, saying that she worried about what would happen in adolescence if obedience was such a problem now.*
>
> *The clinician asked Kari why she didn't pick up her room. Kari said it was "too much." Through a system of baskets, breaking down the task to manageable units ("now pick up all the blocks"), and a series of rewards for a job well done, Kari and her mom got along much better. Kari proudly brought in her star chart of successes at the next visit. Initiative replaced guilt when she was able to do the job.*

BEHAVIORISM AND SOCIAL LEARNING THEORY

Theorists in this group see the environment as the major force shaping child development and behavior. The proponents of behaviorism postulate that only behavior that is observable can be studied (i.e., not motives, beliefs, unconscious forces) and that the environment is a source of behavioral change.[24] The environment supplies patterns of reinforcement or reward that shape and determine the child's behavior. The child becomes "conditioned" to respond in a certain way. The child's association of certain stimuli and responses shapes behavior in increasingly complex patterns over time. Behaviors that are rewarded stay; those ignored or punished disappear or are "extinguished" with predictable regularity. Environment is the pivotal force in development in this theory, so behavioral problems and solutions come from patterns of reinforcement in the environment.

Social learning theory evolved from strict behaviorism[25,26] and highlighted the importance of modeling behavior that is observed to elicit positive responses from the environment. Children learn within the context of specific social structures that model behavior for imitation. Structure changes prompt development. Bandura, a major force in this perspective, has modified his own work to place at the center the child's own cognitive processes in shaping how he behaves and develops.[27] The newest name for this approach, social-cognitive, emphasizes the child's ability to abstract the rules and patterns of behavior rather than simply imitating models. The child then reconstitutes these in a personal way of understanding and acting. Children become more selective in what and whom they use as models, in line with an increasing sense of self and self-efficacy. Bandura now sees children very active mentally in constructing models and developing behavioral patterns on their own. They are like student artists who study the paintings around them, picking up ideas and techniques, but then painting an original.

Behavioral theories have prompted a great deal of applied research, as well as clinical intervention strategies. These include conditioning children to consequences (reinforcers), both positive and negative, associated with their behavior. Programs targeted to get rid of undesirable behaviors through withdrawal of privileges or through punishment rely on these behavior modification techniques.

Modeling of behavior, in role-playing and in real life, becomes a positive force in shaping behavior, particularly for those older than preschoolers. Programs for discipline, for eliminating fears of medical treatments, and for managing bedwetting are founded on these principles. Many programs for children with mental retardation or autism depend heavily on these techniques to eliminate disruptive behaviors, help prompt communication, and teach simple skills.[28]

Strict behaviorism, however, does not take into account a child's inner life, emotions, motivations, and style in adapting to new circumstances and demands. Minimal weight is given to the child's own internal processes of maturation that prompt new behaviors and leave others behind. Also, many behaviors emerge without environmental prompts, in spite of incredible environmental barriers and with a complete lack of models for that behavior. Bandura's broadening perspective is no doubt in response to such observations of the internal processes that allow a child to take in the world but to come out with a unique set of behavioral patterns and to negotiate development in unique ways. Finally, the environment in which children develop is much more complex than a series of reinforcers or even a series of models. The view of learning theorists on the environment itself may be too narrow.

Behaviorist techniques are attractive to clinicians because they can be prescribed for almost any condition or situation brought by a troubled parent. And in many circumstances the techniques work, provided that one has typical children and typical circumstances. Caution should be taken, however, because these techniques are directed at changing behavior alone and do not regularly address the basis for that behavior. Children's behavior has meaning, no matter how seemingly maladaptive or disruptive. The clinician should attend to what that behavior is revealing before prescribing a "cure" for it. Failures of these behavioral techniques to change behavior are seated in the complex interactions between a child and care provider, inappropriate environmental expectations, or needs that go beyond the immediate. The clinician should probe these possibilities as part of a complete clinical intervention, not simply provide a "behavior mode" solution.

Social learning perspectives (Box 2-3) push the imperative to look broadly at a child's environment when disruptive behavior emerges, suggesting the possible roles of inappropriate models, atypical social situations, or unusual focus on the child. A therapeutic intervention to change the environment often changes the seemingly maladaptive behavior of the child. One should evaluate closely what forces the environment is providing before labeling the behavior deviant.

> *Marci, a 5-year-old girl, was placed in foster care after her mother, an alcoholic, was found to be neglectful. Her foster mom was troubled that Marci continued to take and hoard food months after the placement. "Food is always there and she was never starving. Even when she came to us, she was too fat."*
>
> *The erratic care and attention given by Marci's birth mom probably set up an anxiety in Marci about getting what she needed. Overeating and hoarding seem like sensible responses to that experience. (In my experience, hoarding may go on for years of even the best of care.) Merely punishing Marci's behavior was not appropriate until her anxiety was addressed and trust in the environment was established.*

Behavioral techniques require the close and consistent linkage between a behavior and a consequence. Inconsistency in response doesn't allow that linkage to be established and may even establish that behavior in concrete because of intermittent reinforcement.

BOX 2-3	KEY POINTS—BEHAVIORISTS-SOCIAL LEARNING

Only behavior itself can be studied, changed, altered.
Developmental change is prompted from without. The environment is essential.
Environment provides reinforcers for behavior, positive and negative; a behavior that continues has been reinforced somehow.
Children (may) imitate what they see; environmental models are important to learning.

> Mrs. Johnson wanted Jared to sleep in his own bed, not hers. She would put him back and tuck him in for several nights and then give up for a week or two. Jared learned that if he kept coming in, his mom would just give up. "I'm so tired by then," she said.

The younger the child developmentally, the closer the link must be between the behavior and the consequence for the child to learn. Delayed praise or punishment does not work for children younger than 6 chronologically or developmentally. For children younger than 2 the link has to be nearly immediate for the child to learn. Finally, positive reinforcers are much more powerful in shaping human behavior than negative ones; rewards work better than punishments.

CONSTRUCTIVIST VIEWS: PIAGET, ET AL

In this broad school of thought, devoted primarily to cognitive development, the roles of nature and nurture, the child and the environment, are given equal weight. Children are viewed as using their evolving physical and mental capabilities to actively engage the environment in processes of observing and acting on it. Through this ongoing process children construct ever-higher levels of knowledge, capabilities, and action patterns, mental and physical. Environmental forces have different impacts at different ages because the child's inner processes are critical to the outcome and change over time. The environment can, through differing levels of input, either impede or support the rate of development, but the sequence in development is universal. The child and his milieu have reciprocal roles in development with constant interaction and modification between them.

Piaget (1896-1980) developed his view of the active role of the child through detailed observations of children, attending as much to their errors in problem solving and the patterns of exploration as to their successes.[29-32] These "mistakes" told him how children reason about and understand their world. His observations led to the belief that a child's mental processes are qualitatively different than those of adults and that the processes go through distinct stages of mental development. A child's way of acting upon the world, physically and mentally, shifts radically between these stages (Table 2-2).

Piaget's insights dramatically changed the dominant behaviorist schools in America through his premise that the child is an active learner rather than a passive recipient or target of environmental forces. Such concepts as the importance of discovery and exploration to the child, now the foundation of early education, come from his work. Our whole view of cognitive and moral development has been shaped by this perspective on child development.

As we watch children, we can now see how active they are in exploring whatever is in front of them, making combinations of two or more objects, and developing explanations of the world around them based on their views of it. The funny things little kids say often reveal their beliefs about the world, beliefs that they have constructed through perceptions mulled over in a very active mental life.

Testing the development of children is easy when we have this perspective; we set the stage, and they demonstrate (provided they are well and not in a negative, upset state). The

TABLE 2-2 ■ Piagetian Stages of Development

Stage	Approximate Age	Ways of Understanding the World	Basic Concepts to be Mastered
1. Sensorimotor	Birth-2 yr	Through direct sensations and motor actions	Object permanence; causality; spatial relationships; use of instruments, etc.
2. Preoperational	2-6 yr	Mental processes that are governed by the child's own perceptions and linkage of events; no separation of internal and external reality	Sense of animism; egocentrism; idiosyncratic associations; transductive reasoning
3. Concrete operational	6-11 yr	Can reason through real and mental actions on real objects; can reverse changes to the world mentally to gain understanding; can reason using a stable rule system; understands some patterns	Mass; number; volume; linear time; deductive reasoning
4. Formal operations	12 yr and older (variable)	Abstract thought; can reason about ideas, impossibilities, and probabilities; broad abstract concepts	Mastery of abstract ideas and concepts; possibilities; inductive reasoning; complex deductive reasoning

parents' role is to set the stage every day and to provide opportunities, emotional support, safety, and encouragement. This is in contrast to the misguided directives to "teach," "stimulate," and "prompt." Piagetian perspectives call on us to free the child to explore and discover.

Recent observations indicate that Piaget may have underestimated the capabilities of infants and toddlers. Also, familiarity with the tasks used to test these cognitive structures, as well as past teaching and practice, seem to enhance performance more than previously thought. Boundaries between the stages may be blurred, based upon teaching and experience.[33] Cross-cultural observations support Piaget's ideas about the universals of cognitive development in young children, but the mental structures of older children and adults seem to vary across the globe, seemingly in response to the particular cognitive demands placed by a specific environment. Finally, the Piagetian stage theory has been abandoned by some in favor of a more continuous view of mental development in children (Box 2-4). Children roll along rather than bounce from one stage to another.

Moral Development: Neopiagetian Perspectives

Piaget applied his theories to moral development with the description of two stages, divided at about age 10. At the younger stage, children see rules as immutable, handed down by an authority and requiring obedience to the letter. The seriousness of a crime is judged by the

BOX 2-4	KEY POINTS—PIAGET, ET AL

Children are active in determining their own development. They are natural experimenters if given the opportunity and support to explore.

Learning occurs in stages that differ qualitatively in how children reason, act upon, and learn about the world around them.

Mental structures, including the interpersonal ones, are built through interaction between the child and the environment.

The sequence of development is universal, although the rate may vary across domains, cultures, and settings.

damage or the extent of the violation, not by motivation. After age 10, children appreciate that people have different perspectives on what the rules that guide conduct are or should be and that these might be changed. Piaget's work led the way for Kohlberg's theory, which also uses stages to describe the generic characteristics of children's moral problem solving, the way in which they reason about moral situations.[34] Children and adults all over the world seem to solve moral dilemmas along this generic continuum, although the context and values may vary by context and culture. Those in industrial societies and those exposed to higher education advance through the stages faster, and many go farther along the continuum than do those in simpler societies, in which judgments remain at about stage 3. This application of Piagetian theory gives insight on the child's capabilities, which in turn guide our expectations for discipline, adherence to rules, and the formation of values within a given family.

ECOLOGICAL SYSTEMS APPROACH

Emerging as a new perspective on child development, the work of Bronfenbrenner has called attention to the systems of care and nurturance, relationships that shape a child's development and behavior.[35,36] In this view a broad and interlocking set of systems influences the developmental processes (Box 2-5). Table 2-3 describes these. No longer is the child viewed as influenced by the interface with family, peers, and school alone. Rather, the whole sociopolitical and cultural environment has profound impact on one hand and incredible potential for intervention on the other. Beginning in infancy and increasing dramatically as they age, children shape those environments, making critical choices about even which environments will touch their lives (e.g., Will it be the soccer team or basketball? Will I do drama or be on the debate team?). Bronfenbrenner's work on day care sparked his views. The whole milieu in the emergence of day care, from its availability and components down to the interaction with caregivers, brought this model to the fore. In related work, Michael Rutter and colleagues have called attention to the tremendous impact of the school milieu on children.[37] Such forces as the media, violence, cultural diversity, and the prevalence of computers and the Internet shape development in many ways, for good and ill. These are the systems that shape an individual child's development broadly, but powerfully.

TABLE 2-3 ■ Ecological Systems that Influence and Determine Child Development[35]

System	Description	Examples
Microsystem	Direct, reciprocal interactions between adults and children; also includes others who influence those directly acting on the child	Parents, siblings, care providers, teachers
Mesosystem	Environments that serve as connections between individuals in the microsystem	Home, school, day care
Exosystem	Social settings that affect children, but do not contain them; community-based organizations, services, and forces that influence the child-family microsystem; and informal community supports for families	Health and welfare services, workplace policies and programs, social networks, financial aid, jobs, recreational opportunities for families
Macrosystem	Cultural values, laws, customs, resources, and the priority that children and children's issues have in the community	Day care standards, educational standards and expectations, laws

BOX 2-5	KEY POINTS—ECOLOGICAL SYSTEMS

Development is determined by interactions between the child and his family.
Interface between child and family changes constantly in response to internal and external forces.
Societal structures have powerful effects on the child, primarily by altering the interaction between parent and child.
The child's own behavior and development alter the caretaking milieu.

The essence of this ecological systems theory is that all the outer systems mediate their effects through the alteration of the microsystem that surrounds the child, the interaction and care within the family. For example, homelessness, isolation, job stress, and lack of health care all influence the interaction between parent and child through depression, lack of focus, tension, lack of time for the child, and physical hardship. Depression in parents profoundly affects even young infants, as we will see. The components of a health care system will change how and what a parent does in health care and in attention to development. Religious beliefs may determine how many children are in a family or what kind of discipline is used. These, in turn, will act through alterations in the parent-child interface. School conditions alter how children interact with each other, as well as the way teacher and child re-

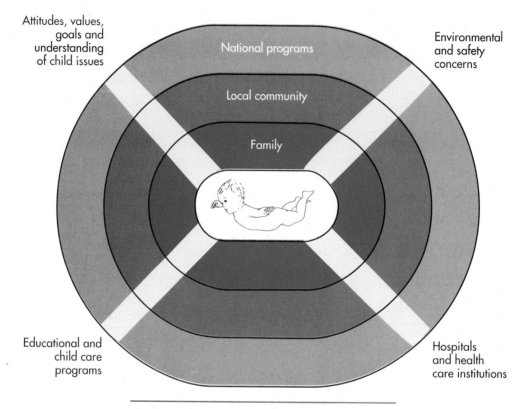

Attitudes, values, goals and understanding of child issues

Environmental and safety concerns

National programs

Local community

Family

Educational and child care programs

Hospitals and health care institutions

Fig. 2-1   Spheres of advocacy in pediatric practice.

late. This theory implies that the whole system is in constant change, including the child. The impact of each factor will vary, depending on the developmental status of the child and all the other factors in this system.

To the pediatric clinician, it is no surprise that a child develops in a context with many complex layers. Many issues in behavior and development have their genesis in the child's surroundings in the broadest sense. This perspective does prompt the necessity to have an understanding of these dynamic systems if we are to provide effective advocacy and intervention. An ecological systems approach mandates a broad perspective on pediatric care.

Bronfenbrenner's work parallels the advocacy perspective put forward in this volume since the first edition (Fig. 2-1). If all these systems influence health and development of the child, the pediatric clinician's role may include care and advocacy based on any or all of these systems. One cannot care for children without taking these systems into account. At one level, these systems become the patient.

MULTIPLE INTELLIGENCES

Howard Gardner, in looking at the way that humans process information, has described seven different ways of learning.[38] Called "multiple intelligences," these clearly varying dif-

TABLE 2-4 ■ Multiple Intelligences

Intelligence	Description
Linguistic	Sensitivity to language; language-based functions
Logico-mathematical	Abstract reasoning, manipulation of symbols, detection of patterns, logical reasoning
Musical	Detection and production of musical structures and patterns; appreciation of pitch, rhythm, musical expressiveness
Spatial	Visual memory, visual-spatial skills, visualization
Body-kinesthetic	Representation of ideas, feelings in movement; use of body, coordination, goal-directed activities
Naturalistic	Classification and recognition of animals, plants
Social	Sensitivity and responsiveness to moods, motives, intentions, and feelings of others
Personal	Sensitivity to self, feelings, strengths, desires, weaknesses and understanding of intention and motivation of others

ferences in a child's "hard wiring" identify strengths and vulnerabilities that influence how a person functions. Each type is neurologically based with its own developmental course (Table 2-4). Gardner dismisses the notion of general intelligence entirely. Schools base their teaching and assessment upon linguistic intelligence, but a child with strengths in other areas may not be successful in that particular milieu. Gardner's theories allow the framing of many difficulties with learning as learning "differences" rather than learning "disorders." His view is that we miss a lot of human potential when we fail to allow these other mental abilities to blossom.

Little research exists to substantiate this theory, and some observations indicate that these abilities may not be so distinct. However, these insights focus on the individuality of each child. Children failing in one domain should be encouraged to develop other areas in which their unique ways of learning may be successful. Identifying these varying competencies to parents allows them to see positives in their child, abilities that may flower later than others because of the differential rate of development of these multiple areas.

TEMPERAMENT

The way a child develops, not just the what, has been the focus of clinicians and researchers since the seminal work of Chess and Thomas.[39-40] The study of temperament has broadened our view of the range of differences between children. *Temperament can be defined as those stable, individual differences in emotional reactivity, activity level, attention, and self-regulation.* Temperament in childhood is a strong predictor of behavior problems in children and of adjustment and personality issues in adulthood.

TABLE 2-5 ■ Temperament Dimensions	
Dimension	**Description**
Activity level	Amount of physical movement during sleep and awake periods
Rhythmicity	Regularity of physiological functions, such as sleep, hunger, elimination
Approach-withdrawal	Nature of the initial response to new stimuli
Adaptability	Ease or difficulty with which reactions can be modified
Persistence–attention span	Length of time that an activity is pursued
Intensity of reaction	Energy level of the responses regardless of quality or direction
Distractibility	Effectiveness of extraneous environmental stimuli in interfering with ongoing behavior
Threshold of responsiveness	Amount of stimulation (e.g., light, sound, touch) necessary to draw a discernible response from the child
Quality of mood	General emotional tone of the child's response and interactions

The standard dimensions of child personality are shown in Table 2-5. Clinical appraisal of these dimensions can be done informally in a primary care setting over time, but has been standardized by Carey and McDevitt (see Appendix).[41] These all have an age-linked grounding so that we do not expect a toddler to have the same activity level as a grade school child, for example. A child is characterized on these dimensions in comparison with other children his age. Although standardized on typically developing children, these same dimensions can be applied, with care, to those with atypical development. Adjusting for the developmental rather than chronological age is one consideration.

Characterizing a child's individuality on these dimensions allows the clinician to assist parents in seeing the child's unique needs and in developing behavior management strategies that are likely to be successful. For example, a child with low adaptability will need help in anticipating and coping with change. A high-activity child will need to wind down before bed. Good advice follows from a clear understanding of individual characteristics.

Temperament Cluster

The way in which these characteristics cluster strongly influences the perception and reality of difficulty in child rearing. In western societies (i.e., where this has been studied in large populations) the population has been described with three characteristics:
- Easy (40%). Regular routines, cheerful and adaptable
- Difficult (10%). Irregular, slow to accept change, and tending to respond negatively
- Slow to warm up (15%). Inactive, mild, low-key responsiveness, negative or neutral mood and slow adjustment.
  The rest (35%) have a mix of characteristics.

Behavioral issues are predicted by temperment. Difficult babies are four times as likely as easy infants to have preschool and school difficulties. Slow to warm up children are likely to have adjustment difficulties in middle childhood and beyond.

Developmental tasks themselves will be approached differently based on temperament. A quiet child who is slow to warm up may try his first steps hesitantly, even late, but demonstrate a relatively well-coordinated gait once he makes the leap to independent walking. Clinical assessment of developmental tasks should take a child's temperamental characteristics into account. Box 2-6 lists points to keep in mind about temperament

The concept of temperamental match or "goodness of fit" between parent and child is often the source of interactional difficulties and behavioral complaints. For example, a quiet, low-intensity boy who withdraws initially in new situations may be regarded by his dad as a "sissy." A high-intensity girl with a negative mood that is also highly persistent may have trouble making friends. She may be regarded by her parents as antisocial, ungrateful, and generally difficult, particularly if the parents are gregarious, flexible, and generally low key. In these circumstances the clinician must help families see these differences and respond with altered expectations.

The concept of temperament has inspired much research since the 1970s. A new thrust in the area is the problem of the biological-genetic origins of these characteristics. Twin studies, cross-cultural studies, and family studies confirm this link. A subarea of these efforts of intriguing interest is the evaluation of behavioral phenotypes that are associated with specific genetic conditions (e.g., Williams syndrome, Lesch-Nyhan syndrome).

Temperament is remarkably stable from infancy to adulthood in most cases. Some constellations of temperament are more likely to create problems at different points in development, but the trait itself does not change significantly. A slow to warm up baby is often easy to manage but may, as a school-age child, have difficulty handling the multiple and changing demands of the school-age years, for example.

Without a strong understanding of how temperament influences behavioral and developmental issues, the clinician will have a hard time evaluating behavior, behavior problems, and difficulties that children and families face in all the systems that change their lives.

BOX 2-6   KEY POINTS—TEMPERAMENT

Temperament is the stable pattern of reactivity and responsiveness. It is the foundation for personality.

Temperamental characteristics influence all aspects of development and behavior.

Certain clusters of temperamental characteristics are associated with an increased likelihood of behavioral concerns, discipline problems, and adjustment difficulties at particular points in development.

Lack of fit or a mismatch of temperamental characteristics is often the source of difficulties for child care provider.

CROSS-CULTURAL ISSUES

Most studies of child development are done in Western, industrialized cultures, often among affluent, well-educated people, who are the people most available for research. These studies represent a small portion of the human family and a small part of the evolutionary patterns of the care of children. These views of humankind, the foundation for most theoretical perspectives, are necessarily narrow unless we look beyond our own borders for broader perspectives on the universals of human development.

The study of human development in varying cultural contexts has emerged as an important area of research, particularly in the last half of the twentieth century. Systematic studies were initially targeted to characterize populations as either ahead or behind the dominant American culture in terms of developmental norms, observations that quickly dropped over the edge into racism. Fortunately, the thrust of recent research has been to look at the connections between certain child-rearing patterns and the antecedent and resultant psychological processes in children and adults within that culture.[42] By looking at the adaptations prompted by the forces that the environment offers, we come closer to defining the universals of human development, as well as the limits of adaptability. These insights inform our understanding of our own culture and our own child care traditions and prompt us to respect and value the richness in the subpopulations that we serve.[20,43-45]

Definitions

Culture is the enduring psychological structure that is common within a population. This encompasses shared beliefs, customs, traditions, values, and sense of self and one's place in the universe. Culture shapes the types and patterns of communication as reflected in the language, the proper interpersonal distance, and even who talks to whom. Culture goes beyond costume. Culture as an underlying guide for the business of life may be held more tightly by those in foreign circumstances or by those in the throes of social change. Even when non-Western populations change their dress to jeans and a T-shirt, they don't change their core selves, at least in the short term. Box 2-7 summarizes some important concepts of culture.

BOX 2-7	CROSS-CULTURAL ISSUES

Culture is the complex internal psychological structure that determines values, sense of self and others, and expected patterns of behavior.

Culture determines ideas about health and illness, personal responsibility in health and disease, and the nature of healing.

Cultural practices in child rearing and in health are most often successful in the environments in which they arose. They may be maladaptive in another setting.

Cross-cultural differences are present in newborns, reflecting long-term genetic, intrauterine, and even perinatal factors.

Traditional practices should be respected and built upon unless they are harmful or clearly maladaptive in the current environment.

Parents and Children

Culture moves bidirectionally from birth onward.[46,47] The health and behavior of newborns vary around the world.[48] In many comparative studies using identical assessments, the modal behavior of the newborn changes around the world, although in all cultures, newborns exhibit the same range of behaviors. This probably reflects differences in genetic endowment, the intrauterine environment, and birth care practices. However, the behavior of the infant in turn changes the way in which the baby is handled and cared for within and across cultures.[44]

Traditional child care practices are the outgrowth of the demands of the environment in which they arose, the characteristics of the infants themselves, and those characteristics that are needed and valued in adults in that culture. For example, among the Gusii of Kenya, a very solicitous pattern of early physical care, including attentiveness to cleanliness, skin health, and nutrition no doubt was adaptive in a culture where high infant mortality was related to bacterial infections coming in through the skin. In contrast, social interaction with the infant is restrained and stylized.[49] Energy expended in this direction would have taken energy away from growth, a more important imperative in that context. Further, adult interaction among the Gusii is restrained in intensity and is governed by strict rules in form and content. Babies learn even the subtleties of these practices in the minute regulation of these early interactions with care providers.[44] A good mother feeds her baby well, keeps him or her clean, and early on trains the child to obediently do as told to contribute to the household economy. No need exists here to foster independence in thinking or in action; to do so sets a child at odds with the demands of fitting into this peasant culture. With one of the highest growth rates in the world, this population's strategies for child rearing are a success in the context of the environment in which they evolved. They may not be completely adaptive in the current context because this culture, like all others today, struggles with the forces of social change.

Another view of what constitutes a good mother is provided by studies of the child-rearing patterns of Japanese mothers in the United States and in Japan. Japanese mothers see their job, usually quite below a conscious level, as taming the feral nature of the infant into a dependent and responsible member of a family. Feeding may be done when the infant is barely awake as the mother organizes every aspect of the child's life, keeping the child quiet, fed, and growing. In contrast, white American moms see success as increasing independence of their completely dependent infant. The early introduction of solids, the baby's sleeping by itself, and toilet training are all landmarks in the quest for autonomy, a value that Japanese moms would find anathema. The requirements of the environments in which these values and practices arose clearly were different. Neither pattern is wrong or inferior, but each is adaptive at least in the historical and cultural context. These cross-cultural examples help us in seeing some of the differences closer to home.

The many groups that make up America bring their own ideas and beliefs to the raising of their children. A child health care provider can support them in doing their best only with a culture-sensitive perspective, respecting differences and having some information on some of the core cultural values that prompt specific practices in child rearing. This is a rich area of research that cannot be fully reviewed here. The wise clinician will expand these basic ideas with more information on the groups with which he or she regularly works. Some basic group concepts and examples are presented in the following section.

Hispanic Americans. This large and growing group has variation in culture within it with origins from diverse areas, such as Puerto Rico, all the regions and subgroups of Mexico, and several Latin American countries. The degree and duration of acculturation vary widely. However, some important commonalties to recognize are the following:

■ Family is of central importance. Sense of self is defined by place in the family. Sense of worth depends on meeting familial obligations. A mother's sense of worth is determined by the health, particularly the growth, of her children and on the well-being of her husband.

 When Maria went home from her son's first visit to the doctor, at 4 days of age, she had decided to bottle feed. The baby had lost weight. Even though the doctor said all babies did that, she was sure her husband would blame her. She wanted a "gordito," a little fat one.

■ Obedience and sociability are of greater value than school achievement, independence, and autonomy in children.
■ In this patrilineal society, men make the important decisions. Women often need to ask their mates before deciding anything of importance for a child.
■ Children are highly valued and indulged when young. Discipline for little ones is sparse, but for older children, particularly boys, it is often severe.
■ The distinction in appropriate behavior and standards based upon gender is very strong.

 The Martinez family refused to let their daughter Elena play in the school band because practice got out late and she would have to walk home alone. Jorge, their son, played basketball at night even though he was 3 years younger. "He can take care of himself," the parents said.

■ Traditional beliefs about hot and cold diseases and cures, the evil eye as a source of illness in children, and illness carried in the air survive even in families that also adhere to modern medical beliefs. Traditional cures and the ministrations of traditional healers are often given simultaneously with modern medicine.

Amoxicillin was prescribed for pneumonia in Baby Sosa. The family didn't give the antibiotic because the instructions said to keep the medicine in the refrigerator. Pneumonia is a cold disease, so a cold medicine was wrong. The family gave the baby hot tea instead.

Black Americans. This divergent group brings cultural traditions primarily from west Africa, but they are mixed with adaptations caused by the long and varying interface with the dominant white culture. Socioeconomic and urban-rural distinctions may be even more prominent than those based upon culture. But some specific characteristics may still be evident in many individuals and families.

- Resiliency and strength are valued in children. "Spoiled" or "bad" are often positive terms to describe a child, reflecting in part the value of being strong, determined, strongly attached to the parent, and going after the parent's attention.

 Mrs. Johnson brought her 9-month-old son in, saying he "was bad" because he seemed to cry every time she was out of his sight.

- Traditional cultures with origins in west Africa were matrilineal, and a lot of decision focus remains with the women. Grandmothers and senior women in the community have always been a powerful force and remain so. This role has increased in current times with the high proportion of single-mother families.
- Religious traditions are a powerful community force. Support for families often comes from these institutions.

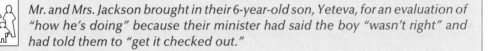 *Mr. and Mrs. Jackson brought in their 6-year-old son, Yeteva, for an evaluation of "how he's doing" because their minister had said the boy "wasn't right" and had told them to "get it checked out."*

- Early independence in children is often valued, particularly among boys.
- Exuberance in expression, dress, talk, and interpersonal interactions is a positive value.

Ethiopian families coming recently to this country are from a different racial group and bring very different beliefs. They are close to their own traditional ideas about child rearing, health, and healing that include medicines, evil eye beliefs, and others. They are a people who have suffered famine and war in the immediate sense. They may share very few characteristics with other Americans of African ancestry.

Asian Americans. This group includes people from Japan and China, as well as Vietnam, Laos, Cambodia, Indonesia, and the Philippines. Clearly, traditions vary widely, as do socioeconomic factors and the degree of assimilation. The following are some broad, common themes of several groups:

- Children are seen as very independent. The goal of parenting is to mold them into an interdependency with family and tradition.
- Men make important family decisions, but women are almost always completely in charge of the direct rearing of children.

- A woman's sense of self-worth may be almost entirely wrapped up in the success of children, particularly educational success.
- Teasing and poking fun at children are seen as appropriate ways of shaping child behavior.
- Restraint and formality in nonfamilial interactions are expected. An overly familiar health care provider may create discomfort and a suspicion that the provider doesn't really have the expected position and status.

 Dr. Atkinson said, "Hi, call me Mel. I'm the new doctor here. How're you doing?" as he gave Alvin, a 10-year-old, a high-five and gave a friendly clasp to Mr. Lee's shoulder. The Lees all stared in silence.

- Psychological processes are poorly conceptualized, and mental distress is often presented in somatic terms. Healing often involves physical and social, as well as psychological cures.

 Mrs. Wong brought in her daughter Cynthia, a sixth grader, because of recurrent abdominal pain. Cynthia, a strong scholar and track star, who was active in student government, looked glum and had lost a lot of weight. Her mom wanted "tablets to fix her up."

Native Americans. This large, heterogenous group comes from both nomadic and agrarian traditions, so some ideas about community, interpersonal space, and male-female roles would be expected to vary. However, some beliefs across groups are more similar to each other than to other cultural groups.

- Each person is seen to have his or her own life path, so imposition upon another violates that freedom. This leads to differences in views on discipline and child rearing in general.

 Mr. and Mrs. Running Bear called to say that they were canceling for now the surgery on their son John's knee. John said he wanted to go home when they arrived in the hospital. They said it was John's choice.

- A proper life is one that fits in with the forces of nature rather than conquers or fights nature. Going along with issues sometimes is seen by outsiders as unwarranted passivity.

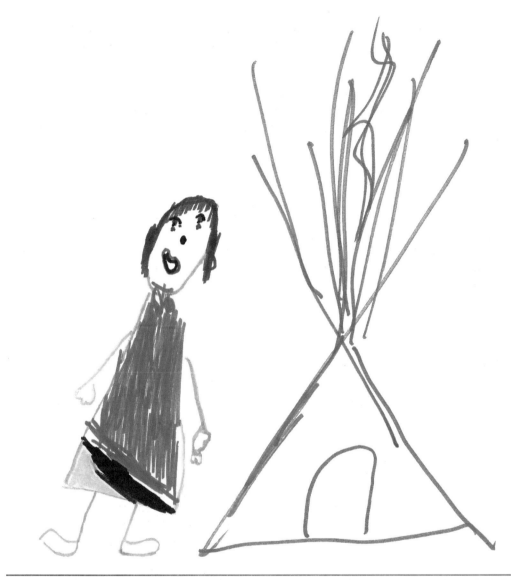

An 8-year-old Native American girl in foster care outside of the tribe draws her birth mother alone, next to a traditional Plains teepee and wearing a long, leather dress. Her mother actually lives in town and abhors the signs of her native culture (original in colored markers on white).

Michael's parents refused the laser removal of his birthmark, even though they thought it ugly. They also thought it meant he was marked for something special.

- These are matrilineal societies by and large, and one's place is set by that lineage. Maternal uncles and others may play important roles in the life of a child.
- Eye-to-eye contact, getting to the point of a meeting without introduction, and greeting and touching an unfamiliar person are considered rude. Loud or gregarious talk is offensive. Patient pauses give openings to speak.
- Illness is considered an imbalance between the individual and the universe. Healing involves restoration of that balance.

 The doctor said that chronic diarrhea in Jerrod was due to an infection the family caught while camping last summer. Jerrod's parents felt that the feud they had with their own parents was really the cause.

Non-Hispanic White Americans. The dominant Euro-American culture is influenced by social, political, religious, and even geographical forces. A few prominent, underlying beliefs that touch on child rearing and that distinguish this large group from those now considered minorities may give perspective.
- Children are viewed as completely dependent at birth. Good parenting involves moving kids to increasing levels of independence quickly. Prolonged dependency is poorly tolerated.
- The characteristics of the individual and the promotion of individual achievement are factors that underlie parent goals. Sense of self is defined by the realization of these individual goals, not those of the family or community.
- Individuals who are moderately aggressive are usually successful in realizing their own goals. Too much aggression is a bad thing.
- Weakness, illness, and disability all contain some element of personal failure.
- Understanding and insight are important in the conduct of everyday affairs. Child rearing involves a lot of talk, discussion, review, and evaluation. Choices are important.
- The possibilities for an individual are boundless. Dependence on family is a weakness. Although many long for the traditional life of an extended family nearby, most families expect to live far from their family of origin.
- Science and technology can solve all ills. Anything can be fixed.

 Darren's parents continued to search for treatments for his learning disabilities in spite of improved behavior and better school performance. They were hoping for "all A's."

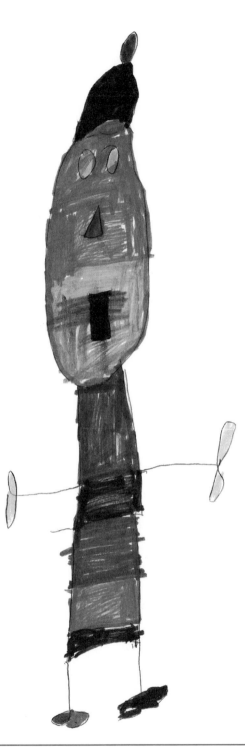

A Hutterite girl of 8 draws herself in her regular daily dress, which is very traditional and stylized. Her long, multilayered shirt and her stiff scarf and bonnet cover her hair and head. No ears or hair is an accurate portrayal of her appearance (original in very bright colors on white).

Approach To Cultural Understanding

All parents want the best for their children so that they will grow, thrive, and develop into contributing members of their society and culture.[50] The strategies and behaviors to accomplish this vary widely, and some of them may be poorly adaptive in the present context. While respecting these underlying goals, we will sometimes be called on to confront practices that are at odds with our own beliefs or that seem to be harmful.

When confronted with an issue that seems to be touched by cultural differences, the clinician should state the concern clearly and then elicit the patient and family's views.

 Dr. Jordan expressed his concern about José's weight: "José's weight gain is very slow; he is thin for his age, and I am concerned. I'd like to know more about what he has actually been getting to eat each day so I can better understand what can be done to help. I know you are concerned and I'm sure you have some ideas about what's going on. I'd also like to hear what you've tried so far to help him grow."

In evaluating how to respond to particular practices, the clinician should consider the following:

■ If the practice is good for the child or is neutral, don't try to change it. If asked, give an honest opinion or view on whether it is of value. Use it as a chance to learn more about the basic values and practices of the culture, not just as a curiosity.

 Baby Maria had a cord around her neck with a small pouch attached. Dr. Milan asked what it was and was told it was meant to protect her from the evil eye. He asked the parents to explain their belief to him.

■ If the practice is having a negative impact on the child or preventing the implementation of an approach that would be helpful in the present setting, explain that impact by "contexting" your advice.

 Hy Lui had cupping scars all over his back, results of the traditional healing for pneumonia. Dr. Sorenson said that modern medicine now has a more specific cure for this disease that doesn't cause pain and scarring. He indicated that warmth and tapping the chest are still seen as helpful but that the cupping causes undue pain.

■ If the practice is clearly harmful, identify the belief or value that is at its genesis and validate that goal. Then explain the harm to the child that you identify. Tell what you see as the result or consequence of the practice. Clearly state what you think should happen and try to connect that action to the shared goal. Involve key decision makers (who may not

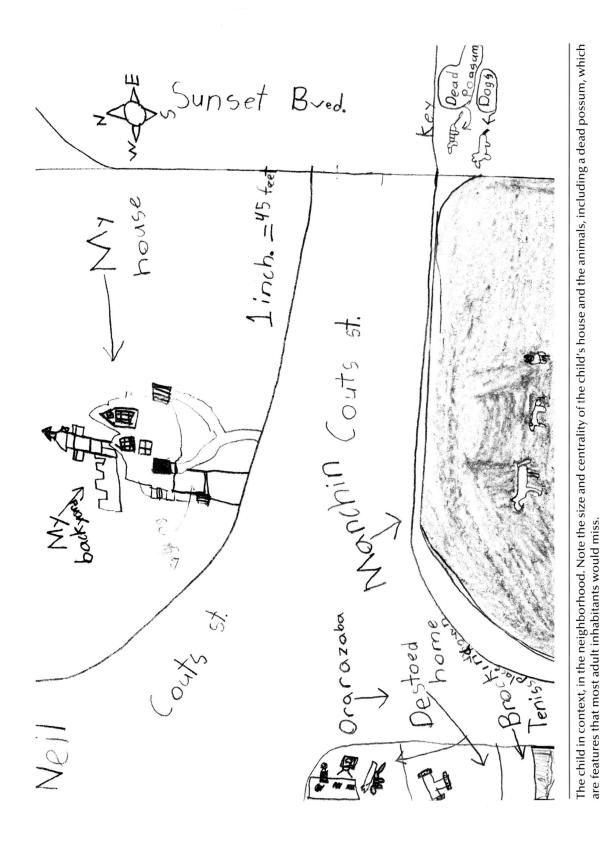

The child in context, in the neighborhood. Note the size and centrality of the child's house and the animals, including a dead possum, which are features that most adult inhabitants would miss.

TABLE 2-6 ■ Perspectives of Human Behavior

Age	Theories of Development			Skill areas		Possible Psychopathology
	Freud	Erikson	Piaget	Language	Motor	
Birth-18 mo	Oral	Basic trust vs. mistrust	Sensorimotor	Body actions; crying; naming; pointing; shared social communication	Reflex, sitting; reaching; grasping; walking, mouthing	Autism; anaclitic depression; colic; disorders of attachment; feeding and sleeping problems
18 mo-3 yr	Anal	Autonomy vs. shame, doubt	Symbolic preoperational	Sentences; telegraph; unique utterances; sharing of events	Climbing; running; jumping; use of tools, using toilet, early self care	Separation issues; negativism; fearfulness; constipation; shyness, withdrawal; aggressiveness
3-6 yr	Oedipal	Initiative vs. guilt	Intuition, preoperational	Connective words; can be readily understood; tells and follows stories, questions	Increased coordination; tricycle; jumping; writing	Enuresis; encopresis; anxiety; aggressive acting out; phobias
6-12 yr	Latency	Industry vs. inferiority	Concrete operational	Subordinate sentences; reading and writing; language reasoning	Increased skills; sports; recreational cooperative games	School phobias; obsessive reactions; conversion reactions; depressive equivalents; anxiety; attention deficit hyperactivity disorder
12-17 yr	Adolescence (genital)	Identity vs. role confusion	Formal operational	Reason abstract; using language; abstract mental manipulation	Refinement of skills	Delinquency; promiscuity; schizophrenia; anorexia nervosa; suicide
17-30 yr	Young adulthood	Intimacy vs. isolation	Formal operational	Reason abstract; using language; abstract mental manipulation	Refinement of specialized skills; sports skills peak	Schizophrenia; borderline personality; adjustment disorders; development of intimate relationships; difficulties with relationships
30-60 yr	Adulthood	Generativity vs. stagnation	Formal operational	Reason abstract; using language; abstract mental manipulation	Refinement of skills	Depression; self-doubts; career development issues; family, social network; neuroses
>60 yr	Old age	Ego integration vs. despair	Formal operational	Some loss of skills; decreased memory, focus	Loss of functions	Involutional depression; anxiety; anger; increased dependency

include the parents at all) from the patient's community in the negotiations. Use all "I" phrases ("I am concerned because . . ."). Acknowledge the care and passion that are behind adherence to the practice while clearly advising against the practice itself.

Child development is powerfully influenced by the cultural context in which it occurs. Culture goes much deeper than language, dress, and specific practices. These all reflect underlying psychological structures. Differences between groups lead to different methods for the job of raising children. Health, disease, and healing are viewed in distinct ways that influence the experience of a health care encounter. Without an understanding of the cultural element that a family brings to that setting, it is difficult to find solutions supporting health and development that are likely to be fully accepted and adopted. Further, without a cultural perspective, we miss much of the richness and vibrancy that families bring to our professional lives.

SUMMARY

As clinicians, we do not have to commit to one theoretical perspective. No single school has all of the answers, nor can any theory explain the richness of even one child's behavior completely. Table 2-6 lays out some of the crossovers that surface in the comparison of three of these perspectives. Every age carries themes and issues that distinguish each stage from the next. Included are the major language and motor milestones for each age so that you can "hang your hat" on the milestones with which you may be familiar. Developmental difficulties and frank psychopathology appear at various ages and emerge from the basic developmental processes operant at that time. Although severe forms of most of these difficulties are rare, they represent to some degree a failure or a delay in coping with various developmental issues. The march of a child (and family) through these stages is surrounded by cultural, sociopolitical, economic, historic, scientific, and artistic forces that color, shape, determine, and are determined by each child's unique course. This makes human development one of the most complex processes imaginable. And we are privileged to see it unfold, one encounter after another, day in and day out.

At this point, an abundance of knowledge about a child's development can inform and enrich these encounters. The pediatric clinician will do well to pack some of this wealth of information into a "mental black bag" every day as he or she goes "into the field," that is, the office, so the knowledge can be used in close interactions with children and their families.

REFERENCES
1. Kagan J: *The nature of the child,* New York, 1984, Basic Books.
2. Cole M, Cole SR: *The development of children,* ed 3, New York, 1996, WH Freeman and Co.
3. Elkind D: *A sympathetic understanding of the child: birth to sixteen,* ed 3, Boston, 1994, Allyn and Bacon.
4. Berk L: *Infants, children and adolescents,* ed 3, Boston, 1999, Allyn and Bacon.
5. Gesell A, Ilg F: Infant and child in the culture of today (1943). In Gesell A, Iig F, editors: *Child development,* New York, 1949, Harper & Row.
6. Gesell A: *The embryology of behavior,* New York, 1945, Harper & Row.
7. Gesell A: The ontogenesis of infant behavior. In Carmichael L, editor: *Manual of child psychology,* New York, 1946, John Wiley & Sons.

8. Gesell A, Amatruda C: *Developmental diagnosis,* ed 2, New York, 1965, Harper & Row.

9. Watson JB: *Behaviorism* (1924), New York, 1970, WW Norton & Co.

10. Pavlov IP: *Conditioned reflexes,* London, 1927, Oxford University Press (translated and edited by GV Anrep).

11. Illingworth RS: *The development of the infant and young child: normal and abnormal,* London, 1966, Williams & Wilkins.

12. Knobloch H, Stevens F, Malone A: *A Manual of developmental diagnosis: the administration and interpretation of the revised Gesell and Amatruda developmental and neurologic examination,* Hagerstown, Md, 1980, Harper & Row.

13. McGraw M: *The neuromuscular maturation of the human infant,* New York, 1943, Columbia University Press.

14. Bayley N: *Bayley scales of infant development,* New York, 1994, Psychological Corp.

15. Freud S: Three contributions to the theory of sex. In Brill AA, translator: *The basic writings of Sigmund Freud,* New York, 1905, Modern Library.

16. Freud S: *Collected papers,* vol 2-5, New York, 1959, Basic Books.

17. Hall C, Lindzey G: *Theories of personality,* ed 2, New York, 1975, John Wiley & Sons.

18. Emde R: Individual meaning and increasing complexity: contributions of Sigmund Freud and Rene Spitz to developmental psychology, *Dev Psychol* 28:347, 1992.

19. Erikson EH: Identity and the life cycle. In Klein GS, editor: *Psychological issues,* vol 1, New York, 1959, International Universities Press.

20. LeVine R: *Culture, behavior and personality,* Chicago, 1973, Aldine.

21. Thompson C: Cultural pressures in the psychology of women. In Mullahy P, editor: *A study of interpersonal relations,* New York, 1950, Hermitage Press.

22. Mahler MS, Pine F, Bergman A: *The psychological birth of the human infant: symbiosis and individuation,* New York, 1975, Basic Books.

23. Erikson EH: *Childhood and society,* ed 2, New York, 1963, WW Norton & Co.

24. Skinner BF: *About behaviorism* (1927), New York, 1974, Alfred A Knopf.

25. Bandura A: Influence of model's reinforcement contingencies on the acquisition of imitative responses, *J Pers Soc Psychol* 1:589, 1965.

26. Bandura A, editor: *Psychological modeling,* Chicago, 1971, Atherton, Aldine.

27. Bandura A: *Self-efficacy and the exercise of control,* New York, 1997, Freeman Press.

28. Lovas OI: *Behavioral treatment of autistic children.* Morristown, NJ, 1973, General Learning Press.

29. Piaget J: *Play, dreams and imitation in childhood,* New York, 1951, WW Norton & Co.

30. Piaget J: *The origins of intelligence in children,* New York, 1952, WW Norton & Co (translated by M Cook).

31. Piaget J, Inhelder B: *The psychology of the child,* New York, 1969, Basic Books (translated by H Weaver).

32. Ginsburg H, Opper S: *Piaget's theory of intellectual development,* Englewood Cliffs, NJ, 1969, Prentice-Hall.

33. Dasan PR, editor: *Piagetian psychology: cross-cultural contributions,* New York, 1977, Gardner Press.

34. Kohlberg L: Development of moral character and moral ideology. In Hoffman ML, Hoffman LW, editors: *Review of child development research,* vol 1, New York, 1974, Russell Sage Foundation.

35. Bronfenbrenner U, Ceci S: Nature-nurture reconceptualized in developmental perspective: a bioecological approach, *Psychol Rev* 101:568, 1998.

36. Bronfenbrenner U, Ceci S: *The Ecology of human development: experiments by nature and design,* Cambridge, Mass, 1979, Harvard University Press.

37. Rutter M et al: *Fifteen thousand hours: secondary schools and their effects on children,* Cambridge, Mass, 1979, Harvard University Press.

38. Gardner H: *Frames of mind: the theory of multiple intelligence,* New York, 1993, Basic Books.
39. Chess S, Thomas A: *Temperament and development,* New York, 1977, Brunner Mazel.
40. Chess S, Thomas A: *Origins and evolution of behavior disorders,* New York, 1984, Brunner Mazel.
41. McDevitt SC, Carey WB: *The Carey temperament scale,* Scottsdale, Arizona, 1995, Behavioral Developmental Initiatives.
42. Barr RG et al: Crying in !Kung San infants: a test of a cultural specific hypothesis, *Dev Med Child Neurol* 33:601, 1991.
43. Greenfield PM, Suzuki L: Culture and human development: implications for parenting education, pediatrics and mental health. In Siegel I, Renninger K, editors: *Handbook of child psychology,* vol 4, ed 5, New York, 1998, Wiley.
44. LeVine RA et al: *Child care and culture: lessons from Africa,* Cambridge, England, 1994, Cambridge University Press.
45. Werner EE: *Cross-cultural child development: a view from the planet earth,* Monterey, Calif, 1979, Brooks-Cole.
46. Leiderman PH, Tulkin SR, Rosenfeld A, editors: *Culture and infancy,* New York, 1977, Academic Press.
47. Werner EE: A cross-cultural perspective on infancy, *J Cross-Cult Psychol* 19:96, 1988.
48. Dixon S et al: Perinatal circumstances and newborn outcome among the Gusii of Kenya: assessment of risk, *Inf Behav Devel* 5:11, 1982.
49. Dixon S et al: Mother-infant interaction around a teaching task: an African-American comparison, *Child Dev* 55:1252, 1984.
50. LeVine RA: Human parental care: universal goals, cultural strategies, individual behavior. In LeVine RA, Miller PM, West MM, editors: *Parental behavior in diverse societies,* San Francisco, 1988, Jossey Bass.

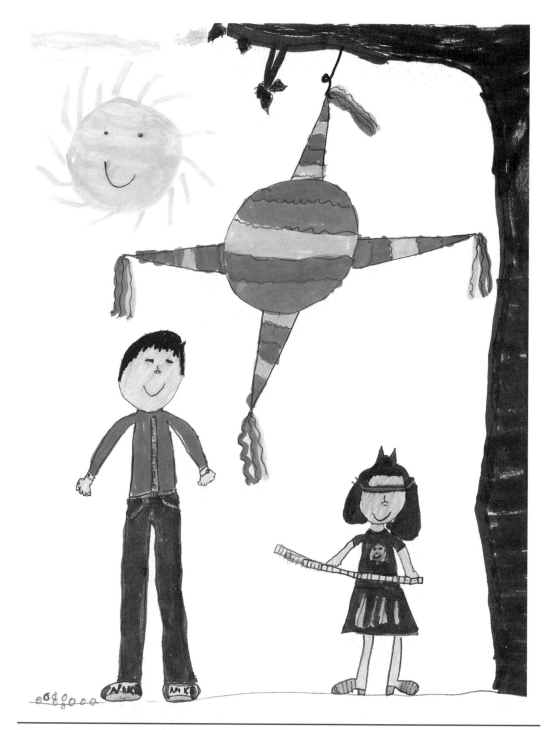

Cross-cultural perspectives. A Mexican American girl, age 11, shows herself ready to go after the piñata with a smiling dad nearby. Cultural traditions anchor childhood memories.

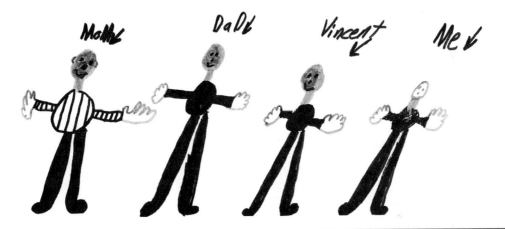

A 9-year-old boy shows himself with his family. Large hands, even grounding show positive self-image. The beginnings of actual proportion of figures versus the child's perceptions of power and importance are clear. By Quinn Loendorf.

"I think you should ask the patient what's wrong with him or her, not the parent. The parent is not sick. The kid is sick. He knows more of himself than anyone else understands. A patient. Thanks. Karen." A child reminds the doctor about the importance of talking to children. (This statement was discovered on a bench in a teaching clinic after all the patients had been seen. It was wrinkled and rolled in a ball. Courtesy of Dr. John Kennell.)

THE DEVELOPMENT-BASED OFFICE: DOING MORE WITH EACH VISIT

■ **Martin T. Stein**

KEY WORDS

Interview
Transactional-Educational Model
Dual Patient
Verbal and Nonverbal Communication
Process and Content
Explanatory Model
Active Listening
Transference

Families are the focal element of life's circumstances and the primary context within which life is experienced, especially for children.[1] Pediatricians tend to focus on the child's symptoms, developmental skills, and behaviors and spend less time assessing family strengths, stresses, and life-event changes. By incorporating the parent(s) and the child as equal partners during the clinical **interview,** the clinician will discover important information about a family's strengths and potential stressors, such as marital discord, depression, and economic and social uncertainties, along with specific data about the child's place in the family and community. The family-directed interview model supports the notion, confirmed by research and clinical experience, that the developmental potential for most children is affected by the environment in which they live.[2,3] Family-directed interviewing also encourages data generation about the child's home environment, which has been shown to have an important impact on a child's development.[4]

THE ENCOUNTER AS A PLANNED EVENT

The clinical practice of preventive pediatric care is built on a **transactional-educational model.** When the clinical interview is directed in a manner that provides an educational experience for the parents, child, and clinician, expanded gains emerge from the encounter. By *planned orchestration* of the style and content of the interview, a new dimension is added to the practice of pediatrics, making it both more effective and more rewarding. The manner in which questions are asked, the types of questions asked, the direction of the questioning (to the parent and the child), and the actual interaction with the child are critical components of the interview. They control not only the informational data base but also what the parent and child become mindful of in the broader context of growth and health.

THE PHYSICAL LAYOUT

The potential for an "educational experience" during a pediatric office visit begins before the actual clinical interview. The physical and social ecology of a medical office that serves the needs of children requires forethought in planning and continuous modification. An appreciation that personnel, space, color, and design can interact to create a positive, health-promoting atmosphere may generate interesting ideas that allow the office environment to enhance child development, parent-child-clinician interactions, and assessment of health and development.[5] The pictures or children's drawings selected for the walls, the availability of crawl and walk space, the toys in the reception area, and the educational material made available to parents and children are at first seemingly unrelated decisions, but they create a unique theme in each office. A special message will be given to families even as they enter the door of the practice that this is a place for children and families, that children are expected to explore, and that developmental concerns are front and center at this practice.

Whether a new office or clinic facility is being planned or modification to an established office seems possible, two questions are useful: "How can we plan to use the available space in a manner that is consistent with the developmental needs of the children and parents who will come to the facility? Can the design promote comfort, relieve anxiety, nurture the parent-child relationship, and maintain a learning and educational milieu?" Priorities, budgets, and available space will vary among settings, but a core group of developmental principles are applicable to most pediatric offices, including the following:

■ *A busy waiting room is like a neighborhood park.* Parents can observe their children learning to play and interact with other children. Toys, books, or a wall board equipped for drawing will make these interactions more interesting for parents and children. The waiting room might also serve as an after-hours meeting place or informal classroom.

■ *The waiting area should allow for movement and play of children.* Flooring, walls, and furniture should consider the developmental requirements of children at various age groups. Safety, clean lines, and cheerfulness are key elements. Avoid overstimulating, noisy, or trendy decor. Doors should shut off main traffic areas.

■ *Furniture and play objects can be safe, but still engaging and instructive.* A concern for a safe environment should not create a sterile office. Providing a space for containment of busy toddlers and a separate area for teens is ideal. Smaller, semicontained areas set a quieter and more contained tone for families.

■ *Pictures of children and their families or drawings created by children* in the practice invite children to feel comfortable in the office and encourage conversations about the pictures' content among parents and other children.

■ *A fish tank in the waiting room* may help alleviate anxiety and fears that many children experience when visiting a physician's office.

■ *Table and chairs designed for toddlers and young children* and placed in the reception area may encourage a child to separate from the parent and independently open a book or play with a puzzle. Anxiety may be momentarily decreased as the child learns to manage a fear independent of the parent.

- *Available paper and marking pens or a chalkboard* will encourage children to draw pictures that may help them redirect fears about their symptoms, an illness, or the unrecognizable concern they have observed in their parent. These drawings can be shown later to the clinician; they may provide valuable insight into the child, family, or illness (see Chapter 26).
- *The observation of children and parents together by the office personnel* allows for the collection of data about developmental and interactional issues. Mechanisms in place to periodically assess these important "naturalistic" observations by an experienced office staff can be invaluable.
- *Televisions can be distracting* to the parent and give an unintended message that viewing should fill in life's empty spaces. Monitoring appropriate content is an added burden.

AN INTERACTIVE MODEL

It is apparent that the clinician acquires information (both outside and inside the examination room) from the parent and child and generates a broad, sociomedical data base. The parent and older child receive information from the clinician that focuses on diagnosis, treatment, and education. During the interview, parent-child interactions provide the clinician an opportunity to assess developmental skills of the child, as well as parenting skills and the dynamics of family interaction[6] (Fig. 3-1). When clinicians encourage the kind of interchange that allows this educational dynamic to occur, the rewards of the clinical interview can be a shared learning experience. Careful engineering of this process can provide long-term gains in an understanding of the family and a clearer focus for care and guidance.

THE DUAL PATIENT

The pediatric interview encompasses the notion of the **dual patient.** The parent and child are the patient, both as individuals and as an interactional unit. We do not see any of them as "clients."

Although most of the historical facts during an interview will come from the parent, the child often provides important clues through verbal and nonverbal interactions. In addition, the interview should provide information and supportive care of the "third patient," the interaction between the child and the family unit, through direct questioning of the partici-

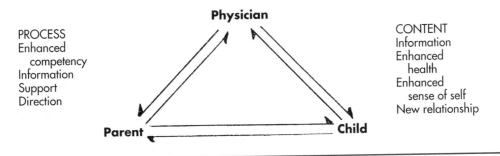

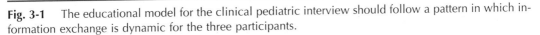

Fig. 3-1   The educational model for the clinical pediatric interview should follow a pattern in which information exchange is dynamic for the three participants.

pants and observation of that interaction. A frequent shortcoming of the pediatric interview is that the physician, rather than actively involving the child, communicates exclusively with the parent. In the 3-year-old, expressive and receptive language skills provide the child with the ability to communicate symptoms and concerns to the clinician. If you find yourself talking more than half the time, it usually means you aren't getting what *you* need from the interview.

Questions should be directed to children with age-appropriate words and eye contact that will encourage the child's participation. A direct interaction with a child of any age acknowledges the important contribution any individual child has on his own rearing, health, and development. An appreciation of the dual patient directs the clinician's attention to concerns of both the parent and the child and to the important role that the interaction between them really plays. This approach enhances traditional pediatric advocacy for the needs of the child. (See Chapter 16, the 4-year-old health supervision visit, and subsequent chapters for examples of a coordinated parent-child interview.)

NONVERBAL COMMUNICATION

Information from the clinical interview is derived from two major sources: **verbal and nonverbal communication** (Box 3-1). Interactional behaviors—how the baby is held, fed, stroked, spoken to, looked at, and so on—are also part of the nonverbal data base. Similarly, the relationship between an older child and parent should be observed and assessed during the interview. Observations about communication style and content regarding discipline and self-help skills (e.g., undressing and getting onto the examination table) can provide important clues about parent-child relationships, as well as developmental capacities. Children who are delayed or whom the parents perceive to need care appropriate for a younger age will show this behavior during the interaction. In fact, motor, social, adaptive, and individual temperament skills can be assessed in the young child by observing the child's activity while the parent is providing the medical history, provided the room and your focus are set in that direction.

Nonverbal data are as real as verbal statements and therefore should be incorporated into the medical evaluation. Often they give clearer and added information. These observations should be written in the medical record and be given diagnostic status when appropri-

---

BOX 3-1	VERBAL AND NONVERBAL COMMUNICATION: MAJOR INFORMATION SOURCES

Verbal information refers to the data that patients tell us about themselves, the core of the traditional medical history.

Nonverbal information refers to those observations we make about the style, timing, emotive ambience, flow of the interview, and even what's *not* said. Facial expressions, posture, movements of the extremities, and the quality and tone of speech are examples of important observations that frequently provide clues to critical aspects of a child's life and family environment. Clinicians often neglect this source of important information, making their data gathering less efficient and less accurate.

ate (e.g., the sad child, rule out depression; the parent with multiple tics and a halting voice, consider parental anxiety; the active and difficult to comfort infant, keep in mind an active infant temperament). They should be incorporated into the problem list to ensure appropriate attention during follow-up care. In practices that have a child behavior checklist or a parent-family psychosocial screening instrument (see Appendix) that is filled out before the office visit, nonverbal observations can be compared with the parent's written observations. Confirmations and discrepancies may provide useful clinical information.

Nonverbal cues given by parents and children are a component of the **process** portion of the interview as compared with the **content** portion. Although the process of an interview is interwoven with the content, it is helpful for the clinician to be aware of the two components as separate.[7] In that way, verbal data can be understood within the context of nonverbal statements that were generated simultaneously by the parent or the child and that were monitored by the sensitive clinician. For example, a 2-month-old infant's mother, who demonstrates her anxiety as she states her concern about multiple minor somatic symptoms, is understood more clearly when observation of nonverbal clues suggests maternal sleep deprivation or depression following the birth of the child.

POSITIONING THE PARTICIPANTS

Certain aspects of the interview environment controlled by the clinician determine the quality and quantity of data that will be obtained. The architecture of the clinical space may be guided by knowledge that the word *interview* derives from *between* and *seeing*. By implication, the process of interviewing is a mutual communication of thoughts that can be influenced by the nature of the space between clinician and patient.[8] The following are things to consider to create the best interview environment possible:

- The clinician and parent should be positioned at the same level to ensure eye contact and to prevent a subservient positioning effect.
- The decision to conduct the interview in a sitting or standing position will change with the type of visit.
- For a new patient or a new problem that requires an extensive history, sitting down with the parent and child may encourage greater information exchange, as well as allow the clinician to pay more attention to nonverbal cues.
- For an established patient with an acute illness the history may be taken while the parent and clinician are standing.
- A young child who is ill may remain in the arms of the parent.
- The placement of chairs in an examination room and the proximity of clinician and patient influence the style and content of the interview.
- A desk between a practitioner and the parent and child can be a barrier to optimal communication.
- Picking up a chair and moving it closer to a parent may facilitate the exchange of information; the act itself may enhance a therapeutic relationship.

Some clinicians prefer to examine the child while taking the history. Although this may be a necessity on occasion when time is very limited, simultaneous interviewing and physical examination run the risk of shortchanging both aspects of data collection. The clinician is not free to establish eye contact with the parent or to communicate effectively with the child. Critical nonverbal data will be missed if the parent feels rushed or believes that what she says is subsidiary to what the clinician finds on exam. In contrast, most information is from a history given with verbal and nonverbal cues. The placement of the child also determines the quality and tone of the interview (Table 3-1), and the following factors should be kept in mind:

- Infants less than 6 months of age should be placed in the parent's lap if possible. Some infants less than 6 months of age will not settle down when placed on the table, and most infants will do better to at least start the examination in the parent's lap.
- With children between 6 months and 2 or 3 years, because of the emergence of stranger awareness and the accompanying need to be close to the parent, interviews are conducted most efficiently while the child is sitting on the parent's lap. This position is reassuring to the child. The physical examination can be performed in the same position with a cooperative child of this age. A child younger than 2 years of age should not have to cope with direct eye contact from the clinician while being examined. This distancing through gaze avoidance by the clinician will reassure the child.
- When the clinician is interviewing parents of an older child, the child may be occupied with a request to draw a picture of her family. Not only a distracting maneuver, the family

TABLE 3-1 ■ Pediatric Examination: A Developmental Approach

Age (Approximate)	Developmental Stage	Approach to Physical Examination
0-6 mo	**Symbiotic** (not fearful of strangers)	Usually easy to examine infant on table; start with least invasive parts of examination (abdomen, cardiac, pulmonary nodes, etc.).
6 mo-3 yr	**Separation-individuation** (fear of strangers initially followed by the toddler clinging to parent)	Examine while standing parent holds the child or while infant is in parent's lap; approach the child gently; use of toys, peekaboo games, keys, flashing otoscope may be helpful.
3-6 yr	**Preschool age: age of initiative** (a period of fantasy play and increasing verbal ability)	Communicate with child in simple language; explain procedures and ask child to participate in examination; make use of child's interest in fantasy.
6-12 yr	**School age: age of industry** (a period of cognitive growth; growing interest in and ability to understand cause and effect)	Recognition of child's ability to understand procedures leads to cooperation; an explanation of body functions and results of assessments are helpful.
12-17 yr	**Adolescence: age of identity** (heightened awareness of body and its perceived effect on others)	Respect privacy during examination; careful explanations help.

picture may provide helpful insights into the child's visual-motor skills and psychological development. It directs expected anxiety into an activity in which the child is in charge and enables the child to regain control of the circumstances to some degree (see Chapter 26). For discussion of sensitive areas for many children older than 4, the parent should be interviewed alone while the child is weighed, measured, allowed to draw, or engaged in other diagnostic activities. Emotional tone, if not the content, is picked up by even small children.

■ The adolescent patient should be interviewed separately from the parent as a way to show appreciation of the teenager's separate identity and to encourage the development of a trusting relationship between adolescent patient and clinician. Parents of an adolescent may also need help in realizing their child's maturation and increasing independence (see Chapters 20 to 22). The clinician's behavior models that acknowledgment.

To maximize the quality of the interview of a child at any age, the clinician should be at the same level as the child. For the tall clinician the importance of positioning is especially important when interviewing young children and parents. A younger child should be allowed to scan the physician at a distance first and become familiar with her. Eye-to-eye contact is an intense, invasive interpersonal maneuver and may be very threatening to the child younger than 2 years old or to a child of any age if the contact is presented early in an interview. A friendly interchange with the parents first allows the child to size the clinician up before the interaction.

VERBAL AND EMOTIONAL COMMUNICATION WITH CHILDREN

When interviewing a child who has achieved interactive language skills at about 3 to 4 years of age, the physician can speak directly to the child to ask questions and to listen carefully to responses. It is helpful to remember that receptive language development is often ahead of expressive language. A 2-year-old may understand as many as 300 words, but expression may be limited to 50 to 100 words. Children may reveal information of which the parent is either unaware or has suppressed. In addition, allowing the child to participate in the interview provides an opportunity to assess language development and auditory functioning. Furthermore, it provides the child with an experience of participating actively in the visit to the physician, which may encourage a sense of responsibility and participation in personal health and medical care. It may also provide a model for parents in listening to and respecting the opinions of the child. Beginning with the health supervision visit for the 4-year-old (see Chapter 16), the clinician has the opportunity to conduct the interview with child and parent in a parallel fashion. This rich clinical experience requires a knowledge of age-appropriate developmental skills and a comfort level of communicating simultaneously with an adult and child. The rewards are tremendous.[9,10] This adds minimal time and a much-expanded clinical data base.

The clinician's interactions with the child during the interview and physical examination provide an opportunity to model certain behaviors for the parent. For example, the physician's holding, rocking, and stroking the infant while talking to the parent can give the young, uncertain mother a chance to observe effective soothing techniques. Providing firm discipline to the uncontrolled toddler with a concise and authoritative statement can help the parent experience the effect of appropriate limit setting and discipline. These chance events, when a behavioral or developmental issue naturally comes up, open up "teachable moments"[11] that become part of the real output or gain of the encounter itself.

Giving a 5-year-old the choice of using the left or right arm for an immunization or a tuberculin skin test may illustrate to the parent the value of providing some kind of option for the child facing something that is really nonnegotiable. In addition, the clinician may demonstrate to the parent the powerful effect of reflecting on a child's feelings when an emotional response is intense. For example, to the tearful youngster about to undergo a painful procedure, the physician might say, "You're worried that the stick is going to hurt, aren't you?" The altered emotional response to these "feedback" statements is often dramatic and encourages further communication about the child's feelings.[12] In general, clinicians should be sensitive to the effect that their behaviors vis-à-vis the child have on the parent's behavior and style of child rearing. These models are more effective than any amount of formal instruction or critiques of the parents' own behavior.

Sensitivity to verbal cues and emotional experiences during a clinical encounter may introduce unexpected opportunities that lead to an understanding of the parent-child relationship. In addition, it may provide insight into the important relationship between the child, parent, and clinician. These events, characterized as "critical incidents,"[13] require clinical vigilance. They may be fleeting and awkward, as seen in the case study, "Jake: A Teachable Moment."[14]

Jake has been a healthy child before his health supervision visit at 18 months old. As you enter the examination room, you observe Jake playing on the floor with a plastic toy that has several movable parts. He appears engaged and intent on mastering the toy. You also notice that his fine motor skills are mature for his age when you observe Jake drawing. Jake appears not to notice you when you enter. Shortly after you begin to gather information from his mother, Jake's activity level and focus change dramatically. He starts hitting the toy, screams "bad. . . bad," and throws the toy into a wall. He starts to cry, resists his mother's attempt to hold him while she provides reassuring words, and hits her with his hand several times. His mother begins to cry and says, "He was such a good baby. In the last few months, he's a different child—selfish, angry, and always throwing a tantrum." You are faced with several options at this point:

1. *Quickly perform a physical examination, check the growth chart, and order immunizations (and a blood lead and hematocrit if appropriate).*
2. *Talk to Jake's mother about tantrums and the need for discipline. Provide a handout on toddler development and discipline.*
3. *Attempt to engage Jake with words and a toy (i.e., sit down on the floor and play with the toy and say something like: "Gee, this is a great toy. I can make the door open so the boy can go inside."). Alternatively, address Jake and say, "It's real hard to come to the doctor!" or, "You are real upset at the doctor's office." Follow these words with silence and wait patiently for Jake's response.*

The first option brings closure to the office visit but does not address Jake's be-havior. The second option demonstrates recognition of a problem and expands the mother's knowledge about toddler behaviors and approaches to discipline. The third option illustrates immediate recognition of a "teachable moment." The pediatric clini-cian chooses to model an age-appropriate response to a tantrum through action and lan-guage. Engaging the child formulates the scene to the child's reality. The pediatrician's language is direct and brief; she tries to mirror the child's feelings with a few words and waits for a response. This technique, known as "active listening," encourages Jake's mother to learn that she can interact with her son at these difficult moments by feeding back to him the feelings he is experiencing. The physician's modeling the behavior can be followed by the information exchange illustrated in the second option.

STRUCTURING THE INTERVIEW

Structuring the well-child medical interview is helpful in ensuring complete data collection, as well as in providing a framework for controlled digressions. An opening statement should include an introduction by name if this is the first visit. A concerned, friendly, and empathetic atmosphere can be established by a warm introduction and immediate eye contact with the parent. Some clinicians find that an extended hand assists in the development of a new medical relationship. For health supervision visits, a brief statement about the goals for the visit may be helpful at the beginning of the interview. This can be followed by asking, "What areas of your child's health would you like to discuss during this visit?" A similar question might be directed to the older child. This approach, early in the visit, ensures that the parent or adolescent will have an opportunity to state the agenda for the visit; it allows the clinician an opportunity to structure the visit in a format that includes that agenda.

The content of the health supervision interview depends on the child's age and sig-nificant developmental themes. Specific chapters in this book provide guidelines for each age. To encourage a developmental perspective for the well-child visit, questions and edu-cational information should be organized around the major issues at a particular age. In this manner, specific goals can be established for each visit. For example, the visit when the in-fant is 6 months of age highlights the emerging motor skills of grasping and reaching out. Advice about solids (especially finger foods), toys, and poison prevention should be pro-vided to parents in the context of specific current and anticipated developmental skills. Choosing a central concern or theme gives the visit more cohesiveness and less of a feeling of an assembly line or check-off list. The chapters in this book on each health supervision visit prepare clinicians for this task. The contents of the clinical interview, both data gather-ing and instruction, for each age will be outlined in subsequent chapters.

Parents appreciate a summary statement after the history and physical examination. When the child's health and development is satisfactory, the physician should report that finding positively, emphatically, and with enthusiasm. The parent should be congratulated on the care and health of the child. These supportive statements encourage a high level of self-esteem with regard to parenting skills and strengthen the relationship between parent and clinician. When a problem has been uncovered and discussed during the content portion of the visit, reviewing the problem briefly during the summary statement may be helpful. This should include an assessment of how serious the clinician judges the problem to be and the plan he advises. Options for the parents and child should be clearly stated. The parents may raise an important question or concern when their options are reflected back to them.

Each well-child visit should terminate with a *closing statement* that allows the parent and older child to express an uncovered problem or concern. "Was there anything else you wanted to bring up?" may encourage the surfacing of an emotion-laden problem that the parent or older child is able to express only after a feeling of trust has been established by the end of a visit. These *out-the-door (OTD) questions* as the visit is about to end may be frustrating in a busy clinical setting. However, they frequently reflect significant parental concerns.

> *After completing a health supervision visit for a 2-week-old, the pediatrician, with one hand on the doorknob, was told, "Oh, by the way . . . my 3-year-old has trouble with her bowel movements." A quick screening history revealed significant constipation for a year and a paucity of language development associated with apathy and social withdrawal during that time. She had not grown during the year. As the father described the history, the pediatrician visualized a midline anterior neck scar. When it was revealed that a cyst had been removed before the onset of constipation, the diagnosis was apparent. An iatrogenic thyroidectomy was the result of an excision of a thyroglossal duct cyst with most of the child's thyroid tissue imbedded in the lining of the cyst. A diagnosis of severe hypothyroidism (TSH = 950; $T_4 < 1$) was the result of an "out-the-door" question by a concerned parent.*

If time for an adequate response is not available, a statement such as "It sounds like something we should talk about when we both have more time together" may be followed by arranging the next available appointment if the concern is of a nonemergency nature. Although the clinician should not feel obligated to answer all OTD questions, interest and concern can be expressed with an immediate, appropriate follow-up arrangement as part of a new contractual agreement.

Each clinician develops a personal style for interviewing that optimally encourages the establishment of a helpful and healthy therapeutic relationship with children and parents. If education, guidance, and developmental monitoring are the objectives of well-child visits, a flexible, empathetic, and compassionate approach is helpful to ensure optimal communication between the clinician and the family. Awareness of tools available to the clinician in constructing the interview will create a form and foundation for the art of medicine.

Open and Closed Questions. Open-ended questions (e.g., "How is your baby doing?" "What's new with the baby's development?" "What do you like about your baby?") generate more spontaneous, less-structured responses. They allow the parents to bring up problems of greatest concern to them. They acknowledge the parents' responsibility in establishing priorities in the interview. The interview should start with these. Open-ended questions allow the child or the parents' **"explanatory model"**[15] of the illness or problem to come out. The explanatory model is the culturally dependent perspective of an illness that the family brings to the medical encounter. This is the first step in meeting the family's needs for understanding an issue. Open-ended questions can be followed by closed-ended questions that are focused, specific, and more concrete (e.g., "Is the baby sitting up without support?" "How is breast feeding going?" "Are you getting any help with child care?"). These provide important concrete data and shift the control of the interview to the interviewer. The clinician's explanatory model and agenda for the interview can be brought out by the careful use of these questions. Some cultural groups may have an initial negative response to an open-ended question at the initiation of the interview because they may be used to a more formal health encounter with the physician being more directive. Putting the open-ended question into context can help, such as saying "I like to hear a parent's concerns first."

 Pauses and Silent Periods. When emotionally difficult issues are discussed, the use of silent periods is extremely beneficial. It allows the patient time to collect thoughts and to express feelings. It carries with it the message that you care enough about the patient to take the time to listen to her deepest concerns about the child and family. This is not wasted time.

 Repetition of Important Phrases. When a patient makes a statement that appears significant from either verbal or nonverbal cues but stops the communication abruptly, the clinician may choose to repeat or interpret an important phrase that was mentioned. This encourages further exploration, clarification, or modification by the patient.

The mother of a 6-month-old infant was told that her child, who had previously exhibited normal development, demonstrated signs of spasticity. When the meaning of this finding was discussed with her, she said that she had worried about her son's breathing problems at birth. A period of silence was followed by a statement from the clinician: "You worried about the baby's breathing at birth?" The mother was then able to express her concern about the need for ventilation and oxygen supplementation during the perinatal period and her ongoing fear that it would affect her child's brain development.

 When parents say outrageous or alarming things, the clinician should just repeat their comment back in an even voice without comment. The ball is then passed to the parent to explain, clarify, or expand the startling comment. The clinician can then gather the wits to respond appropriately. The use of an "I" phrase is usually the best way to begin a response to an alarming statement (e.g., "I'm really concerned about what you've just said" or "I think that's a pretty powerful statement").

 Active Listening. **Active listening** refers to the process of giving undivided attention to what a person is saying through words and body language. It requires, above all, the ability to concentrate. The assumption underlying active listening is that the patient will provide most of the important information spontaneously, verbally or nonverbally, if given an opportunity and the encounter is set up correctly. The clinician who listens actively uses open-ended questions, pauses, silences, and repetition of important phrases. Such an empathetic listener can discover, through a unique, interpersonal style, a way that brings about a succinct and accurate acceptance of the patient's feelings. This understanding of the patient's feelings is communicated through facial expressions, posture, hand movements, and head nodding. Active and empathic listening can decrease a patient's anxiety, increase trust in the clinician, encourage greater patient participation in the interview process, yield more information, and increase the clinician's satisfaction in the relationship.[16] It is a skill that can be learned and is one of the most effective and efficient ways to build a complete data base. Henry Louis Gates Jr.[17] has observed that "the art of the interview. . . paradoxically depends at once upon the presence of the interviewer *and his or her absence, silence, or invisibility.* The role of an interviewer is somewhat that of a catalyst in a chemical equation: elemental and essential, yet destined to disappear." Most mistakes have to do with too much talking.

Transference. Primary pediatric care is based on the development of a long-term relationship with families. When continuity of health care is provided in this framework, a special relationship develops between the caregiver and the patient. In pediatric practice, parents usually have significant respect and admiration for their child's physician; it is the foundation for a trusting, long-term relationship. This relationship is the single most powerful tool in effecting change for the child. It is also one of the rewards of primary care. At the same time, and to various degrees, as a result of this close and special relationship, a parent may respond to the pediatrician as someone who is symbolically and psychologically identified with another important person in his own life, past or present. For some mothers, the symbolic attachment may be a father or a mother, and for others, an uncle or other important person in their lives. This **"transference"** phenomenon may surface only at times of deep emotional expression, such as overwhelming joy, relief, and admiration for the clinician after a successful therapeutic intervention. It may also be the unconscious source of hostility directed toward the clinician by the parent of a child with a chronic, functionally disabling illness. An appreciation of parental reactions mediated by transference may assist the clinician in providing more appropriate and helpful responses during medical interviews and in understanding some aspects of the interaction. In addition, it may sometimes allow for an understanding of strong personal feelings experienced by the clinician. This insight does not get rid of transference in an interaction, but acknowledges it, uses it for the healthy energy it provides, and keeps in check the less helpful aspects of its presence. Monitoring of the clinician's own emotional response allows awareness of this phenomenon and use of it to advantage.

Analyses of pediatric interviews through videotape records have documented those clinical skills to which parents are most responsive. Process and outcome measures, such as parental understanding of a diagnostic label and compliance with a medical regimen, have been measured and correlated with specific traits of clinicians that yield optimal results. Effective interviewing skills go a long way toward optimal results. Dr. Barbara Korsch,[18] a pioneer in pediatric interview research, suggests that the following traits produce the most effective medical encounters:

■ Pay attention to the *concerns of patients.* Three open-ended questions will elicit *most* parental concerns for the child with a problem:
  1. Why did you bring Johnny to the clinic today?
  2. What worried you most about him?
  3. Why did that worry you?

- *Acknowledge the parent's expectation* for the medical visit and the parent's explanation of the child's problem, the explanatory model. Parents may bring to the visit their own explanatory model of illness and health. It is important to bring that model to the surface and show the parents that you understand their perception, whether it is similar to or different from your own.
- Parents need an *explanation of the diagnosis and cause.* If the medical explanation is inconsistent with the parents' own understanding, the clinician should try to reconcile the difference. For example, the parent who believes that the child acquired a cold from rain exposure may be assisted by the statement, "The cold was caused by a virus he acquired rather than by your taking him out into the rain."
- Nurture the *doctor-patient relationship.* Be relaxed, friendly, positive, and warm in manner.
- *Limit medical jargon.* This is often a protective barrier for yourself. Jargon can be used to establish power over another or to hide ignorance when you feel threatened. Rather than hide behind words, try to deal with the situation directly.
- Most parents prefer a *friendly, professional attitude* rather than an authoritative, business-like stature or an overly casual or familiar manner.
- *Attend to parental anxieties* as manifested by nervousness and tension during the interview. Examples of responses are the following: "You look nervous to me today . . . is there something you want to bring up?" "You don't seem to accept my explanation of his sore throat."

These skills can be acquired during medical training or in pediatric practice. As with most aspects of learning, supervision is extremely helpful in gaining insights into interviewing techniques. A one-way mirror provides an opportunity for observing interviews. A videotape of a patient encounter can be played back in front of the student and teacher. Videotaping has the advantage of allowing comments periodically when the tape is stopped and replayed. Medical centers with teaching programs usually have video facilities that can be used by pediatricians in practice as a form of continuing education.

Communication is the high technology of the twenty-first century. But without computers, satellites, or forms of artificial intelligence, the primitive art of communication during the medical interview remains a powerful and effective way to gather data, teach, and develop the specifically human way of connecting with another human being empathetically and therapeutically. We owe it to ourselves and to our patients to develop these skills optimally.

CULTURALLY SENSITIVE INTERVIEWS

In developed countries, cultural diversity is the rule rather than the exception. Although most of the general principles of effective medical interviewing reviewed in this chapter are applicable when there are culturally derived differences between a clinician and patient, such differences may pervade the encounter at many levels. Patcher has defined culturally sensitive pediatrics as "care [that] *respects the beliefs, attitudes, and cultural life-styles of patients* [italics mine]. It acknowledges that concepts of health and illness are influenced by patients' ethnic values, religious beliefs, linguistical considerations, and cultural orientations."[19] A culturally sensitive pediatric clinician discovers ways to blend ethnomedical interpretations of a child's developmental skills and behaviors with a biomedical understanding. Culture, however, does not dictate the beliefs and behaviors of a child or parent in a specific way, but rather acts implicitly to guide a patient's decisions.[20] (See Chapter 2.)

Some clinicians may be frustrated by a false impression that, to accomplish an effective medical interview that also nurtures a therapeutic relationship, a clinician must possess specific information about a family's cultural beliefs and practices. Certainly, knowledge about some customs is useful, such as the reason for limiting direct and sustained eye contact in some Asian cultures; an appreciation of "mal de ojo," the evil eye belief found in many Hispanic cultures where symptoms are perceived as arising from feelings of malevolence or jealousy;[21] and the use of physical punishment for misbehaving children practiced by many parents in disparate cultures. However, two clinically useful techniques will guide and assist medical encounters across cultures without an extensive knowledge of specific customs and beliefs.

EXPLANATORY MODEL FOR SYMPTOMS[22]

All patients have a culturally based model for understanding health status at times of health and disease. Their interpretation and explanation of symptoms may be different from the assumptions of the clinician. Through a process of specific questions, the family's explanatory model of health and illness will emerge (Box 3-2).

MINIETHNOGRAPHY[20]

In the process of an empathetic, respectful interview with the parents and child, the pediatric clinician should strive to understand cultural and personal meanings and interpretations of the child's development and behaviors. When the patient is seen in the context of continuity of care, defining a miniethnography for a child and family over time is a clinically and personally rewarding exercise. Other family members and interpreters

---

BOX 3-2	QUESTIONS FOR A HEALTH-BELIEFS HISTORY[19,22]

What would you call this problem?
Why do you think your child has developed it?
What do you think caused it?
Why do you think it started when it did?
What do you think is happening inside the body?
What are the symptoms that make you know you know your child has this illness?
What are you most worried about with this illness?
What problems does this illness cause your child?
How do you treat it?
Is the treatment helpful?
What will happen if this problem is not treated?
What do you expect from the treatments?

BOX 3-3	GUIDELINES FOR THE BILINGUAL MEDICAL INTERVIEW

Always use an interpreter (ideally a trained professional rather than an *ad hoc* interpreter) unless you are fluent in the family's language.

Try to match the individual interpreter to the individual patient and clinical setting. Reassure the parent or child regarding confidentiality.

Avoid technical terms, jargon, lengthy explanations without breaks, ambiguity, idiom, abstraction, figures of speech, and indefinite phrases.

Use clear statements planned in advance with language appropriate for the interpreter and expect to spend twice the usual time.

Be prepared to obtain information via narrative or conversational modes.

Ask the interpreter to comment on nonverbal elements, the fullness of the parent's or child's understanding, and any culturally sensitive issues.

Learn the basic language and common health-related beliefs and practices of patient groups regularly encountered.

Modified with permission from Putsch RW: *JAMA* 254:3334, 1985.

may be essential in the development of a meaningful history. Box 3-3 gives guidelines for a bilingual medical interview.

ELICITING INFORMATION

At its best, the clinical interview yields information that will elaborate on a particular diagnosis or parental concern. The priorities set by the clinician, nurse, or telephone receptionist can enhance or suppress important information. After an appointment is made for a health supervision visit, a receptionist might routinely offer the following suggestion: "You might think about your concerns before the appointment. The doctor is interested in your child's development and behaviors. Some parents find it helpful to make a short list of concerns before the visit." In the office, a medical assistant or nurse should inquire about specific concerns while preparing the child for the visit. Parent and child questionnaires for health supervision visits can also be used to enhance each visit.[9]

Two studies suggest strategies for more effective acquisition of data and strengthening of the relationship between the child's clinician and parents by inquiring about specific behavioral concerns. The Pediatric Symptom Checklist (PSC) (see appendix) was developed as a screening test for psychosocial dysfunction among school-age children seen in general pediatric practices.[23] While in the waiting room, the parent is asked to complete a 35-item list of symptoms by approximating their occurrence as never, sometimes, or often, scored 0, 1, and 2, respectively (see Appendix). A total of 28 points or more constitutes a positive screen. Comparison studies of the established Children's Global Assessment Scale given blindly to the same sample of children revealed that about 15% of middle class–school age children would screen positive compared with 24% of economically disadvantaged children. Using 28 points as a positive screen, the sensitivity of the test is 95% (5% false negatives) and the specificity is 68% (32% false positives).

While screening checklists in clinical practice are limited by their tendency to oversimplify complex developmental issues, they have the advantage of bringing clues to the child's behavior into the pediatric encounter for elaboration. In addition to the PSC, investigators have developed other parent-generated checklists for preschool behavior problems[24] and school-age behaviors.[25-27] The Eyberg Child Behavior Inventory asks a parent 36 questions on behavioral problems common among children from 2½ to 11 years old; the test has excellent sensitivity and specificity.[28] A recently published instrument, the Family Psychosocial Screening test, was designed for use by pediatric primary care clinicians to assess family function with regard to specific behaviors, including depression, substance abuse, parent abuse as a child, and other risk factors for developmental and behavioral problems in children.[29]

Epidemiological studies indicate that up to 15% of school-age children have a disorder of psychosocial dysfunction and that pediatricians identify only a small percentage of these disorders during most office visits.[30] Some clinicians may find the Pediatric Symptom Checklist and other behavior screening instruments helpful in setting the agenda for health supervision by giving the parent (and child) the message that behavioral concerns are appropriate and that discussion is encouraged during the visit. A behavioral screening test can be used as a springboard to initiate the dialogue and therapeutic alliance necessary to explore behavioral concerns.

RECOGNIZING HIDDEN AGENDAS

Parents who bring children to a physician for an illness visit are frequently motivated to come to the office because of a concern that is not immediately apparent. The "secondary diagnosis" often originates from a behavioral, psychosocial, or developmental uncertainty that the parent may be unaware of at the time of the visit or one that seems inappropriate to bring to the attention of the child's clinician. The real concern must be uncovered or it will prompt additional, unnecessary office or emergency room visits.

Bass and Cohen[31] investigated ostensible and actual reasons for seeking care in a pediatric office practice. Over a 3-month period they asked parents involved in 370 sick visits, "What are you concerned about?" When the parent responded with a physical symptom, the next question was "Is there anything special about the (fever, cold, or infection) that causes your concern?" In the 370 office visits, 34% of the parents expressed a fear not verbalized initially that appeared to worry them about a more serious condition than could be anticipated from the ostensible reason for the visit (Table 3-2).

These parental concerns reflect fears and anxieties about the child's health that provide insight into family functioning and parental perceptions that are critical to the growth and development of the child. Parents in 10% of the visits saw the child as "vulnerable" because of a previous illness or event in the life of the child, a family member, or a close friend.[32] Providing the parent with a brief opportunity to express any hidden agenda may be therapeutic in itself. The clinician then has a window of opportunity to place the symptom in perspective and, when appropriate, reassure the parent about the health of the child and the limited duration of the current illness. When these fears create significant or chronic parental anxiety, a future visit is necessary.

TABLE 3-2 ■ Actual* Reasons for Visits to Pediatric Provider

Reason	Patients (370 visits)
Vulnerable child syndrome	39
Parent thought the worst	30
Parents' fear of cancer or leukemia	10
Authority figures raised concerns	10
Illness lasted "too long"	9
Death of relative or friend	8
Travel or moving	7
Symptoms of "vital organs"	7
Absent parent	5
	125 (34%)

*Actual reasons as opposed to ostensible reasons for the visits.

These explorations in causality are the rewards of sensitive interviewing. For the child and family, the therapeutic value is as important as unraveling the pathophysiology of a cardiac murmur. The long-term benefit comes from the relationship that begins to be built when clinicians give parents the message that their concerns are important and worthy of the physician's time.

REFERENCES

1. Schor EL: Families, family roles and psychological diagnoses in primary care, *J Dev Behav Pediatr* 9:327, 1988.
2. Cohen SE, Parmelee AH: Prediction of five-year Stanford Binet scores in preterm infants, *Child Dev* 54:1242, 1983.
3. Werner E, Honzik MP, Smith RS: Prediction of intelligence and achievement at ten years from twenty-month pediatric and psychological examinations, *Child Dev* 39:1063, 1968.
4. Casey PH, Bradley RH: The impact of home environment on children's development: clinical relevance for the pediatrician, *J Dev Behav Pediatr* 3:146, 1982.
5. Weinstein CM, David TG: *Spaces for children: the built environment and child development*, New York, 1987, Plenum Press.
6. Allmond BW Jr, Tanner JL, Gofman HF: *The family is the patient*, ed 2, Baltimore, 1999, Williams & Wilkins.
7. Rosenthal R et al: *Sensitivity to nonverbal communication: the PONS test*, Baltimore, 1979, Johns Hopkins University Press.
8. Lipkin ML Jr, Putnam SM, Lazare A: *The medical interview—clinical care, education, and research*, New York, 1995, Springer-Verlag.
9. American Academy of Pediatrics: *Guidelines for health supervision III*, Elk Grove Village, Ill, 1997, American Academy of Pediatrics.

10. Green M, editor: *Bright futures: guidelines for health supervision of infants, children, and adolescents*, Arlington, Va, 1994, National Center for Education in Maternal and Child Health.
11. Zuckerman B, Parker S: Teachable moments: assessment as intervention, *Contemporary Pediatrics* 14:41, 1997.
12. Gordon T: *Parent effectiveness training*, New York, 1970, PH Wyden.
13. Pantell RH, Lewis CC: Communicating with children in the hospital. In Thornton SM, Frankenburg WK, editors: *Child health care communications: enhancing interactions among professionals, parents and children*, Skillman, NJ, 1983, Johnson & Johnson.
14. Stein MT: Preparing families for the toddler and preschool years, *Contemporary Pediatrics* 15:88, 1998.
15. Klineman A, Eisenberg L, Good B: Culture, illness and care, *Ann Intern Med* 88:251, 1978.
16. DiMatteo MR, Prince LM, Hays RD: Nonverbal communication in the medical context: the physician-patient relationship. In Blanck PD, Buck R, Rosenthal R, editors: *Nonverbal communication in the clinical context*. University Park, Pa, 1986, Pennsylvania State University Press, pp 74-98.
17. Gates LG Jr: Forward. In West C: *Restoring hope*, Boston, 1997, Beacon Press.
18. Korsch BM, Freemon B, Negrete VF: Practical implications of doctor-patient interactions and analysis for pediatric practice, *Am J Dis Child* 12:110, 1971.
19. Patcher LM: Practicing culturally sensitive pediatrics, *Contemporary Pediatrics* 14:139,1997.
20. Johnson TM, Hardt EJ, Kleinman A: Cultural factors in the medical interview. In: Lipkin ML Jr, Putman SM, Lazare A, editors: *The medical interview: clinical care, education, and research*, New York, 1995, Springer-Verlag, pp 153-162.
21. Roberts JM: Belief in the evil eye in world perspective. In Maloney C, editor: *The evil eye*, New York, 1976, Columbia University Press, p 223.
22. Kleinman A: *Patients and healers in the context of culture*, Berkeley, Calif, 1980, University of California Press, p 106.
23. Jellinek MS, Murphy JM: Screening for psychosocial disorders in pediatric practice, *Am J Dis Child* 142:1153, 1988.
24. Willoughby JA, Haggerty RJ: A simple behavioral questionnaire for preschool children, *Pediatrics* 34:798, 1964.
25. Rutter M, Tizard J, Whitmore K: *Education, health and behaviour*, New York, 1970, Wiley.
26. Conners CK: Symptom patterns in hyperactive, neurotic and normal children, *Child Dev* 41:667, 1970.
27. Goyette CH, Connors CK, Ulrich RF: Normative data on revised Connors Parent and Teacher Rating Scales, *J Abnorm Child Psychol* 6:221, 1978.
28. Boggs SR, Eyberg S, Reynolds LA: Concurrent validity of the Eyberg Child Behavior Inventory, *J Clin Child Psychol* 19:75, 1990.
29. Kemper KJ, Kelleher KJ: Family psychosocial screening: instruments and techniques, *Ambulatory Child Health* 4:325, 1996.
30. Costello EJ: Primary care pediatrics and child psychopathology: A review of diagnostic treatment and referral practice, *Pediatrics* 78:1044, 1986.
31. Bass LW, Cohen RL: Ostensible versus actual reasons for seeking pediatric attention: another look at the parental ticket of admission, *Pediatrics* 70:870, 1982.
32. Green M, Solnit AJ: Reaction to the threatened loss of a child: a vulnerable child syndrome, *Pediatrics* 34:58, 1964.

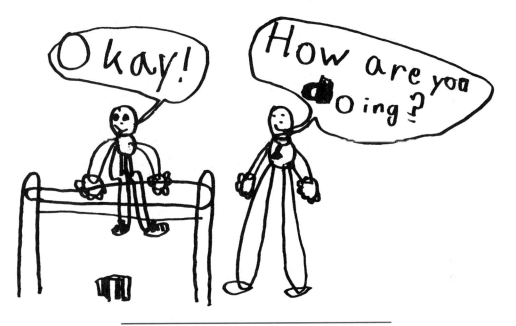

"Talking to my doctor." By Ryan Hennessy, age 7½.

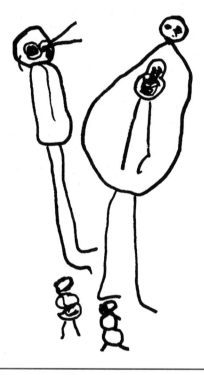

Father shoots kisses at the (pregnant) mother. Two other kids are there (underneath). By Colin Hennessy, age 4.

CHAPTER 4

THE PRENATAL VISIT: MAKING AN ALLIANCE WITH A FAMILY

■ Suzanne D. Dixon

KEY WORDS

Psychological Changes
Father's Involvement
Birth of a Sibling
Risk Factors for Attachment
Fetal Behavior
Breast Feeding

Debbie and Mark Hanson, soon-to-be parents, come in at the end of a busy day, having requested an interview to see if they would like you to take care of their baby, who is expected in 6 weeks. Debbie wants to know if you support breast feeding and have evening hours for working mothers. She says she has a list of questions and wants to know if you have any books or pamphlets. Mark expresses no immediate concerns and appears uncomfortable in the office. He says he is worried about being late for his second job helping in his dad's store.

The period of time before an infant's birth is a time of readjustment, concern, anxiety, and some adaptive stress in a family's development. This time is the true start of the unborn child's physical and psychosocial development. It is, therefore, the time for the pediatric clinician to begin work. The American Academy of Pediatrics endorses the practice of making prenatal interviews part of pediatricians' practices and encourages them to become more involved with prenatal anticipatory guidance.[1] This type of prenatal encounter offers the unique opportunity to begin to build a strong working relationship with a family, as well as to support the necessary psychological development that is demanded by the birth of a child. A unique body of information can be gathered at this time. The prenatal visit offers the opportunity to make an impact on the child's family, even before the infant's birth. It establishes your territory, your style, and your perspectives.

PERINATAL RISK: THE CLASSIC APPROACH, PEDIATRIC STYLE

The data base established in the prenatal period should include an assessment of perinatal risk to the unborn child, as well as familial occurrence of inherited disease, history of prior reproductive casualty or success, exposure to toxins, pregnancy events, and the medical history of the parents. These factors are shown in Box 4-1. Most of this data can be gathered by questionnaire with follow-up of any issues. Pediatric concern for these issues emphasizes to the family the continuities in prenatal and postnatal life, allowing for a focused medical assessment of the child to come.

All expectant parents will have concerns about the physical well-being of their unborn child; your questioning is far more likely to be an assurance of your ability to address the issues than to be a source of new worries to a family. These data allow you to provide an accurate assessment of prenatal factors that may influence the development of the child and to provide some preventive intervention. Because genetic disease recognition is more common and gene therapy is increasingly promising for a variety of disorders, a detailed family profile is even more vital now than before.

The pediatric perspective on these issues may vary somewhat from the obstetric and may call for renewed emphasis on issues that have impact on the infant. For instance, the tuberculosis screening test may be seen by the obstetrician as not having the great priority that it does for the pediatric clinician, with whom the specter of neonatal tuberculosis exposure looms. Hepatitis B carrier status in a mother requires immediate action by the child's clini-

---

BOX 4-1   PERINATAL MEDICAL RISK FACTORS

History of prior pregnancy loss or infertility
Prior preterm delivery, threatened preterm delivery
Pregnancy complications, such as infections, bleeding, trauma, and high blood pressure
Occupational exposures, risks
Drug exposure, prescribed and illicit
Smoking
Alcohol use
Unusual or highly restricted diet, malabsorption syndrome
Thyroid disease, diabetes mellitus
Hepatitis B or HIV, disease or carrier status; unknown status
Poor weight gain
Inherited disease, such as hemoglobinopathies, neurological disorders
Prenatal identification of concerns, such as low alpha-fetoprotein (AFP)
Prenatal ultrasound abnormalities including abnormal growth
Family history of perinatal or early neonatal illness or death
Prior birth interval <18 months
Multiple fetuses (e.g., twins, triplets)
Maternal age <15 or >35 years
Maternal chronic illness (e.g., renal disease, cardiac disease, colitis)
Breast abnormalities, past surgeries, or past difficulties with breast feeding

cian after birth and in the months following. The pediatric clinician will emphasize dietary counseling by highlighting the importance of good nutrition for the success of lactation and the intrauterine development of the infant. The public is aware of the danger of illicit drug exposure to the pregnant woman, but the pediatrician's specific concern may be the catalyst for maternal treatment or change.

The list of concerns is expected to grow with an increased emphasis on environmental toxins. For women involved in occupations outside the home, the factors associated with occupational risks should be addressed. This ascertainment of physical risk and the preventive potential is certainly a part of the important work to be done in the prenatal interview. Some questions about topics such as smoking, drug use, and depression should be asked again, directly, and with some context. The questioning might go like this: "It's important that I know clearly what has been part of the pregnancy so I can check everything I need to when your baby arrives." This creates a convergence of motivation around fetal health for the family and the child's physician.

Smoking cessation is particularly important for long-term child health. Although most women do cut down or stop smoking during pregnancy, many will start again after the baby's birth. Pediatric support for improved fetal growth in the absence of smoking should continue with encouragement to stay smoke-free after delivery. In addition to the reduction in the risk of sudden infant death syndrome (SIDS), the decreases in respiratory illnesses should be highlighted to both mom and dad. Alcohol and drug histories should be taken in the same way as a smoking history, as issues that affect the infant's health and ones that the health care provider can mobilize help to address as needed. Vulnerability to go back to drug use increases late in pregnancy and after the birth of the baby. Families should know that all these issues are pediatric concerns and that they and the baby deserve help if they need it to deal with substance abuse issues. A nonjudgmental attitude and an even tone of voice help in discussions about these difficult concerns. Even if all the information isn't forthcoming at the first encounter, the stage is set to bring up the issues at a later date.

EXPANDING THE HORIZON: PSYCHOLOGICAL ADAPTATION

The prenatal pediatric interview is too limited if it stops merely with the data base concerning physical risk appraisal. Parents are particularly open to the establishment of a new relationship with a clinician as they reorder their views of themselves and their relationships with others.[2] Data are gathered with incredible efficiency at this time because of the energy a family brings to the situation and how close the adults' needs and feelings are to the surface during pregnancy. The dialogue between clinician and parents becomes a therapeutic alliance around which health and optimal development of the child may be built. It is this alliance that will allow the pediatric clinician's effective care of the child in the days after birth and throughout childhood. It is the foundation of care.

An anticipatory or preventive model is clearly presented in this setting, offering a format for future encounters as you establish your territory of concern and your range of care, which involves psychosocial aspects of development, as well as physical concerns in the care of the child. Parents can look you over to see if your approaches are in line with their expectations; a "misfit" between clinician and parents can thus be avoided.

PSYCHOLOGICAL ADJUSTMENT TO PREGNANCY

The **adaptive psychological changes in** the adults have important implications for the unborn patient. The mental turbulence, an adult developmental crisis, at this time is both normal and adaptive in mobilizing the family to meet the needs of the unborn child.[3] Excessive stress may alter the family's ability to make these important developmental changes. Severe psychological stress may directly affect fetal growth, normal fetal development, and perhaps psychological structures of the child.[4] The loss of a close loved one during pregnancy is a particularly high-risk situation as the energy for attachment to the unborn is drawn off into this other "disattachment" process. Stress between spouses or between expectant parents and grandparents may be seen to some degree in every pregnant family while individuals reorder relationships. Extremes in conflicts may draw energy away from the adaptive changes that are a necessary part of every pregnancy. Indeed, the lack of a female support system may be one of the most significant risk factors for any mother undergoing pregnancy.[5,6] The isolated, unsupported family represents a high risk for both psychosocial and physiological adjustments during gestation and beyond.[7] The whole family and the pregnancy context must be taken into account if one is attempting to assess a child's full well-being.

Pregnancy is a time of psychological turmoil for every family and has been described as "a developmental crisis"[8-10] (summary of research). Energy is mobilized, reordered, and directed around the unborn child in a process of attachment.[6,8,11] Anxiety, conflict, tension, and fears all are normal and necessary emotional components of even the most uncomplicated gestations for mothers, fathers, and other family members.[12-15] It is a time for both parents to take on new roles and identities.[10,16] Shifts in attention, time allocation, and monetary resources follow from the process of changing priorities within the whole family unit.

This process begins by a turning inward[9] and a reassessment of old relationships, particularly those between the expectant parents and their own parents. The search, either conscious or unconscious, for a role model and the need to be dependent again are all bases for this renewed focus on one's own parental relationships. Whether the grandparents of the unborn child are perceived as positive or negative, whether they are present or not, does not diminish their central psychological place in this adjustment process. Parents must work through this relationship with their own parents with each new pregnancy.[2,8] Exploration of the place of grandparents is a vital part of understanding the developing family.[10]

THE DEVELOPMENTAL COURSE OF PREGNANCY

A predictable developmental course of adjustment has been described through interviews with pregnant women[6,8] conducted as they dealt with the four major developmental tasks outlined in Table 4-1. These tasks are (1) seeking a safe passage; (2) finding an assurance of acceptance of the child by significant others; (3) binding or bonding to the unborn child; and (4) learning to give of oneself.

First Trimester

In the first trimester the inward preoccupation of the mother is largely focused on her changing body. The new body sensations, most of them unpleasant, serve to repeatedly verify the presence of pregnancy. These conflicting sensations press to resolve any old feelings of an-

TABLE 4-1 ■ Psychological Stages of Pregnancy	
First Trimester	Self-focus Becoming attached to the idea of pregnancy Pregnancy as a change in the mom—"I am pregnant" Ambivalence about the ability to handle the demands of a(nother) child Realignment of parenting issues, relationships of the past Anxiety about loss, fetal damage, or mishap Emotional lability
Second Trimester	The fetus experienced as a separate entity; increased awareness of the fetus Dreams and fantasies about the unborn child Making changes, readjustments, plans Maternal sense of well-being Nest building Increased dependence Interest in traditions, belief systems Sense of pride in the pregnancy; seeking acceptance by others Information seeking
Third Trimester	Preparing to give up the fetus; disattachment from the idea of being pregnant Seeking safe passage through the labor and delivery; making plans Attachment to the idea of being a parent Fears of damage to self, the partner, and the infant Looking for help and support Vulnerability to renewed alcohol, drug use Sleep changes Vivid dreams
Later	Introversion Cognitive slowing, daytime sleepiness Focus on details Fatigue, anxiety Putting things in order, cleaning, sorting

ger, guilt, remorse, and disbelief that may linger around the pregnancy.[17] The baby is not yet a real person to the family, although the mother may become attached to the *idea* of being pregnant. The fetus is viewed as a change in the mother rather than as a separate individual. Most mothers report feeling tense, edgy, nervous, irritable, and occasionally depressed.[16] For mothers with a history of spontaneous abortions, previous infertility, and other perinatal problems, these feelings are deepened and complicated by fear of loss and failure.

Second Trimester

With the onset of fetal movement in the second trimester, a marked shift in psychological processes takes place. The mother starts to become attached to the child as an individual. This natural process of change is suspended while the results of genetic testing are awaited, with the possibility of a termination still present. Families push away an attachment and often hide the pregnancy if this decision is left hanging. Dreams and awake fantasies about the unborn child begin at this time. These may be positive or really frightening. Both are normal, a rehearsal for whatever does come. No good data exist yet as to whether the prenatal identification of the gender of the child changes these fantasies, speeds attachments, or narrows the range of fantasies. Parents may need to bring all these imaginary babies into the open to feel less fearful.

In general, most expectant parents increase their efforts to solidify ties with friends, community, and extended family at this time. Renewed interest in traditions, religious affiliations, and hobbies are all signs of these processes. "Nest building" (i.e., the thinking about and preparing a place for the baby) is a positive sign. Even in the absence of concrete preparations for the infant, parents may be involved in important internal preparations for the infant's arrival. Indeed, for some families and cultures, physical preparations may be prohibited or viewed as dangerous. However, even in these cases, mothers will be preoccupied with making plans for the infants and themselves.[18] Most older children, even toddlers, now begin to show behavioral changes that indicate their awareness that their relationship with mother is changing, even if they haven't been told or cannot understand the concept of a new baby. Unexpected behavioral problems may arise because of shifts in family relationships, discussed or not discussed.

Third Trimester

The work of the third trimester is that of seeking a safe passage through the turmoil of labor and delivery. Interest in getting the birth over and reluctance to face what is ahead are present. The focus is on labor and delivery.[19] An increase in apparent passivity and introversion peaks at 7 to 8 months in the pregnancy. This is combined with underlying fear and anxiety. Parents who have a pattern of coping with stress by drugs or alcohol may be vulnerable to renewed use during this time. Sleep may be erratic, may be lighter, and may change electrophysiologically as well as behaviorally[20] to be in line with the needs of the infant.[21] Sleep is disrupted by dreams of the unborn infant,[13] as well as by shifts to a shorter sleep cycle and lighter sleep. Psychological nest building continues through a process of inward direction of thoughts and ideations—positive, and at times, very negative. Cognitive changes also occur; women focus on microscopical details, appear somewhat disorganized, and are preoccupied at this time. Prenatal interviews late in the third trimester may not be as successful as those held earlier. Educational programs done very late in pregnancy also appear to be less effective, perhaps because of these shifts in mental or cognitive focus. Parents may not even remember infant care advice presented at this time.[22]

FATHERS—WHAT ABOUT DAD?

Although research in this area is sparse, the adjustment process for fathers in pregnancy is very real.[10,12,14,23] Fathers' reactions often may be delayed and less intense, but appear to be similar to those of mothers-to-be. An initial response of either (or both) joy and excitement or anger and disappointment follows the public announcement of the pregnancy. Emotional distancing, introspection, and jealousy are often the father's second-trimester experiences. A shift toward attachment, protectiveness, and involvement are part of the late pregnancy changes. A father must work through his sense of loss of the relationship he once had with his wife, including the sexual aspects.[24]

The third trimester may bring specific new anxieties about the child and the delivery. In addition, the actual cost of caring for a child may push some fathers to seek extra work and to develop new strategies for financial future planning. Some fathers will seek work to balance the anxiety that the impending delivery brings.[25] Mothers may misinterpret this as "fleeing."

Do fathers make any difference to the delivery and well-being of the infant? Unequivocally yes! Research has shown that in families in which the father is involved and present for labor and delivery, everything goes better. Mothers go through labor more easily, and deliveries are smoother. Indeed, the actual effectiveness of childbirth preparation classes may be through the medium of father participation.[26] In the Parke et al[26] study, 95% of the fathers reported the delivery as a positive experience. The father's presence at a cesarean section prompts greater involvement with the infant in the neonatal period and even into the first months of life. Fathers also have a role in aiding older children in their adjustment to pregnancy.[27] In one study, fathers increased the time spent with the older child on the average by 34%, and the time allocation was positively related to the ease of the older child's adjustment.[26] The best predictor of breast-feeding success is the support of the spouse. Paternal education about breast feeding, even among low socioeconomic status (SES) groups, changes knowledge, attitude, and support.[28] A father's attitude in this matter is vital.[29]

A **father's involvement** with the pregnancy and delivery bodes well for the family's adjustment. It is well worth the effort to actively encourage and support involvement of the father in the child's life before birth. A specific invitation to the father by the office receptionist at the time an appointment for a prenatal interview is made goes a long way in affirming the father's positive contribution to the child's well-being.

Mark Hansen's apparent discomfort (see beginning of chapter) during the prenatal visit is an important observation that invites a positive intervention by the clinician. The clinician might congratulate him on taking the time to attend, particularly given his job pressure. Specific questions about his expectations for the delivery and his hopes and plans for the first weeks after the birth might draw him in. Few fathers readily volunteer much without an outreach.

In summary, *pregnancy demands an important transition in adult development for both mothers and fathers,* a process that is not complete at the time of the infant's birth or beyond. The parents who come in for the prenatal interview will not be the same as those the clinician will meet after the delivery. The pediatric clinician can anticipate the strength of the infant to mold some of the uncertainties, anxieties, and mild, often adaptive, disorganization seen in most families at this time. Strong, reassuring support from the clinician will be the foundation of the relationship with the parents. This, in turn, is the strongest tool for monitoring and care.

ATTACHMENT—ASSESSMENT OF RISK

Some families are more at risk for a poor attachment of the infant, which in turn can result in poor child care down the line. *Early attachment is defined as a strong affectional connection with another person that endures over time.*[30] Although most families will make a strong relationship with the infant, the few that will need additional help should be identified early, if possible. Intervention, including a recommendation to reach out to family members and close friends, along with the support given by the primary health care provider and professional referrals, can prevent long-term consequences of an impoverished emotional environment for the child. Extra vigilance is needed when factors place an individual family at risk. Some of these are shown in Box 4-2.

BOX 4-2	PRENATAL RISK FACTORS FOR ATTACHMENT

Recent death of a loved one
Previous loss of or serious illness in another child
Prior removal of a child
History of depression, serious mental illness
History of infertility, pregnancy loss
Troubled relationship with parents (i.e., the grandparents)
Financial stress, job loss
Marital discord, poor relationship with the other parent
Recent move, no community ties
No friends, no social network
Unwanted pregnancy
No good parenting model
The experience of poor parenting
Drug and/or alcohol abuse
Extreme immaturity

OTHER CHILDREN

Adaptation to the impending arrival of a competitor is a hurdle for any young child.[15] The **birth of a sibling** requires readjustment of the child's views of himself and of his place in the family. The nature of that change depends on the child's own developmental level and temperament. The parents' own adjustment processes make a child aware of a change in a family long before he is aware of its source. In fact, concealment of the pregnancy not only is impossible, but leads to an increase in the anxiety the child may be experiencing because of all of the changes that are occurring. The young child needs to be reassured often of the parents' unwavering love and the security of life. The child needs to know what will happen to him or her. For a child younger than 3 years of age, whose capacity to understand future events and whose world is largely confined to family and home, the birth of a sibling will be difficult. If changes are needed (e.g., change in beds), they should be done early to allow for accommodation. Pressure to toilet train at this time may lead to a prolongation of the process unless the child is really ready. Those younger than 3 years old rarely should be told about the pregnancy until the second or even early third trimester.

Young children may enjoy feeling the baby move in utero, accompanying mother for checkups, looking at books, or playing with dolls, although no data suggest that these activities ease the adjustment. Rehearsal of the specific plans for a child at the time of the delivery is helpful to a young child so that he or she knows what to expect. Mild regressions and an increase in demands by the child are positive signs of a child's sensitivity to the pregnancy and offer testimony to the child's attachment to his parents. Parents should be congratulated for this evidence of a positive emotional response. Pushing the child to "grow-up, act like a big boy" probably will make the older child become more clingy, irritable, and demanding. There is no reason to expect that having to share one's parents with another child will be greeted with enthusiasm, at least not during some period of adjustment. This is true no matter what the spacing interval is between children. It's a developmental crisis for the child that can be handled with support. The central issue in the adjustment is the parents' continuing psychological availability for the older child.

Parents may have significant feelings of loss in their relationship to the older child with the anticipated arrival of another and wonder if they have enough time, energy, and love to share with another child. They may need to grieve this loss in order to move to another level of parenting. A sense of urgency about that relationship with the older child and a feeling of pressure to do all that the parent can before the birth of the next child may be a source of additional tension in a family. The pediatric clinician should consider this family process as the basis for renewed behavioral problems, mild developmental regressions, or even an increase in phone calls to the office. Addressing the adjustment issue directly may get to the heart of the matter. These issues run counter to the pulling away, inward turning of mothers at this time. An expectant mother is a new and changeable person with whom the older child must adjust. Observations in Africa suggest that this preparation time may be even more stressful for the child than the period following the birth.[18] The same psychological shifts occur in the United States.

In the third trimester, parents can introduce books that deal with the birth of a sibling. Children's questions about the event should be answered clearly and honestly, bearing in mind what might be the *basis* for the specific question from the child's perspective (e.g., separation, loss of possessions, special shared activities), as well as the child's developmental level. Medical details are usually of less interest to the child.

ATTENDANCE AT THE BIRTH

Some families will ask about a sibling's presence at the birth. Research on the effects of this experience is sparse. A consideration of the child's capacity to deal with fears and fantasy must be brought forward. The clinician may ask the parents to consider the following as they think about their older child's perspective:

- Will the intensity of the emotion be overwhelming or frightening?
- How will the child respond to an unexpected event as well as the expected events?
- Who will be present with the *exclusive* job of support for the older child, to monitor this child's responses, answer questions, and give the child permission to leave?
- Are the parents willing and able to prepare the older child insofar as they can?
- Does the child wish to attend the birth, and will there be a chance for him to change his mind?

Hospital visitation after the infant's birth may ameliorate some of the child's worries about separation. Acceptance of the new baby should not be the goal of this visit; the reassurance of maternal availability and intactness should be. No evidence shows that a hospital visit decreases any of the expected negative behaviors at home. That rivalry appears to have to run its course.

WHAT IS THE FETUS UP TO?

Helping a family learn about the developing new life in terms of the fetus' response is a way to draw members into the idea of the infant as an important interactive participant in their lives. At least part of the visit should be a "did you know . . ." recounting of **fetal behavior** capabilities. This sets the stage for the newborn's arrival, when these interactional capabilities will be observed directly.

Specific studies of the fetus give an enhanced view of the emerging behavioral capacities during gestation. These insights, shared with parents, may help the process of attachment and give the parents a sense of the evolving interactional capacities of their child. These capacities are summarized by Hepper,[31,32] and examples are given here:

■ The infant is very sensitive to motion and position by the fifth month, making postural adjustments and anticipating maternal moves in patterns. He may be very still while mom is active only to start to "dance" when mom rests.

■ Responsiveness to sound develops early, at around the fourth month, so the infant has plenty of time to learn to recognize the parents' voices. Babies have real memory of familiar sounds, music, and voices.

■ Babies respond to maternal stress and attention, both acutely and chronically. Changes in heart rate, physiological reactivity, and cortisol secretion all testify to this.

■ Habituation, the ability to cut down responsiveness after repeated exposure to a stimulus only to renew attention when the stimulus is changed, is evidence of early perception of differences and learning. This is evident at 28 weeks at least.

■ Recognition of music regularly played during gestation is evident in newborns by heart rate and behavioral alerting, but no evidence proves that one can induce musical skill or perfect pitch through this early exposure. Infants can learn to recognize stories if these are read several times per day during fetal life.[32,33]

■ Vision comes in later than other senses, but responsiveness to outside light is evident by the twenty-sixth week. Shining flashlights on the outside of the abdomen of the mom doesn't enhance intelligence, alertness, or any other skill, although the fetus will respond, either positively or negatively.

■ The fetus's olfactory sense allows him to respond positively to smells to which he has been exposed in utero (e.g., cumin, garlic). His heart rate changes after birth, testifying to his olfactory memory. He's absorbing his own culture even before he's born!

These observations add strength to the pediatric perspective on good pregnancy health. The baby is developing the capacity to actively engage the outside world through the growth of vital brain and body systems. These systems are influenced in the long term through improved nutrition and health. Pediatric advocacy begins here with the affirmation of good nutrition, healthy lifestyle and habits, and the reduction of stress, as well as regular care. Hearing these perspectives from the unborn infant's health care provider may be just the push needed for the mother to start or maintain the best in pregnancy health. Even late in the pregnancy, a change in health habits can make a difference in outcome for the child.[35]

STRESS AND SUPPORT

Families under stress bring additional risk to the developing fetus. Among others, Van Den-Bergh[36] has shown that increased levels of maternal stress result in increases in fetal activity and less optimal perinatal profile. Fetal well-being is affected by support from and integration into the community, probably through the medium of reduction in stress. Social issues during pregnancy and the health parameters of the infant are strongly related, so the former are clear pediatric concerns.[37] Family well-being and support really are a pediatric concern and should be part of the factors addressed in the prenatal interview. This in turn sets the stage for the ongoing appraisal of the family as part of the child health evaluation throughout childhood, the essential microenvironment for growth and development. This territory of concern is defined by the issues discussed in the early days of the relationship between the child health care specialist and the parents.

IMPROVED DEVELOPMENT THROUGH BREAST FEEDING

Breast feeding will go a long way toward enhancing infant health and development.[38] The decision to breast feed is usually made in the prenatal period, so it's important for the prenatal visit to provide information and particularly motivation on this issue from the child's perspective. Strategies that have proven successful in increasing breast feeding have been laid out by the Best Start program.* This involves building on the motivating factors of improved infant health (of which most women are well aware) and the mom's own desire to be the best mom possible and have a strong bond with the infant. Information about the benefits of breast feeding is rarely the missing piece in making the decision. Affirmation of the positive motivators, however, goes a long way to support breast feeding.

Psychological barriers (Box 4-3) that counter these for many women should also be addressed. Although each woman has her own issues or her own angle on these barriers, they fall into predictable categories that can be specifically and briefly addressed. Notation of these prenatally allows the pediatric provider to address these early insights into the basis for problem solving after the baby is born. At that time, the *real* concerns will be less available. The clinician can offer specific information and help about the supposed difficulties This is done without being prescriptive or dogmatical and can be very brief. This short, targeted intervention to counter the mental barriers is a better use of time than providing a list of breast-feeding benefits. Encouragement to attend breast-feeding classes and identification of community resources should follow. Breast-feeding intervention done prenatally can positively influence attitudes, as well as knowledge, and can lead to improved rates and duration of breast feeding. The attitude and support of the primary health care provider are just behind spousal support in assuring breast-feeding success.

---

*Best Start Social Marketing, 3500 East Fletcher Avenue, Tampa, FL 33613.

BOX 4-3	BREAST-FEEDING ISSUES*

Motivating Factors in the Choice to Breast Feed

Infant Health

Most women know that breast feeding adds protection from disease for infants, but most are not as aware of the reduction of illness in the long term or of the developmental advantage.

Mother-Infant Bonding

Women want a special, long-lasting bond and closeness with the infant; they want to give the infant what no one else can give.

A Special Time

Women enjoy the forced quiet time, the relaxed feeling, the warmth and pleasure that comes with breast feeding.

Affirmation of Womanhood

Women realize their physical potential and have a sense of pride at doing this, see it as a sign of maturity and responsibility.

Maternal Health

Few women are aware of the long-term benefit to themselves in terms of reduced rates of breast cancer, osteoporosis, and arthritis.

Psychological Barriers to Breast Feeding

Lack of Confidence

Fear of inability to produce enough milk of high enough quality. Overemphasis on the need for a good diet that women cannot afford or prepare. Belief that this is hard to learn. Misinterpretation of the baby's cries. Touches on lack of self-confidence.

Embarrassment

Fear of breast exposure in public or even in the home, making husband jealous, prompting "disgust" in other women.

Loss of Freedom

Belief that breast feeding will cut down on an active social or work life, that she will never get to use a baby sitter, that the baby will be spoiled by breast feeding. Often disguises a fear of bonding or fear of that bond becoming too close caused by the need to work outside the home or pressure by the father of the baby to rejoin social life, unchanged by baby.

Dietary and Health Practices

Belief that breast feeding requires a strict adherence to a special diet, giving up spicy foods and fast foods, foregoing smoking or alcohol or drug use, getting extra sleep, or staying "too relaxed," which seem impossible. Perception that birth control pills cannot be used while breast feeding. Perception that one isn't healthy enough to breast feed.

Influence of Family and Friends

The father of the baby or the grandparents overtly or covertly discourage breast feeding or give faulty advice.

Fear of Pain

Perception that breast feeding will be painful or disfiguring.

From Best Start: *Best Start training manual,* Tampa, Fla, 1997, Best Start.

DATA GATHERING
Setting the Stage

Each clinician will have a unique style of doing prenatal interviews, and this will vary according to parental factors as well. However, this encounter can be maximized by at least beginning with a set format. Many pediatric clinicians may be slightly uncomfortable at first without the presence of a child; a set agenda will help to ameliorate this discomfort.

Group pediatric prenatal visits are a new option for some practices, often attached to childbirth, breast-feeding, or sibling preparation classes. These sessions offer the opportunity to answer questions and to efficiently review your own philosophy and practice plan. Information can be given to the group, and productive discussion can take place. Many families respond to the group support, which can lay the foundation for group health supervision visits. All such group formats should include some private time with each couple to address particular concerns and to begin to establish an individual relationship. Following are guidelines for a prenatal visit:

■ Allow about 30 minutes for the interview if possible.
■ Invite both parents to participate at a time that is convenient for both of them and for you. The ideal time appears to be 4 to 8 weeks before birth. The end of morning or afternoon office hours may provide the necessary quiet time in a pediatric practice.
■ Provide at least two comfortable adult chairs in the office setting and provide these in a position where eye-to-eye contact is possible.
■ Ask the parents to fill out a medical history before the interview and review it before your interaction with them.

Observational Data

■ Note who comes and why.
■ Assess the interaction between the parents as they enter the room for the interview process.
■ Be aware of the general affect; some degree of anxiety and apprehension is expected.
■ Determine the degree of comfort with the pregnancy through behavioral and verbal clues of both the mother and the father.
■ Note the patting of the abdomen by the pregnant woman as an indicator of a positive attitude.
■ Note the use of pronouns or names for the unborn child and the type and quantity of questions asked.

What To Ask

The format of questions outlined in Table 4-2 allows the control of the interaction to flow from the clinician to the parents.

A discussion of the specifics of your contract with the family should include the following: your availability and backup plans, the schedule for seeing the infant in the neonatal

TABLE 4-2 ■ **Questions To Be Asked in Prenatal Visit**

Question	Objective
How are you feeling?	Lay the territory to include parents' well-being; assess response to the situation overall.
Ask how the pregnancy has gone; expand to cover medical events, life stresses, etc., as noted on the medical history form and your own individual outline (i.e., a pregnancy history from a pediatric standpoint)	Gather data for objective risk factors and the parents' perception of them as well assess general response to the pregnancy and the perception of the pregnancy as high risk (whether it is by medical criteria or not).
Turn to the father and ask how the pregnancy has gone for him.	Assess the father's perceptions and concerns about his wife and baby and his own adjustment to the pregnancy.
Was this a planned pregnancy?	Assess the place of the child in the relationship, parents' adjustment to pregnancy, and degree and nature of adjustment for child's health.
Do you have other children at home? What are their ages and sexes? Have you cared for an infant before? What was that experience like?	Assess the family structure; note the child's place in it; assess experience and expectations for infant care; note locus of control (i.e., do parents see themselves in control of this event?); assess preparedness and give general information on the subject; open opportunity to give information or your own preferences about the delivery event, which may tap in on particular anxieties or fears in the third trimester; assess unrealistic or rigid expectations; when appropriate, assert that you think that the parents are in charge.
How do you plan to feed the baby? (Expand to include a diet history during pregnancy, preparation for nursing.)	Assess realistic planning for the baby and advise; reaffirm parents' control of this option; emphasize the importance of nurture in general; offer the opportunity for parents to say how they feel about the situation; assess maternal nutrition vis-à-vis the infant; assess specific breast-feeding preparations; do not push a decision if the family is not ready.
If the infant is a boy, will you have him circumcised? (Address question to father).	Assess individuation of the baby; bring the father into the decision-making process; open this topic for a two-way discussion, providing objective information on circumcision (i.e., the lack of clear medical indications) and the procedure itself.[39]

TABLE 4-2 ■ Questions to be Asked in Prenatal Visit—cont'd

Question	Objective
Have you purchased a carseat?	Show interest in safety and caretaking; assess the parents' anticipation of the needs of the infant.
How long have you lived in this area? Where do most of your family live? Who will be available to help you after the baby comes?	Assess family support systems; assess the re-alignment of old relationships; tap in on parents' relationship to their own feelings.
Do you have other responsibilities outside the family?	Assess the mother's other areas of responsibility and stress; assess what realignment of these is anticipated; some areas of ambivalence and concern may be discussed.
Are both of you working outside your home? What are your job plans? Do you have any ideas about the time you will return to work? Are you attending school? Have you made plans for the infant's care?	Assess the psychosocial situation of the family; assess parents' perceptions of their roles in career or education and as parents; assess realistic planning for infant care.
Do you have any worries about your infant? Most parents do have some concerns about the child. Would you like to share any of those with me? Is there anything in your past history that makes you think you have some special worries about your child?	Open discussion of concerns directly; but also use this setting to discuss normalcy of feelings and perhaps deeper concerns; provide information about common fears, fantasies, and dreams during a normal pregnancy.
For families with other children: How are your other children reacting to your pregnancy? What things have you done to prepare them for the birth? Most parents have some worries about how they'll manage to have enough time and love for more than one child. Do you share any of these concerns? What are the specific arrangements you've made for the older child at the time of the baby's birth?	Assess the realignment of family relationships; assess the plans for readjustment around the care of the infant; assess the maternal and paternal feelings toward the attachment to their children who have already been born.
Do you have any questions?	Set a model for pediatric visits (i.e., you are open to questions and waiting for parents to take lead).

period and beyond, some general statements about your own philosophy of pediatric care, and your fee schedule and payment options.

Special Referrals

■ Call or write a note to the obstetrician regarding special concerns from a pediatric perspective.
■ State terms of your own availability at the time of the birth (e.g., another clinician may provide care for the baby in the hospital in some circumstances).
■ Recommend prepared childbirth, breast-feeding, or other parenting classes if these have not already been attended.
■ Refer patient to social service agency or public health nurse for diagnostic aid and support system, if indicated.
■ Make nutrition referral if indicated by nutritional history or economic needs.

Anticipatory Guidance

■ Encourage open discussion between parents of the subjects addressed in the interview.
■ Advise the parents that it may be wise to plan to get help (e.g., a relative, friend, or employee) in the immediate postnatal period, but to limit visitors for about 2 weeks.
■ Encourage class attendance or reading as a supplement to, but not a substitute for, your own care.
■ Reassure parents that fears, fantasies, and feelings of loss of control are normal, adaptive, and a good indicator of care.
■ Emphasize good nutrition and safety planning for the infant and congratulate the parents on advance planning and responsibility in initiating the interview process.
■ Emphasize that it is important to approach the birth with some flexibility so that unforeseen events (e.g., anesthesia or a cesarean section) can be weathered with adaptation and grace.
■ Emphasize planning for sibling response.

A summary statement about your understanding of the interview's content and process will allow a resolution of differences or highlight areas of omission. For example, "Although you had a little concern at the beginning of the pregnancy with bleeding, things have gone very well since. We'll send off thyroid studies on the baby right away, just to be sure, given your thyroid problem. We'll be sure to get you the help you need to breast-feed. Dad, think about the circumcision question. Let me know what you both decide."

Your Record

Make your own assessment of this family's strengths and vulnerabilities.
■ Write down temperament or style characteristics in the parents
■ Make note of the social support
■ Make note of any risks to attachment
■ Note things of special interest, as shown in the following examples:

Example 1

Debbie and Mark (see case at beginning of chapter) are attractive young parents-to-be.

Strengths (+):   Married 3 years
Strong extended family
Interested in learning about the baby
Committed to breast feeding

Vulnerabilities (−):   Debbie's mom died last year. Girl will be named for her.
Economic. Dad has two jobs. No boy's name. Dad does wood-working. Family history + congenital heart disease.

Example 2

Lydia: Shy, but strong minded. Rigid expectations; clear questions. Bilingual. *Not* on welfare (proud of it). Single: Father of baby not involved. Wants a girl.

Strengths (+):   Good parenting model
Support from family
Good job

Vulnerabilities ( ):   First trimester drug use. In recovery group.
Still smoking a bit
Needs to return to work in 2 weeks
Family history of early infant deaths; ? cause

REFERENCES

1. American Academy of Pediatrics, Committee on Psychosocial Aspects of Child and Family Health: The prenatal visit, *Pediatrics* 97:141, 1996.
2. Brazelton TB: *On becoming a family: the growth of attachment,* New York, 1992, Delacorte Press-Seymour Lawrence.
3. Liebenberg B: Prenatal counseling. In Shereshefsky PM, Yarrow LJ, editors: *Psychological aspects of a first pregnancy and early postnatal adaptation,* New York, 1973, Raven Press.
4. Yamamoto KJ, Kinsey DK: Pregnant women's ratings of different factors influencing psychological stress during pregnancy, *Psychol Rep* 39:203, 1976.
5. Kennell JH: The physiologic effects of a supportive companion (doula) during labor. In Klaus MH, Robertson MO, editors: *Birth, interaction and attachment,* Pediatric Round Table Series, Skillman, NJ, 1982, Johnson and Johnson Baby Products Co.
6. Rubin R: Maternal tasks in pregnancy, *J Adv Nurs* 1:367, 1976.
7. Egeland B, Sroufe LA: Attachment and early maltreatment, *Child Dev* 52:44, 1981.
8. Bibring GL, Valenstein AF: Psychological aspects of pregnancy, *Clin Obstet Gynecol* 19:357, 1976.
9. Deutsch H: *Psychology of women,* New York, 1944, Grune & Stratton.
10. Zwelling E: Psychological responses to pregnancy. In Nichols F, Zwelling E, editors: *Maternal-newborn nursing: theory and practice,* Philadelphia, 1997, WB Saunders.
11. Leifer M: Psychological changes accompanying pregnancy and motherhood, *Genet Psychol Monogr* 95:55, 1977.

12. Bittman SJ, Zalk SR: *Expectant fathers,* New York, 1978, Hawthorn Books.
13. Heymans H, Winter ST: Fears during pregnancy, *Isr J Med Sci* 11:1102, 1975.
14. Hott JR: The crisis of expectant fatherhood, *Am J Nurs* 76:1436, 1976.
15. Legg C, Sherick I, Wadland W: Reaction of preschool children to the birth of a sibling, *Child Psychiatry Hum Dev* 5:3, 1974.
16. Caplan G: *Emotional implications of pregnancy and influences on family relationships in the healthy child,* Cambridge, Mass, 1976, Harvard University Press.
17. Uddenberg N, Fagerstroom CF, Hakanson-Zaunders M: Reproductive conflicts: mental symptoms during pregnancy and time in labor, *J Psychosom Res* 20:575, 1976.
18. LeVine RA et al: *Child care and culture: lessons from Africa,* Cambridge, England, 1994, Cambridge University Press.
19. Stainton MC: Parents' awareness of their unborn infant in the third trimester, *Birth* 17(2):92, 1990.
20. Petre-Quadens O et al: Sleep in pregnancy: evidence of fetal sleep characteristics, *J Neurol Sci* 4:600, 1967.
21. Sanders L et al: Primary prevention and some aspects of temporal organization in early infant-caretaker interactions. In Rexford EN, Sanders LW, Shapiro T, editors: *Infant psychiatry,* New Haven, Conn, 1975, Yale University Press, pp 187-204.
22. Handfield B, Bell R: Do childbirth classes influence decision making about labor and postpartum issues? *Birth* 22(3):153, 1995.
23. Parke RD: Fathers. In Bruner J, Cole M, Lloyd B, editors: *The developing child series,* Cambridge, Mass, 1981, Harvard University Press.
24. Holtzman LC: Sexual practices during pregnancy, *J Nurs Midwifery* 21:29, 1976.
25. Obrzut LE: Expectant fathers' perception of fathering, *Am J Nurs* 76:1440, 1976.
26. Parke RD et al: The father's role in the family system, *Semin Perinatol* 3:25, 1979.
27. Earls F: The fathers (not the mothers): their importance and influence with infants and young children, *Psychiatry* 39:209, 1976.
28. Sciacca JP et al: A breastfeeding education promotion program: effects on knowledge, attitudes and support, *J Community Health* 20:473, 1995.
29. Freed GL, Fraley JK, Schanter RJ: Attitudes of expectant fathers regarding breastfeeding, *Pediatrics* 90:224, 1992.
30. Bowlby J: *Attachment and loss,* vol I, *Attachment,* New York, 1969, Basic Books.
31. Hepper PG: Fetal habituation: another Pandora's Box? *Dev Med Child Neurol* 39:274 and 343, 1997
32. Hepper PG: Fetal psychology: an embryonic science. In JG Nijhuis, editor: *Fetal behavior: development and perinatal aspects,* New York, 1992, Oxford University Press.
33. Fifer WP, Moon CM: The effects of fetal experience with sound. In Lecaunet JP et al, editors: *Fetal development: a psychological perspective,* Hillsdale, NJ, 1995, Lawrence Erlbaum Associates.
34. DeCasper AJ et al: Fetal reactions to recurrent maternal speech, *Inf Behav Dev* 17:159, 1994.
35. Dixon SD et al: *Economic, social and medical risk profiles of pregnant, addicted women with and without case management services,* Sacramento, Calif, (in press), State of California, Department of Drug and Alcohol Services.
36. Van DenBergh BRH: Maternal emotions during pregnancy and fetal and neonatal behavior. In JG Nijhuis, editor: *Fetal behavior: development and perinatal aspects,* New York, 1992, Oxford University Press.
37. Gorski P: Perinatal outcome and the social contract: interrelationships between health and humanity, *J Perinatol* 18:297, 1998.
38. American Academy of Pediatrics, Rubenstein C: What pediatricians really think about working mothers, *Working Mothers,* April, 1990 (Reprinted in *AAP News,* May, 1990.)
39. Wallerstein E: *Circumcision: an American health fallacy,* New York, 1980, Springer.

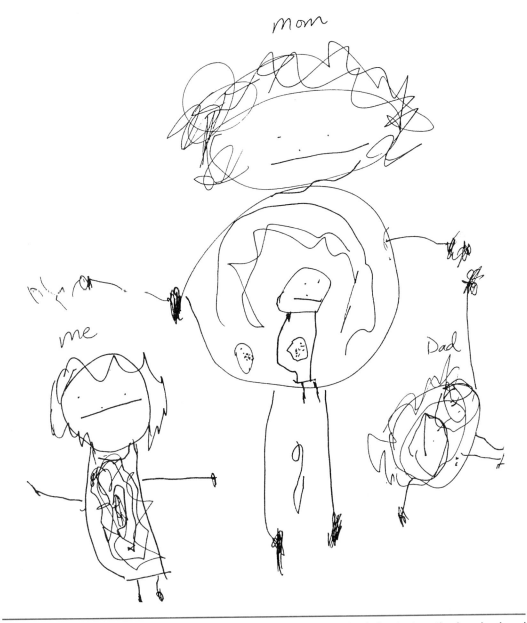

A 4-year-old girl seems uncertain about her mother's pregnancy. The father is described as aloof, and his job keeps him away from the family for extended periods.

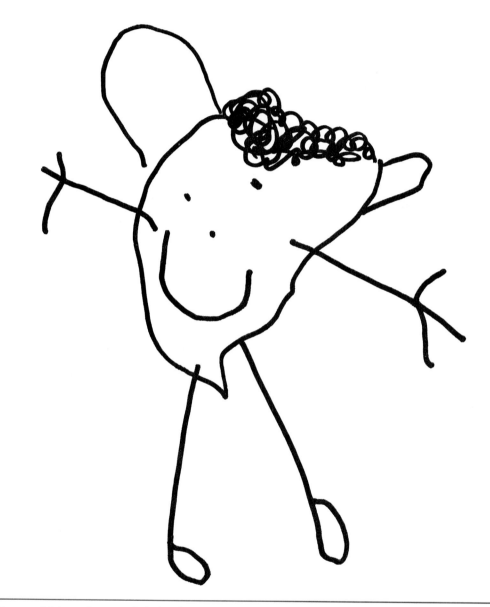

A 3-year-old draws her new little brother. His big ears and curly hair are clearly impressive. His bright-eyed, reaching out to the world is more accurate than his sister knows (original in pink marker).

CHAPTER 5

The Newborn Examination: Ready To Get Going

■ **Suzanne D. Dixon**

KEY WORDS
Attachment
Perceptual World
Six States of Consciousness
Reflex Behaviors
Habituation
State Organization
Motor Behaviors
Primitive Reflexes
Hospital Practices
Cesarean Section
Recovery Process
Discharge Planning

Jessica, born without complications, was to be examined at 1 hour of life. Her body was relaxed under the warmer, her hands and feet bluish. Her respirations were even. She scanned the environment with head to one side, fingers in her mouth. When her father spoke, she startled, and her eyes shifted toward him. Gradually she turned to find his face and then stared intensely at him, until her eyes crossed. She closed her lids briefly and then found his face again. Her father said he was in love already. Then she turned pale, moved restlessly, and spit up mucus. Jessica's father jumped back and called for the nurse.

The full-term human infant enters the world fully equipped to negotiate the dramatic physiological changes and behavioral adjustments required for postnatal life. These capacities enable him to begin the job of learning about his world and participating in his central interactive setting, his family.[1] The newborn does not just function on a reflex level; primitive reflexes only attest to neurological adequacy and provide a behavioral base on which he builds social and cognitive structures.[2,3] These structures emerge through direct interaction with the environment. The neonate is fully capable of participation in the social world with abilities to discriminate and direct selective attention toward those around him.

The goal of the newborn physical examination is augmented by a strong behavioral component to assess the full range of infant competencies and to monitor the process of postpartum adjustment. The infant's behavior reflects both his genetic makeup and his intrauterine experience.[3] We get an opportunity to look at both groups of factors when we evaluate the neonate. In addition, the initial visit with the newborn and his family offers the opportunity to participate in and perhaps facilitate the initial getting acquainted period for baby and family. In that sense, this is both an intervention and an assessment. The clinician enters into the system of the family through the shared evaluation of the infant. The first step toward **attachment** and parenting requires assurance that the infant is intact and is successfully negotiating the postpartum adjustment. The newborn examination offers the opportunity to assure the family of the infant's intactness, but also to assist in helping the parents learn about their baby. Being able to productively play with an infant is one of the rewards for the pediatric clinician as well.

In the current era the initial examination is often the discharge examination. This means that the agenda is broadened to an appraisal of whether the infant and mother are ready to leave the hospital and its supports. If they are, the clinician must decide what is the best follow-up plan. This requires a broad appraisal of physiological and behavioral competency.

BEHAVIORAL COMPETENCIES—THE SENSES

The newborn's sensory capacities are far greater than was previously believed.[4] Not only are these capacities well developed in each sphere of perception, but a substantial degree of coordination between senses is evident, even in the neonatal period. Or, as stated by Bower,[5] "The newborn lives in a unified **perceptual world** with some degree of intersensory coordination." The examination offers the chance to evaluate these.

Vision

The full-term neonate's visual system is intact at all levels.[6] The human infant can see faces and objects when they are presented in his *best focal distance, 8 to 12 in.,* although his depth of focus may actually cover a wider range. Lens mobility is limited but improves rapidly. Retinal structures, especially rods, are well developed at birth. Foveal structures are less well developed, and central focus is less than in older children and adults. Acuity is limited primarily by retinal immaturity. *Acuity and improved accommodation proceed rapidly* in the first 4 months. Extraocular movements allow for *slow tracking of objects* up to 180 degrees horizontally, perhaps briefly vertically, but not diagonally; this skill develops in the last quarter of the first year. Infants are *very sensitive to light,* perhaps more so than adults, and will open their eyes only in light that is considered dim by adult standards. Automatic visual scanning occurs even in conditions of darkness.[6] The infant clearly *has the capacity to see in three dimensions,* as evidenced by a primitive reaching and the ability to blink as an object approaches, even controlling for other inputs.[5] This defensive response is more elaborate and less automatic than a reflex behavior and attests to the integration of visual and motor systems.

Additional laboratory studies have shown that infants demonstrate differential attention to visual displays with the following characteristics:

- High contrast
- Curved lines over straight
- Bright colors rather than dull colors
- Many elements as opposed to few[6,7]
- Infants increasingly scan for edges and contrasting interfaces.

Color preference has been studied in the same way, but the results are equivocal because color is inevitably confounded by brightness, and infants do prefer moderately bright objects. Infants probably can discriminate red, green, and yellow, but not blue, when intensity is controlled.[8]

The *human face* draws much attention from the human newborn. Even as neonates, infants will preferentially look at their mothers' faces even without sound or smile, although the concept of complete facial recognition is controversial. By 12 weeks this capacity is clear, and the face is the most salient sight to the baby.[6]

The human newborn can successfully *imitate* an interesting visual display, such as the mother sticking her tongue out, even at 1 day of age.[9] This capacity implies marvelous intersensory and motor coordination. The infant must be in a quiet, alert state and allowed enough time to process the interesting display held out for imitation.

The importance of visual input for the infant is illustrated by derangements in the visual system. An impairment of vision, such as that present with cataracts, may prevent the development of *functional* pattern vision if it is not corrected during the first 6 months of life; subtle residuals of newborn visual compromise have been noted in children who have this condition even for 1 week. Without binocular input for even short periods of time, long-lasting impairment may result. Frank cortical blindness in the case of severe esotropia is the extreme of a continuum of perceptual compromise when vision is unavailable. The infant is vulnerable to alterations in vision even up to the third year of life. Early detection and remediation is imperative.

A newborn's visual capacities can be demonstrated at their fullest only when the infant is in a quiet, alert state and all distracting stimuli, even his own motor movements, are minimized. Visual performance may be limited to brief periods and may be overridden, especially early on, by physiological events (e.g., bowel movements, hiccups). Visual processing is one of the most complex neonatal abilities and may be difficult to demonstrate in all infants all the time.

The newborn's higher visual processing can be seen by observing the whole face and body when visual stimuli are presented. When attentive, the infant may initially startle slightly and then shut down body movements to focus on the visual display. Facial muscles will lift, and palpebral fissures will widen, giving the baby a bright, softened look. Brief periods of attention will cycle with periods of inattention, gaze aversion, and possibly even sleep.[2] The infant thereby will limit the duration and the complexity of the visual events to be handled at any point in time. Gaze is the capacity under the infant's control from early on. Maturation and recovery from birth or illness are characterized by increasing duration of these alert periods and the ability to respond to increasing complexity of stimuli. Infants who readily habituate to visual stimuli and show a strong preference for novelty are more likely to show more advanced development.[10] The ability to attend to salient features is supported by mothers who draw selective attention to objects in the environment for visual scanning.

Audition

The infant can hear and is responsive to sounds even in the uterus, as described in Chapter 3. The ability to clearly direct attention to auditory input may even be seen in 28-week-old premature infants,[11] and this ability may be much better developed than the visual system in these small babies. Although fluid is present in the middle ear for days after birth, the full-term newborn is attentive and responsive to sound environment, although with a slightly higher threshold.

The infant will respond to a pleasant auditory signal, such as a voice or soft rattle, in ways similar to his visual alerting response—an initial alerting startle, a brightening of expression, and a diminishing of body activity. The infant may turn his eyes and then his head toward the sound after a short delay and will often search for the source of it. Female voices in highly modulated tones (i.e., "baby talk") produce the most consistent orientation response. Adults in general speak to infants in short bursts of 5 to 15 seconds, the same time unit that produces this differential auditory attention. Lower tones, such as those produced by male speakers, produce a quieting response in a newborn who is upset. Short bursts of modulated human speech produce a greater behavioral response than unpatterned speech or speech of a greater or lesser duration. Selective attention is paid to the basic elements of human speech, the phoneme or consonant-vowel combination,[12] with particular attention to one's own language beginning in early infancy.

Clearly, by 1 month of age, and often in the immediate newborn period, an infant can distinguish between mother's voice and another's, as demonstrated through differential quieting and sucking responses. The infant will work harder sucking to receive the reward of a taped recording of the mother's voice than for that of another person. A baby will often quiet immediately on hearing mother in the room. Soft, low-pitched lullabies and particularly human heart tones produce decreased activity and decreased crying in the newborn. Even while continuing to cry, the infant coordinates his cry and movements with the lullaby within seconds, eventually quieting. Lullabies around the world have the same rhythms that appear soothing to infants. In contrast, "game songs" (i.e., lively, fast, and repetitive short verses as in "This Old Man") produce either alerting or behavioral disorganization.[13] The sound of his or her own cry or other newborns' cries produces dramatic increases in distress and crying.

The now classic work of Condon and Sander[14] has shown that a newborn readjusts ongoing body movements to the voice patterns of those speaking around him and will do so more consistently if the speaker is his or her mother or at least someone speaking in the family's native language. Pure tones, runs of babble, and other nonspeech tones do not produce this differential response. Early interactional synchrony attests to complex integration of the newborn's behavior, auditory and motor, as well as to the in utero learning that has occurred.

Infants fail to respond to auditory stimuli if it is loud (e.g., hand clap), aversive (e.g., "white noise" in a nursery), or if confounded with other stimuli (e.g., loud voice with an overly animated, close face). The infant shuts out these adverse auditory events very successfully and may even appear to have impaired audition under these conditions. The clinician can be fooled by this inattention. A gentler approach (less background noise, soft sounds, and no competing visual display) is needed to bring out these auditory capacities.

Early hearing is vital to the development of language as well as to emotional health, which involves the ability to self-soothe and to anticipate change in the environment.[15] The parent-child interaction is distorted and less positive when one of the partners is deaf, although the use of facial expression in adult native signers adds some emotional depth to the interaction.[16] Early remediation through amplification and cochlear implants is now available. These are strong bases for the recommendation of universal hearing screening in newborns.[17]

Although major hearing loss can be identified by the infant's failure to respond to the human voice as evidenced by at least heart rate change, there is no way to completely screen behaviorally. Risk factors are only present in half the cases of hearing loss. Formal screening of all newborns is needed if we are to detect serious hearing loss that can impact development, which has a prevalence of 1 in 500 to 1 in 1000.

Some infants will be more responsive to sound than others; visual displays will produce greater behavioral attention with other infants. These individual differences may be noted even in the newborn period and will highlight the special behavioral profile of an individual child. Some infants are listeners and some are lookers.

Taste and Smell

Studies have demonstrated that infants have a well-developed sense of taste. Their taste buds are of greater number and are more widely distributed than those of an adult. Even while in utero, infants can demonstrate an alteration in sucking frequency when sugar is introduced into the amniotic fluid. Sensitivity to sour tastes is present at birth, whereas sensitivity to salty and bitter tastes develops postnatally,[18] at about 4 to 6 months of age. Complex patterns of taste preference, as opposed to sensitivity, are shaped by experience during the first year of life. The infant is preprogrammed to avoid aversive tastes that in nature are largely poisonous and to seek out those that are sweet and differentially nourishing. Facial expression of infants presented with varying tastes are similar to adults' expressions in the same circumstances.[19] Breast milk is sweeter than formula and may be preferred on this basis. Although some infants are more sensitive to the varying tastes in breast milk based upon maternal diet,[20] it is the rare infant who truly alters his nursing pattern because of the presence of a particular taste. Behavioral changes in nursing are rarely related to maternal diet.

Smell is well developed in newborns and is of great importance in orientation to the environment.[21,22] The infant can successfully localize odors and may demonstrate preference through differential turning away and orienting toward unpleasant and pleasant odors, respectively. Associative learning, linking smells with other events, shows the importance of olfaction in learning about the world.[23] Infants as young as 5 days of age can differentiate by smell alone the breast pad of their own mother from that of other mothers.[22,24] Parents, in turn, can recognize their own infant's smell after only 1 hour of exposure,[25] suggesting that each infant has his own odor signature, and one that is the easiest identifier for the parent to learn. Smell is thought to play an important role in familiarization with parents immediately after birth. Infants placed at birth on the thigh of their moms will crawl up to the breast aided only by smell.[26,27] When touch and smell are linked, the infant shows very strong preference for familiar and rewarding odors.[28] This is another reason to keep the infant close and to avoid artificial scents.

PHYSIOLOGICAL STABILIZATION

The ability to maintain breathing, heart rate, and temperature and to modulate peripheral perfusion improves over the first days of life with varying speed and smoothness. Infants stressed by difficult labors, deliveries, or postnatal perturbations generally have more trouble with these transitions. Slightly preterm infants, 36 to 38 weeks, and large-for-gestational-age (LGA) babies with glucose irregularities take longer to stabilize. Skin color, skin perfusion, and the degree of acrocyanosis and its increases with stress are important to characterize and monitor for continuing improvement. The response to and recovery from undressing, handling, reflex assessment, and even social interaction give us an indication of the infant's vulnerability, margin of tolerated stress, and maturity. These vital observations can be made incidentally as part of every exam, adding no more time but giving important information on the infant's individual resilience. Infants still grappling with organization at this physiological level will not be as available for auditory and visual alerting tasks because these processes seem to be organized on a hierarchical level.[29] Feeding difficulties are more common in youngsters who are less mature or who evidence stress at this level of organization.

STATE BEHAVIOR

Infants exist in at least **six states of consciousness:**[30]
- Quiet sleep
- Active sleep
- Drowsiness
- Quiet alert state
- Active alert-fussy
- Crying

They move through these states in cycles with some regularity (Table 5-1). Responsiveness to some outside stimuli, physiological processes (e.g., heart rate, breathing) and even **reflex behaviors** based on motor tone vary with these cycles.

The clear characterization of each state and the regular movement from one state to another testifies to a neurological competency and maturity. The intact newborn can resist outside disturbances during sleep and even awake states by shutting out these intrusive events. Noises, lights, and even painful stimuli will be behaviorally and electrophysiologically ignored with successive presentation.[2] This process is called **habituation.** The adaptive, protective nature of this capacity is obvious. The infant protects his own vulnerability to noise and light stimuli through a process of selective inattention. In the active state, repeated stimuli that are exactly the same are successively ignored. When a new stimulus of even a

TABLE 5-1 ■ States in the Newborn

State	Activity	Muscle Tone	Heart Rate	Respirations
Quiet sleep	Eyes closed, no eye movements, still with occasional startles	Steady, tonic	Regular	Regular
Active sleep	Eyes closed with globe movements Random movements of low level facial movements, wiggles	Low	Variable	Irregular
Drowsy	Flat face, eyes closed, dully open, or partially open Writhing movements, variable	Low, variable	Variable	Variable
Alert	Face bright Eyes open, following Motor movement mostly absent	Steady	First a rise, then lower than baseline	Regular
Irritable	Negative face, avoidance maneuvers, squirmy, brief whimpers, or fussy vocalizations	Slight increase	Variable	Irregular
Crying	Crying, motor activity at high level	Increased	Slightly elevated	Irregular, with crying

Modified from Prechtl HFR: *The neurological examination of the full term newborn infant*, Vol 63, *Clinics in developmental medicine*, London, 1975, MacKeith Press and Brazelton TB, Nugent JK: *Neonatal behavioral assessment scale*, Vol 137, *Clinics in developmental medicine*, London, 1995, MacKeith Press.

slight variation is presented, the infant will again redirect attention toward the altered, now moderately novel, stimuli. Habituation, then, can be an outcome measure by which we assess the infant's sensitivity to minor changes in his environment. These are some of the techniques used to evaluate the infant's ability to discriminate between similar stimuli. These may include changes in visual acuity, auditory perception, smell, taste, and position sense. Renewed attention, often associated with heart rate changes (an initial slowing, followed by an increase), testifies to the infant's ability to detect change in his environment and direct his attention to this "new" information. He is preset to differentially attend to these new learning opportunities.

The first hours and days of life are characterized by disruption of the regularity of state changes seen in late gestation. An alert period of about 40 to 70 minutes in the term, nondrugged neonate after birth is followed by a period of 3 to 5 hours of deep sleepiness. Brief, drowsy arousals occur until the newborn is about 18 to 24 hours old. Renewed wakefulness and obvious hunger with frequent feedings are the norm for the next 24 to 72 hours. Babies often feed every 1½ to 2 hours during this period. The state cycle stabilizes when the mother's milk comes in, with wakefulness every 2 to 3 hours. Infants discharged at 24 hours or less may be perceived at home later as ill, unhappy, and certainly uncooperative unless the clinician draws attention to this normal pattern of adjustment in state.

Neurologically intact infants under the care of one caretaker will show progressive gains in state cycle stabilization. Many infants will remain somewhat irregular and unpredictable as part of their individual temperament profile and the slope of their recovery after birth.[1] Infants older than 3 days (and very sleepy ones before that) will benefit from a little help in establishing a regular wake-sleep cycle through the care of a regular caregiver responding to the subtle cues of early wakefulness, wiggles, and brief eye openings. Feedings at that stage are usually more successful than those attempted after a crying bout. Crying is a late sign of hunger.[31] Regular feedings, variations in illumination and sound, and close body contact with another human being all work toward a stabilization of **state organization.**[32] In contrast, constant illumination, continuous noise, many caregivers, and an irregular response to restlessness, crying, and distress (all characteristic of a hospital nursery) will make it more difficult for the infant to get organized with sleep, feeding, and alertness. We do neither mothers nor healthy infants any favors by bringing the babies to the nursery "so mother can sleep." This is an added delay in postpartum adjustment that is to be avoided if at all possible. It confounds the process for both and may make sleep and feeding areas of concern when they go home. Because infants in a rooming-in situation cry very little, the risk is small that other mothers who are in the same unit will lose sleep.[33] Full rooming-in should produce a quiet unit.

MOTOR BEHAVIORS

Motor behaviors are built on a set of **primitive reflexes** originating in the brainstem (Table 5-2). These reflexes are indicators of general neurological integrity, and each has its own developmental course (Table 5-3). These reflexes are based on muscle tone, which, in the normal infant, varies with the state of consciousness. Therefore in addition to noting the presence, absence, or asymmetry of these reflexes, the clinician should assess active and passive tone within the context of several states, in sleep and wakefulness. The physician should also be aware of state throughout the motor examination. Relative hypotonia and hypertonia are each appropriate in different states of consciousness, but the persistence of these through several states is worrisome. For example, plantar and palmar grasp should be sluggish in active sleep, when tone is diminished, but brisk in a cry state when tone is increased.

Learned behaviors are built on these reflexes. For example, the reflexive suck becomes specific for the breast or the bottle early in the first days of life. It becomes coordinated to milk flow characteristics of each and becomes part of a complex pattern of behavior between a mother and infant. The tonic neck reflex enables the infant to watch his hand movements so that gaze and reach become linked—the first step toward volitional reach. Reflexes provide an opportunity for the infant to interact with the environment so that experiences can begin immediately and are the beginning of both cognitive and affective growth.[34] This software package helps the infant start exploring and experimenting with the world.

The most obvious activity in which the reflexes form the basis of learned behavior is breast feeding. The infant must organize root, suck, and posture to get the nipple correctly in his or her mouth, extract milk efficiently, accommodate to the mom's anatomy and milk flow characteristics, and coordinate breathing.[35-37] Some infants take more time to get this all together than others. Some infants get off track more easily than others with the use of

TABLE 5-2 ■ Reflexes of the Normal Full-Term Infant

Reflex	Normal Response*
Deep tendon reflexes	
biceps	Brisk response without spread
knee	Crossed adductor response without knee jerk
ankle	Ankle clonus up to 10 beats
Palmar hand grasp	Closure over finger
Plantar grasp	Plantar flexion of toe and forefoot
Babinski	Toe extension, with or without initial flexion
Moro	Extension and abduction of the arms followed by flexion and adduction; cry may or may not be present.
Tonic neck reflex	Increased tone, leg extension on side of head direction, flexion in contralateral arm and leg; this response is the basis for asymmetries in tone and reflexes when the head is not in midline
Placing	Extension of leg with dorsal stimulation
Stepping and walking	Range from minimal weight-bearing to several brisk steps with plantar stimulation

*Asymmetries that are consistent and demonstrated when the head is in the midline are always abnormal.

TABLE 5-3 ■ Ontogeny of Neonatal Reflexes and Tone

Reflex and Muscle Tone	Age of Emergence	Age of Disappearance
Tonic neck reflex	35 wk, peak at 44 wk	7-8 mo
Moro	28 wk incomplete, 37 wk complete	3-6 mo
Head turn in prone	37 wk	Variable
Palmar grasp	28 wk	2 mo
Trunk incurvation	28 wk	4-5 mo
Placing, stepping	37 wk	2-4 mo
Ankle clonus, up to 5-10 beats	33-35 wk (?)	1 mo
Pupillary response	32 wk	Never
Flexor tone, lower extremity	32 wk	>1 yr
Flexor tone, upper extremity	36 wk	? >1 yr

Modified from Volpe JJ: *Neurology of the newborn,* Philadelphia, 1971, WB Saunders.

pacifiers and artificial nipples. Those who have been sucking and biting in utero as evidenced by hand or lip sucking blisters or a tight chomp of the jaw, may have to unlearn these habits to be good nursers. They need assessment, support, and remediation. Until the patterns are in place, it's best to avoid pacifiers or artificial nipples if possible. Helping the mother to see that this is a learning process and providing bedside appraisal and help will go a long way to ensure nursing success. Because breast feeding is good for development,[38,39] as well as disease protection, it is well worth paying attention to the progress of this learning activity for the infant.

The execution of *"random" movements* gives clues to neurological competency, maturity, and style. Careful observation of these movements in the course of the examination add to the data. Persistent jitteriness and tremulousness, especially in both asleep and alert states, attests to a neurological immaturity, perinatal stress, or metabolic abnormalities. Jerky movements in arcs of 45 degrees are less worrisome in the full-term infant. Ankle clonus greater than two beats and many startles throughout the regular pediatric examination or with minimal handling are of similar concern in the term infant. However, these motor abnormalities do not carry predictive significance beyond the newborn period. These should be monitored over a period and should be taken as clues indicating the possibility of other adjustment difficulties rather than as being diagnostic or prognostic in themselves.

All in all, the infant's perceptual and behavioral repertoire is geared toward initiating and maintaining positive interactions with his world. All of his capacities enable him to reach out, to become active in eliciting responsive care. These are shown in Table 5-4.

BIRTH EXPERIENCE

The impact of perinatal events on the development of the family unit is profound. Labors that are attended by supportive people, particularly the father, tend to be shorter and less fraught with complications.[40,41] The mother's experience of labor and delivery are much more positive in these circumstances. Clear knowledge of the events of labor and delivery allows family members to feel that they are in control of this natural process and gives an enhanced feeling of competency. Prepared childbirth training offers help on several levels, such as educating, laying out expectations, calming fears, and offering the support of a group of parents. Childbirth education may be the beginning of a parenting community. Certainly, labors are shorter and medication is needed less often after these preparations.

The role of a knowledgeable support person, a *doula,* has been shown to be helpful in smoothing the course of labor. Close physical contact with the mom seems to be particularly effective.[42]

Long labors and epidural anesthesia can produce a rise in temperature that may be misconstrued as a pathological fever. This sets up the need for medical intervention, separations, and discharge delays. Delivery room practices that keep the infant and parents central, that respect the infant's physiology and adjustment needs, and that facilitate the infant's spending as much time as possible, as early as possible, with the parents, are the best. The clinician should examine all practices with these priorities, not the institution's, in mind.

The impact of these practices was first highlighted by Klaus and Kennell[43] in work exploring the development of *mother-infant attachment.* The rigid concept of critical time be-

TABLE 5-4 ■ Clinical Assessment of Capacities of Newborns: Trends in the First Days of Life

Capability	Trends
Vision	Follows face without voice in arc of 30 to 180 degrees horizontally when quiet and alert; face "softens"; shuts down motor activity when attention is directed at a visual display (e.g., face of examiner); hand and mouth activation with pleasant visual display; blinks at looming object (e.g., stethoscope). Eyes open and scan in dim light. Spends more time looking at high contrast.
Audition	Eyes shift to positive sound source; turns to soft sounds (e.g., soft rattle, voice); shuts down motor activity to listen to pleasant sound; ignores, startles, or cries in response to loud sounds (e.g., clapping).
Smell	Aversive response to strong smell (e.g., alcohol wipe near nose). Knows parents' smells.
Taste	Increase of sucking of sucrose vs. water.
State regulation	Has increasingly regular wake-sleep patterns; goes to sleep with aversive maneuvers on general examination (e.g., circumcision, PKU stick); has clear, although brief, quiet-alert times; progressively easier to waken for feedings or wake periods.
Physiological stability	Gradual moderate skin color changes during the course of the examination; increasingly less mottling, acrocyanosis; heart and respiratory rate vary with state changes (not during examination and in medical record); increasing tolerance for a pediatric examination without showing signs of stress (e.g., color changes, gaze aversion, abrupt state change to cry or sleep).
Vestibular	Responds to rocking with quieting; opens eyes when held upright in a dim room; turns head to direction of an upright spin.
Motor	Observe posture and active tone within context of state (e.g., hypertonia to some degree while crying; hypotonia is normal in sleep).
	Observe tremulousness (mild to moderate appropriate in cry states) and jerky movements.
	The greater the arc of movement of the arms, the greater the maturity of the child.
	Assess primitive reflexes.
	Asymmetries and marked extremes call for repeat assessment and perhaps further evaluation.

PKU, Phenylketonuria.

tween parents and infants hasn't been substantiated, and some are frankly critical.[44] However, the basic importance of **hospital practices** and how they influence the early development of families certainly is now well established.[45] The pediatric primary care clinician should keep the broad picture in mind and help establish priorities within the bounds of the best medical practice.

Birth is the beginning of a relationship and, as in any human relationship, it is as variable as the people involved. Sensitivity to the feelings of parents, both positive and negative, will allow the infant's physician to support this "getting acquainted" as it proceeds in its own individual way. Adaptation to the medical needs may require that parents realign priorities; the clinician should guide and assist in this process.

Cesarean section, especially if it is unanticipated, may result in feelings of failure and unmet expectations on the part of parents. In addition, infants delivered by cesarean section may be drowsy, slow feeders, and poorly responsive to their parents' attempts at early social interaction. Mothers indeed may feel more pain from the incision and have a more prolonged recovery course than mothers of infants born by vaginal delivery. Infants delivered by cesarean section often require more time and patience getting themselves behaviorally organized in the immediate newborn period, but long-term detrimental effects on health or development have not been seen in populations of infants who have not experienced perinatal distress. The good news is that fathers may be even more involved with infant care after a cesarean section birth,[40] and this has long-term positive consequences.

Babies belong with their parents in all circumstances except critical illness in infant or mother, and even then contact should occur as soon and for as much time as possible. Advantages of this contact include better and easier breast feeding,[33] more positive attachment behaviors by the moms,[46] less distress in the infant,[47] and perhaps some protection from sudden infant death syndrome (SIDS), although this may be mediated through enhanced breast feeding.[48] Close physical contact enhances physiological stability and growth. Any separation should be considered a perturbation in the parent-child relationship and should not be considered casually.

Medication given to the mother during labor and delivery affects the infant's behavior, ranging from hypotonia after epidural, spinal anesthesia, and magnesium administration, to frank depression of respirations if inappropriate medication is given immediately before delivery.[49] Even a small amount of drugs may make a mother less alert for her early interactions with her infant, and the infant may be poorly responsive to her. Breast feeding may take a little more time to get started.[50] If drugs have been used, the clinician should note some of the behavioral changes related to the delivery events. This sets the stage for monitoring the expected changes and the **recovery process** with the family in the hours and days ahead as the infant becomes increasingly well organized.[50]

Minor Illnesses

Infants of diabetic mothers tend to be drowsy and hypotonic, have long latency for response during the neurodevelopmental examination, and may have only brief periods of alertness. Some of these behavioral abnormalities are also seen in infants with *hyperbilirubinemia,* particularly those undergoing phototherapy. No systematic studies of *polycythemic infant* behavior have been done, but many clinicians have observed that these infants tend to be lethargic, even without demonstration of frank hyperviscosity or with correction of their hematocrit levels. Infants born of mothers with pregnancy-induced hypertension (PIH) may be behaviorally disorganized, even if not undergrown. They need more patience in the first days of life, allowing for more behavioral recovery. Breast-feeding initiation is often slower in these situations, usually because of both maternal and infant factors. Weight loss in some of these infants may be at the higher range of normal, perhaps related to relative fluid retention around birth.

Circumcision

Circumcision is a stressful event that predictably alters the infant's behavior, both during and after the procedure.[51] This is especially true if the circumcision is done without anesthesia. Parents should anticipate that their son may be sleepy after the procedure and may need a little more prompting with feeding. These behavioral alterations appear to be self-limited. The dorsal penile nerve block provides a safe and effective local anesthesia during a circumcision,[52] decreasing, but not eliminating, the recovery period.

Procedures and Pain

Neonates feel *pain* with the same sensitivity as older humans.[53] Their response may be less localized and may even be delayed until the procedure is complete. "Behavioral meltdown" in terms of physiological instability is more likely to occur after, not during, a painful procedure. Physicians tend to ignore or undermedicate young infants.[54] Full and complete pain relief should be given the neonate, commensurate to what adults receive. They need additional monitoring and support after a painful event.

Special Features

Minor or major physical deformities may strongly influence a parent's response to the infant. Every effort should be made to correct these early, if possible. Disfiguring features may be a severe impediment to attachment, and prompt discussion and attention are necessary. Even without an abnormality, the baby's appearance plays a central role in his meaning and place in the family. Parents interact more with attractive babies[55] and attribute competence to an attractive infant.[56] The clinician should pay close attention to remarks about who the child resembles, whose eyes (temper, feet, ears, etc.) he has. These linkages may surface later in attributions of the child's behavior.

Early perceptions of an infant have long-term consequences, affecting parenting behavior.[57,58] Further, seemingly benign events in the perinatal period may haunt parents and truly alter their relationship with the child. They may harbor feelings of the infant's vulnerability long after seemingly small difficulties, from the clinician's perspective, have resolved (e.g., neonatal jaundice). This is an example of a "ghost from the nursery"[59] that can haunt families for years.[60] A perceived or threatened loss of the child or of an aspect of the child seems to be the pivotal event in the development of the "vulnerable child syndrome."[61,62] Although any family can acquire this psychological burden, those with many prior losses, unsupported parents, and higher socioeconomic status and education seem more prone to it. This results in a ". . . disturbance in the parent-child relationship related to the parents' difficulty in supporting age-appropriate . . . separation and individuation"[62] (see Chapter 14). The clinician should be careful to give direct information about level of concern, course of recovery, and any possible sequelae for the infant. The parents should be engaged as fully informed partners in watching the stabilization and recovery in their infant from even a minor alteration in expectations. These neonatal events should be reviewed with families in the second 6 months of life as a primary prevention activity.

THE NEWBORN EXAMINATION
What To Observe

The infant's examination should, with rare exception, occur at the mother's bedside with both parents present. This is an intervention as well as an assessment. You should narrate your observations as part of the ongoing interaction with the family. You are there to assess the infant's neurobehavioral health and individuality. Some of the things to note are the following:

■ Examination as a minor stressor for the infant—the infant's response to the procedure and the examiner can be used as an indicator of robustness, stability, and maturity. The exam should be ordered with a gradient from the least stressing (e.g., observation of color and breathing) to the most (e.g., the Moro reflex).

■ Where is the infant? In the nursery, in the bassinet, held by whom? Who's active in care?

■ The nurses' and parents' handling of the infant—this is determined by both the caretaker and the infant. Is this infant treated very tentatively or very vigorously? What do the nurses say about the infant?

■ Your own responses to the infant—as a consistent examiner, you are registering whether this is a frail infant, an attractive one, an alert one. Do you like the baby? Why or why not?

■ Nursing record—check for sleep and crying, heart rate and breathing regularity, response to procedures (e.g., bath, phenylketonuria), and difficulties with caretaking. Experienced nurses know which infants "have it together" and which ones need more support. These observations are critical for **discharge planning** with a family.

■ Parents' impression and handling of the infant—what do they say and do with the infant? What are their descriptions of the baby? Whom does the baby resemble?

■ Maternal (and paternal) fatigue, stress, and ill health—is the mom moving around the room and calling friends and relatives or does she look like she's pasted to the bed? Is she crying? Can she ask questions of you or is she entirely focused on her own issues? Is the dad there, involved, supportive?

What To Ask

Questions to be asked and the objectives of each question are presented in Table 5-5.

TABLE 5-5 ■ Questions To Be Asked During Newborn Examination	
Questions	**Objective**
How are you? How did the delivery go? Did things go as you had planned?	You care about parents as people; assess whether expectations were fulfilled.
How is he/she the same/different than you expected?	Assess perceptions of the child; note any discrepancies with your own.
Do you have any special worries or concerns about him/her?	Answer concerns.
Ask about any maternal medical concerns (e.g., maternal fever, ABO or Rh incompatibility).	Assert the locus of control with them.

What To Assess[2]

Begin assessment at the mother's bedside, lights dim. Narrate your findings to the parents. Keep the following in mind:

- Conduct a general examination, but reorder it from least intrusive to the most intrusive maneuvers. Observe the infant's color change, breathing, and awakening as you do your assessment, starting with uncovering and undressing.
- Interrupt what you're doing if the infant becomes alert. When the infant is alert, present an object, such as a ball, the stethoscope, or other toy at his focal distance, 8 to 10 inches. Move object slowly, horizontally, and vertically, to assess infant's tracking and whole performance in visual alertness processing. The baby should stop moving, and his or her face should brighten.
- Repeat the visual assessment using your face and then using face and voice together. (The combined stimulus is more compelling than the single one for term infants; stressed and immature infants may find the combined stimulus too complex and therefore aversive.) The baby will show you that you have exceeded your limit by turning away, looking away, gagging, or with color change. You and the parents will have learned the infant's limits and signal system.
- With the infant held securely above eye level, swaddled as needed, talk softly to him or her. Wait for the response. Having an alert look, turning the eyes toward you, and then turning the head toward you is the expected response, if given time and a positive auditory cue.
- Repeat this with one or both parents on the other side. Watch them fall in love when the infant turns to their voice rather than yours. Point out recognition of them.
- During this time, note the infant's irritability, changes of motor tone with state of consciousness, and the amount of tremulousness and startles. This assessment gives you an idea of the infant's maturity, neurological integrity, and physiological stability. This first assessment provides a basis of comparison for subsequent assessment, allowing you to

monitor the infant's recovery. Very physiologically fragile infants will be less available socially than those who are more organized at that level.

■ A full neurological examination with careful assessment of active and passive tone and the presence, character, and vigor of the reflexes should be done. This is a stressor; watch how the infant copes with it, signals distress, and recovers from the distressing maneuver, including how long recovery takes.

■ During periods of crying (e.g., after the test of the Moro reflex), carefully observe and assess the infant's self-quieting maneuvers and the amount of effort needed by the examiner to quiet the infant. This level of need will be replicated at home. Some infants need more help to settle down than others. These infants should be described as "feisty, strong-minded" or other positive terms. Less perturbable infants should be described as "calm." Mildly hypertonic infants with brisk responsiveness are often experienced as "strong." Mildly hypotonic infants may be described as "relaxed."

■ The infant walk and step are reflexes that are powerful in showing the parents how much a person the infant is. Don't skip these.

■ Put a gloved finger in the infant's mouth to assess oral-motor organization. An infant who is poorly coordinated, bites, or puts his tongue up will need extra help with feeding.[36]

■ Cuddle the infant in the crook of the arm and at the shoulder. The infant should mold in but also maintain bend control. If not, an alteration in tone should be investigated.

■ Clinicians should see themselves as a barometer of the infant's behavior. If one feels that an infant is behaviorally vulnerable, he or she probably is, and the parents will feel that too. If the child is particularly attractive, it may be because the infant is exceptionally well organized.

DISCHARGE DECISIONS

The timing of discharge for mother and infant is a decision that has to take into account maternal, infant, interactional, and family issues.[63] The mother must be *sufficiently recovered* to take independent care of herself and her infant. She must also have a safe place to go, with adequate food and shelter for herself and the infant, factors that may be inappropriately taken for granted. Real task support by someone with child care experience is ideal.

The infant must be psychologically stable, having negotiated the postnatal physiological and behavioral transitions. The baby must be able to signal needs, have those signals understood by care providers, and be able to feed well, which means that an experienced professional has seen the infant feed well at least twice and that the mom also feels comfortable with the feeding. Both mom and infant should demonstrate good nursing technique. The baby should awaken to feed, and elimination should be proceeding normally. The baby should be responsive to interactions with the environment as an index of neurological intactness. *Parents should be instructed in routine care* such as handling a spit up, taking the temperature, and getting the infant correctly into a car seat.

A follow-up plan should be solidly in place. A checkup within the first week of life should be routine, often coordinated with a home health visit. Problems, including breast-feeding difficulties, jaundice, and poor weight gain emerge and are more easily solved in the first week to 10 days of life. Criteria and provisions for emergency care should be explicitly laid out. Assurance of transportation should be part of that.

Mothers should not be discharged without the infant unless the child is in need of critical care that will be ongoing. Similarly, infants should stay with their moms if mom needs to stay, unless her situation is critical. Federal law now guarantees at least a 2-day stay for a vaginal delivery, 4 days for a cesarean section. However, good medical care demands that the individual needs of each family be kept in mind. These needs include behavioral readiness of the baby and the mother to thrive outside the hospital or birthing center. This is a joint decision between the clinician and the parent(s).

SPECIAL REFERRALS AND TREATMENTS

Good medical management is, of course, the first necessity. Behavioral assessment and care must be delivered in this context.

Children born of diabetic mothers or of mothers who received medication during labor and delivery, those born after long labors or labors complicated by PIH, those who are semi-preemies of 36 to 38 weeks, or those born by cesarean section are expected to have a more prolonged recovery, with mild hypotonia, lethargy, and drowsy states. The primary care physician should anticipate and not ignore these behaviors. They may herald or mask significant metabolic problems (e.g., hypoglycemia), the presence of sepsis, or just immaturity. These infants require increased vigilance for these medical problems. Secondary difficulties such as poor feeding, jaundice, and mild dehydration may ensue from the behavioral abnormalities. The parents' initial perceptions of their child are shaped by these early difficulties. The clinician can place these transient behaviors in perspective, as part of a normal recovery process. Extra efforts to alert the infant, especially around feeding, will require bedside demonstration and extra nursing help.

Swaddling, quiet rooms, and dim lights are helpful to all infants, but especially to those experiencing drug withdrawal or drug effect, prenatal alcohol exposure, and any other events that result in a hyperirritable, hyperresponsive state.

Even mild hyperbilirubinemia and phototherapy lead to significant alterations in infant behavior. These drowsy, floppy, or jittery infants appear to be poorly responsive to caretaking maneuvers, even into the second week of life, after discontinuance of the phototherapy. The behavioral changes in the child should be explained to the parents, and assurance of their transiency made.

Wake-sleep cycle regulation for the infant is facilitated by close interaction with a single caretaker. Rooming in is beneficial for babies and parents, almost without exception. A differential response to the infant, day and night, facilitates the infant's organization. Babies should be with their mothers unless either of them is seriously ill.

SUMMARY

The initial newborn examination is an opportunity to assure parents that the infant is physically and behaviorally intact. Congratulations are in order for producing a lovely baby. This reassurance and an added sense of competency as being reproductively sound are necessary to begin the work of caring for and caring about the infant. It's time to introduce the real, individual infant to the family by showing the baby's unique characteristics and abilities. Unmet expectations for the delivery, or the infant, or any intercurrent concerns are to be put in clear perspective so that they can be reconciled. Parents' choices in care options within the boundaries of the best care should be respected. The infant's temperament and individuality should begin to be understood in the context of the assessment, by the clinician and by the parents. Finally, plans for ongoing care should be set up based on an understanding of all the individuals involved.

REFERENCES

1. Brazelton TB: *Infants and mothers: individual differences in development,* New York, 1969, Delacorte.
2. Brazelton TB: *Neonatal behavioral assessment scale,* ed 2, London, 1984, Spastics International Medical Publications.
3. Brazelton TB: A window on the newborn's world: more than two decades of experience with the Neonatal Behavioral Assessment Scale (NBAS). In Meisels S, Fenichel E, editors: *New visions for the developmental assessment of infants and young children,* Washington, DC, 1996, Zero to Three.
4. Lewin R, editor: *Child alive,* Garden City, NY, 1977, Anchor Press.
5. Bower TGR: *The perceptual world of the child,* Cambridge, Mass, 1977, Harvard University Press.
6. Bronson G: The postnatal growth in visual capacity, *Child Dev* 45:887, 1974.
7. Miranda SB: Visual abilities and pattern preferences of premature and full term infants, *J Exp Child Psychol* 10:139, 1970.
8. Adams RJ, Maurer D, Davis M: Newborn discrimination of chromatic from achromatic stimuli, *J Exp Child Psychol* 41:267, 1986.
9. Melzoff AN, Moore MK: Imitation of facial and manual gestures by the human neonate, *Science* 198:75, 1977.
10. Borenstein MH, Sigman MD: Continuity in mental development in infancy, *Child Dev* 57:251, 1986.
11. Volpe JJ: *Neurology of the newborn,* ed 2, Philadelphia, 1995, WB Saunders.
12. Marean G, Werner L, Kuhl P: Vowel categorization by very young infants, *Dev Psychol* 28:396, 1992.
13. Lopez S: *The effect of the lullaby and game song on the behavior of the newborn,* doctoral dissertation, LaJolla, Calif, 1991, University of California-San Diego, Department of Music.
14. Condon WS, Sander LW: Synchrony demonstrated between movements of the neonate and adult speech, *Child Dev* 45:456, 1974.
15. Kuhl PK et al: Linguistic experience alters phonetics perception in infants by six months of age, *Science* 255:606, 1992.
16. Goldin-Meadow S: Language development under atypical learning conditions. In Nelson K, editor: *Children's language,* Hillsdale, NJ, 1985, Earlbaum.
17. American Academy of Pediatrics Joint Committee on Infant Hearing: Position statement, 1995, *Pediatrics* 95:152, 1994.
18. Mennella J, Beauchamp G: Maternal diet alters the sensory qualities of human milk and the nursling's behavior, *Pediatrics* 88(4):737, 1991.
19. Izard C: Innate and universal facial expression: evidence from developmental and cross-cultural research, *Psychol Bull* 115:288, 1994.
20. Mennella J, Beauchamp G: Early flavor experiences: when do they start? *Zero to Three* 14(2):1, 1993.
21. Self PA, Horowitz FD, Paden LY: Olfaction in newborn infants, *Dev Psychol* 7:349, 1972.
22. Porter RH et al: Breastfed infants respond to olfactory cues from their own mother and unfamiliar lactating females, *Inf Behav Dev* 15:85, 1992.

23. Sullivan RM et al: Olfactory classical conditioning in neonates, *Pediatrics* 87:511, 1991

24. MacFarlane A: Olfaction. In *The development of social preference in the human neonate,* Ciba Foundation Symposium No. 33, 1975.

25. Edelman AI, Kartz M: Olfactory recognition: a genetic or learned capacity, *J Dev Behav Pediatr* 13(2):126, 1992.

26. Varendi H, Porter RH, Winberg J: Does the newborn baby find the nipple by smell? *Lancet* 344:989, 1994.

27. Righard L, Alda MO: Effect of delivery room routine on success of first breastfeed, *Lancet* 336:1105, 1990.

28. Leon M: Touch and smell. In Field TM, editor: *Touch in early development,* Mahwak, NJ, 1995, Lawrence Erlbaum.

29. Brazelton TB, Nugent JK: *Neonatal behavioral assessment scale,* London, 1995, Mac Keith Press.

30. Prechtl H, Beentema D: *The neurological examination of the full term newborn infant,* Philadelphia, 1975, JB Lippincott.

31. American Academy of Pediatrics: Breastfeeding guidelines, *Pediatrics* 100:1035, 1997.

32. McKenna J, Moska S: Sleep and arousal, synchrony and independence among mothers and infants sleeping apart and together: an experiment in evolutionary medicine, *Acta Paediatr Scand* 397:94, 1994.

33. Yamauchi Y, Yamanouchi I: The relationship between rooming-in/not rooming-in and breastfeeding variables, *Acta Paediatr Scand* 79:1017, 1990

34. Piaget J, Inhelder B. *The psychology of the child,* New York, 1969, Basic Books.

35. Weber F, Woolridge M, Baum J: An ultrasonographic study of the organization of sucking and swallowing by newborn infants, *Dev Med Child Neurol* 28:19, 1986.

36. Lawrence R: *Breastfeeding: a guide for the medical professional,* St Louis, 1989, Mosby.

37. Shelley WG et al: Coordination of sucking, swallowing, and breathing in the newborn: its relationship to infant feeding and normal development, *Br J Disord Commun* 25:311, 1990.

38. Lucas A et al: A randomized, multicenter study of human milk versus formula and later development in preterm infants, *Arch Dis Child* 70:141, 1994.

39. Feldman W, Feldman M: The intelligence of breastfeeding, *Lancet* 347:1037, 1996.

40. Parke R: *Fathers,* Cambridge, Mass, 1981, Harvard University Press.

41. O'Driscoll K, Meagher D, Boylan P, editors: *Active management of labor,* St Louis, 1993, Mosby.

42. Klaus M, Kennell J: *Maternal-infant bonding,* St Louis, 1976, Mosby.

43. Klaus M, Kennell J, Klaus P: *Mothering the mother: how a doula can help you have a shorter, easier and healthier birth,* Reading, Mass, 1993, Addison Wesley.

44. Eyer DE: *Mother-infant bonding: a scientific fiction,* New Haven, 1992, Yale University Press.

45. Kennell J: The time has come to reassess delivery room routines, *Birth* 21(1):49, 1994.

46. Prodromidis M et al: Mothers touching newborns: a comparison of rooming-in versus minimal contact, *Birth* 22(4):196, 1995.

47. Christensson K et al: Separation distress call in the human neonate in the absence of maternal body contact, *Acta Paediatr* 84:468, 1995.

48. McKenna JJ: The potential benefits of infant-parent co-sleeping in relation to SIDS prevention: overview and critique of epidemiological bedsharing studies. In Rognum TO, editor: *Sudden infant death syndrome: new trends in the '90s,* Scandinavian University Press, 1995.

49. Walker M: Do labor medications affect breastfeeding? (Literature review), *J Hum Lact* 13(2):131, 1997.

50. Nissan E et al: Effects of maternal pethidine on infants' developing breastfeeding behavior, *Acta Paediatr Scand* 84:140, 1995.

51. Dixon S et al: Behavioral effects of circumcision with and without anesthesia, *J Dev Behav Pediatr* 5:246, 1984.

52. Kirya C, Werthmann MW: Neonatal circumcision and penile dorsal nerve block: a painless procedure, *J Pediatr* 96:998, 1978.

53. Anand KJS, Hickey PR: Pain and its effects in the human neonate and fetus, *NEJM* 317(21):1321 and 1347, 1987 (commentary by A. Fletcher).

54. Porter F et al: Pain and pain management in newborn infants: a survey of physicians and nurses, *Pediatrics* 100(4):626, 1997.

55. Langlois JH et al: Infant attractiveness predicts maternal behaviors and attitudes, *Dev Psychol* 31:464, 1995.

56. Stephan CW, Langlois JH: Baby beautiful: adult attributions of infant competence as a function of infant attractiveness, *Child Dev* 55:576, 1984.

57. Broussard E, Sergay M, Hartner S: Further considerations regarding maternal perception of the firstborn. In Hellmuth J, editor: *Exceptional infant*, New York, 1971, Brunner-Mazel.

58. Korner A: The effect of the infant's state, level of arousal, sex and ontogenic stage on the care giver. In Lewis M, Rosenblum L, editors: *The effect of the infant on the care giver*, New York, 1974, John Wiley & Sons.

59. Fraiberg S: *The magic years*, New York, 1959, Scribner.

60. Forsyth B, Canny P: Perceptions of vulnerability 3½ years after problems of feeding and crying in early infancy, *Pediatrics* 88:757, 1991.

61. Green M, Solnit AJ: Reactions to the threatened loss of a child: a vulnerable child syndrome, *Pediatrics* 34:58, 1964.

62. Thomasgard M, Meltz WP: The vulnerable child revisited, *J Dev Behav Pediatr* 16:47, 1995.

63. American Academy of Pediatrics, American College of Gynecologists: *Guidelines for perinatal care*, ed 4, Elk Grove Village, Ill, 1997, American Academy of Pediatrics.

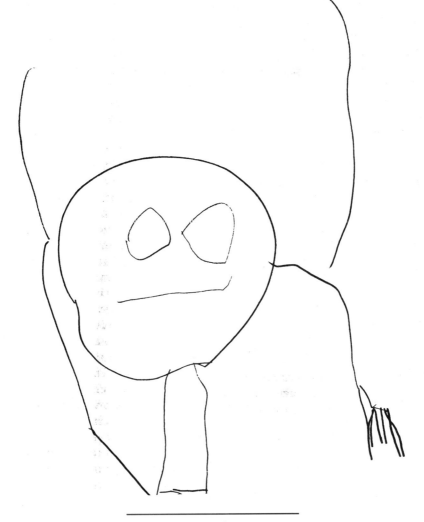

"A baby." By Heather R., age 3½.

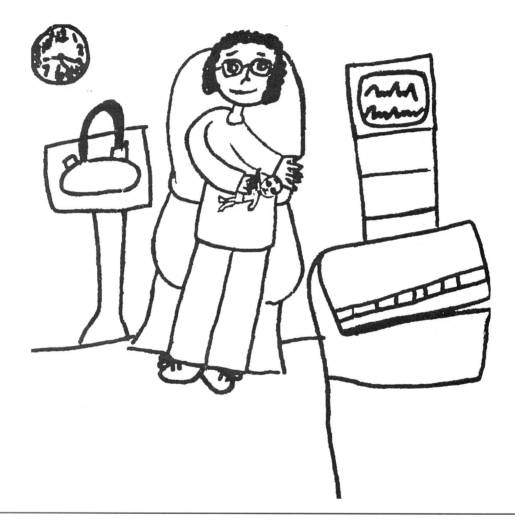

A nurse takes care of a small premie amid the machines, strange sink, and other equipment in the neonatal intensive care unit. By Carly Riehl, age 10.

CHAPTER 6

NEONATAL INTENSIVE CARE UNIT: SPECIAL ISSUES FOR THE AT-RISK INFANT AND FAMILY

■ Suzanne D. Dixon
■ Yvonne Vaucher

KEY WORDS

Preterm Infant's Behavior
Developmental Course
Discharge Planning
Special Care Parenting
Grief Reaction
Neonatal Intensive Care Unit Environment
Multiple Births
Strategy for Treatment and Follow-up

Jason Merrill, born 5 weeks ago at 31 weeks' gestation, has an adjusted age of 36 weeks and is now ready for discharge home from the neonatal intensive care unit (NICU). His parents, Carolyn and Bill, have been very involved with his care since he was born. They seem to be a competent, professional couple who have waited a long time for this infant, have visited daily, and have asked many good questions throughout the hospitalization about his condition. Although they did meet the respiratory therapist as scheduled to learn about the home monitor and to review cardiopulmonary resuscitation (CPR), a discharge conference has had to be rescheduled twice, and their visiting has decreased in the last week. The nurses report they have no more expressed stored breast milk to give Jason. When the parents came in last night, they became very angry about the dust on the bassinet and the milk around Jason's mouth. The neonatologist asks you for help handling this "difficult family" and to see what you can do about the breast milk and the discharge conference.

NEONATAL INTENSIVE CARE

The advent in the 1940s of intensive care for the ill or high-risk infant began an era of dramatic change for the neonate, the family, and the health care provider. With increasing technological sophistication, we have pushed back the limits of viability, improved the chances of survival, and increased the incidence of multiple births.[1] Families are exposed to the NICU

109

environment for longer and longer periods of time during the increasingly complex care of babies who are smaller and smaller. In the course of this progress, we have also learned a great deal about the neurological development of the immature child, the behavior and developmental course of the preterm infant, and the impact of intensive care itself on the infant and family.[2-7] Through these insights, we now have the opportunity to provide care that is not only more effective but also less stressful for infant and family. We have become more aware and respectful of the special needs of these fragile individuals. We have refocused on the family as the ultimate intervention in the support of the high-risk infant so that nurture of the family's competencies has become part of the care mission. Medical issues contribute to the long-term prognosis, particularly of very-low-birth-weight infants, but the ability of a parent to be responsive to the high-risk infant remains the best predictor of outcome over the longer term. We now have insights and supports parents can use to learn about and care for their high-risk infant. The role of the health care provider has expanded to include not only the technical aspects of care but also assistance to the family through the crisis of an early or complicated birth. This assistance is directed at helping parents to gain skill in the special care needs of their child and to access the community resources that they will need after discharge and over the longer term. These tasks involve understanding the behavior of the high-risk infant, the parent perspectives, the NICU environment, and the special follow-up care that is required for special populations.

PREMATURE INFANT DEVELOPMENT

The **preterm infant's behavior** and **developmental course** will not be the same as that of the infant born at term, no matter how smooth the postnatal course is. Although behavioral expectations should be adjusted for the degree of prematurity (i.e., the adjusted age) as the best approximation, differences can be anticipated. Some of these are the following:

- *Motor tone and posture will be altered.* Many will have a pattern of passive hypotonia (i.e., floppiness or offering little resistance to passive movement). This may be accompanied by active hypertonia and brisk reflexes, especially of the lower extremities. Predominance of extension postures is present in many infants throughout the first year. Although most of these infants will resolve these differences by the second year, some will maintain an imbalance in tone that will be seen as subtle movement or postural differences.[8]

- Much development that depends on posture and tone may take a different, often delayed, path if external support is not provided to these children. *Shoulder girdle weakness* and *shoulder retraction* (i.e., shoulders rolled back) may mean that the infant has difficulty with self-quieting behaviors, such as hand to mouth, and will need special help to settle in a tucked, flexed position. Without support to bring the hands forward, the natural hand regard and midline play opportunities will be diminished. This may appear as delay in cognitive abilities or visual-motor irregularities unless intervention is provided to bring the hands forward to midline. This can be accomplished by attention to positioning and provision of trunk support.

- *Truncal hypotonia* results in the infant's actively resisting prone activities that are vital to learning. These babies need physical support (e.g., rolled towel under the chest) and inducements (e.g., a toy or face in front) to enable them to tolerate prone positions or to assist them with sitting.

■ *Alterations in wakefulness and sleep* may continue even beyond the first year. An undifferentiated drowsy state at about 28 weeks gradually evolves into wake and sleep at about 32 weeks, becoming clearer over time, with emergence of active and quiet sleep at about 36 weeks.[9] Increasing periods of alertness can be seen by 36 weeks. Full-cry states become available to the infant after 35 to 36 weeks. However, even at term, the prematurely born infant is likely to continue to have irregular sleep, variability in quality of alertness, and more time in a drowsy or irritable state. These difficulties are lessened if the special care environment has quiet and dark times, if the infant is not disturbed for blocks of time, and if intrusive levels of light and sound are avoided. Parents often perceive the lack of wakeful interaction as rejection and sleep difficulties as evidence of subtle damage or poor parenting. These misconceptions need to be directly countered with realistic explanations of the evolution of social availability in this group.

■ *Subtle visual difficulties* are more common in this group, including astigmatism, refractive errors, and strabismus.[10] Loss of peripheral vision occurs following photocoagulation for retinopathy of prematurity. Careful visual follow-up and periodic reassessment should continue throughout early childhood even without obvious abnormalities or visual complaints. Additionally, significant visual impairment precludes valid use of the usual developmental tests.

■ *Alterations in motor tone,* as well as anatomical changes resultant from the placement of endotracheal tubes, place this group of youngsters at risk for difficulties with feeding and swallowing early on and for articulation problems later because of structural and functional changes in the mouth and palate. Orthodontic care may also be needed.

■ *Recurrent otitis media* may also result from these differences in structure and function in the mouth, pharynx, and airway.

■ *Sensitivity to pain, touch of the feet, and scars from procedures* may be a source of discomfort and later unusual, aversive responses. Some infants, for example, dislike their feet touched, perhaps an association with repeated heel sticks.

■ *Limited energy and oxygen reserves* result in slowed growth, particularly in children with bronchopulmonary dysplasia and congenital heart disease, and may result in additional delays in motor activities because of decreased muscle mass and strength.

■ The emphasis on feeding and growth that is appropriate in the first year or two in this group may result in *long-term feeding issues* with origins in the baby, the parents, and the interaction between them. Feeding struggles are difficult to resolve. Oral aversions and oral-motor dysfunction appear to be linked to prolonged intubation and delays in initiating oral feeding.

■ The preterm infant needs *additional calories, minerals, and protein* throughout the first year to grow.[11,12] Nutritional requirements are even greater if the child is chronically ill. This may run counter to a family's adherence to a low-fat, low-salt regimen.

■ The infant's *self-protective behavior* of avoiding or ignoring intrusive stimuli may mean that the infant sends signals to care providers that are seen as confusing or counterintuitive. For example, gaze avoidance sends the message, "Leave me alone, I'm better off without you." Confusing behavioral signals, interactional availability only in short segments, and unpredictability of behavior may remain even after the baby is "well."

All the differences of these preterm and high-risk youngsters, as well as other ones that track with individual conditions, mean that the jobs for the parents and the health care provider are inherently altered. The roles change for all parties in these cases.

The primary care clinician has dual therapeutic opportunities in interactions with a child and family under these circumstances. As important as monitoring the infant's changing capacities as he or she recovers and grows is the chance to observe and support the parents' growth into the role of caretakers of a vulnerable, special needs infant.

ROLES IN THE CARE OF THE SPECIAL NEEDS BABY

The single most important variable in long-term developmental outcome for these vulnerable children may be the responsiveness of the parents to the child during the first year of life.[13] With the exception of severe insult directly to the central nervous system (e.g., severe intracranial hemorrhage or meningitis), chronic hypoxia, or extremely low birth weight, the developmental outcome depends less on medical events and perinatal circumstances than it does on the family's ability to meet the needs of the individual child, as summarized by Sameroff.[14] Maternal education and socioeconomic status (SES), both highly predictive of the type and amount of support and input the mother gives the child and sometimes reflective of some genetic factors, are the best predictors of outcome after 2 years of age in the majority of cases. Enhancement of the interaction between parent and child through education and support is the avenue that will positively influence development.

This is not surprising, given what we know overall about children. If a parent can learn to provide contingent and consistent interactions and appropriate responsiveness for a high-risk infant, the chances for learning and long-term developmental adjustment are augmented. If a parent continues to be unable to read the child's signals and fails to meet the child's needs on either a physical or behavioral level, the child experiences the world as non-contingent and chaotic[15]; emotional and cognitive growth are undermined in this circumstance. The parents' effectiveness in dealing with their own child leads to stronger attachment and improved parental self-esteem.

ROLE OF FAMILY

In most circumstances, the primary care clinician can do little about the particular perinatal insults that the child sustains except to ensure optimal perinatal medical care and referral as needed. However, the primary care physician may be in a better position than a neonatologist or other medical specialist to view the broad picture of this infant and family. Often less involved with the technology of neonatal care, the primary care clinician can offer a broader perspective and can see beyond the walls of the special care nursery, beyond all the machines, technology, and bright lights to the strengths and vulnerabilities in the child and the family. He or she can offer perspective and common sense in **discharge planning.**

> *Ms. James, a single mother, had an angry, distrustful look as she approached her son's open warmer for the first time. Then she said, "he's too small" and asked, "who's in charge?" The nurse came forward and extended an invitation to touch the baby. She shook her head "no." When asked, she said she had no questions.*
>
> *Instead of becoming irritated or getting pulled into a struggle, the clinician should recognize the passion and strength behind these actions and comments. The job will be to create a relationship so that energy can be directed to the care of the baby, not to irritating the staff.*

Special care parenting demands that the parents see the infant as he or she really exists, with both strengths and weaknesses. This implies a clear and shared view of the child's physiological and behavioral capacities at a particular point in time. From this view, the primary care provider can guide the family in supporting the development of the individual child and in accessing the special follow-up services that will be needed. This approach implies the clinician's responsibility for restoring a sense of competency and confidence in parenting in a family in which these factors have been assaulted by the less-than-optimal circumstances of the child's birth.

Most neonatal units actively try to include families in care. Depending on geography and training, the primary health care provider may be more or less involved in the management of the acute neonatal illness but will always be involved in the important work of helping a family rebuild around the needs of a particular child after discharge. That work involves attention to details, such as the following:

- Families must have the knowledge and skills to provide physical care of the infant. If this is beyond their capabilities, specialized care must be mobilized. The goal of this care should be to assist families in assuming more responsibility over time.
- Judgment about the infant's needs should come from the nursing staff in the NICU with information from the primary health care provider. A home health nurse can provide insights about the home environment.
- Families must be able to focus on the needs of the child. Although this is a core requirement for all parenting, it is even more critical for a fragile baby who signals needs poorly. Serious mental illness, ongoing substance abuse, extreme poverty, domestic violence, or mental deficiency are some of the barriers that must be faced in making realistic discharge plans. Young teen parents require special appraisal of their caretaking capacities.
- Families must have access to care that is acceptable to them and adequate to the needs of the infant. This means in-home telephone, reliable transportation, health insurance, and culturally sensitive and linguistically compatible ongoing care. A discharge without these in place is likely to lead to less than optimal, if not dangerous, circumstances. Don't send the baby and mother home without them.

PREMATURE PARENTS

The parents of a preterm infant are "premature" too, having a baby that they did not fully expect with demands for care that usually go beyond their own abilities to provide. They themselves have not completed the developmental work of pregnancy (see Chapter 4), and, in addition, they must put energy into the resolution of the complex feelings of guilt, anger, anxiety, depression, and shame that emerge as a consequence of their infant's birth. The predictable course of response to the loss of a loved one (even an imagined person in this case) has been described in classic works.[16,17] The initial responses of *denial and anger* give way to depression and guilt and, finally, resolution. These same stages of **grief reaction** are apparent in the parental response to an infant born prematurely or with neonatal illness. Parents truly have lost a valued person in the form of the hoped-for or imagined child. They must resolve that grief in order to attach themselves to the *real* child who is now before them. They must begin accepting this less than perfect child while simultaneously letting go of the idealized child. They may require extra time to even see the infant as a separate person if the baby has been born very early. And they cannot be expected to attach to the infant until they sense a good chance for survival.

 Mrs. Martin was wheeled in to see her daughter, born at 26 weeks' gestation, for the first time. She had barely looked pregnant. She sat immobilized and refused to touch the baby. She said she was tired and asked the busy nurse to get her a glass of water.

This mom is still in the stage of pregnancy experienced as a change in self, an egotistical phase that is normal (see Chapter 4). Unfortunately, the baby's extremely premature birth interrupted these normal processes of pregnancy. Mrs. Martin probably can't even believe that this has happened. She hasn't even considered the process of delivery at this time. She will need time and lots of support to see the baby as a separate individual and to focus on the baby, not herself.

Even if survival is assured, parents may also need to cope with the long-term loss of a normal child when chronic disease or neurological disability results from the preterm delivery. Parents may also face the actual death of their child; this is more likely in the case of multiple gestation, in which extreme prematurity is associated with an increased antepartum and intrapartum, as well as neonatal loss.[18-21]

THE CLINICIAN AND THE PARENTS

Clinicians should monitor the process of grief resolution and attachment and not be surprised at the turbulence and seemingly inappropriate responses or anger that may be leveled at them or others. These are healthy, expected reactions that testify to the ongoing recovery process. Over the long run these feelings will mobilize emotional energy that will enable the family to reorganize around the real child and his special needs. Short-term counseling may be necessary to achieve resolution of this process in some cases. Many anxious calls, trivial questions, requests for laboratory values, and reluctance to be discharged from the hospital or leave the office are manifestations of this turmoil. Withdrawal from the situation as discharge nears speaks to anxiety that seems overwhelming (see opening case). One should avoid answering these demands or concerns at a superficial level only; they must be seen as opportunities to support a parent's recovery of competence and self-esteem and as part of the larger, core process of becoming a family. The defense mechanism of *intellectualization* of medical aspects of care is another frequent response in middle class and professional families. Avoid being drawn into prolonged technical discussions, intellectual nit-picking, or arguments. Chasing specific concerns can lead to frustration until one pulls back to identify the underlying and unvoiced worries.

Fathers are more often active in the care of their premature infants than are fathers of full-term infants. Pressed into extraordinary service early and frequently in the hospital, they remain more involved with care later.[22] In addition, in families in which the father is supportive and involved, the mother visits more often and participates more regularly in the infant's care.[23] The smart primary care clinician will cultivate a real involvement of fathers of high-risk infants as an effective way to infuse energy into the whole family system. Grandparents and other family or community supports also can add balance and energy. The clinician should look broadly for sources of help that can be mobilized. Rarely can a nuclear family manage entirely on its own.

IMPACT OF NEONATAL INTENSIVE CARE UNIT ENVIRONMENT

The caretaking requirements of the small baby create an environment so different from the intrauterine one that it in itself provides a source of additional morbidity. Data suggest associations between that environment and acute physiological fluctuations.[24-27] These, in turn, appear to alter important clinical and central nervous system parameters, including intracranial pressure changes, cerebral autoregulation, brain oxygenation, hypoxemia, apnea, and bradycardia.[28,29] In the past, investigators have examined the sensory characteristics of NICUs along with infant behavioral and physiological responses to the caretaking activities in this environment.[25,30-33] The **NICU environment** may provide both sensory overload and deprivation.[33,34] These studies found that infants experience a bombardment of stimuli from sheer numbers of different caregivers and procedures each day. At the same time, however, very little social contact and long intervals of social isolation may also be present. From the infant's view, this may be experienced as a chaotic, nonresponsive milieu. The auditory environment may be aversive; shutting an isolette door is as loud as a rock band up close. Constant mechanical noise from equipment adds to the auditory stress. Soft talk to the infant may be minimal. Constant bright lights, noise, lack of diurnal variation in light and sound, and abrupt changes in position with handling are important, stressful factors present in the NICU that were not part of intrauterine life.

DEVELOPMENTALLY SUPPORTIVE CARE

Caretaking can be altered to counter some of these aversive factors.[35-38] Procedures and examinations can be scheduled so that quiet sleep times are uninterrupted, improving behavioral organization and growth. Diurnal variation in lighting and noise reduction serve to minimize physiological stress for the immature infant. Gentle, gradual movements and soothing and holding after procedures also improve organization. Some activities that support this process are shown in Box 6-1.

BOX 6-1	COMPONENTS OF INDIVIDUALIZED CARE PLAN FOR FRAGILE BABY

Baby-specific care plans posted on each bedside. These include schedule issues, behavioral cues, likes and dislikes, stressors and facilitators.

The baby's specific nonverbal vocabulary—how does he or she signal positive or negative responses?

Isolette covers to allow quiet, undisturbed rest

Protected times for rest—posted and enforced

Swaddling or positioning in a supported, flexed, or prone posture.

Nesting within an isolette, using cloth rolls, slings to provide tactile input or containment

Tapes of soft music or parental voices played *periodically* in the isolette

Personalized isolette with pictures, small toys

Family visiting plans stated and posted. Nurses may want to "save" feeding, bathing and treatments for these times if possible.

The name of the two or three nurses who serve as primary nurses and know the family and the baby best

The baby's name clearly posted and used in the record and in conversations

The baby's own clothes and blanket if the infant is stable

This responsive care provision requires that the bedside nurse interpret the baby's behavioral and physiological cues and fit care around them. It also means that the nurse has the power to orchestrate the baby's day for optimal well-being. The physician should respect and support this new role for the primary nurse as an interface and buffer for the infant. Not only is it good for the baby, but it is a model for parents to emulate. They too have to learn to respect these behavioral cues as they become increasingly active in the infant's care. They too must see that the necessities of life get done, but in a way that is responsive to the fluctuating needs of the individual child. Whether developmentally supportive care actually improves long-term outcome remains unproven at this time.[39,40]

BABY BODY LANGUAGE

The infant uses body language to signal both positive and negative responses to various life experiences. Even a short period of observation during the nursery rounds, treatment sessions, or examinations will demonstrate many of these, which are listed in Boxes 6-2 and 6-3.

The behavior of the premature infant can be confusing to even an experienced caregiver.[41] Facial expressions have a limited range, body movements may be few, and cries nonexistent or irritating.[42] The latency of responses may be so long that it is difficult to connect one activity with the response. Social interactions that are so exciting with a full-term infant may cause the premature infant to turn away, become mottled, to hiccup, or even to stop breathing.[43] The baby may actively avoid eye contact, sending a very negative message to those who would like to interact. At other times an unremitting irritability seems to resist all the usual consoling and comforting measures. All these behaviors run counter to what is

BOX 6-2	BEHAVIORS THAT SAY "YES"

The following behaviors signal that the baby can handle, enjoy, and gain from the current interaction with the environment:

   A relaxed posture, neither hypertonic nor limp
   Easily flexed hands and feet
   Grasping movements with the hands and feet opening and closing rhythmically
   Mouthing and sucking movements when looking or listening
   Eyes widening, face lifting, lips making an oval
   Short, quiet vowel sounds—cooing
   Attending to visual or auditory stimuli—looking or listening carefully
   Decreasing bodily movements, wiggles, to quietly attend
   Turning toward the phenomenon, even with long latency
   Improved color—no mottling, duskiness, or pallor over baseline
The caretaker should continue, monitoring for signs or distress or overload.

BOX 6-3	BEHAVIORS THAT SAY "STOP, PLEASE"

The following behaviors often signal that the interaction with the environment is overwhelming, adversive, or overly costly for the infant's coping abilities:

   Extension postures—arms out, legs straightened, neck stretched
   Arching back
   Gaze avoidance
   Turning away
   Splayed hands and feet
   Grimace, lip retraction
   Furrowed brow, a worried look
   Spitting up, gagging, onset of hiccups
   Sudden limpness
   Increasing pallor, mottling, cyanosis
   Irregular breathing, apnea
   The caretaker should respond by backing off, by cutting down some aspects or intensity of the interaction, and by supporting and waiting for recovery.

usually expected of infants. Without some special knowledge and some techniques to make sense of the premature infant's behavior, caregivers may feel ineffective, frustrated, angry, and perplexed. Conversely, if the health care team can interpret some of the confusing messages and help a family to develop effective caregiving patterns, parenting competency and confidence will be enhanced.

What is experienced as aversive stimuli will vary from infant to infant and will change as the infant matures. Aversive stimuli tend to be those that are overwhelming or involve high levels of input, such as bright lights, noise, rapid movements, two or more simultaneous inputs (e.g., movement of the infant and speech directed at him or her). In addition, aversive responses emerge with rapid changes in input, even if the level of input is low. *Transitions* between one activity (e.g., feeding) and another (e.g., vital sign checks) may produce considerable disruptions. Even the transitions to sleep or to wakefulness may be prolonged and accompanied by much physiological instability.[40] Times of change in activity are vulnerable times; aversive behaviors are likely to emerge at these times. Support for the infant *through* the activity is needed if instability in behavior is to be avoided.

Ruth finished her shift in the care of Jonathan, now 31 weeks, with a session of chest physiotherapy. He seemed to do well, got his diaper and shirt changed, and was tucked in. As she was charting, the cardiac monitor went off with a significant apnea and bradycardia (A & B) event. The next time, she held Jonathan quietly for 10 minutes after his care session while she did her charting, and no instability was present.

KANGAROO CARE AND THE IMPACT OF TOUCH

The positive role of human touch on the preterm infant is illustrated by the demonstrated benefits of skin-to-skin care of the immature infant.[44,45] The infant is placed prone-upright on the bare chest of the mom or dad and covered on the dorsal surface by a blanket for some or all of the time intensive care services are received. This kind of care has no minimum weight requirement or specific time limit. It can be used for infants on ventilators. They don't get cold. This approach can have a very positive impact on care and outcome. Benefits that have been linked to kangaroo care are shown in Box 6-4.

Parents who can participate in this intimate care of their infant get a real sense of their own value and importance to the child. Only moms can specifically thermoregulate

BOX 6-4	BENEFITS OF KANGAROO CARE

Decreased apnea
Decreased bradycardia
Less irritability
Improved oxygenation
Improved weight gain
Improved temperature stability
Improved breast feeding

for their infants, adjusting skin temperature to the baby's needs, but skin-to-skin contact with dad can also produce significant benefit, including temperature stability. A speeded recovery for the child, as well as firsthand knowledge of the care of their own infant, follows from this care.

PARENTS IN NEONATAL INTENSIVE CARE UNIT

The special care nursery may add to parents' stresses by overtly, or inadvertently, giving the message to parents that they cannot take care of the baby or that something they did caused the baby's difficulties. "Experts," such as nurses, therapists, and physicians, must take over because the parents "have failed." The mother feels this sense of failure especially acutely, believing her own body has failed to protect the fetus from adversity. Parents are left with little confidence and little energy to assert themselves, to learn new skills, to make decisions, or to get to know their infant. Even in the best of circumstances the special care nursery environment itself exacerbates these feelings. This does not imply that nurses or physicians are insensitive to parents' needs; rather, it shows that the high technology and overwhelming care requirements for sick and premature infants give these unspoken messages to families. It takes a lot of work to move away from these feelings. In addition, nurses must attach to their infant charges if they are to give the best of care, and this may lead to unconscious competitiveness with parents. As a result, parents, especially mothers, may feel both emotionally and physically inadequate even if nothing specific is said or done to prompt such feelings. Thus, both technology and the necessary substitute caretakers compete with and undermine the parents' abilities to become part of their infant's life.

The lack of opportunity to be alone with their child or to engage in any sort of care-taking without the surveillance of the nursing staff adds stress for parents. Only 2% of human contact in the NICU experienced by the infant was from the parents, according to one careful study,[34] although this obviously depends upon the availability of the parents and the willingness of the staff to encourage physical contact between the baby and family. Most families may experience direct and indirect financial and time pressures associated with the care of their infants. Spending days to weeks to perhaps months in the special care nursery requires extraordinary adaptive skills at a time when parents are least able to muster these resources. Sparse visiting, lack of telephone calls, lack of initiative, or angry accusations are more often adaptive responses to these circumstances and competing demands at home rather than a measure of disattachment to the child or lack of appreciation of the expert care. The clinician and the NICU staff can help to interpret these behaviors correctly to one another and display considerable patience with families, granting the family latitude and time in which to recover.

MULTIPLE BIRTHS

The number of **multiple births** is increasing, related to fertility treatment, which in turn is more commonly related to delayed child bearing. More than one fourth of NICU admissions now are multiple births, and these are usually premature infants. Multiple gestation increases the chance of a high-risk delivery, low-birth-weight babies, a prolonged stay in the NICU, the likelihood of the family facing at least one serious neonatal complication, and the likelihood of neonatal death.[46]

Even in the case of term or near term twins, the situation has higher risk and places higher demands upon the parents. The process of attachment to two babies at the same time is more complicated than to one. For some period of time, ranging from hours to weeks, families respond to these youngsters as one unit. The process of individuation in response and care comes on gradually in healthy circumstances and waxes and wanes. Increasing levels of recognition of individual differences, beginning with appearance and moving to behavioral characteristics, is the added dimension that should be monitored by the health care provider caring for multiples. The health care provider's sharing observations of differences between the babies may help this process along.

Attachment difficulties get more complex if there is a discrepancy in size and vigor between the babies. Data would suggest a general tendency to spend more time with the more fragile, usually lower weight baby. This child is likely to be both more irritable and more demanding. The health care provider can assist the family in the difficult task of balancing efforts, being sure that the one who "needs the least" doesn't get left out and that both infants' bids for attention are well tended.

Multiple gestations increase the chance of a neonatal death, either prenatally (e.g., twin-to-twin transfusion, intrauterine growth retardation [IUGR]), in the course of early care, or postnatally because of complications of illness or sudden infant death syndrome (SIDS).[18] The bereavement causes parents to pull back from the process of attachment to the surviving child(ren). Fear of loss of the surviving child is a natural impediment to attachment because we don't attach to that which we think we will lose. Parents are appropriately guarded in their full psychological commitment to the survivor(s). Supportive care, including acknowledgment of the loss (no, the survivor doesn't "make up for" the loss of the other), patience, and a longer time frame are needed here. A mental health referral may be necessary to assist in this complex psychological adjustment.

BEHAVIORAL CHANGE WITH MINOR ILLNESS

Children who experience relatively minor complications of the perinatal period, such as minor IUGR,[47] hyperbilirubinemia,[48] or maternal diabetes,[49] sustain alterations of behavior that may affect their ability to interact maximally with their families in subtle ways. The child perpetuates the parents' perception that things are not quite right, that extraordinary care is required that may be beyond their limits of providing,[50] or that the infant is unresponsive to their caregiving.[51] Epidural anesthesia may alter tone to the extent that oral-motor skills are compromised and breast feeding gets off to a slow start. Evaluations for sepsis, leading perhaps to an NICU observation, blood work, perhaps an IV, or maybe a delay in discharge, all seem minor to the clinician, but may have lasting effects on the parental perception of their infant's well-being. Maternal analgesia may also alter responsiveness so that feeding and social interaction are altered transiently.

> *Mrs. Scottfield and her baby are scheduled for discharge. She continues to have difficulty with feeding her 3-day-old term daughter. It had been a long labor, with some terminal fever and a sepsis evaluation for the baby, who now had a heparin lock in her left hand for medication. A large cephalhematoma distorted the baby's head, and she was very sleepy. The nurse noticed a poorly coordinated suck when she placed a gloved finger in the baby's mouth. The baby fell asleep at the breast after about 5 minutes. She awoke, irritable, about an hour later. Mrs. Scottfield was in tears.*

Even in these minor circumstances, the clinician should anticipate some extra hurdles for parents to overcome in spite of the clinician's own perception that things are just fine. Although this situation is not at the level of those in the NICU, clear recognition of the fragility in the circumstances overall will prompt extra care and vigilance now and in the months ahead.

VULNERABLE CHILD SYNDROME

The family's perception of the child is not always directly related to the severity of the perinatal illness. Even conditions that the clinician may regard as relatively minor, insignificant, or transient may set the groundwork for a permanently altered perception of the child by the family. Green and Solnit in their now classic description[52] have highlighted the important dimensions of the "vulnerable child syndrome." In this circumstance a child with an imagined or real illness in early life is the target of an altered attachment by her parents. The parents develop a long-term sense of the child as particularly susceptible to illness, injury, or loss. The child is viewed as fragile and incapable of age-appropriate behavioral expectations, particularly in areas of independence. This perception of vulnerability leads to ongoing intrafamilial stress, an alteration of interaction between the child and the parents, and inability either to allow age-appropriate autonomy or to set limits. In our own work in a rural region of sub-Saharan Africa, the residual effects of this early impediment to attachment had long-term nutritional consequences; our observations parallel those in the United States.[53] It appears that consequences of perceiving one's offspring as vulnerable in early life are universal. The clinician must be sensitive to this perception in the newborn period as a basis of many later problems (e.g., problems with sleep, eating, discipline, and school phobias).

> *Mrs. Donaldson brought in her 4-year-old because of behavior problems at home and in the preschool. She said he "never minds me" and is aggressive with the other kids. He "never sleeps—not his whole life." She says he is slow in development and needs medicine. She attributes it all to his "terrible birth, when he almost died." She brings in a picture of him in the NICU. He doesn't look ill at all to the clinician. The medical record notes that he was a child born by cesarean section with a brief period of transient tachypnea and a negative evaluation for sepsis.*

A continuing ascertainment of parents' views of the child will help the clinician be sure that these are in line generally with the realities of the child's situation and that these perceptions change appropriately with time. Maintaining a vulnerable outlook in the face of improvement or normalization defines this syndrome. If family members cannot reframe their view of the child with cognitive input from the clinician, a mental health referral may be needed.

GETTING READY TO GO HOME: DISCHARGE PLANNING

As discharge approaches, parental anxiety increases sharply.[54] The demands of unrelenting care, the lingering sense of inadequacy, and the fear of further damaging the infant while at home all contribute to this. This may be manifested as decreased visiting, anger, accusations, or the proposal of impediments to discharge. The clinician should recognize the need for the family to withdraw and consolidate before this new step, support the process, but still hold firm on the discharge plan with as specific a course as possible.

The family needs to know what the baby must be able to do to demonstrate readiness for discharge, such as the following:

■ Tolerate all feedings by mouth
■ Be gaining weight and maintaining body temperature in an open crib
■ Have no significant apnea and bradycardia
■ Complete discharge assessments (e.g., eye exam and hearing screen)

The family then knows that discharge is not at a specific date, gestational age, or weight. Rather, it depends on the child's own maturation and recovery. If a date is given, the result will be disappointment, failure, and anger if the date changes, as it often does.

Preparing a discharge notebook for all instructions, appointments, important telephone numbers, and critical observations helps to channel parents' anxious energy into a useful mode. Reflection on these feelings of anxiety and inadequacy as normal and as a testimony of caring will help parents put the feelings into perspective.

The *explicit* agreement of *frequent, scheduled* calls and visits appears to generate earlier independence in a family than does an ad hoc arrangement. Parents need permission to call back to the NICU for advice. The primary care nurse is usually in the best position to do this. A gradual transition rather than an abrupt change is usually helpful. A conference at discharge should be concrete, focused on short-term goals, expectations, and specific care plans. The primary care physician may lead this conference; if that isn't possible, the clinician should attend or receive a written summary of the session. A more expanded "debriefing" with the primary care provider should be set up 6 weeks to 3 months after discharge.

Social service evaluation for ill neonates' families should be routine in the NICU and should also be offered to other families who seem unable to make progress in the adaptation process after discharge. Parent-to-parent connections with families with similar challenges can be very positive. Practical skills, access to service information, and emotional support are all valuable. The clinician should facilitate such encounters because families are usually unable at this time to do much resource acquisition themselves.

Parenting groups, particularly for children with specific problems of known outcome (e.g., Down's syndrome) may be helpful to families during this adjustment phase.

PRACTICE SESSIONS

To learn the infant's signal system, parents must spend time in the nursery, watching and participating in care. The parents can be asked to monitor their own infant's response to the environment, caregiving, and support (Box 6-5).

Nurses should share their own observations and care techniques and note how they change over time. However, the goal here is not just to provide excellent care, but also to support the parents in the process of discovery about their own infant. Parents have made it with their at-risk infant when they see the baby as a special individual with communicative intent—a person who can be known and understood. Parents can reach this level only after they are sure that the infant will survive and are confident that they can cope with the child's practical care needs. Skills in CPR, monitor use, medication administration, and so forth should be seen as building tools for the parent-child relationship, as well as skills required for infant survival. Competency in skills enables parents to see their infant as manageable, understandable, and lovable. It is only with those feelings that true attachment can occur.

BOX 6-5	BEDSIDE OBSERVATIONS FOR CLINICIANS AND PARENTS

Observe the infant's state
Can you see the cycles of sleep?
Can you tell when the infant is waking?
What soothes the child's upsets?
What are the child's responses to sight? To sound?
What things are aversive, and what are positive?
What kind of movement and posture are positive, and which are stressful?

DEVELOPMENTAL APPRAISAL

It is clear that we should make adjustments in our neurodevelopmental expectations commensurate with a child's postconceptual age rather than chronological age, beginning with a correction in the physical growth chart and how we label an office visit. Families should be reminded of this correction to adjust their expectations accordingly. For the infant who weighed less than 1500 g, this adjustment should last for at least 2 to 3 years. For higher-birth-weight babies, the adjustment should continue for at least a year.

Mr. James brought in his 6-month-old son for a health supervision visit. The dad was worried because Derek wasn't doing anything that his cousin, also 6 months of age, did. Derek was 2 months premature. Dr. Ellis said, "This will be like a 4-month visit for Derek, given his prematurity." She then corrected the growth chart, pushing back the current measurement by 2 months. This put Derek's growth within the normal range for his adjusted age. Mr. James seemed to relax immediately.

BOX 6-6	DEVELOPMENTAL ABNORMALITIES

1st Year*:   Cerebral palsy
Severe sensory abnormalities
Significant visual compromise
Severe hearing loss

2nd Year: Speech and language difficulties
Early cognitive delays
Subtle visual and hearing difficulties

3-5 years: Fine motor difficulties
Behavioral regulation difficulties
Hypo- or hyper-responsive behavior (i.e., ADHD)
Motor and behavioral "immaturity"

6-8 Years: Learning disabilities
Sensory processing problems
Visual-motor difficulties
Minor degrees of compromised motor coordination

*Likely appearance time frames.

Formal appraisal of development should be at regular intervals through specialized programs that offer the time to do comprehensive assessment of development. Appropriate referrals to community-based services can be done. This follow-up should be continued until school age. Across this time period, the likelihood of the emergence of particular problems changes. The early motor difficulties are rarely missed; the cognitive, organizational, and linguistic concerns are more difficult to pick up in a general office setting (Box 6-6). They may require specialized evaluation tools.

The best window in a primary care setting on developmental competencies overall is an observation of free play, particularly at about 8 to 9 months of corrected age. Several observations that will help assure the clinician of appropriate development are shown in Box 6-7. It may be useful and efficient to change the format for this visit entirely to look at development as the central focus.

If the clinician's observations raise concern in this unstructured setting, a more formal appraisal using an assessment tool is warranted. The physician should be familiar with appropriate screening instruments (e.g., Knobloch and Gesell). Major developmental delays and hearing abnormalities should elicit referrals for early *intervention* before 1 year, if not earlier.

SLEEP DIFFICULTIES

Children cared for in the bright light and continuous sound environment of the NICU will maintain immature state patterns for the first several months after discharge. It will be

BOX 6-7	EVALUATION OF HIGH-RISK INFANT AT 9 MONTHS (CORRECTED AGE)

Baby should sit unsupported
Good mouthing of toys
Transfer of toys should be present
Pincer grasp should be developing and used in play
Child should turn to a sound behind his back
Stranger wariness should be present with going toward mom present
Jabber and babbling should be evident with good voice quality and sounds strung together
Gestures and early imitation should be present (e.g., "Bye bye," "pat-a-cake")
Child should point at objects or show them to another person
Some kind of movement should be present: creeping, scooting, twisting, rolling

more difficult for these infants to settle down for sleeping; they may have long periods of irritability when awakening and falling asleep; and they may find it difficult to come to a quiet-alert state for sustained periods.[55] However, once removed from the stressful NICU environment, the baby will demonstrate increasing competency at state regulation in a quieter, more predictable environment, although full normalization of sleep pattern is rarely achieved in the first year. A quiet radio and a dim light may help the baby make the transition from the NICU environment. Sleep disorders are more common in toddlers who had perinatal difficulties,[56] and these may persist. Difficulty with making transitions from one activity to another may also be impaired well beyond discharge from the nursery. Fragility makes transitions particularly troublesome. These are predictable and are not diagnostic of either poor parenting or neurological damage in themselves. Irritability and sleep difficulties should *start* to decrease at 3 to 4 months of adjusted age in most children. The individual child should be monitored for increasing regularity and predictability in sleep, using the infant's own behavior as a baseline for comparisons.

HEARING ISSUES

Premature or ill infants show a high incidence (2% to 4%) of hearing disorders.[57] These difficulties can rarely be detected in office settings; they require formal assessments. A brainstem auditory evoked response (BAER) should be done near discharge, followed by visual reinforced audiometry or other behavioral audiometry when the child is sitting stably, at about 9 months. The role of otoacoustic emission (OAE) techniques for this population is unclear at this time. Even normal results of these early tests do not rule out a subtle high-frequency or progressive hearing loss that will affect school learning. Recurrent or resistant otitis media secondary to palatine dysfunction may also contribute to later hearing loss. Another preschool test of hearing is advised if any speech or language difficulties persist. An audiologist who has experience with infants and young children is necessary for accurate results.

DATA GATHERING AT DISCHARGE

It is assumed that the primary care clinician has been observing or has reviewed the course of the infant and is aware of the resolved or lingering medical concerns. Specific plans for these need to be laid out in concrete, short-term schedules. A formal discharge summary should be made available to the primary care clinician and the family before discharge.

What To Observe

Following are examples of observations and discussions that should be a part of the preparation for discharge:

■ The clinician should discuss with NICU nurses the infant's awake and sleep pattern. The regularity of these state changes is an indicator of neurobehavioral integrity and maturation. It also gives a base on which to evaluate at-home change.

■ The clinician should observe the parents while they are feeding and handling their infant. Competence and confidence should be evaluated. Supportive comments and suggestions should be offered. If this is not possible, notes or conversations with this information should be gathered ahead of time.

■ The clinician should work with the NICU staff to identify specific training needs, such as gastric tube feeding and cardiopulmonary resuscitation (CPR). This training should should be documented as completed before discharge.

■ The infant record should indicate increasing stability of breathing, consistent feeding, steady weight gain, and increasing alertness and activity. The parents should be able to describe these processes and identify the infant's individual characteristics.

■ The exact feeding patterns, particularly regarding breast-feeding transitioning, should be clearly laid out at discharge.

What To Ask

Questions to be asked when the infant is to be discharged from the special care nursery are presented in Table 6-1.

Examination

It is essential that the primary care clinician and the family examine the baby *together* before discharge or shortly thereafter. The clinician should observe the baby first in sleep, through gentle talking, moving, undressing, and examining, and narrate the reading of the infant's behavior, both positive and negative. Parents should be asked to comment as well, so that everyone is seeing the *same* infant. The level of stimulation that the infant tolerates should be noted. Signals of overstimulation, physiological instability, and fatigue should be met with a rest period, a pulling back of stimulation, and a period for recovery.

If the infant becomes alert, the clinician should demonstrate the baby's alerting and orienting to voice, then to a face, and then both together. If overload occurs, this should be pointed out to the parents as evidence of the child's limits. Considerable support for ex-

TABLE 6-1 ■ Questions To Be Asked at Special Care Nursery Discharge	
Question	Observation
How is the baby doing?	Level of attachment—are the parents answering with a shrug of bewilderment, with a list of laboratory values, or with personalized, accurate observations of their infant's response to them?
Is the baby ready for discharge?	Assess the parents' understanding of readiness issues; gather data from their perspective about the infant.
Are *you* ready to take (name) home?	Assess readiness and response—expand to include specifics of readiness, special needs; assess parental adjustment.
Who will be at home to help?	Assess support systems, intrafamilial concerns, level of father's involvement; assess sibling and family needs.
Do you feel comfortable with (name)?	Evaluate feelings of inadequacy; reassure parents of normality of anxiety; evaluate specific areas in which parents' skills are inadequate.
Do you have any questions about the infant's hospital course?	Open the discussion for any questions about the perinatal events; be honest about your level of concern vis-à-vis these events.
What things would you like to see happen before you take (name) home?	Establish locus of control with parents; develop a plan to meet these wishes if possible, explain if not.

tremities, head, and trunk and temperature control may be needed to demonstrate the brief periods of alertness. The *cost* to the infant or difficulty the infant experiences for these periods should be noted so that this may be observed at home, hopefully to track an improving course.

The general pediatric examination, including a detailed neurological evaluation, should proceed. Any areas of abnormality, as well as encouraging signs, should be clearly stated in an ongoing narrative of what the clinician is evaluating and what is observed, normal and abnormal. The clinician should carefully describe behaviors that will represent the next step in improvement—for example, increasing periods of alertness, decreased color change with undressing, and more ability to quiet self.

A summary statement by the clinician should open a discussion with parents about the evaluation. For example, "Joey is able to really take in more of the world around him these days, and his sleep pattern is getting more regular. His legs still seem a bit tight, however, and getting a full feeding in without a break is still hard for him." An unrushed pause and encouragement may be needed for parents to bring out their own observations and concerns. It is not to be expected that all issues or concerns will be laid out and discussed at this time; rather, this discussion sets a pattern for ongoing developmental surveillance, an honest partnership in observation and care and an individual perspective.

ANTICIPATORY GUIDANCE

The planning for discharge begins on admission as the clinician interprets the issues, weighs them for families, and lays out a **strategy for treatment and follow-up.** This plan is expanded, revised, and updated through the child's course. A formal conference or at least a phone call should occur at least every 2 to 3 weeks thereafter.

Problems that are expected should be discussed with families. A specific list of conditions or complications should be given to parents, with a chance to ask questions or get clarification.

A comprehensive conference should be held before discharge that lays out specific plans, contacts, and appointments in detail. Written materials should always be provided to parents. The goal of this conference is to review the hospital course, to make plans for follow-up, and to review any treatment plans. The following are examples of specific components to include in the conference:

- A readiness assessment should include input from all disciplines and an assessment of behavioral maturity, as well as physiological stability.
- Parents should be told that certain problems specifically related to the infant's condition at birth as a sick neonate *will not* recur (especially intraventricular hemorrhage [IVH], air leak, etc.). Many parents continue to worry that these neonatal problems could recur or be chronic, but they never ask!
- A notebook with all the infant's needs, resources to meet those needs, warning signals, appointments, medications, and telephone numbers of specialists and staff can be most helpful. Most parents remember few specifics without such an aid. Highlight one or two resources, including the primary care pediatrician, to work with the parents in coordinating multiple services.
- Appropriate community agency referrals should be initiated or noted even if services may not be needed immediately. Few parents are able to do this on their own.
- The NICU staff may designate one nurse to follow up with a call in 1 or 2 days to ease the family's transition to home.
- An explicit invitation to visit the NICU after discharge is also helpful as parents attempt to separate from the nursery, the staff, and the support that has been so vital.
- The parents should have demonstrated competency in every aspect of their infant's care. They should have rehearsed what will be needed in emergencies. Instruction in infant CPR and appropriate emergency action will relieve fears rather than generate them.
- A telephone should be in the house. Guarantees of heat, electricity, and basics should be reviewed in some cases.
- Videos, dolls, and pamphlets should supplement, not replace, *direct* teaching in this and other areas.
- Families should have transportation plans laid out for both emergency and planned visits. Adjustment of the car seat, taxi vouchers, and other issues should be addressed.
- An iron-deficient infant is an irritable infant. Premature infants require additional iron supplementation up to 1 year of age. Anemia is a *late* sign of iron deficiency, which has been shown to have adverse effects on development even before anemia surfaces. Appropriate vitamin and iron supplementation should be initiated even in the absence of frank

anemia. Check the hematocrit value at discharge and periodically throughout the first year.

■ The clinician should describe the infant's growth, behavior, and development by the *adjusted age* so that neurodevelopmental expectations are realistic. Always do this correction at the beginning of each encounter.

■ Parents often need to be reassured that their "sleepy" premature infant will become more alert and interactive with maturity. Until they understand this, their infant's apparent response to them (to sleep) is very discouraging. The irritability that may follow it can also be predicted. Parents need to understand these aspects of typical behavior for their atypical infant.

■ Be sure an accurate head circumference is done at the time of discharge. A growth chart including head circumference should be started and values added at the adjusted age at each visit.

■ Parents should be encouraged to stay overnight, if possible, before discharge, or they may be accommodated for a period of time in nearby lodging if they are going to a rural or remote area.

SETTING THE COURSE: MAKING MINI-OBSERVATION PLANS

The construction of a developmentally supportive care plan should be part of every discharge plan. This should be developed with and guided by the nursing staff, who have come to understand the baby's capabilities and limits. The primary care clinician will pick one or two areas of concern or immaturity in the infant and set very small improvement goals with the family at discharge and continuing across the first year. For example, if the infant sleeps erratically, the parents might be asked to keep a sleep record to see if this improves in regularity over a period of 2 to 4 weeks. Or, if the infant has difficulty handling the stress of bathing, the parent and the clinician can devise supports (e.g., swaddling half the body) so that the child can begin to at least tolerate, if not enjoy, the experience. By setting *specific short-term* goals, the parents and the clinician can gain a sense of progress and recovery. The parents' energy can be actively engaged in making and supporting progress. Specific notes on the target area should be noted in the medical record so that the clinician can mark progress or problems at the next visit. The high-risk child will not follow the development pattern of the "normal" child. The clinician makes benchmarks of change for each child. This allows parents to focus on their individual child rather than on comparisons with children taking a typical course.

Hurdles

Soothing. The irritability of many high-risk infants is a major hurdle that often emerges some weeks after discharge, often at 6 weeks adjusted age. This is sometimes referred to as *"super colic."* The development of effective soothing techniques and the avoidance of overloading situations will ameliorate but not obliterate this process. Swings, swaddling, front pack carrying, and pacifiers all may help. Respite care is often needed. Many babies settle more easily on the chest or lap of a caretaker, so additional carrying and quiet cuddles may be easier and better for all concerned.

Breast Feeding. The transition to full breast feeding is a process that takes weeks to months. Some babies never adapt to feeding directly at the breast but can continue to receive the benefits of breast milk if the mother is willing to bottle feed her expressed milk. Even if full breast feeding doesn't occur, any amount of breast milk will be of value to the premature infant in disease protection, brain development, and balanced nutrition. A gradual course of decreasing formula supplements should begin before discharge, and a realistic feeding plan laid out clearly. The mother should increase pumping to eight times daily for a period of 7 to 10 days before discharge to increase her milk supply. The preterm infant should be able to nurse at breast before discharge for part of a feeding or for all of some feedings. A recommended approach for each feeding should be:

■ Breast feed at breast
■ Supplement with pumped breast milk
■ Pump for next feed to keep up supply; store appropriately

Hearing and Vision Assessments. The baby's vision and hearing should be monitored throughout early childhood. The first follow-up appointment for each area should be planned at discharge (Box 6-8). Parents should be told that this is routine and does not imply a special concern for their child. Specialized follow-up services are needed beyond what the primary care clinician can do.

Home Visits. Home visiting, sometimes including a predischarge or postdischarge visit, is helpful if done by the NICU staff or others who knew the infant in the hospital. Discharge plans become realistic, and teaching can be focused. Follow-up and compliance are increased at least threefold when a visit is made.

Planned Review

A review of the perinatal course should be added to the 6-week to 3-month visit if a discussion has not been opened by the parents before that time. Confusion about diagnoses, conditions, treatments, and expected follow-up is often identified at this time. Clarification may

---

BOX 6-8	ASSESSMENTS

Hearing
Discharge hearing screen (BAER or OAE) with follow-up BAER if abnormal 6 to 9 months adjusted age: VRA when sitting
Further follow-up if abnormal speech-language development or frequent otitis media.

Ophthalmology
If premature baby weighs less than 1500 g, examine before discharge: complete visualization of retina
Ophthalmology follow-up for astigmatism and refractive errors at 1-2 years

head off the vulnerable child syndrome (mentioned earlier in this chapter), increase compliance, and alleviate fears.

The 8- to 9-month visit should be expanded to allow for a play observation and a structured developmental assessment. (See Box 6-7.) A complete neurological examination should be done at 1 year at minimum.

Special attention should be paid to a receptive and expressive language assessment at 2 to 2½ years. Oral-motor dysfunction may also result in speech articulation difficulties that may be evident throughout the preschool period. A preschool examination should place added emphasis on visual-motor tasks (e.g., figure copying). Disabilities in this area should trigger *immediate, specific* testing, not just a standard intelligence test.

REFERENCES

1. Guyer B et al: Annual summary of vital statistics—1997, *Pediatrics* 102:1333, 1998.
2. Hille ETM et al: School performance at nine years of age in very premature and very low birth weight infants: perinatal risk factors and predictors at five years of age, *J Pediatr* 125:426, 1994.
3. Chapieski ML, Evankovich KD: Behavioral effects of prematurity, *Semin Perinatol* 21:221, 1997.
4. Vohr BR, Msall ME: Neuropsychological and functional outcomes of very low birth weight infants, *Semin Perinatol* 21:202, 1997.
5. Whitfield MF et al: Extremely premature (≤800 g) schoolchildren: multiple areas of hidden disability, *Arch Dis Child* 77:F85, 1997.
6. Lucas A et al: Breast milk and subsequent intelligence quotient in children born preterm, *Lancet* 339:261, 1992.
7. Singer LT et al: Maternal psychological distress and parenting stress after the birth of a very low-birth-weight infant, *JAMA* 281:799, 1999.
8. Drillien CM: The incidence of mental and physical handicaps in school age children of very low birth weight, *Pediatrics* 27:452, 1961.
9. Ardura J et al: Development of sleep-wakefulness rhythm in premature babies, *Acta Paediatr* 84:484, 1995.
10. Page JM et al: Ocular sequelae in premature infants, *Pediatrics* 92:787, 1993.
11. Lucas A et al: Randomized trial of nutrition for preterm infants after discharge, *Arch Dis Child* 67:324, 1992.
12. Bishop NJ, King FJ, Lucas A: Increased bone mineral content of preterm infants fed with a nutrient enriched formula after discharge from hospital, *Arch Dis Child* 68:573, 1993.
13. Achenbach TM et al: Nine-year outcome of the Vermont intervention program for low birth weight infants, *Pediatrics* 91:45, 1993.
14. Sameroff AJ: Longitudinal studies of preterm infants. In Friedman S, Sigman M, editors: *Preterm birth and psychological development,* New York, 1981, Academic Press.
15. Lozoff B et al: The mother-newborn relationship: limits of adaptability, *J Pediatr* 91:1, 1977.
16. Bowlby J: *Attachment and loss—loss: sadness and depression,* vol 3, New York, 1980, Basic Books.
17. Lindemann E: Symptomatology and management of acute grief, *Am J Psychiatr* 101:141, 1944.
18. Vance JC et al: Psychological changes in parents eight months after the loss of an infant from stillbirth, neonatal death, or sudden infant death syndrome—a longitudinal study, *Pediatrics* 96:933, 1995.
19. Frischer L: The death of a baby in the infant special care unit, *Pediatr Clin N Amer* 45:691, 1998.
20. Wallerstedt C, Higgins P: Facilitating perinatal grieving between the mother and the father, *JOGNN* 25:389, 1996.

21. Cuisinier M et al: Grief following the loss of a newborn twin compared to a singleton, *Acta Paediatr* 85:339, 1996.
22. Parke RD: *Fathers,* Cambridge, Mass, 1981, Harvard University Press.
23. Minde K et al: Mother-child relationships in the premature nursery: an observational study, *Pediatrics* 61:373, 1978.
24. Gorski PA, Huntington L: Physiological measures relative to tactile stimulation in hospitalized preterm infants, *Ped Res* 23:210A, 1988.
25. Linn PL, Horowitz FD, Fox HA: Stimulation in the NICU: is more necessarily better? *Clin Perinatol* 12:407, 1985.
26. Long JG, Lucey JF, Philip AGS: Noise and hypoxemia in the intensive care nursery, *Pediatrics* 65:143, 1980.
27. Long JG, Philip AGS, Lucey JF: Excessive handling as a cause of hypoxemia, *Pediatrics* 65:203, 1980.
28. Brazy JE: Effects of crying on cerebral blood volume and cytochrome aa;s3, *J Pediatr* 112:457, 1988.
29. Perlman JM, Volpe JJ: Episodes of apnea and bradycardia in the preterm newborn: impact on cerebral circulation, *Pediatrics* 76:333, 1985.
30. Gaiter JL: Nursery environments: the behavior and caregiving experiences of full-term and preterm newborns. In Gottfried AW, Gaiter JL, editors: *Infant stress under intensive care,* Baltimore, 1985, University Park Press, pp 55-81.
31. Gorski PA et al: Direct computer recording of premature infants and nursery care, *Pediatrics* 72:198, 1983.
32. Gottfried AW et al: Physical and social environment of newborn infants in special care units, *Science* 214:673, 1981.
33. High PC, Gorski PA: Recording environmental influences on infant development in the intensive care nursery. In Gottfried AW, Gaiter JL, editors: *Infant stress under intensive care,* Baltimore, 1985, University Park Press, pp 131-155.
34. Gottfried AW: Environment of newborn infants in special care units. In Gottfried AW, Gaiter JL, editors: *Infant stress under intensive care,* Baltimore, 1985, University Park Press, pp 23-54.
35. Als H, Gilkerson L: The role of relationship-based developmentally supportive newborn intensive care in strengthening outcome of preterm infants, *Semin Perinatol* 21:178, 1997.
36. Nyqvist KH, Lutes LM: Co-bedding twins: a developmentally supportive care strategy, *JOGNN* 27:450, 1998.
37. Parker SJ et al: Outcome after developmental intervention in the neonatal intensive care unit for mothers of preterm infants with low socioeconomic status, *J Pediatr* 120:780, 1992.
38. Feldman F, Eidelman AI: Intervention programs for premature infants: how and do they affect development? *Clin Perinatol* 25:613, 1998.
39. Ariagno RL et al: Developmental care does not alter sleep and development of premature infants, *Pediatrics* 100:9, 1997.
40. Als H et al: Individualized developmental care for the very low birth weight preterm infant, *JAMA* 272:853, 1994.
41. Frodi AM et al: Fathers' and mothers' responses to the faces and cries of normal and premature infants, *Dev Psychol* 14:490, 1978.
42. Lester BM: Developmental outcome prediction from acoustic cry analysis in term and preterm infants, *Pediatrics* 80:529, 1987.
43. Gorski PA: Premature infant behavioral and physiological responses to caregiving interventions in the intensive care nursery. In Call JD, Galenson E, Tyson R, editors: *Frontiers of infant psychiatry,* New York, 1983, Basic Books, pp 256-263.
44. Anderson GC: Current knowledge about skin-to-skin (kangaroo) care for preterm infants, *J Perinatol* 11:216, 1991.

45. Messmer PR et al: Effect of kangaroo care on sleep time for neonates, *Pediatr Nurs* 23:408, 1997.
46. Leonard CH et al: Outcome of very low birth weight infants: multiple gestation versus singletons, *Pediatrics* 93:611, 1994.
47. Als H et al: The behavior of the full term yet underweight newborn infant, *Dev Med Child Neurol* 18:590, 1976.
48. Telzrow RW et al: An assessment of the behavior of the preterm infant at 40 weeks gestational age. In Lipsitt L, Field TM, editors: *Infant behavior and development: perinatal risk and newborn behavior,* Norwood, NJ, 1982, Ablex Publishing Corp, pp 85-96.
49. Yogman MW et al: The behavior of newborns of diabetic mothers, *Infant Behav Dev* 5:331, 1982
50. Newman LF: Parents' perceptions of their low birthweight infants, *Paediatrician* 9:182, 1982.
51. Brazelton TB: *On becoming a family: the growth of attachment,* New York, 1981, Delacorte.
52. Green M, Solnit AJ: Reactions to the threatened loss of a child: a vulnerable child syndrome, *Pediatrics* 34:58, 1964.
53. Dixon S et al: Perinatal circumstances and newborn outcome among the Gusii of Kenya: assessment of risk, *Infant Behav Devel* 5:11, 1982.
54. Brazelton TB: Early intervention: What does it mean? In Fitzgerald HE, Lester BM, Yogman MW, editors: *Theory and research in behavioral pediatrics,* New York, 1981, Plenum Press.
55. Sigman M, Parmelee AH: Longitudinal evaluation of the high risk infant. In Field TM et al, editors: *Infants born at risk: behavior and development,* Jamaica, NY, 1979, Spectrum Publications.
56. Bernal JF: Night waking in infants during the first fourteen months, *Dev Med Child Neurol* 15:760, 1973.
57. American Academy of Pediatrics Task Force on Newborn and Infant Hearing: Newborn and infant hearing loss: detection and intervention, *Pediatrics* 103:527, 1999.

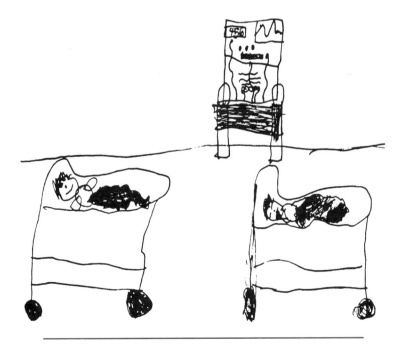

"Babies in nursery with machines." By Ryan Hennessy, age 8.

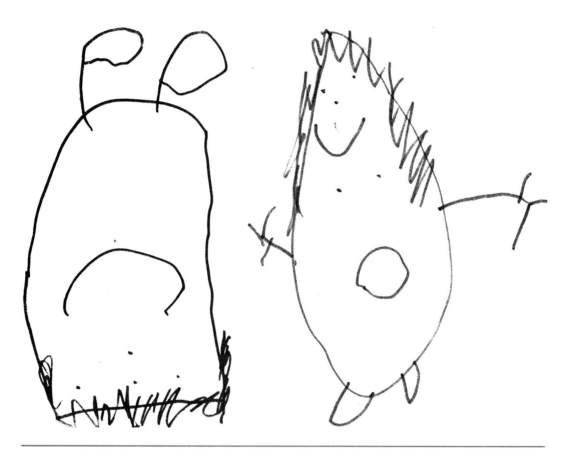

A 4-year-old draws his parents topsy-turvy. Many families feel that way with the arrival of a new child.

CHAPTER 7

FIRST DAYS AT HOME: MAKING A PLACE IN THE FAMILY

■ Suzanne D. Dixon
■ Martin T. Stein

KEY WORDS

Postpartum Adjustment
Breast Feeding
Maternal Depression
Sibling Rivalry

Mrs. Ferris brings in her 3-week-old son, Ethan, for a weight check, carrying him in a plastic carrier. This full-term infant has been gaining slowly with breast feeding. He awakens very quickly when unwrapped on the examining table and immediately starts to cry. Mrs. Ferris sits quietly, mechanically getting out a new diaper for the infant. She appears pale and tired and is less well dressed than usual. Melissa, her 3-year-old, plays with the examining room toys, throwing a small car across the room. Her mother jumps up quickly and scolds her. Melissa dissolves into tears and then sucks her thumb. You notice that Melissa has on diapers. Mrs. Ferris says she's thinking of starting bottle feeding. She looks tearful.

The early neonatal period after hospital discharge is usually filled with turmoil and adjustments for all members of the family. These individuals must struggle to fit themselves and the infant into a family unit that has irrevocably changed. The infant is working too, using capacities for learning and adaptation to fit into the caretaking unit. He must capture other family members and build a secure web of sensitive caretaking. The baby's physical and psychological needs are met by those members who will learn to understand the infant's signals and generate appropriate responses. Each infant's particular temperament, physiological stability, stamina, and behavioral characteristics determine how those needs are met. *The parents' perception of the child, as it is formed during this time, is a powerful predictor of their own interaction with the child over the long term; this, in turn, has major consequences for the child's development.* Parental self-esteem and sense of competence in the parenting role are influenced dramatically by the events of the first months. Feelings of competency energize the overall work of parenting. This is an important time for the child and all the family members.

The clinician's role during this first month is critical to monitor and support the development of synchrony in the family unit while evaluating the infant's growth and physical well-being. It is expected that this process of **postpartum adjustment** will not be without turmoil. Turbulence is evidence of healthy developmental work. More serious difficulties occur in families whose members are not free enough of other concerns to make a place for the infant and a new role for themselves. Particularly when no extended family members are available, the clinician has a special role of support and guidance. The clinician may have to provide extra energy to help refocus the family on the particular needs of the infant and, indeed, of all the family members.

The family must get on track with the infant. This is done through the generation of successes in each member's care of the infant. Through sensitive observations and through some thoughtful suggestions on seemingly small matters of management, the clinician can ensure that everyone, including the infant, grows during the adjustment process. It is in the course of this daily care that psychological realignment is accomplished.

INFANT SOCIAL DEVELOPMENT

The infant begins life fully equipped to interact with the environment.[1] Evidence of the baby's actively participating in social interactions includes movement in rhythm to the human voice,[2] selective orientation to mother's milk by 6 days of age,[3] and a visual fixation on the human face that is different from that of any other kind of stimuli.[4-6] The infant's early behavioral repertoire includes socially directed behaviors used both to elicit and to terminate interactions.[7] Directed gaze is important to the bonding between infant and family in the U.S. culture.

Generally the baby's eyes widen and brighten as they fixate and track the parents' movements and scan their faces. This has a powerful, positive effect on the adults, locking them into a relationship with their child. Gaze aversion, conversely, is often actively used by the infant to either avoid or take a break from an interaction. In addition to gaze the infant can demonstrate readiness for interaction with body language (e.g., smooth, cyclic movements of extremities or slowing down of body movements, open hands, and mouthing). Behaviors that signal withdrawal from caregivers, either to modulate the level of input or to avoid insensitive or overwhelming interaction, include back arching, pulling away, hand to head, increased body tension, and diffuse jittery movements of extremities. Parents may need to have these behaviors identified as communication from their infant, particularly if the infant has difficulties locking in with the parents. Additionally, attentive mothers and spectral analysis can distinguish different types of cries by the time the infant is 2 days of age. These types of cries include those for hunger and those expressing pain.

Smiling is a powerful social "tool," progressing from a reflexive activity to a responsive activity elicited by external events (e.g., a human face, gaze, or voice) to spontaneous behavior produced to elicit response from others at the age of 6 to 8 weeks.[8] Newborns prefer high-pitched voices from either mothers or fathers. Parents from different cultures with different languages instinctively use high-pitched voices when communicating with an infant in the first month of life.[9] The laugh appears by 4 months of age as a response to external stimuli and delightfully draws social attention and amazement from caregivers. Baby talk, including feeding sounds, cooing, and then babbling, is another mode of initiating interactions. These soft vocalizations come out of a positive social interaction sometime in the first month. By the second month, most infants will engage in verbal "dialogues" with their mothers, using these sounds. This unfolding of patterns and building of a relationship begins in the first days of life.[10,11]

The infant's interactional pattern emerges with each parent over the first days and weeks of life.[10,11] During this acquaintance period the family members develop reciprocal relationships, often rhythmic, smooth, and modulated with mothers and more evenly intense and positive with fathers.[12] This "waltzing" or "turn-taking"[13] can be observed in periods of engagement that increase in frequency and duration during the first weeks.[14] Balanced harmony is largely dependent upon the parents' contingent responses and their sensitivity to the child's visual, verbal, and motor cues. Individual variation in both infant and parental temperament is a significant factor in the development of the style and form of this interaction, but not in its basic structure. Its appearance attests to the basic foundation of all other aspects of development to follow. The infant participates in these by developing predictable patterns of behavior; the parent participates by being a good observer and reading the infant's cues closely. Caretaking activities are the matrix upon which this synchrony is built. Being successful with the infant's care and being able to see pattern and meaning in the infant's behavior enable the parents to grow in their role and to meet the child's physical and psychological needs.[10] Close physical contact early on enhances the attachment process both immediately and down the line.[15]

The breast-feeding situation in particular emphasizes the basic interactional nature of the infant's behavior within a family. Each partner brings characteristics to this interaction (Table 7-1). The infant is born with reflexes, but these must be quickly adapted to the feeding interaction. The infant's temperament, state regulation, physiological variables, and behavioral organization all contribute to that process. Likewise, the mother's nutrition, hydration, psychological state, and rate of recovery enter into the equation. In a variable time of adjust-

TABLE 7-1 ■ Interactional Nature of Breast Feeding

Infant Characteristics	Maternal Characteristics
Reflexes	Nutrition
Temperament	Hydration
State regulation	Psychological state
Physiological variables	Recovery stage
Behavioral organization	Concepts of parenting
Residual of recovery from delivery influences	Extent and use of support
Neurological maturation	Psychosocial history
	Residual of pregnancy, delivery circumstances
	Role models

ment for both partners, rhythms and behavioral patterns of individuals are melded into a successful interaction. Through this medium, both partners learn about themselves, as well as the other. Personal, cultural, and group differences are evident here as they are in other situations of interaction. The clinician should be *very* familiar with the practical advice and support required for successful **breast feeding** (Box 7-1). Unfortunately, this is not always the case. Most professionals feel they need to learn more.[16] Within that context, the foundation for later interactions is laid down, as well as the nutritional basis for physical growth. The success that is realized with optimal nursing energizes the whole interactional system.

The American Academy of Pediatrics recognizes that support of nursing has not only nutritional, immunological, and infectious disease consequences but psychosocial ones as well (Box 7-2). The first 2 weeks of life are the toughest as these patterns are set. Mothers may feel that they have been reduced to a milk machine at this point. The clinician can help them see this broader perspective, as well as provide practical management advice. The setting of family priorities (feeding for the infant, rest and good nutrition for the mother) may have to be explicitly explored.

For mothers who decide not to nurse their infants, the basic interactional synchrony must be the basis for feeding. Feeding time should provide close physical contact and attention to the infant's behavioral cues and contingent responsiveness. Nurture in the broadest sense should be the outcome here as in breast feeding. Even greater vigilance is needed if these broader needs will be consistently met because this kind of physical and emotional contact is not automatic with bottle feeding. Obviously, bottle propping is never appropriate.

Observation of the mother feeding the infant in the office offers the best opportunity to assess the synchrony that is developing between mother and infant. In addition, direct observation offers opportunities for support, specific suggestions, and direct reflection on the baby's behavior. This situation provides a very economical way of observing the interaction between mother and infant. It should be a set part of the examination at least once in the first 2 weeks of life and more often if the adjustment process seems to be progressing slowly or with difficulty. An effective way to observe nursing without altering standard office routines is for the office nurse or medical assistant to suggest that the mother nurse the baby after measurements are taken, while waiting for the clinician, as the history is initiated. The clinician is then able to observe nursing. A planned office visit within the first week enables the clinician to intervene if difficulties are identified. A delayed first office visit often means that a preventable problem with feeding or an opportunity for better adjustment has been lost. Optimally, the visit should be planned within 1 week after hospital discharge for new parents and no longer than 2 weeks for those with prior experience. In communities where home-visitation programs are available,[18] office visits in the first few weeks may be adjusted to coordinate with the home visit.

POSTPARTUM "BLUES" AND DEPRESSION

Parental adjustments to a new baby do not come automatically, nor do they emerge in a neutral emotional atmosphere. Some turbulence occurs in most families. Having postpartum "blues" is a normal, transient phase in the adaptation process. Most women experience some sadness in a mild form during this time that is related to exhaustion, physical depletion, and

BOX 7-1	KNOWLEDGE ABOUT SUCCESSFUL BREAST FEEDING FOR PEDIATRIC CLINICIANS

As a result of earlier discharge after delivery, health professionals are being called on to evaluate newborns within the first few days of life. The following specific criteria will help clinicians accurately assess the success of early breast feeding and provide timely intervention to prevent excessive infant weight loss or diminished maternal milk supply.

Schedule of Feedings

An infrequent or otherwise inappropriate feeding schedule is a common, preventable cause of insufficient milk. The mother must be prepared to nurse her baby whenever the infant signals readiness to feed, such as increased alertness, sucking motions, or rooting. Crying is a late sign of hunger.

Breast-fed newborns should nurse approximately 8 to 12 times in 24 hours, usually taking both breasts at each feeding. A breast-feeding mother should nurse her baby every 1½ to 3 hours during the early postpartum weeks. A single longer night interval of 4 or 5 hours between feedings is permissible. Nonnutritive sucking on a pacifier should be discouraged until a consistent pattern of acceptable weight gain has been established. Nondemanding babies should be aroused to feed. The intrafeeding interval in days 2 to 4 of life and at any time of a growth spurt may be *very* short, an hour or so.

Duration of feedings should be approximately 15 minutes per breast, during which the infant suckles actively with short pauses. Infants are unlikely to obtain sufficient milk by sucking less than 10 minutes per breast in the early weeks of life. Conversely, marathon feedings that last more than 50 minutes are usually indicative of ineffective nursing. Older breast-fed babies often nurse very efficiently, taking the bulk of their feeding in only 5 to 7 minutes per breast, although they may nurse longer for comfort. Very short feedings may mean that the infant only gets the thin foremilk. The caloric, fat-rich hindmilk follows the mother's sense of let down. It is this milk that results in real weight gain.

Infant Behavior and Appearance

Reports of the infant's behavior during and after nursing can provide important clues about the quality of feedings. Well-fed infants should act satisfied after feedings and sleep contentedly. Hyperbilirubinemia in breast-fed infants is a common marker for inadequate breast feeding, a condition known as "breast-feeding jaundice."

Once milk has come in, a mother should hear her baby swallow regularly during feedings and see evidence of milk in the baby's mouth. These observations are somewhat subjective, however, and do not always correlate with objective measures of milk intake.

Generally, a breast-fed baby should appear satisfied after nursing and sleep contentedly until the next feeding. Persistent crying or excessive need for a pacifier often signifies infant hunger and suggests that little milk was obtained during feeding.

Modified from Neifert M: *Early assessment of the breastfeeding infant*, Marianne Neifert, MD, Lactation Program, 1719 E. 19th Avenue, Denver, CO 80218.

BOX 7-1	KNOWLEDGE ABOUT SUCCESSFUL BREAST FEEDING FOR PEDIATRIC CLINICIANS—cont'd

Infant Behavior and Appearance—cont'd

Exaggerated physiological jaundice in a breast-fed infant is a common marker for inadequate breast feeding. Whenever unexplained, unconjugated hyperbilirubinemia is present in a breast-fed infant, evaluation of the infant's nutritional status is warranted. The baby is probably getting insufficient milk to push the bilirubin out via the gut and kidneys. Strategies to improve the effectiveness of breast feeding should be implemented whenever "breast-feeding jaundice" is diagnosed. Formula supplements may be necessary to provide adequate nutrition, but breast feeding need not be interrupted.

Infant Elimination

A newborn's pattern of voiding and stooling provides one of the most sensitive historical indicators of the adequacy of milk intake. Always inquire about infant elimination patterns.

Shortly after milk comes in, a thriving breast-fed newborn should void colorless urine at least 6 to 8 times daily. With inadequate infant intake, mothers often report a "brick dust" appearance in the diaper caused by precipitated urate crystals. Dark yellow, scant urine or visible urate crystals beyond 3 to 4 days of life strongly suggest that a breast-fed infant is not obtaining sufficient milk.

Beginning about the 4th or 5th day of life, well-nourished breast-fed infants typically pass sizable (not a small stain), loose, yellow "milk stools" after most feedings. Between about 4 days and 4 weeks of age, a thriving breast-fed baby should pass at least four such "milk stools" daily, often resembling a mixture of cottage cheese and mustard. Dark transition stools, infrequent movements, or scant volume of stools in the young breast-fed infant are common indicators of insufficient milk intake. However, beginning around 1 month of age, stooling frequency may gradually diminish in breast-fed infants, although stools remain soft and easily passed.

BOX 7-2	KEY POINTS FROM POLICY STATEMENT ON BREAST FEEDING

Human milk is the preferred food for all infants, including premature and sick newborns, with rare exceptions.

Promote and support breast feeding enthusiastically. In consideration of the extensive published evidence for improved outcomes in breast-fed infants and their mothers, a strong position on behalf of breast feeding is justified.

Although economic, cultural and political pressures often confound decisions about infant feeding, the AAP firmly adheres to the position that breast feeding ensures the best possible health, as well as the best developmental and psychosocial outcomes for the infant. Enthusiastic support and involvement of pediatricians in the promotion and practice of breast feeding is essential to the achievement of optimal infant and child health, growth, and development.

From American Academy of Pediatrics: *Pediatrics* 100:1035, 1997.

hormonal changes. Contributing factors are sleep deprivation caused by demanding caregiving responsibilities, as well as changes in role and body image. Household and other child-care duties may be overwhelming. While letting go of the former relationship of "two," the couple begins to incorporate this "third person" who generally upsets most established home routines and patterns, such as mealtimes, talk times, social activities, and sexual patterns. Being home all day and delaying career or academic pursuits often adds to the ambivalence and role conflict many women experience. Economic uncertainty also may compound the stress. The single mother's difficulty during this time may be heightened by her sense of aloneness if supporting individuals or groups are not available. Existing family stresses usually get worse rather than better at this time.

As a result of these factors, new mothers must cope with many unanticipated feelings.[19] They are often overwhelmed by the chaos this new baby seems to have created. During their "baby blues," women may feel unusually dependent on others or even intimidated by would-be supporters.[20] The clinician may be caught up in the adjustment process as the new mother turns to him as a resource. Many women are confused and embarrassed by their inexplicable crying, indecisiveness, and fatigue during these first few weeks. Clinicians may be frightened, feel awkward, or be uncertain about how to respond to this excessive dependency and emotionality unless they see it as a transient process of normal adult development. Clinical features of severe depression are immobilizing indecision, impaired cognitive functioning, irritability, and changes in sleep and appetite. The usual onset is within the 30-day period after birth. Most new mothers resolve these feelings by 6 to 8 weeks postpartum. Ongoing success as a parent with renewed self-esteem will aid in the resolution of the turbulence. Help and frequent acknowledgment of maternal competencies are the tools that are available for the pediatric caregiver to assist this process.[21] Encouragement to reach out to support systems will enable the family to cope. Mothers with postpartum depression may recover faster if they participate in group health supervision visits than if they receive individual pediatric care.[22]

Mrs. Ferris' own behavior and her responses to her 3-week-old son and 3-year-old daughter are an opportunity for effective pediatric intervention. The pediatrician comments, "A new baby and a toddler are an enormous amount of work. . . . How has it been going for you?" Mrs. Ferris' tears begin to subside when she talks about her feelings of inadequacy as a mother, her sense of isolation from her husband and friends, and her sleep deprivation.

The pediatrician listens without immediate suggestion. She engages the toddler with a toy, tells her what a big sister she has become, and lifts her to the examination table while encouraging her participation as an observer during the exam. The normal physical and developmental examination is narrated to assure Mrs. Ferris that her baby is healthy. The notion of temperament is introduced as the clinician demonstrates soothing measures.

Mrs. Ferris is then informed that "feeling blue" is experienced by many mothers during the first month after delivery. That the feeling is usually transient and responsive to interventions is emphasized.

> *The pediatrician then assesses nursing by observing the baby at mother's breast. In a now calm environment, effective latching-on and sucking appear adequate. The mother's fluid intake, need for more sleep, and plans for recruiting available social support from her family friends are reviewed.*

Persistent or severe symptoms of depression (in 10% to 20% of new mothers) require psychiatric referral, clearly beyond what can be provided in a primary care setting. Mothers may experience a prolonged depressive state accompanied by sleep disturbances, anorexia, constipation, agitation, and a sluggish affect. They may develop an altered way of thinking, such as talking about past, present, and future events in a negative or unrealistic way that expresses a radical departure from the prenatal personality. The mother's ability to function may be significantly impaired. Suicidal ideations, delusions, and hallucinations may be uncovered, both by specific questioning, or by following an unusual response to a routine question. These mothers may require significant respite care, as well as psychiatric referral. Most studies report high rates of recovery from the acute phase of this illness. Mothers with the following characteristics are significantly more vulnerable to severe depression or psychosis in the postpartum period:

- A history of psychiatric illness
- A history of drug abuse
- A recent loss (e.g., death of parent)
- Isolation, with other major life stressors

Parents of preterm, ill, or disabled children also are more vulnerable during resolution of grief. Because the pediatric clinician may be the mother's only source of medical contact in the first month postpartum, these symptoms may only surface during pediatric health supervision visits with specific questioning and with a sensitivity to these issues. It becomes the pediatric clinician's responsibility to identify the need for further evaluation, referral, and possible treatment. If the mother requires psychotropic drugs, the pediatrician should evaluate the extent of the drugs' excretion in breast milk.[23,24]

Maternal depression and mental illness are a pediatric issue.[21] Although the mother's well-being is clearly at risk in this circumstance, the baby's is too. Even brief periods of depressive behavior have profound effects on the infant's behavior.[25] A prolongation of symptoms may have long-lasting effects on the child.[26,27] This may be indirectly caused by the lack of reciprocal interaction with the infant.[11] Many adverse child-rearing conditions may affect the infant through the medium of maternal depression.[28,29] The pediatric clinician cannot afford to ignore this condition in parents if she wants to support optimal development in the child.

REACTIONS OF OLDER SIBLINGS

Sibling rivalry is a predictable, normal, and healthy response to the birth of a new brother or sister. In most families it demonstrates that the older child is appropriately attached to the parents and is able to respond to a perceived threat to the parent-child relationship. In this context the emergence of behaviors that reflect sibling rivalry should be viewed in a positive way. Ambivalence toward the baby, evidenced by the ongoing shift between positive and negative behaviors, is to be expected. Indeed, its absence may be worrisome. Sibling rivalry is not a disease, but a manifestation of psychological health and an impetus for developmental progress. Behavioral manifestations of sibling rivalry can take several forms, such as the following:

- *Aggressive* behavior is directed most commonly toward the mother, but also may be directed toward the baby, father, playmates, self, or toys. Aggressive behavior most often occurs when the older sibling is a toddler. Accelerations in this tension probably will occur when the new baby becomes increasingly socially engaging at 4 to 5 months of age and becomes mobile during the last half of the first year. Open hostility may be mollified to more subtle intrusive behaviors directed at the younger child, such as pulling the pacifier out of the baby's mouth.

- *Naughtiness,* or doing things contrary to family rules, occurs frequently at the times when the mother is busy with the baby. This strategy serves both to increase the tension in the household and to verify the continuing power of the toddler to alter the behavior of those around him. A careful history of when these behaviors occur may highlight to the family for the first time that these are not "random," but dependent on a particular situation.

- Some children are *overly compliant,* or overly solicitous to the infant. Perhaps the child fears being totally replaced if she misbehaves, so the child becomes "extra good" to ensure her place in the family, or she is so frightened of her own aggressive and angry feelings that she holds them tightly in check. This may become a costly strategy.

- *Regressive and dependent behaviors* are usually seen in the form of clinging and demanding. Other possible regressive behaviors include sleep disturbances, stuttering, thumb sucking, bed wetting, and baby talk.

Behavioral manifestations of sibling rivalry are often moments of psychological turmoil that reflect a child's limited and primitive response to change in family structure. These generally decrease, but may not entirely disappear, during the year following the new sibling's birth. Over this period the child becomes confident of a new place in the family, with its status and privileges. Additionally, the older sibling usually develops a relationship with the younger child.

The arrival of a younger sibling can evoke positive behavioral changes, as well as the negative ones, even in the early, get-acquainted period. Dunn and Kendrick[30] report gains in the older child's independence and mastery, particularly with regard to self-help skills (e.g., dressing and feeding). The child may gain skills and a growing sense of competency through the participation in "her" baby's care. She may be able to reflect on her own growth and development as she sees the baby's emerging capabilities. The older sibling may try out new ways of dealing with the little stranger, initiating and maintaining interactions in which she bears the burden of greater understanding. She will learn to laugh at the antics of the baby and grow in confidence as she learns to make the infant laugh, play games, and imitate. This is an opportunity for growth if such behavior is understood and supported.

FACTORS THAT INFLUENCE RIVALRY

Some factors are correlated with a *positive* response to the infant. Enhanced signs of affection and interest in the baby are correlated with same sex pairs in children whose mothers allow the older child to participate in the baby's care and discuss the baby's needs and behavior with them. However, an overemphasis on behaving "like a big girl (boy)," with demands for more grown-up behavior, is costly for the child. It is a high price to pay for continuing parental love. It does not allow for the working through of inevitable negative feelings or the recuperative process of acting like a baby oneself. Breast feeding the second baby does not compound stress for the first child.[31]

Certain factors have been shown to intensify an older child's *negative* responses at the time of the sibling's birth:

■ An intense, close relationship between the first child and the parents before the baby's arrival is correlated with the child's increased hostile and aggressive behaviors.

■ Extremely withdrawn behavior is more likely in children whose mothers experience severe postpartum exhaustion or depression.

■ Evidence is conflicting regarding the effects of child spacing on the sibling's response, that is, whether or not a narrow age gap intensifies rivalrous behavior.[32,33]

The child's own issues and coping strategies differ at varying ages, but an adjustment period appears at all ages. Temperamental characteristics (see Chapter 2) are also a major contributor to the nature and intensity of a sibling's response to the birth of a baby.[34] Children who are adaptable to new situations, with positive or mild behavior changes when separated from a parent, usually have a similar behavioral response to the birth of a newborn. Temperamentally challenged siblings who are less tolerant of change in routines and novel situations are more likely to have sleep problems and clinging behaviors and to lack a positive interest in the baby.[35]

In response to the pediatrician's request, "tell me how Melissa has responded to new situations since Ethan's birth," Mrs. Ferris remarked that her daughter experienced change with difficulty. Separation experiences were intense and drawn out. When her bedroom was moved to prepare for the baby, she had frequent crying episodes followed by withdrawal and a sullen appearance. The pediatrician saw this as an opportunity to frame Melissa's behavior following the birth of Ethan in the context of her temperament. When Mrs. Ferris was informed that Melissa's response to change was a reflection of her innate temperament (low adaptability and difficulty with novel situations), she was relieved to know that it was not a result of her parenting alone. She was also more responsive to the use of behavior modification as a way to prevent or redirect Melissa's responses to the newborn.

Severe responses in younger children may be markers of a long-standing family adjustment problem, not just that associated with the infant's birth. The pediatrician or clinician may be the only professional to see the family at this time of crisis when the issues are very close to the surface. He then is able to suggest a more extensive evaluation of the family as a whole.

Several *parental* factors affect the parents' own response to the child's behavior. These include the parents' ambivalence toward the new baby, guilt in feeling less attached to the new baby, and mourning over the loss of the previous family structure. Parents may be surprised, embarrassed, or disappointed to see the older child's rivalry after their concerted prenatal efforts to prevent it. Certainly, the parents' physical exhaustion in caring for the new baby diminishes their ability to meet the other child's needs physically and psychologically. It is not surprising that the relationship between mother and firstborn changes after the arrival of the second baby. Second-time mothers show less affection for, spend less time with, and have more confrontations with the firstborn[31,36] after the birth of the infant. It is no wonder that birth order has a profound effect on child development.[37,38]

SUPPORT FOR THE NEW FAMILY

Families and cultures show wide variations in the type, extent, and duration of support given to a new family. Support systems may functionally include emotional support, baby care or advice, or homemaking tasks. The baby's father,[39] extended family (especially grandparents), friends and neighbors (with or without children of their own), and various members of the health care team may be part of the support structure. Many studies show that the number of friends a new mother has is correlated with her success in parenting, attesting to the power of this network.

The amount and kind of support may be constructive or undermining. Some new parents may resent the intrusion, the "taking over" of their perceived role. Sometimes support systems offer divergent and even contradictory advice, leading to the new parent's sense of confusion and anxiety in feeling caught in between two "authorities." Other new parents feel fearful and overwhelmed when the support systems are withdrawn (e.g., when the grandparents return to their own home). Some visitors may take away more energy than they leave; the clinician would do well to inquire about the cost-benefit ratio of the supports. In general, the availability and use of this social network—with the family and in the community—should be supported.[40]

Subcultural differences in role expectations are evident in the way families work out the patterns of activity when a new infant arrives (see Chapter 2). In some situations, the grandmother takes over—to do less would make a mother feel abandoned. In others, relatives are expected to supply large amounts of food and clothing. Most cultures have a period of at least 1 to 2 months postpartum of relative seclusion and care of the new mother, whose sole roles are to recover and to feed the neonate. Every family needs this protected time to gain strength and to do the necessary mental reorganization. Cultural and economic issues may dictate what form this time period takes. Parents asked to return immediately to work without this protected time may protect themselves against "too close" an attachment[41] and may be reluctant to invest in breast feeding. Clinicians should actively encourage use of some protected time at the first or second office visit.

DATA GATHERING
History

To take the history, begin with open-ended questions about the infant—"What new things is the baby doing?" "In what ways can you tell that the baby knows you?"—and proceed to others issues, such as the following:

- Ask more focused questions regarding hearing (Does the baby turn to sounds?), seeing (Does the baby enjoy seeing things?), and feeding behavior (How does the baby act while being fed?).
- Ask about irritability episodes and soothing preferences. What seems to work best to settle the baby down? What upsets the baby? How can you tell if he doesn't like something or is enjoying something?
- Activity patterns. How predictable is he? How regular are his sleep patterns? Is he easily awakened? How long are his alert periods? Does he like his bath?
- Open-ended questions regarding the parents' adjustment are important also: How are *you* feeling? How are *you* dealing with all this? Are *you* eating and sleeping well?).

If any concern appears in content or affect, have the mother describe what happened yesterday in detail. If she has a minimal response, explore further by stating possible feelings the mother may be experiencing ("Many moms describe this time as so exhausting and discouraging that they feel overwhelmed, frightened by the responsibility. Some have feelings of regret or even negative feelings about having the baby. Have you experienced any of these feelings?").

Ask about the father's reactions and involvement. Does he hold and feed the baby, change diapers, help with housework? What does he think the baby is like? This is best done directly by inviting father's participation in health supervision visits.

The clinician also should evaluate the siblings' responses. If only positive responses are given, be suspicious, although some sibling adaptive behaviors may not manifest until months after the birth of a baby. Give permission for the parent to discuss possibly negative behaviors with you now or in the future ("Most children show some negative reaction to the new baby at some point. This is a normal response to feeling somewhat replaced."). If negative behaviors are described, pursue how these are perceived and handled by the parent.

The availability and use of support systems should be specifically explored, including the emotions that surround those reports. Ask, "How does your family feel about the baby? How is having grandparents around, positive or negative, on a scale of 1 to 10? Are there any friends or neighbors with kids you can depend on? Who is cooking, cleaning, shopping?" The alone and isolated mother or couple is at high risk for difficulties in the adjustment to parenthood.

Observation

Social Development
Be sensitive to the rhythms of interaction between parents and child. Point out to the parents the infant's body language during the history taking and examination. This is a wonderful opportunity to inform parents about their infant's ability to communicate with them. Note the baby's responsiveness to parents. How easily is the infant consoled? How well does

the baby maintain eye contact? The clarity of the baby's cues is important. Are needs and moods easy or difficult to read? Note the parents' sensitivity to the baby's cues. Do they pick up on the baby's subtle behaviors that require parent readjustment? How do they console the infant? Note comfort in handling the baby. Keep in mind individual and cultural differences in the parents' sensory mode with the baby (e.g., talking, touching, eye contact, and grooming behavior).

The feeding situation offers an excellent opportunity to observe social development and interaction between baby and parent. Note maternal affect, latency to respond to questions, and the amount of physical and verbal activity on the parents' part. Note any slowing of movement or responsiveness or evidence of fatigue.

If the older child is in the room, observe interactions with the baby and parents. Note any affect changes in the child and the parents' response to him. If the father or grandparents are present, note their interactions with the baby and the mother and other children. Who holds the baby? How do they respond to the baby's distress (e.g., bowel movement, crying)? Is dad helpful and consoling? Does anyone talk for mom (e.g., giving history, asking questions)? Provide a positive comment about the value of an extended family's presence during the office visit.

Examination

Direct the parent to sit with the baby on her lap to maximize your opportunity to observe their interactions. The infant should turn to a voice. Interact (play, smile) with baby to evaluate response, as well as to model behavior. Observe visual and auditory responses in this context. Comment aloud about baby's social behavior and individuality. Encourage parent to hold and talk with baby often at home. Explain that narrating activities with the baby encourages and promotes language development. Give reassurance that baby cannot be "spoiled" at this age. Holding will, in fact, decrease crying overall.[42] Quick responses to cries, effective soothing, and close human contact lead to less crying in the second year and fine developmental progress in general.

Ask mother specifically about her mood, feelings, and behavior. Allow the mother to cry and use touch if it seems comfortable. Attempt to restore confidence (e.g., "You're doing a good job; it takes a while to adjust to this baby and to get to know one another"). Enhanced self-esteem energizes new parents. Even minor concerns (e.g., diaper rash, mild jaundice) may impinge upon the parents' feeling of competence. Clinicians should be careful to put problems in a clear perspective and to be unequivocal in their praise and support of positive things about the infant, both physical and behavioral. Be explicit about your availability to discuss feelings further. If the mother seems sad, ask specifically about hallucinations or feelings of doing harm to self or others. If these are present or if the sadness appears more severe than seen in normal postpartum "blues," referral is indicated.

Reactions of Older Siblings

If an older sibling is present, acknowledge and focus on him first. Ask specific, separate questions of the older child rather than only asking, "Do you help with the baby?" Give praise for any recent developmental achievements the parent may have mentioned or any helpfulness shown toward parent and baby. Ask about the child's interpretation of the baby (e.g., "Does she cry a lot? Is she not as much fun as you thought she'd be?").

Explain to the parents the positive aspects of their older child's behavioral changes. For example, you might say, "Although I'm sure it's frustrating to see your older child behaving this way, it's actually very healthy behavior. He is clearly demonstrating that he is attached to you and highly values his relationship with you." Reassure them that no matter what preparation was made before the baby's arrival, children will have hurt and resentful feelings; this is real and natural. The goal is not to minimize the negative behaviors, but to help the older child get through and gain from this experience. Some of the ways to help that happen are the following:

- Acknowledge the adjustment process all second-time parents experience when learning to juggle their availability with the needs of two or more children. It takes time for families to settle into new patterns and rhythms. For many selected families, books for parents and children regarding these issues can be helpful (see Resources for Parents, Chapter 27).
- Encourage parents to continue "special time" with the older child alone on a daily basis; a realistic time frame may be 10 to 15 minutes. Emphasize the importance of physical affection or "snuggle time."
- Encourage parents to discuss the new baby's needs and behavior with the older child and to allow participation in the baby's care. Children often benefit from duplicating these activities with their own dolls; these play experiences should be encouraged.
- Plan structured activities for the older child during the baby's bath and feedings so that an attractive distraction is available for the older child.
- The child should not be expected to share all toys, even if she has outgrown them. Reserving some items that are hers alone and providing a special place in which to keep them are important. Sharing parents with the baby on a permanent basis is hard enough.
- Urge parents to minimize changes in the older child's life for a while. This is especially important for an older sibling who is temperamentally slow to adapt to change. Such changes as moving to a new bed or new room or starting nursery school should ideally occur a few months before the baby's arrival or after some weeks of adjustment.
- Displaced aggression can be released through play (e.g., with modeling clay or foam ball and bat). As long as the younger child cannot defend himself, hitting should not be allowed and leaving the two alone should be avoided. The intensity of the parents' message that children must not hurt others is a most powerful factor in helping children learn to appreciate others' feelings.
- The need to be tolerant of regressive behavior should be stressed. Most parents will be reassured to learn that most lapses in developmental achievements are temporary.

Support for New Family

If the father is present, be sure to include him rather than directing comments, eye contact, and questions only to the mother. Direct some questions to him specifically (e.g., "What do you think about this baby? How do you handle his fussy periods? How is the baby affecting your sleep, your work?").

If the grandparent holds the baby for the majority of the visit, ask the mother to hold the baby during the examination in order to allow an opportunity to observe interaction and comfort in handling. If the father or grandparent entirely dominates the visit, the clinician will need to more overtly direct some questions to the mother. Solicitous and supportive inquiry should be the goal. Judgmental comments or rigidly preconceived ideas of optimal family interactions should be avoided. Appreciation of the individual path that each family takes to adjust to the new baby enriches the clinician's professional life. Members of each family should be given appropriate support while they mark their own trail.

REFERENCES

1. Mehler J, Dupoux E: *What infants know: the new cognitive science of early development,* Cambridge, Mass, 1994, Blackwell.
2. Condon WS, Sander LW: Neonate movement is synchronized with adult speech, *Science* 183:99-101, 1974.
3. MacFarlane JA: Olfaction in the development of social preference in human neonates. In Ciba Foundation: *Parent-infant interaction,* Ciba Foundation Symposium No. 33, pp 103-133, New York, Elsevier, 1975.
4. Bower TGR: The visual world of infants, *Sci Am* 215:80, 1966.
5. Pascalis O et al: Mothers' face recognition by neonate: a replication and extension, *Inf Behav Dev* 18.79, 1995.
6. Walton GE, Bower NJA, Bower TGR: Recognition of familiar forms by newborns, *Inf Behav Dev* 15:265, 1992.
7. Stern D: The infant's repertoire. In Stern D: *The first relationship: infant and mother,* Cambridge, Mass, 1977, Harvard University Press.
8. Hetherington EM, Parke RD: Emotional development. In Hetherington EM, Parke RD, editors: *Child psychology: a contemporary viewpoint,* New York, 1979, McGraw-Hill Book, pp 215-218.
9. Kuhl PK et al: Cross-language analysis of phonetic units in language addressed to infants, *Science* 277:684, 1977.
10. Brazelton TB, Cramer BG: *The earliest relationship,* part III, Reading, Mass, 1990, Addison-Wesley.
11. Klaus MH, Kennell JH, Klaus PH: *Bonding: building the foundations of secure attachment and independence,* Reading, Mass, 1995, Perseus Books.
12. Dixon SD et al: Early infant social interaction with parents and strangers, *J Am Acad Child Psychiatry* 20:32, 1981.
13. Brazelton TB, Koslowski B, Main M: The origins of reciprocity: the early mother/infant interaction. In Lewis M, Rosenblum L, editors: *The effect of the infant on its caregiver,* New York, 1974, John Wiley & Sons, p 59.
14. Hill V, Eriks J: Turn-taking in the caregiver-infant interactional system. In Barnard K, editor: *Nursing child assessment satellite training: learning resource manual,* 1980, pp 44-49.
15. Anisfeld E et al: Does infant carrying promote attachment? An experimental study of the effects of increased physical contact on the development attachment, *Child Dev* 61:1617, 1990.
16. Schanler RJ et al: Feeding strategies for premature infants: randomized trial of gastrointestinal priming and tube-feeding method, *Pediatrics* 103:434, 1999.
17. American Academy of Pediatrics: Breastfeeding and the use of human milk, *Pediatrics* 100:1035, 1997.
18. American Academy of Pediatrics: The role of home visitation programs in improving health outcomes for children and families, *Pediatrics* 101:486, 1998.

19. Cooper PH, Murray L: Postnatal depression, *BMJ* 20:316, 1998.
20. Barber V, Skaggs M: *The mother person,* New York, 1975, Schocken Books.
21. Seidman D: Postpartum psychiatric illness: the role of the pediatrician, *Pediatr Rev* 19:128, 1998.
22. Rice RL, Slater CJ: An analysis of group versus individual child health supervision, *Clin Pediatr* 36:685, 1997.
23. American Academy of Pediatrics: The transfer of drugs and other chemicals into human milk, *Pediatrics* 93:137, 1994.
24. Briggs GG, Freeman RK, Yaffe SJ: *Drugs in pregnancy and lactation,* ed 5, Baltimore, 1998, Williams and Wilkins.
25. Zuckerman B, Beardslee WR: Maternal depression: an issue for pediatricians, *Pediatrics* 79:110, 1987.
26. Weisman MM et al: Children of depressed parents, *Arch Gen Psychiatry* 44:847, 1987.
27. Tronick EZ, Als H, Adamson L: The infant's response to entrapment between contradictory messages in face-to-face interaction, *J Child Psychol Psychiatry* 7:1, 1978.
28. Beardslee WR et al: Depression among adolescent mothers: a pilot study, *J Behav Dev Peds* 9:62, 1988.
29. Beck CT: The effects of postpartum depression on child development: a meta-analysis, *Arch Psychiatr Nurs* 12:12, 1998.
30. Dunn J, Kendrick C: *Siblings,* Cambridge, Mass, 1982, Harvard University Press.
31. Dunn J, Kendrick C, MacNamee R: The reaction of first-born children to the birth of a sibling: mothers' reports, *J Child Psychol Psychiatry* 22:1, 1981.
32. Dunn J, Plomin R: *Separate lives: why siblings are so different,* New York, 1990, Basic Books.
33. Schubert HJP, Wagner ME, Shubert D: Child spacing effects: a comparison of institutionalized and normal children, *Dev Behav Pediatrics* 4:262, 1983.
34. Boer F, Dunn J: *Children's sibling relationships: developmental and clinical implications,* Hillsdale, NJ, 1992, Lawrence Erlbaum.
35. Dunn J: Temperament, siblings, and the development of relationships. In Carey WB, McDevitt SC, editors: *Prevention and early intervention: individual differences as risk factors for mental health of children,* New York, 1994, Brunner-Mazel, pp 50-58.
36. Weiss JS: *Your second child,* New York, 1981, Summit Books.
37. Maccoby E: *Patterns of child rearing,* Stanford, Calif, 1976, Stanford University Press.
38. Najonc RB, Markus GB: Birth order and intellectual development, *Psychol Rev* 82:74, 1975.
39. Parke RD: *Fatherhood,* Cambridge, Mass, 1996, Harvard University Press.
40. American Academy of Pediatrics: The pediatrician's role in family support programs, *Pediatrics* 95:781, 1995.
41. Brazelton TB: *Touchpoints: your child's emotional and behavioral development,* Reading, Mass, 1992, Addison-Wesley, pp 12-13.
42. Barr R et al: Carrying as colic therapy: a randomized controlled trial, *Pediatrics* 87:623, 1991.

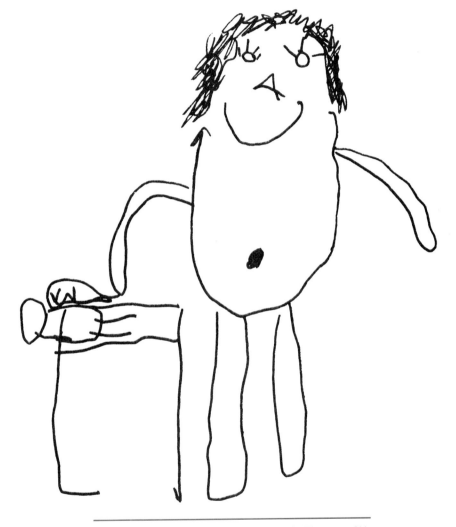

"Mom changing baby's diaper." By Eric Ries, age 6½.

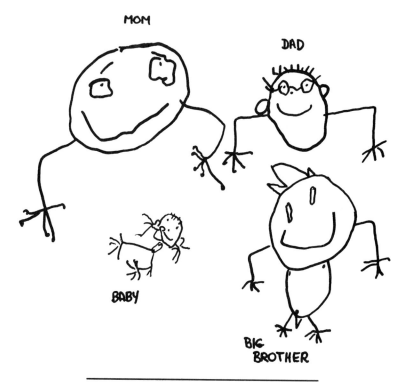

"Our family with our baby." By boy, age 4¾.

GETTING ON TRACK: MONTHS ONE AND TWO

■ **Martin T. Stein**

■ **KEY WORDS**

Psychosocial Deprivation
and Growth Failure
Nutrients and Nurturance
Catch-up Growth
Infant Colic

> *Cody's mother hovered anxiously over the scale as the nurse weighed the baby. She wanted to be sure she got the number right to place in the baby book. She asked the nurse if she should start cereal, especially to get the baby to sleep all night.*

FOCUS OF DEVELOPMENTAL WORK

The period of an infant's life bounded at one end by the first month and at the other by the third month represents an early transitional time. Having adjusted to the neonatal period (including postpartum physiological changes and the new extrauterine environment of family), the second month of life is often a settling-in time for infant and parents. Physical growth takes on a new proportion. As the face fills out, the chin "doubles up," and the thigh folds multiply, the baby's rapid growth seems to organize the parents' attention on growth measurements at this stage. Feeding the baby consumes much of the mother's time, coupled with concerns about the adequacy of the diet. At the same time the moments just before, during, and after meals provide opportunities for optimal social and verbal interactions. By the middle of the second month, the parents recognize the infant's ability to smile in response to their smiles. Mutual gaze becomes a powerful form of social interaction. More frequent periods of visual tracking and the onset of reproducible cooing sounds enhance this milestone. When feeding is managed in a secure setting and the parent is emotionally available for social interactions, physical and psychological growth is assured.

Meeting the infant's nutritional needs in terms of appropriate growth requirements becomes the work of this period of infancy. Developmental setbacks at this time usually affect either the quality of the feeding experience (e.g., infant colic or family emotional conflict) or outcome (e.g., failure to thrive).

GROWTH ASSESSMENT

From birth until the age of 6 months, infants experience the most rapid rate of growth of their life (with the exception of fetal growth). This is true for length, weight, and head circumference (Fig. 8-1). Several decades ago, doubling of birth weight occurred by 5 months of age; today it is not uncommon to record a twofold increase in birth weight before the fourth month. For the breast-feeding infant, successful weight gain from about 2 weeks to 2 to 3 months should approximate 1 ounce per day. Brain and linear growth are also rapid and predictable at this age. Of course, other organ systems are growing and maturing in function simultaneously.

As child health clinicians, we monitor development as a manifestation of ongoing maturation of the central nervous system and the quality of parent-infant interactions. In the same way, physical growth can be monitored as a reflection, at one point in time, of the nutritional adequacy provided the infant and the psychological stability of the environment in which the infant grows.

From studies of emotionally neglected infants in foundling homes, the devastating effect on physical growth from less than optimal tactile, auditory, and visual stimulation has been observed. These infants were given formula (by bottle propping) but were rarely held, spoken to, or engaged visually. The effect was growth failure and an affect that appeared depressed. These infants suffered not only from caloric deprivation,[1] but also from the necessary complement of psychosocial stimulation apparently required for optimal growth.[2] If this state were diagnosed early and remediated psychosocially, these infants could experience catch-up growth and thrive physically and emotionally. Behavioral changes precede by several days the onset of weight gain regardless of the caloric intake.[3]

Psychosocial deprivation and growth failure among infants remind us that adequate physical growth requires sufficient **nutrients and nurturance.** When an infant is growing along the expected curve on a standard growth chart, it provides some degree of objective evidence that both diet and social interactions are adequate. Conversely, early signs of growth failure are clinical signals to assess not only the diet and potential organic illness, but also the manner in which the baby is fed, the temperament of the baby and the mother (see Chapter 2), and the psychosocial state of the family. Growth failure in early infancy has devastating effects on parental feelings of competence. Conversely, good growth vitalizes the whole nurturing environment.

The behavior of the small-for-gestational-age infant or that of the infant who postnatally becomes underweight is altered. These infants remain hyporesponsive and stay irritable or drowsy for prolonged periods. They may show frank gaze aversion, arching, turning away, or marked physiological instability. These characteristics, in turn, induce feelings of incompetency or disengagement in parents. These infants can be unrewarding for parents even beyond the neonatal period.[4]

Standard growth curves should be utilized in clinical practice to assess physical growth. Accurate measurements of weight, length, and head circumference (occipitofrontal measurement) are plotted on these curves at each visit, as shown in Fig. 8-2. Growth curves are of tremendous value in clinical practice. They can reassure an anxious parent about the adequacy of growth. In some sense they are like report cards of parenting adequacy. Clini-

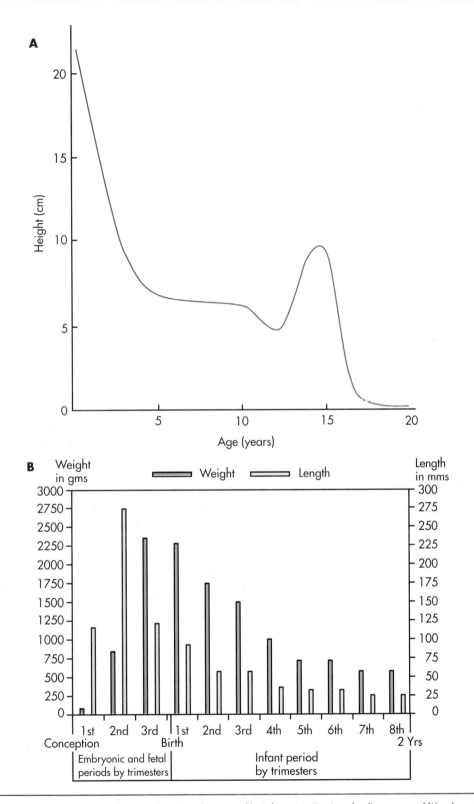

Fig. 8-1 **A,** An incremental curve showing the rate of height gain. During the first years of life, the growth rate is more rapid than in other periods. **B,** Average increment in weight and length by trimesters. (From Valadian I, Porter D: *Physical growth and development: from conception to maturity,* Boston, Little Brown & Co, 1977.)

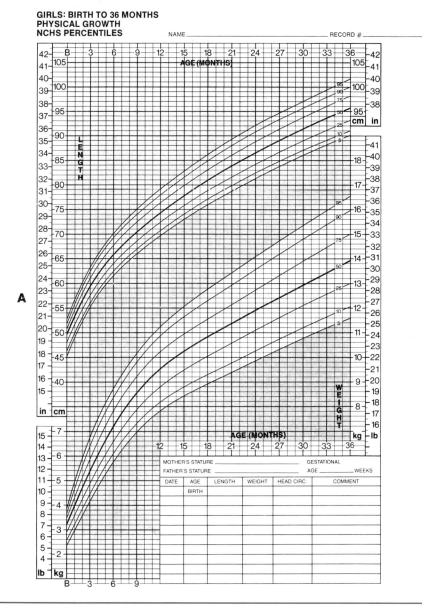

Fig. 8-2 A standard growth curve: birth to 36 months. **A,** Length and weight. (From Center for Health Statistics Report No 3, Supplement NCHS Growth Charts, 1976. Hyattsville, Md, Public Health Administration, 1976. Department of Health, Education and Welfare No [HRA] 76-110.)

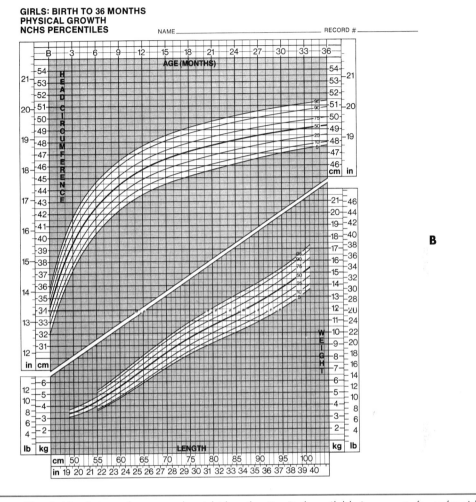

Fig. 8-2, cont'd   B, Head circumference and weight-length ratio. Both available in separate forms for girls and boys.

cians must appreciate, however, that physical growth measurements at any one point generate a bell-shaped curve, with 5% of the normal population heavier, longer, lighter, or shorter than the extremes of the charts. The infant's measurements at one time are not as significant as the rate of growth over a period of time (i.e., the curve of that infant's growth). In this way, cumulative measurements over several office visits are usually more revealing than a single measurement. The stature, weight, and head circumference of the parents may also be helpful in interpreting the infant's growth after 6 months of age.

NORMAL VARIATIONS OF GROWTH IN EARLY INFANCY
Postpartum Weight Loss

Extracellular water loss may account for 8% to 10% of weight reduction from birth weight. Some weight loss results from the conversion of brown fat to glucose that is needed as an energy source. Generally it is greater in breast-fed than in formula-fed babies and in infants born of toxemic mothers. Also, breast-fed babies may take longer to regain the weight (usually 1 week for those infants receiving formula, often 2 weeks for breast-fed babies). Premature babies require even longer periods to regain their birth weight; the smaller the birth weight, the longer the period of regaining. Special growth curves for the preterm infant are available. Most full-term, breast-fed babies surpass their birth weight by 14 days of age.

Intercurrent Illness

A brief period of illness in early infancy (e.g., gastroenteritis) is often associated with both anorexia and an increase in metabolic requirements that yield either a plateau in the growth curve or weight loss. In addition, a breast infection, a systemic illness, or postpartum depression in a lactating woman may have an adverse effect on infant growth. These maternal conditions may cause painful feedings (breast infection), decreased milk production (maternal hypothyroidism), or limited interest in nursing (depression). Too rapid a weight loss for the lactating woman means that she may not be sustaining milk production between meals. The effect on infant growth is the same—as the baby consumes less breast milk for any reason, the supply declines and infant growth diminishes.

An experienced mother (emergency room nurse, second child) brought her 3-month-old breast-fed daughter to the office for a health supervision visit. Following a normal pregnancy and delivery, the child had grown appropriately at the 75th percentile at the 6-week examination. At the current visit, careful measurement revealed no weight gain in 2 months with normal linear and head circumference growth rates. In fact, the child looked well; physical features and developmental milestones were normal. Observation of nursing in the office confirmed an adequate and sustained sucking pattern.

Social history revealed that the father, previously very involved with the family, was out of town for 6 weeks on business. An 18-month-old toddler added to the burden of child care, and the mother was not sleeping well. With normal complete blood count, urinalysis, electrolytes, urea nitrogen, and serum glutamic pyruvate transaminase laboratory determinations in the baby, the mother was instructed to supplement her breast milk with formula and to ask friends for occasional assistance with child care.

At a follow-up visit 1 week later, the mother reported that her sister, a second-year medical student, had remarked that "your face looks like you have an endocrine problem." Myxedema was noted by her internist, and Hashimoto's thyroiditis with hypothyroidism was diagnosed. On thyroid replacement therapy, the mother's milk production apparently increased and the baby thrived.

Postpartum thyroid dysfunction occurs in 5% of women and is vastly underdiagnosed and treated. The onset of symptoms may be subtle and overlap substantially with "overloaded mother syndrome." The pediatric clinician may be the only one to see the mother during this time.

Catch-Up Growth

After a period of growth failure, a healthy infant has the marvelous capacity to accelerate growth rate during recovery. This is seen especially in the weight curve, which is most vulnerable to transient caloric depressions and most adaptable by dramatic **catch-up growth.** Depressions in linear growth in infancy testify to the chronicity of the problem, thyroid disease, or long-standing organic illness (Fig. 8-3). Premordial (before birth) growth failure of a severe nature may not catch up; these children will remain small. This is particularly true of those infants with reduction in length for gestational age.

In a healthy premature infant, postpartum catch-up growth is expected to take place (Fig. 8-4). Growth parameters in this population should be corrected for the degree of prematurity (i.e., postconceptual age for the first 2 years or up to 3 years in infants born at less than 1500 g) to better assess growth velocity and relative gains in height, weight, and head circumference.

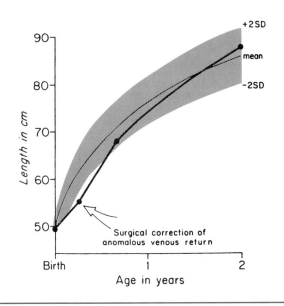

Fig. 8-3 Catch-up growth following corrective surgery in a child with congenital heart lesion associated with growth failure. (From Smith DW: *Growth and its disorders,* Philadelphia, 1977, WB Saunders. Used by permission.)

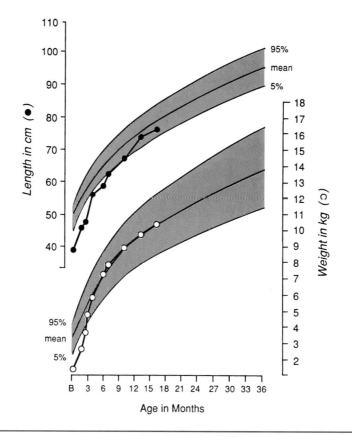

Fig. 8-4 Postnatal growth curve of a 32-week appropriate-for-gestational-age premature infant. The curve demonstrates rapid catch-up growth in a healthy preterm infant.

Too Rapid Weight Gain

Many appropriately nourished infants in the first 6 months of life demonstrate rapid weight gains, often outstripping linear growth. They may appear chubby. Most of these infants, as long as they are not obviously overfed, will decrease their growth rate and "find" their genetic curve between 6 and 12 months of life (Fig. 8-5).[5] If the infant in this category is breast fed every 3 to 4 hours, with longer periods at night (or if formula fed, the baby is consuming no more than 32 oz per day), it is appropriate not to change the diet and to reassess growth after 6 months. Even in many developing-nation populations, these young infants are very "fat" by our expectations, but eventually demonstrate a diminished rate of weight gain. This may be more normal than U.S. growth charts reflect.

Excessive weight gain is usually secondary to an intake of calories that exceeds normal growth and metabolic needs. The etiology of caloric excess may have its source in the parent (providing too much for a variety of reasons) or infant.

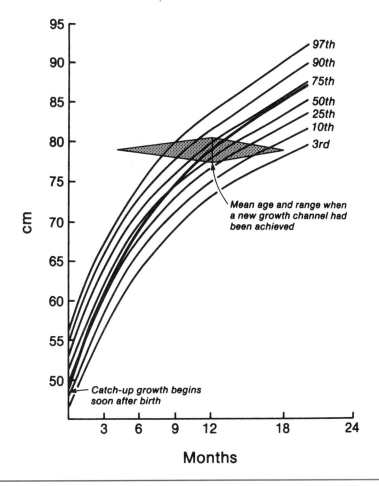

Fig. 8-5   Average linear growth of 18 middle-class, normal babies who had been below the 10th percentile for length at full-term birth but achieved the 50th percentile or better by the age of 2 years, by which time their stature correlated well to that of their parents. The catch-up in linear growth began soon after birth, and a new channel of growth had been achieved by 4 to 18 months. (From Smith DW et al: *J Pediatr* 89:225, 1976. Used by permission.)

Juanita, a single mom with little experience or support, brought in her daughter at 6 months with head still covered, cradled in her arms. The baby's hands were covered with mitts, and she was dressed in a gown tied at the bottom. The baby weighed 22 pounds and appeared pale. As soon as she whimpered, Juanita put a bottle in her mouth.

Juanita was not aware that her baby would enjoy more open space to move and explore. Nor was she sensitive to different reasons for crying. Focused counseling about these issues resulted in varied maternal responses to crying and a more appropriate rate of growth. Babies rated by their mothers as temperamentally difficult and especially negative gain significantly more weight for height than other babies.[6] These babies are probably fed more as a way to quiet their high activity level.

LANDMARKS AND CLINICAL PEARLS OF GROWTH ASSESSMENT

The following are growth landmarks in the first 6 months:

- *A full-term newborn,* determined by gestational age examination (38 to 42 weeks), who weighs less than 2500 g or is less than 45 cm in length is small and has intrauterine growth retardation. Linear growth depression reflects second-trimester growth failure. Absolute or relative underweight babies have usually had late gestation losses.
- *Small-for-gestational-age babies* who have the genetic capacity to catch up to the normal range usually show accelerated growth in the first 6 months. Failure to show catch-up growth in the first 6 months usually means that growth will continue at a slow rate.
- *Following the reacquisition of birth weight,* most babies will grow at approximately 1 oz per day. Weight increases much greater than 1 oz per day often are associated with overweight infants or those undergoing catch-up growth. Premature infants (less than 38 weeks corrected age) may sustain weight gain velocities consistent with expected intrauterine growth, higher than those of the infants beyond 40 weeks conceptual age. Weight gain that is less than 0.5 oz per day usually is inadequate.
- A *head circumference* of less than 32 cm in a full-term newborn represents microcephaly; more than 38 cm represents macrocephaly.
- *Head circumference measurements* in the first 6 months of life usually conform to the following schedule: birth to 2 months, 1 cm per 2 weeks; 3 to 6 months, 1 cm per month.
- *Breast-fed infants who have a decelerated growth rate* after 1 month should draw attention to maternal diet and rapid maternal weight loss during this time (i.e., dieting, illness, or strenuous exercise).
- Occasionally, a baby with a *head circumference* in the usual or upper range at birth rapidly crosses percentile lines in the first few months and is at or above the 95th percentile. When this curve is maintained in the absence of any evidence for increased intracranial pressure, it usually represents familial macrocephaly, a benign condition. Measurement of parental head circumference will suggest the diagnosis.

SLEEP PATTERNS

Sleep-awake cycles after the first month are highly variable and dependent on the infant's temperament, satisfaction with feedings, and the parents' response to periodic awakenings. Early introduction of rice cereal before bedtime does not extend sleep time.[7] This period represents a transitional time between neonatal sleeping, which is characterized by shorter multiple sleep periods and longer sleep time each day, and the more organized central nervous system maturation after the third month, in which each sleep period is longer (see Chapter 9, Figs. 9-1 and 9-2). The 2 standard deviation range of maximum longest sleep time at 6 weeks of age varies from 3 to 11 hours. No wonder parents of infants with shorter sleep times seem bewildered when sharing their infants' nighttime experience with other parents!

Although a child's individual biological determinants dictate most of the variability in sleep patterns at this age, signals from the environment mediate a powerful effect. At as early as 10 days of life, infants who roomed in with their mothers slept longer at night than did those cared for in the hospital nursery.[8]

Infants' and mothers' sleeping together in the same bed bring several potential benefits, such as increased total sleep time for baby and mother, increased frequency and duration of breast feeding at night, and increased sensitivity to each other as indicated by briefly arousing to each other's movement or sounds.[9] The sleeping environment can also have a detrimental effect for infant well-being; bedsharing without breast feeding and combined with maternal smoking increases the risk of sudden infant death syndrome.[10] Other potential environmental risks of bedsharing are a soft mattress, a couch where the infant can become trapped against the back and fall into the crevice created by a seat cushion, the baby's head being covered with a blanket, and the baby's slipping between a mattress and bed frame or headboard. Parents who bedshare should be provided with anticipatory guidance about these safety issues. In many cultures, both in the United States and in other countries, bedsharing with a parent (and often with other family members) is a common practice.[11,12]

Clinical studies suggest that the way a parent responds to an infant at the time of sleep induction and nighttime awakenings sets long-term patterns. Babies who are settled in a crib while partially awake learn to soothe themselves to sleep compared with those infants who are always nursed or rocked into a deep sleep before being placed into the crib.[13,14] Associations with falling asleep may be learned at this early time. If infants experience falling asleep alone in the crib, they can reestablish that experience at predictable times of night awakening and soothe themselves back to a sleep state.

Since 1992, following review of several epidemiological studies, the American Academy of Pediatrics has recommended that healthy infants be placed on their sides or backs to sleep. The data that supported this position pointed to a dramatic decrease in the incidence of sudden infant death syndrome (SIDS) associated with the "back to sleep" position.[15] Following the new recommendation, the prevalence of prone sleeping dropped from 70% in 1992 to 24% in 1996. In addition, the SIDS rate in the United States decreased by almost 50%.[16] Although side and back positions are associated with a decrease in SIDS, the back position is optimal. Firm bedding, breast feeding, and avoidance of smoking also are important in SIDS reduction. Babies sleeping on their backs need to spend awake time in the prone position to strengthen arms and shoulder musculature.[17]

INFANT COLIC

Parents are confronted with intermittent periods of fussiness in their babies at various times during the initial few months of life. Most parents describe a period of manageable irritability beginning at about 2 weeks of age, peaking between the first and second month, and disappearing by 3 to 4 months. Typically the fussy behavior begins in the late afternoon and resolves in the early part of the evening. Most parents find that if they hold, position, gently rock, or feed the infant, the fussy periods resolve into a comfortable sleep.

The predictability and inevitability of these events suggest that such diurnal behavior is part of normal development, probably mediated by the central nervous system. The infant wears out (as do parents!) over the course of the day, becoming increasingly unable to modulate responses to environmental stimuli. **Infant colic** occurs in babies who are breast fed and those who are bottle fed. Boys and girls are affected equally. Premature infants may experience this behavior somewhat later in proportion to their conceptual age and may have this irritability extend to a later age.

When these behavioral outbursts are either more intense or longer in duration (i.e., not limited to the latter part of the day), the term *infant colic* is used. That colic is a more severe form of the diurnal behavior seen in the majority of infants is clear. Why certain infants at this particular age (2 to 3 weeks through 3 to 4 months) express this behavior with more intensity is unclear. Individual temperamental factors seem to be important. The intensive, hyperresponsive, somewhat hypertonic infant can be spotted in the neonatal period as a likely candidate for colic. Before a diagnosis of infant colic is made, the clinician should have an appreciation for normal crying at this age. In a study of 80 infants from middle-class families, crying lasted about 2 hours daily at 2 weeks and progressed to nearly 3 hours daily by 6 weeks in normal infants. It then gradually tapered to about 1 hour daily by 3 months (Fig. 8-6). During this interval, most crying occurred in the evening.[18] With this normal pattern in mind, Wessel's definition[19] of infant colic is helpful. It says that "colic occurs when an infant,

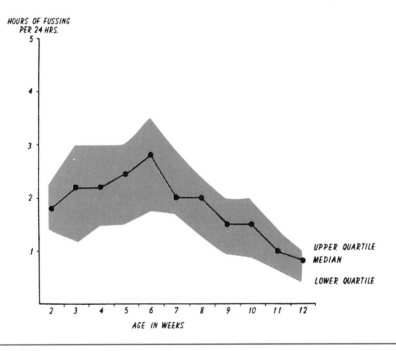

Fig. 8-6 Distribution of total crying time among 80 infants from 2 to 12 weeks old; data derived from daily crying diaries recorded by mothers. (From Brazelton TB: *Pediatrics* 29:582, 1962. Used by permission.)

otherwise healthy and well fed, has paroxysms of irritability, fussiness, or crying lasting for a total of more 3 hours a day occurring on more than 3 days in any 1 week."[20]

Many theories have been suggested to explain early infant colic. It was once thought to reflect maternal anxiety, but it is now clear that although severe colic may produce anxiety in parents, most cases are not caused by an overly anxious parent. Humans (especially women) are biologically programmed to respond to infant cries regardless of individual personality differences; lack of success in calming the infant is experienced as failure. However, high-strung parents tend to give birth to high-strung infants. Colicky infants are born, not made.

Our understanding of infant temperament may provide some insight into the behavior of colicky infants. Temperament refers to an individual's behavioral style of reactivity to external events or stimuli (see Chapter 2). The normal spectrum of infant temperaments is broad. The behavior of babies described with a low sensory threshold and high intensity is similar to those with colic. Babies rated by a parent at 2 weeks of age with a "difficult" temperament were more likely to have longer and more frequent episodes of crying at 6 weeks of age.[21]

Perhaps colic is an early infant behavior response that occurs when a baby with a susceptible, innate temperament is cared for by a parent who is less responsive (or overresponsive) to the infant's behavioral cues and is unable to organize the caretaking environment effectively.[6] In this context, colic is an interactional phenomenon between a baby and a parent. The acoustical characteristics and duration of an infant's cry may be viewed as a graded signal to which a parent may react with a nurturing response (relief of the infant's distress) or a nonnurturing, avoidant response (relief of the parent's distress).[22]

Because these babies are observed to press their flexed hips against the abdomen during the crying spree and then pass audible flatus at the termination of the episode, it has been suggested that these babies have a form of intestinal dysmotility that produces segmental air-trapping secondary to autonomic dysfunction. Supporting this theory is documentation of lower colonic dysmotility in some infants. Another piece of supportive evidence is that early infant colic resolves in most cases by the end of the third month of life, which correlates chronologically with several behavioral aspects reflecting central nervous system maturation. For example, babies at 4 months of age show more organized sleep-wake cycles; several primitive reflexes disappear; and electroencephalographic (EEG) tracings reveal greater organization. It seems reasonable to assume that higher levels of central organization would be accompanied by maturation of the more primitive autonomic nervous system that, in turn, might modify and regulate gastrointestinal tract motility. Research in the psychobiology of stress is beginning to describe links between different levels of reactivity and physiological responses in the cardiovascular, immunological, and neuroendocrine systems.[22] Some circulating hormones (motilin) and neurotransmitters (serotonin) that cause enterospasm have been found to be increased in colicky babies. This conceptual framework suggests that colicky infants may tend to have hyperresponsive gastrointestinal tracts that mirror their behavioral response to external stimuli.

Whatever the cause, infant colic (also known as 3-month colic) resolves by the end of the third month in almost every case. When the colic is mild to moderate, simple measures (discussed later) suffice as the parents learn to modify the behavior through various manipulations. More severe cases of colic require special attention from the child's clinician. If allowed to continue, these difficult periods of crying are taxing on parents (as well as siblings and grandparents). The potential for disrupting ongoing attachment behavior between infant and parents exists. In this context, moderate to severe colic represents an interactional problem and requires astute clinical attention. Box 8-1 illustrates that crying patterns are culturally dependent and are related to fundamental child-rearing principles.

| **BOX 8-1** | **CULTURAL DETERMINANTS OF CRYING IN EARLY INFANCY** |

All normal human infants cry, although they vary a great deal in how much. A mysterious and still unexplained phenomenon is that crying tends to increase in the first few weeks of life, peaks in the second or third month, and then decreases. Some babies in the United States cry so much during the peak period—often in excess of 3 hours a day—and seem so difficult to soothe that parents come to doubt their nurturing skills or begin to fear that their offspring is suffering from a painful disease. Some mothers discontinue nursing and switch to bottle feeding because they believe their breast milk is insufficiently nutritious and that their infants are always hungry. In extreme cases the crying may provoke physical abuse, sometimes even precipitating the infant's death.

A look at another culture, the !Kung San hunter-gatherers of southern Africa, provides us with an opportunity to see whether caregiving strategies have any effect on infant crying. Both the !Kung San and Western infants escalate their crying during the early weeks of life, with a similar peak at 2 or 3 months. A comparison of Dutch, American, and !Kung San infants shows that the number of individual crying episodes is virtually identical. What differs is their length. !Kung San infants cry about half as long as Western babies. This implies that caregiving can influence only some aspects of crying, such as duration.

What is particularly striking about child rearing among the !Kung San is that infants are in constant contact with a caregiver; they are carried or held most of the time, are usually in an upright position, and are breast fed about four times an hour for 1 to 2 minutes at a time. Furthermore, the mother almost always responds to the smallest cry or fret within 10 seconds.

I believe that crying was adaptive for our ancestors. As seen in the contemporary !Kung San, crying probably elicited a quick response and thus consisted of frequent but relatively short episodes. This pattern helped keep an adult close to provide adequate nutrition, as well as to protect the child from predators. I have also argued that crying helped an infant forge a strong attachment with the mother and, because new pregnancies are delayed by the prolongation of frequent nursing, secure more of her caregiving resources.

In the United States, where the threat of predation has receded and adequate nutrition is usually available even without breast feeding, crying may be less adaptive. In any case, caregiving in the United States may be viewed as a cultural experiment in which the infant is relatively more separated—and separable—from the mother, both in terms of frequency of contact and actual distance.

The Western strategy is advantageous when the mother's employment outside of the home and away from the baby is necessary to sustain family resources. But the trade-off seems to be an increase in the length of crying bouts.

From Barr RG: *Natural History* 106:47, 1997.

DATA GATHERING
Observations

As you enter the examining room, observe the interaction between infant and mother (and father, when present). If the infant is being held, observe the comfort of the mother in handling the baby.

- Does the infant seem at ease, tense, unsure of self?
- At the same time, observe the baby's response. Does the infant cuddle easily? Is the baby tense or responsive to mother?
- Do the infant's posture and position appear tense with an increase in extension behaviors?
- Is there evidence of visual engagement between mother and infant?
- How does the mother talk to the baby—rhythmically and quietly or erratically and with a harsh voice?

If the baby is lying on the examining table, similar observations can be made. Does the mother maintain contact with the baby, by touching the infant or by visual contact? Alternatively, it may be important to be sensitive to the situation in which the infant has been left alone in a corner of the examining table while the mother is seated away from the infant. In this case, the clinician might want to consider if the mother is anxious about the examination, overwhelmed by the office procedures, insecure about her mothering abilities, or depressed. Careful assessment of the initial visual and verbal interactions with the mother may yield clues about how she is feeling about herself and about the infant.

The accumulation of these observations will assist the clinician in assessing the individual style, quality, and intensity of the bond between mother and infant; when the father is present, it is remarkable to observe the way in which his presence alters the mother-infant attachment behaviors. In a sense, the family's style of interactional behaviors is available to you for clinical observation at this examination. These observations attain a heightened level of importance when viewed in terms of the requirements for satisfactory growth, particularly in early infancy, in other words, an emotionally nourishing bond between the young infant and its parents.

History

Table 8-1 presents questions that should be asked in taking the history and observations that should be noted during the physical examination.

MANAGEMENT AND GUIDANCE
Undernutrition

Growth failure at this age usually represents insufficient caloric intake. In breast-fed infants, problems in latching on or continuously ineffective sucking are not uncommon; the correct diagnosis is usually apparent from the history of feeding behavior. Observing the baby feed (either by direct observation in office or from a videotape recorded at home) may be helpful to the mother and to the diagnostician. Improving the mechanics of nursing often resolves the problem, such as suggesting pillow support of the baby or mother's arm, helping the mother to encourage the infant to latch on effectively, or

TABLE 8-1 ■ History Taking and Examination

History Taking	
Clinician's Question or Action	**Objective**
How is nursing (or feeding when baby is formula fed) going?	Listen carefully to response to this open-ended question; assess mother's comfort with nursing; is she self-assured or does she show evidence of insecurity?
Does the baby seem satisfied at the end of a feeding? How do you feel when you are nursing?	Assess *maternal* satisfaction with nursing.
How often and for how long do you feed the baby? How do you know when the baby is hungry?	Assess the mother's settling-in with baby's needs and individual rhythms, as well as an estimation of the amount of milk each day.
Tell me about your own diet (for nursing mothers). How much weight have you lost?	Assess lactating mother's diet; mothers who are back to their prepregnant weight at this time may have difficulty sustaining milk supply through the anticipated increase in caloric requirement at about 2 to 3 months.
How do you manage nighttime feedings? How often and for how long is the baby fed . . . In a chair or in bed? Are you getting enough sleep?	Assess feeding regularity and schedule. Is the mother sleep deprived?
When baby is formula fed, ask, "How do you prepare the formula?"	Assess amount of milk at each feeding (calculate daily intake); assess quantity of formula and appropriate concentration.
Can you describe your baby's personality? What is the baby like most of the time?	Assess the infant's temperament and style and the mother's attentiveness and awareness about these aspects of the baby's development.
Does the baby have a fussy time during most days? Can you describe it to me?	Assess colic-like behavior.

TABLE 8-1 ■ History Taking and Examination—cont'd

History Taking	
Clinician's Question or Action	**Objective**
Do you think that your baby cries longer than most infants? What do you do when the baby cries?	Help parent adapt to periods of difficult infant behavior; explain the expected amount of crying.
In the presence of infant colic, "What do you think causes these episodes of crying?" When appropriate, "What does your husband think?"	Assess parent's explanatory model for the behavior; may give clue to most effective therapeutic suggestion for particular family

Physical Examination	
Obtain accurate measurements of weight, length, and head circumference plotted on standard growth curves.	Assess adequacy of growth (vs. overnourished or undernourished infant); demonstrate rates of growth on chart to parent.
Complete physical examination.	Although always important at a health supervision visit, performing a careful physical examination while demonstrating normal findings is particularly important to parents with a colicky baby at this age.
Assess skin texture and turgor, fat folds, and state of hydration.	Evaluate nutrition.
To determine infant temperament, observe the baby at rest on the examining table and during physical examination maneuvers; when weighed and immediately following the diphtheria-pertussis-tetanus (DPT) immunization, infant temperament in response to stress can be observed.	Is this an easy baby? An overly active baby? How did the baby respond after the DPT injection? How did the mother or father respond?
If colic appears likely from the mother's history, rule out during routine physical examination the following: inguinal hernia, corneal abrasion, otitis media, or a thread wrapped tightly around a finger or toe.	Note: These are uncommon causes of paroxysmal crying at this age.

pointing out that it is normal for the baby to suck vigorously, followed by a brief rest period before sucking is resumed.

An insufficient milk supply may be the problem in some nursing mothers. Breast milk insufficiency may be caused by the following:

- Inadequate amount of fluid in the mother's diet—usually a minimum of 2 qt per day is required; more may be needed if mother is exercising moderately.
- Anxiety or depression—oxytocin suppression may result in inhibition of the let-down reflex, which may diminish availability of milk, or prolactin secretion may inhibit milk production. Mild to moderate postpartum depression (see Chapter 7) is usually resolving around this time. Reassurance about the baby's development, coupled with frequent weight checks in the office, may be helpful. For the more severely stressed nursing mother, an appropriate mental health referral, more active involvement of the father (or other member of the extended family), or, *rarely*, formula supplementation may be appropriate.
- Sleep deprivation—observe for signs of fatigue, such as a tired appearance, listlessness, or irritability. Always ask, "Are you getting enough sleep?" Maternal sleep deprivation is a common primary or secondary cause of milk insufficiency and growth failure.
- Excessive weight loss—from dieting, excessive exercise, or depression. Addressing the issue with compassion and knowledge may be sufficient to help the mother address the problem by reorganizing her life-style and focusing on her diet or sleep-wake schedule. Reassurance about the baby's development, coupled with frequent weight checks in the office, may be helpful.

A comprehensive assessment of undernutrition in the breast-fed infant includes a detailed review of the feeding schedule, an evaluation of infant behavior and appearance (see Box 7-1), and examination of the mother's breast for signs of breast engorgement and sore, cracked nipples. An objective office measure of the yield of breast milk during a single feeding time is available (Box 8-2).

Formula-fed babies may not be receiving enough milk at each feeding or may be fed too infrequently, or the milk may be inappropriately overdiluted. Corrective measures are simple once the problem is recognized.

With either breast-fed or formula-fed infants who are undernourished, it may be revealing and often therapeutic to observe the mother feeding the child in the office. Positioning of the baby, maternal-infant eye contact, comfort with feeding, and quality of sucking mechanism are important characteristics that can be observed. Interactional difficulties can be assessed and corrected.

Less commonly, growth failure at this age is secondary to an organic disorder, either one apparent during the newborn period or one that surfaces during the history or physical examination. Laboratory assessment is seldom indicated at this age until after the interactional, mechanical, and nutritional problems discussed earlier are considered thoroughly.

Overfeeding

If the baby's weight curve is greater than 2 standard deviations above the mean, the first step is to repeat the measurements to determine accuracy (especially length). If the data are correct and the baby looks obese, carefully review the feeding pattern of a typical day.

BOX 8-2	OFFICE ASSESSMENT OF UNDERNOURISHED BREAST-FEEDING INFANTS

Maternal Breast Evaluation

Assessment of breast feeding should include historical information about the maternal breasts. The breasts should be inspected whenever risk factors are elicited or when breast-feeding adequacy is in doubt.

Lactogenesis, or the onset of copious milk secretion, typically occurs 2 to 4 days postpartum. Most mothers have no difficulty recognizing the telltale signs that their milk has come in, including increase in breast size, fullness, and firmness. Rarely does lactogenesis fail to occur and infant supplementation become essential.

The leading preventable cause of insufficient milk is failure to accomplish regular, effective milk emptying once postpartum breast engorgement occurs. Many cases of insufficient lactation are associated with a maternal history of unrelieved breast engorgement during the first week. When an infant is unable to empty the breasts effectively, a rental grade electric breast pump can preserve a mother's milk supply while efforts are made to improve her baby's breast feeding.

Once milk comes in, mothers should report that their breasts feel fuller before feedings and softer after nursing. Perceptible pre- and post-feed breast changes suggest that milk is being made and transferred to the infant.

Most women experience slight nipple discomfort at the beginning of feedings during the first few days of nursing. However, *severe nipple pain, pain lasting throughout feedings, or pain persisting beyond one week postpartum is atypical and suggests that the baby is not positioned correctly at the breast.* Improper infant latch-on not only causes sore nipples, but it impairs milk flow and leads to diminished milk supply and inadequate infant intake.

Objective Measures of Milk Yield and Infant Intake

The common practice of using clinical cues to estimate milk consumption during breast feeding can be highly inaccurate. Several techniques are available to more precisely estimate maternal milk yield and infant milk consumption.

Infant feeding test weights represent a noninvasive, accurate method of measuring infant milk intake during a breast-feeding session. The infant is weighed under the same conditions (identically clothed) before and after nursing. The prefeed weight (in grams) subtracted from the postfeed weight equals the volume of milk consumed (in millimeters). A simplified rule-of-thumb for normal milk consumption in breast-fed infants between 2 weeks and 2 months of age is about 1 oz of milk (28.5 ml) per hour. A relatively inexpensive, portable, user-friendly, commercial scale is available for performing accurate infant feeding test weights in the home or office.

Another option for estimating a mother's milk production is to use *a rental grade electric breast pump to empty the breasts at a usual feeding time.* The volume of milk expressed approximates the quantity of milk available to the infant at that feeding. A pump may remove milk either more or less effectively than the baby, affecting the accuracy of pumped volumes in predicting milk yield or infant intake.

Modified from Neifert M: *Early assessment of the breastfeeding infant,* Marianne Neifert, MD, Lactation Program, 1719 E. 19th Avenue, Denver, CO 80218.

Continued

BOX 8-2	OFFICE ASSESSMENT OF UNDERNOURISHED BREAST-FEEDING INFANTS—cont'd

Objective Measures of Milk Yield and Infant Intake—cont'd

Beginning around 2 weeks postpartum, *the oxytocin-mediated let-down reflex becomes well-conditioned, and mothers begin to experience the sensations associated with milk ejection.* Mothers typically report a "tingling," "pins-and-needles," or "tightening" sensation in their breasts in conjunction with spraying milk. The sensations usually begin shortly after the infant starts sucking, but the reflex also can be triggered by hearing one's baby cry. Let-down usually is more dramatic in women with abundant milk, while the response is often blunted in those with diminished supplies. The let-down response can be inhibited temporarily by adrenalin.

Inspection of the maternal breast can reveal lactation risk factors, such as inverted nipples or surgical scars. Periareolar incisions for cosmetic or diagnostic breast surgery may sever lactiferous ducts and impair milk drainage. Abnormal breast development and lack of prenatal changes may be associated with insufficient lactation.

Strategies for Improving Inadequate Breastfeeding

Correct any problems identified with breast-feeding technique or scheduling. Improve the infant's positioning at the breast, increase the frequency of nursings if appropriate, and ensure that infant take both breasts at each feeding.

Prescribe a rental-grade electric breast pump to augment the breast stimulation and emptying provided by the infant. Instruct the mother to pump her breasts simultaneously (using a double collection system) for 10 to 15 minutes immediately after nursings. Residual milk expressed by pump should be used to supplement the infant's sucking.

Ensure that the infant receives adequate nutrition. Use objective measures of breast milk intake (infant feeding test weights or pumped milk volumes) to estimate the quantity of required formula supplement. For malnourished babies, expect rapid catch-up weight gain, usually 2 oz a day for several days, then 1 oz a day.

Provide close infant follow-up and supervision of the feeding plan. Taper supplements *only* if objective measures confirm that maternal milk supply has increased. All too often, infant weight falters again because supplements arbitrarily are discontinued after initial weight gain is achieved.

Have the mother continue pumping after feedings until the baby has weaned from all supplements and is gaining adequate weight with exclusive breastfeeding. Then instruct mother to begin tapering and pumping sessions over the course of a week or two.

Be willing to collaborate with the breast-feeding referral sources in your community to help your patients overcome their breast-feeding problems. Physicians should retain their role as principal coordinator of their patients' care, while utilizing the specialized services of breast-feeding counselors and lactation centers. Other valuable resources include pump rental depots, telephone advice lines, WIC agencies, and mother-to-mother support groups such as La Leche League.

A breast-fed infant who is 1 month old is put to the breast every 2 hours (each time she cries) for at least 12 feedings per day, each lasting 10 to 20 minutes.

Diagnosis: Overfeeding is typically the problem. However, some vigorous infants, who are growing at an appropriate rate, may be frequent feeders without need for intervention.

Therapy: Teach mother other forms of soothing behavior, such as pacifier (after nursing is well established; usually no sooner than 2 weeks of life), swaddling, rocking, and swinging. Explain the nature and adaptive value of two different sucking behaviors—nutritive and nonnutritive. Some babies seem to want to suck more frequently; a pacifier is very helpful in these cases. The mother may need to be taught to respond to other needs in her infant (e.g., boredom) with an expanded range of interactions. Assessment of the infant's temperament and the "goodness of fit" (see Chapter 2) between baby and mother may offer clues to alternative parenting responses during nursing.

A breast-fed infant is nursed approximately every 3 to 4 hours for 10 minutes on each side at most feedings.

Diagnosis: This apparently overweight baby is probably not being overfed. Her appetite is vigorous, and she looks big. If her length is also at or above the 95th percentile, her weight may be appropriate for stature. If not, most of these breast-fed infants will find their genetic growth curve (usually closer to their length curve) after 6 months.

Therapy: Reassurance with education about normal growth. The growth chart is an effective visual aid for parents in this situation.

A formula-fed infant is consuming 40 to 45 oz each day; at 2 months she is given the bottle every 2 to 3 hours.

Diagnosis: Overfeeding.

Therapy: Limit formula to 32 oz a day. Explain baby's nutritional requirements to the mother along with your concerns regarding obesity. Review concept of nutritive and nonnutritive sucking. Suggest pacifier and other tactile soothing techniques. If the baby requires more than 32 oz of fluid a day, suggest a water supplement or, alternatively, diluting one bottle each day with water to yield 16 oz from 8 oz of formula.

Night Feedings

If you discover that the baby is awakening every 3 hours through the night, inquire how the parents respond. Parents who pick up the infant at the moment he awakes may be encouraging a long-term pattern of frequent nighttime awakenings. Point out that even a 2-month-old infant can often settle down unaided when given an opportunity. A short, fussy period will not be harmful. If necessary, a loving pat on the back while the baby remains in the crib may be sufficient to calm the child to sleep. New parents need the reassurance that brief crying periods will be neither emotionally nor physically detrimental to their baby. They will be rewarded by the knowledge that a simple behavioral intervention, initiated and sustained by them, can bring about more restful nights for the baby and parents. Parents can be taught that a young baby's cry for hunger can be distinguished from one associated with pain or the fussy cry characteristic of sleep transitions. As they learn to recognize their own infant's different cries, parents feel more comfortable letting a 2-month-old fuss for a few minutes before self-soothing behaviors bring a return to sleep. On the other hand, mothers who are gone during the day and are committed to sustaining breast feeding may choose to respond to these night wiggles and nurse the baby at that time. This is a parental choice.

Supplemental Bottles

At this stage, many mothers who are nursing successfully choose to continue full-time nursing until after 6 to 12 months, as now recommended,[23] when the infant can sit and learn to drink from a cup. For a variety of reasons, other mothers may choose to supplement breast feeding with either expressed breast milk or formula in a bottle. The mother's returning to work or school, a plan to wean before the infant's readiness to use a cup, the wish to have an occasional evening or afternoon out without the baby, or a desire to plan for an emergency are some reasons women may have for supplementation at this time. It may be helpful to ask the nursing mother about her plans as they affect nursing. Helping her to choose between expressed milk and formula, the clinician can play the role of educator rather than decision maker. When bottle supplementation is desired, waiting until after 5 or 6 weeks ensures the establishment of an adequate milk supply and gives the infant and mother enough time to form the psychological attachment and mechanical know-how to safeguard the future of nursing. *What To Expect in the First Year*[24] is an outstanding book for parents. It provides detailed guidelines for supplementation, expression, and storage of breast milk.

COLIC ("PAROXYSMAL FUSSING")

In treating the infant with colic, the clinician should follow these steps:
1. Begin with *reassurance,* when appropriate, that the findings of the baby's physical examination are normal. Narrating your normal findings for the parents as you examine each body part may be particularly reassuring, such as "the intestinal examination is normal; the bowels feel fine, and all the organs in the tummy feel as they should."
2. Discuss *"fussiness" and crying at this age in terms of normal patterns* (see earlier section). A parent with a colicky baby may find it helpful to see the infant as a variation of what is expected rather than as someone who is abnormal.[25] Showing a parent Fig. 8-6 will support the concept of normal variation for some doubting parents.
3. Assist in the *alleviation of parental anxieties* that may be exacerbating the paroxysms of crying. Suggesting a time-off afternoon for the mother and brief naps during the day when the baby is sleeping may be helpful.
4. *Prevent overstimulation of the baby.* Parents of a colicky baby may be doing too much with the baby, such as too frequent feeding or picking up. Consider the following interventions:
   - Teach soothing behavior, such as swaddling, gentle rocking, or use of a pacifier.
   - Demonstrate to the mother that her fussy infant can be soothed by holding the baby parallel to the floor and gently and slowly moving him back and forth; this may be enlightening.

- Some colicky babies respond to a heating pad or warm water bottle against the abdomen.
- White noise (a hair dryer or vacuum cleaner) placed near the crib is found helpful by some parents.[26]
- A mechanical swing may soothe some of the most fussy infants.
- Formula change is almost never helpful; these babies are not allergic or intolerant of various formulas for the most part. Even the act of changing a formula may result in the mother seeing her infant as more vulnerable.[27] A double-blind crossover study demonstrated that any initial decrease in colic after elimination of cow's milk diminished rapidly, and only infrequently was the effect reproducible.[28] Lactose intolerance is rare at this age.[29] Whether allergic reactions to breast milk occur is controversial. Some nursing babies seem to improve when cow's milk is removed from the mother's diet.[30] Other studies have not supported an association.[31]
- Occasionally, elimination of caffeine, chocolate (xanthine), or stimulant medications consumed by the nursing mother will alleviate episodes of colic.

  Note these interventions have not been studied extensively. They are part of the folklore for colicky babies. They seem to help (parent, baby, or both) in some cases. Two recent reports demonstrate the creativity and caution found in treatment studies:

- When parents played a recording of a baby's favorite music, gave extra attention to the baby at quiet, calm times, and turned off the music and left the room briefly at the start of a crying episode, crying was significantly decreased in colicky babies.[32]
- Babies without colic whose parents were instructed to hold them for an extra 2 hours each day cried significantly less than a control group of babies[33]; when the same research team conducted a randomized, controlled trial of extra carrying time as a form of colic therapy, increased carrying was not effective.[34]

5. *Review feeding practices.* Encourage quiet feeding times when the mother is comfortable with herself and the baby. This may require a darkened room away from the center of activity in a busy house or apartment. Babies who are nursed more frequently overall show significantly less crying and fretting behavior[35] of the episodic or colicky type.

6. *Medication should not be used as a treatment for infant colic.* One exception is in the most severe cases of infant colic, in which the baby's behavior has produced a significant level of parental tension that threatens healthy, trust-building interactions between the child and parents. These situations may be apparent before the office visit as a result of frequent telephone calls about crying and feeding dysfunction. Before medication is used, the measures discussed earlier should have been tried. The use of a mild sedative or antispasmodic preparation for a brief period (a few days to 1 week) in this situation serves to temporarily break the cycle of a crying baby leading to tense parents leading to dysfunctional family. It may allow the parents a period of rest and an opportunity to try out other soothing behaviors with a more comfortable infant. A medication that may be used is hyoscyamine sulfate (Levsin), four to six drops three or four times daily. It should be emphasized that although rare cases are suitable for a brief course of medicine, the majority of fussy babies should not receive medication. Sedatives and dicyclomine should never be prescribed, and simethicone is not more helpful for colicky babies than a placebo.[36]

7. *A positive and optimistic approach is required and beneficial.*[37] Parents must be told that the baby is normal. Some measures can be tried, and improvement and resolution will occur. In all but the most severe cases, this conservative approach is rewarded by improvement. It often means that the parents have discovered new ways to relate to and settle their baby. Frequent follow-up telephone calls are essential, usually helpful, and serve to enhance the therapeutic relationship.

The time invested in the colicky infant and the family is well worth it. The parents will come to understand that this intensity is part of their own infant's style and that this characteristic is one that the child must learn to handle. They must be taught to respect and appreciate this infant's vitality, vigor, and excitement. If these broader perspectives are not achieved at this juncture, the colicky infant will come back to haunt the clinician in another guise (sleeping, feeding, or discipline issues).

> But what am I?
> An infant crying in the night:
> An infant crying for the light:
> And with no language but a cry.
> Lord Alfred Tennyson (1809-1892)
> *In Memoriam*

REFERENCES

1. Whitten CF, Pettit MG, Fischhoff J: Evidence that growth failure from maternal deprivation is secondary to undereating, *JAMA* 209:1675, 1969.
2. Altemeier WA et al: Prospective study of antecedents for nonorganic failure to thrive, *J Pediatr* 106:360, 1985.
3. Rosen D, Loeb L, Jura M: Differentiation of organic from nonorganic failure to thrive syndrome in infancy, *Pediatrics* 66:689, 1980.
4. Brazelton TB: Nutrition during early infancy. In Susking RM, editor: *Textbook of pediatric nutrition,* New York, 1981, Raven Press.
5. Smith DW et al: *Growth and its disorders,* Philadelphia, 1976, WB Saunders.
6. Carey WB, McDevitt SC: *Coping with children's temperament: a guide for professionals,* New York, 1995, Basic Books.
7. Macknin ML, Medendorp SV, Maier MC: Infant sleep and bedtime cereal, *Am J Dis Child* 143:1066, 1989.
8. Sander L, Julia H, Stechler G: Regulation and organization in early infant-caretaker interaction. In Robinson RJ, editor: *Brain and early behavior,* New York, 1969, Academic Press.
9. Stein MT et al: Cosleeping (bedsharing) among infants and toddlers, *J Dev Behav Pediatr* 18:38, 1997.
10. Fleming P et al: Environments of infants during sleep and the risk of the sudden infant death syndrome: results of 1993-1995 case control study for confidential inquiry into stillbirths and deaths in infancy, *BMJ* 313:191, 1996.
11. McKenna JJ: Cosleeping. In Carskadon MA, editor: *Encyclopedia of sleep and dreaming,* New York, 1993, MacMillan, pp 145-148.
12. Lozoff B: Influence of childhood sleep practices and problems. In Ferber R, Kryger M: *Principles and practices of sleep medicine in the child,* Philadelphia, 1995, WB Saunders, pp 69-73.
13. Ferber R: *Solve your child's sleep problems,* New York, 1985, Simon & Schuster.
14. Ferber R: Sleeplessness in children. In Ferber R, Kryger M: *Principles and practices of sleep medicine in the child,* Philadelphia, 1995, WB Saunders, pp 79-89.

15. American Academy of Pediatrics: Positioning and SIDS, *Pediatrics* 89:1120, 1992.
16. American Academy of Pediatrics: Positioning and sudden infant death syndrome, *Pediatrics* 98:1216, 1996.
17. Davis BE et al: Effects of sleep position on infant motor development, *Pediatrics* 102:1135, 1998.
18. Brazelton TB: Crying in infancy, *Pediatrics* 29:579, 1962.
19. Wessel MA et al: Paroxysmal fussing in infancy, sometimes called "colic," *Pediatrics* 14:421, 1954.
20. Barr RG et al: Feeding and temperament as determinants of early infant crying/fussing behavior, *Pediatrics* 84:514, 1989.
21. Barr RG et al: The crying of infants with colic: a controlled empirical description, *Pediatrics* 90:14, 1992.
22. Boyce WT, Barr RG, Zeltzer LK: Temperament and the psychobiology of childhood stress, *Pediatrics* 90:483, 1992.
23. American Academy of Pediatrics: Breastfeeding and the use of human milk, *Pediatrics* 100:1035, 1997.
24. Eisenberg A, Murkoff HE, Hathaway SE: *What to expect in the first year,* New York, 1989, Workman Publishing.
25. Taubman B: Clinical trial of the treatment of colic by modification of parent-infant interaction, *Pediatrics* 74:998, 1984
26. Spencer JAD et al: White noise and sleep induction, *Arch Dis Child* 65:135, 1990.
27. Forsyth BWC, McCarthy PL, Leventhal JM: Problems of early infancy, formula changes, and mothers' beliefs about their infants, *J Pediatr* 106:1012, 1985.
28. Forsyth BWC: Colic and the effect of changing formulas: a double-blind multiple crossover study, *J Pediatr* 115:521, 1989.
29. Barr RG et al: Carbohydrate change has no effect on infant crying behavior: a randomized controlled trial, *Am J Dis Child* 141:391, 1987.
30. Jakobsson I, Lindberg T: Cow's milk proteins cause infantile colic in breast fed infants: a double-blind crossover study, *Pediatrics* 71:268, 1983.
31. Evans RW et al: Maternal diet and infantile colic in breast fed infants, *Lancet* 1:1340, 1981.
32. Larson K, Ayllon T: The effects of contingent music and differential reinforcement on infant colic, *Behaviour Research and Therapy* 28:119, 1990.
33. Hunziker UA, Barr RG: Increased carrying reduces infant crying: a randomized controlled trial, *Pediatrics* 77:641, 1986.
34. Barr RG et al: Carrying as colic "therapy": a randomized, controlled trial, *Pediatrics* 87:623, 1991.
35. Barr RG, Elias M: Nursing interval and maternal responsiveness: effect on early infant crying, *Pediatrics* 81:529, 1988.
36. Metcalf TJ et al: Simethicone in the treatment of infant colic: a randomized, placebo-controlled, multicenter trial, *Pediatrics* 94:29, 1994.
37. Carey WB: Colic: prolonged or excessive crying in young infants. In Levine MD et al, editors: *Developmental-behavioral pediatrics,* ed 3, Philadelphia, 1999, WB Saunders.

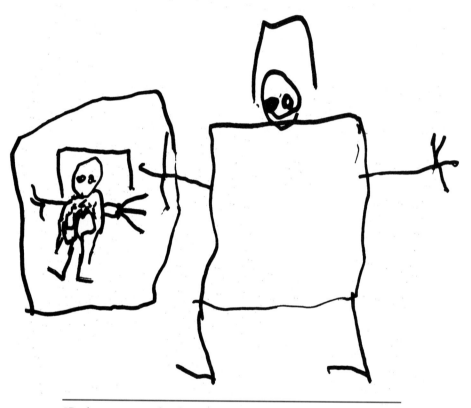

"Dad goes to comfort baby in cradle." By Colin Hennessy, age 4.

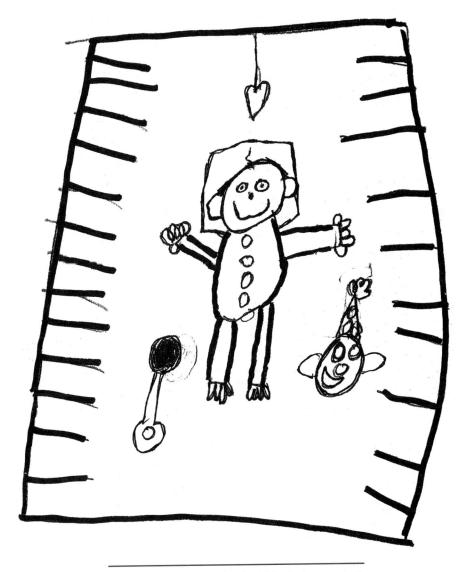

"My brother in his crib." By Abby Roberts, age 6.

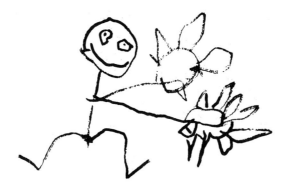

"Smiling kid." By girl, age 5½.

THREE TO FOUR MONTHS: HAVING FUN WITH THE PICTURE BOOK BABY

■ Suzanne D. Dixon

KEY WORDS

Night Awakenings
Social Interaction
Games
Maternal Depression
Social Play
Spoiling
Smiling
Temperamental Differences

> *Mrs. Martin brings in her 3-month-old Anna and asks what formula to buy for the infant. She was previously breast feeding but says the baby does not like to nurse anymore. She is tearful and and says she wonders if it is time she went back to work. She is also concerned because everyone in the supermarket comes up to play with the baby, and he will not go to sleep when they get home; "the whole day gets messed up." She says she has not been sleeping well herself, but the baby "gets along fine without her" all night long. Anna smiles broadly, waves her arms, and pulls the clinician into a nuzzle.*

The child of 3 to 4 months of age is a delightful, cherubic, engaging creature. A big shift in responsiveness, an expanded behavioral repertoire, social needs, and real personality serve to draw people into interaction. A decrease in reflex-determined behaviors and more predictability in routine should free up everyone for the next level of parenting. This new level of organization calls for a change in caretaking and interaction to include social play at a new level. If a mom isn't going along with this shift or isn't having real fun with a baby this age, something is off track. Parents should be enjoying the baby, and this should be a delightful visit for the clinician. The emphasis on the importance of play and social interaction should be the main focus of this visit.

181

STATE ORGANIZATION

By the third or fourth month, the state organization and the wake-sleep cycles of the child have shown increased stability and reliability. Most infants have shifted their longest sleep time to nighttime hours and have developed reasonably set nap times.[1-5] Routines for settling to sleep have usually developed between child and parents, and this predictability gives parents a sense of competence, as well as less fatigue. The child, if left alone, can usually settle back to sleep following the periodic awakenings that occur every 1½ to 3 hours during sleep times. Individual, biologically determined differences are manifested now in these sleep patterns. Some children may be short sleepers and some long sleepers. They are likely to maintain these characteristics through the life span.[3,6,7,8] The infant at this age has two to four naps per day, moving gradually toward two naps throughout the first year and consolidating to one regular nap per day from 18 to 36 months, or longer if a strong environmental push to nap midday exists. This pattern varies a lot. Total sleep time, including night and naptime, decreases gradually across toddlerhood, but the actual amount varies from child to child. As kids give up naps, their nighttime sleep increases.

Regularity in the environment helps with sleep organization; a regular bedtime, a regular ritual, and clear expectations are helpful throughout childhood, including infancy, in facilitating good sleep organization.

Premature infants, even those without serious perinatal complications, will have less regular sleep and will be more difficult to quiet throughout the first year. Some active children are predictably wiggly at night, whereas some children have declared a pattern of difficulty settling to sleep. These children need a little more support from the environment, but *not* qualitatively different interventions.

> *Mrs. Martin comes in looking very tired, complaining that she just can't get Jared "on a schedule" like her other kids were at his age. He's now 5 months old, but was a 34-week preemie with an easy course during a 3-week postnatal hospitalization. He still wakes up frequently at night. His weight gain and development have otherwise caused no concern. Mom still feeds him several times at night.*

Up At Night

Sleep is usually disturbed by periodic awakenings at all ages. Some children are able to quietly settle themselves back to sleep without awakening the parents. These children are said to sleep through the night.[4] Individual differences exist in children, in parents, in families, in household layouts and schedules, and even in cultural expectations.[9,10] In the United States, we usually expect infants to demonstrate substantial independence in the matter of sleeping. Being awakened by an infant at night is a violation of these expectations, of the infant and of the parent who, it is felt, should be able to get bedtime organized. Therefore infants who do not "sleep through the night" are viewed as defective, or at least developmentally delayed, and certainly as a source of stress, if not a sign of "parenting failure." In other cultures, where schedules are more fluid and independence is not a goal in child rearing, "sleep prob-lems" do not exist.[9,11] **Night awakenings** are the usual occurrence in all groups because awakenings are biologically based. The introduction of solid food *does not* result in longer sleep times.[3] Most infants by 3 to 4 months of age do not *need* to be fed during the night to maintain nutrition, although many of them and their parents may choose to do nighttime feedings. Parents can prolong the awakening and sustain this pattern of waking others by re-sponding with an elaborate interaction with the infant at that time. Talk, activities, and game playing all will communicate to the infant that this is a time for play. Quiet comforting, per-haps a quiet feeding, dim lights, and rhythmical soothing (e.g., patting, rocking) will signal the infant that this is the time to sleep.[12]

Sleep at 3 to 4 months of age becomes more vulnerable to outside disturbances (e.g., the telephone ringing). The excitement of the day's activities may infiltrate sleep time, so that settling in for the night or staying asleep may be a new problem when there is a change in routine or household excitement.

Some parents who do not get enough time alone with their infants during the day may choose, consciously or unconsciously, to use the night as a private time to get and stay close. For working parents, those without partners, or parents who've experienced a lot of loss, this is likely to be a separation they cannot stand. They must be willing to invest the time to quiet the infant back down and to realize that this will be an expectation of the infant every night.

No evidence has shown that bringing an infant into the parents' bed is either dan-gerous, psychologically harmful, or even habit-forming at this age.[9,11] This may be the *least* disruptive pattern for some families to manage sleep and is very common, even into the tod-dler years.[13] Some parents may choose to maintain breast milk supply through the pattern of nighttime feedings. Each family must decide a sleep management plan with each child. The clinician should offer information on infancy sleep issues and options and should sup-port families in the development of their own solutions. The age of 4 months is the time to highlight this decision point because a change in the pattern will be much more difficult later. A prescriptive approach is to be avoided, but a choice should be made, either actively or by default (Box 9-1). Consistency in the expectations and the environment is the key from the child's perspective.

READY FOR PLAY
Neurological Maturation

The central nervous system (CNS) changes occurring at this time prompt both shifts in sleep and new social skills. Increases in myelination, synaptogenesis (the establishment of connec-tions between neurons, forming new synapses), and maturation of the electroencephalogram (EEG) demonstrate these processes. Increases in the mobility of the lens in the eye and better optic muscle control mean that the baby can see and track a person close up and across the room and can watch her own hands and their actions in the environment while experiment-ing with distance, size, and depth perception. Refinements in vocalizations and facial move-ments allow a wider range of emotional expressiveness. As noted psychologist Hans Pa-pousek has stated, there is "a marked qualitative change in higher nervous function at the

BOX 9-1	DEVELOPING GOOD SLEEP HABITS IN INFANCY

Be as consistent as possible in *times* of sleep.

Be as consistent as possible in the *place* where the baby sleeps.

Develop a simple *pattern* of putting the baby to sleep.

Put the baby down while she is *drowsy*, not asleep, unless you want to put the child back to sleep all night long through rocking.

Don't give the baby the bottle with which to fall asleep.

Don't respond instantly to every whimper during the night. Give the baby a chance to settle back down.

When you do respond at night, *do it quietly, calmly.* Avoid vigorous play, lots of talk, jiggling, and vigorous diaper changes.

Respond to real crying with calm reassurance, patting, or nursing.

Small infants shouldn't be allowed to "cry it out."

Parents should talk to each other about how they want to handle sleep issues. Underlying assumptions, ghosts from their own pasts, and perceptions of the child's needs may vary widely. Now's the time to discuss it.

third month."[14] This new organizational level enables the child to interact with the family in new and elaborate ways.

Cognitive Growth

New cognitive skills are evident in the infant's ability to momentarily delay gratification and to make linkages in life events. For example, the child of 3 months will stop crying when placed in the nursing position and may hold back on vigorous sucking at breast for a few minutes until the milk letdown begins, content in the anticipation of the reward. The infant may smile while being eased into a front pack, linking that event to an expected adventure, and may flex the hips readily when placed on a changing table. All these behaviors indicate that the child has been mentally active in assimilating events that occur consistently. He is observing patterns of association and can anticipate and wait.[15] These can be observed easily during a dressing, feeding, or play session. Evidence that the child anticipates and expects certain actions and events is usually easily seen or can be identified by history.

Social Skills

The human need and drive for **social interaction** is never more obvious than in the behavior of the 3-month-old infant.[16] The presence of people is more compelling than any other phenomenon.[12] The 2-month-old infant participates in social exchanges; the 3-month-old can actively initiate the interaction with compelling force. These capacities form the foundation for emotional and cognitive life. The infant draws people into play because that is the fuel for the baby's development.[17]

> *Marisa is in her infant seat as you enter the examination room. After a brief, wary look and a subtle startle, she gives you a big grin and some delighted wiggles. She stares at you intensely as you move closer. As you reach for her, she puts her head and arms forward, anticipating a pickup.*

Although studies of parent-infant interactions confirm that infants know their specific parents from the earliest weeks of life,[18] the 3-month-old infant offers very dramatic testimony even to the most skeptical parent. At this age, the child will visually search a room until he finds familiar care providers, will move all extremities in excitement, and will arch forward with outstretched arms to urge them to notice, talk, and touch him. Even the temperamentally quiet infant will stop all activity and increase visual regard in his parents' presence. Vocalizing in different ways, such as squeals, laughs, and phony coughs, serves to initiate and sustain an interaction. The 3-month-old has a whole new series of facial expressions to indicate an expanded range of emotional responses and individual personality: pouting, coyness, disgruntlement, teasing, wariness, appearing to be insulted, fearful, bored, etc. The infant explores the caregivers' faces through looking at the parts, swiping, poking, and pulling. Parents' clothes and skin offer new, safe opportunities to explore the most important part of the environment, the family. These new skills and interests testify to emotional growth.

The Game

In an interactive setting, the infant has incredible abilities to respond to subtle behaviors (e.g., glances away for fractions of a second) or underlying emotional tones (e.g., frustration, tension). The baby is like a sponge for the emotional tones of the environment. Hungry for social interaction, the infant seeks it out by learning to play **games.** The development of "the game"[19] as a concept is strong at this age. The child learns how to prompt predictable exchanges with the caregiver. Verbal, tactile, vestibular, and motor games are the elements through which the child learns about affecting the behavior of others and that his own behavior has meaning and effectiveness.[20] The infant is developing a sense of self.[21] These social game interactions, delivered in the context of caretaking and as individual as the players of the game, are the main event of the infant's day. Responsive caretaking is essential for cognitive and emotional growth.[21,22] The infant needs ready partners for all these games, day in and day out.

Rhythms, styles, content of games, and intensity of interactions vary across individuals, socioeconomic groups, and cultures and subcultures,[23,24] but the basic pattern of game playing with its reciprocal nature, mutually regulated, seems to be a universal pattern of human development.[12,25]

Infants who do not experience this contingent responsiveness have an altered developmental course, either temporarily or permanently. Depressed moms are unable to respond to their infants, and the babies' behaviors offer quick testimony to this missing component of their lives. These infants smile less, frown more, and are more withdrawn and less responsive.[26] This sparse interactional pattern carries over to their behavior with nondepressed adults (e.g., health care providers).[27] Infants of depressed mothers are at risk for developmental compromise.[28]

> *Mrs. Neilson is in the chair by the window in the exam room while her daughter is in the infant seat on the exam table. Mom's face is flat as she says she has no concerns or questions about the baby, that everything is going fine. The baby also has a flat expression and an intense stare as you begin to examine her. She's not very active during the exam and is very still when you pick her up at your shoulder. When she cries, mom quickly puts a bottle into her mouth. You notice that the baby's weight is above the 95th percentile and that there is occipital flattening. Mom would like to be sure that the WIC form is filled out. You can't wait to get on to the next patient.*
>
> *Both mother and baby are depressed. Your own reaction is a good indicator of this altered emotional climate. Pay attention to it. Something's wrong.*

Maternal depression may be the final common pathway of developmental morbidity in circumstances of poverty, family stress, economic decline, etc.; these conditions are known to have an adverse effect on a child's development. Conversely, even depressed moms can learn how to be more responsive in play interactions, and the babies can show behavioral recovery through better eye contact and decreased distress.[27] These observations make it vital to identify and intervene with the parent and infant who are not having fun with each other. Joy in the interaction is a vital observation; its absence is a signal for prompt intervention. This is probably the core evaluation to be done at this stage of infancy.

Infants work hard at **social play.** They are motivated to attend to the social behavior around them and modify their own behavior in response. Familiar people call forth the most attention; unfamiliar adults elicit wariness, an initial unbroken gaze, a tentative bright smile, and then avoidance behaviors, such as gaze aversion and head turning.[18] The baby will make new relationships with regular interaction, so this is a good time to introduce alternate care providers. The baby will hook new adults into a relationship at this age without the stranger anxiety that will come later. Any caretaker should be attentive to the baby in this need for social interaction, as well as for care. The caretaker should be physically nurturing, promptly attentive, and constant. Rarely can a caregiver provide that while caring for four or more infants, which is what occurs in some day-care settings.

"Spoiling" Baby

For game playing to be successful and mutually enjoyable, and to meet the infant's needs for responsive caretaking, some elements are required. The adult must be convinced that these affectionate interchanges are worthwhile. Playing with the infant, holding, massaging, moving, talking to, and nuzzling her are not **"spoiling"** the child (i.e., making the infant more dependent or demanding). Babies at this age don't act with premeditation and can't disobey. In fact, the more that caregivers play with the baby, the more the infant will learn ways to amuse herself. Play is a way of learning, of building basic trust, and of improving self-esteem.[21] Prompt and appropriate responses build self-sufficiency, not dependency. The world is experienced as a safe, responsive, predictable, and exciting place to be. Parents or care providers who continue to "feed and cuddle only" or who leave a baby to "cry it out" don't support development.

Meals Will Never Be Same

The extent of the infant's drive for social interaction is very evident in feeding behaviors at this age. The baby simply cannot resist looking around, **smiling,** cooing, and poking at mom's face during a feeding. Distracted by every sound or sight, the child may even stop nursing just to look around. This is very frustrating for parents, and the danger is that nursing will be discontinued at this time. The mother may interpret the infant's social behavior as indicative of a desire to wean at this time. She herself may not be ready to change her parenting from the "symbiosis" (see Mahler, Chapter 2) of the early newborn period.

> *Mrs. Martin asks what kind of formula to buy because the baby doesn't like breast milk anymore. She says the baby pulls away from the breast whenever anything happens, such as a loud noise from the TV, the cat walking by, or her older brother going through the room. Your notes say that it was Mom's intention to breast feed for the first year.*

An intervention can turn this around. The child's new social interest should be highlighted, as well as the tendency to overdose on excitement if given the opportunity. At least two feedings per day should be in a quiet, darkened room without distractions. Nighttime feedings also will sustain milk supply and maintain a sense of closeness for both mother and baby, although the feedings are not needed for nutritional requirements. Other types of vigorous social interactions should be enjoyed at other times. The social agenda has to be added to the feeding one, with a balance between them. Families should adjust to these new demands and see the interactions and the games with the baby as vital as food. This is a basic change period or "touchpoint" in development.[29]

Overdosing On Fun

The seductive behavior of the 3-month-old infant is hard to resist. The baby's orgasmic smiles, laughs, and total body wiggles are a terrific reward for a few tickles or a play-face expression. Indeed, the investment of effort for the first 3 months is amply paid off in the rewarding baby of 3 to 4 months. Some parents, probably most parents some of the time, will really push the infant beyond the limits of what the child can tolerate. Overstimulation is a very real danger if the infant's body language is not heard, particularly for the neurologically, physiologically, or temperamentally fragile child. The parent must be sensitive to the infant's behavioral cues that she is on "overload" and that play must slow down.[30] This allows an organization of the past experiences, a recovery of attentional energy, and some physiological rest. The required pause may be seconds or hours. Each child manifests stress and overstimulation in different ways. Some children will be more clear in signaling their overload than others. Sensitive adults respond to these behavioral signals and pull back[25]; others need help in understanding the baby's needs (see Chapter 6).

Young children who are brought for long periods to large gatherings, on prolonged trips to large shopping centers, to siblings' schools, or on long car rides may have markedly decreased capacity to handle further stress. Sleep and feeding difficulties are predictable in these contexts. Letting infants at this age "cry it out" may only exaggerate the frenzy at a time when the infant is least able to handle it.[7] Quiet containment by a calm adult helps the infant get back under control. This kind of responsiveness restores energy to the child; it does not "spoil" him. Parents who are upset themselves by the episode should put the baby down or hand him over to another person if they feel out of control.

Infants this age love active play, but "flying baby," roughhousing, bicycle seats, and joggers are not safe at this age. The "shaken impact syndrome,"[31] as well as behavioral overload, can result when these vigorous play activities are used.

Temperamental Differences

Temperamental differences in infants' personalities make some babies' bids for social interaction difficult to interpret. Sometimes the style differences between caregiver and parent are very large. This can lead to poor responsiveness. One infant may signal interactional readiness by serious regard and be overloaded by all but the most gentle play. This child may be perceived as negative, dull, or unappreciative of the parents' efforts at interaction. The parents may even feel that the child doesn't like them. Sensitivity and low-key responsiveness ought to be pointed out, and a subtler style modeled. Reassurances about the child's normalcy and competency must be given.

> *Ms. Galen says she is worried because her baby never smiles at her. She's dropped out of the play group because she's ashamed that her baby doesn't seem as happy as the rest of the infants. She's given up her career to be with the baby and wonders what she's doing wrong; she plays with her all day. Ellie, the baby, regards you very seriously and is very still as you approach. You smile at her without a word or a touch, and she smiles back very tentatively. As you move the stethoscope across her field of vision, her face brightens and she follows it very intently. You feel yourself slowing down with the baby, a welcome relief after a busy morning. Mom scoops her up and starts to bounce and pace. The baby gets fussy. Your notes from the prenatal interview say that Dad is a very serious and busy businessman. Mom did all the talking and was in the local theater group.*

For most infants, classic "colic" has disappeared by this age, but what may not have disappeared is the highly responsive, intense, and overly reactive characteristics in an infant who had a difficult colicky phase. This temperamental profile now is seen as the infant who is easily overwhelmed by exciting days, who handles change in scheduling poorly, and who may have difficulty in falling asleep or restless, disturbed sleep. This may be the embryonic form of the "Difficult Child."[32] Vomiting may follow feedings that are frantic and fast, or feedings may be full of wiggles and distractions. For the clinician, the chief complaint, not the basic issue, has changed. The child's own individual makeup must be understood and appreciated for its value. The need to anticipate and bypass these buildups, give support at time of change in routine, and provide quiet times of winding down is evident now, and such actions will establish patterns that will be needed later.

FAMILY AT 3 MONTHS

Parents should be having fun with their infants at this time, and if they are not, something is wrong with the child, with the parents, or with the interaction between them. The parents should be on or moving toward a new level of parenting, that of attention to the individuality of the infant through playful responsiveness and care. Parents should both enjoy and appreciate the infant as an individual at this time. Feeding in response to every whimper is not enough and should not be the only response. Single parents, parents of ill or preterm infants, overly isolated or stressed parents, or some daycare providers may hold on to the earlier pattern of carrying and feeding as the only responses. Overfeeding or flattening of the back of the head may result and may be the clue to this "development arrest" in family development. Maternal depression will now affect the infant's behavior immediately and profoundly with long-lasting results.[28,33,34] A flattening of responsiveness, lack of joy in the interaction, and lack of social engagement with the baby may be clues that the parent needs a mental health referral.[27,28,33] Often the child health care provider is the only professional who sees the parent at this time and is in the position to make this vital referral.

Siblings may reach a new level of organization at this time as well. The baby is now able to clearly enjoy the older child's antics and bids for interaction, provided these are not too vigorous or overwhelming. The infant will prefer to watch the other child if not overloaded or stressed. The infant's stability of state and the parents' more rested state allow a little more time for the older child's separate time with the parents. The infant should be adding energy to the family at this time in the form of love, delight, and active appreciation of the life around him or her. If not, something is wrong.

Devin, age 3, marches into the exam room ahead of his mom and baby sister as he carries the diaper bag. He says he wants you to check "his baby." He pulls out a small car and shakes it in front of the baby, making car noises. The baby smiles broadly and nearly wiggles out of mom's arms. Mom laughs and says that the baby watches everything that Devin does.

SUMMARY

The visit at 3 to 4 four months is about joy, delight, and fun. This is not a frivolous agenda. When we look at the essential tasks of infancy—the development of trust, a sense of self-effectiveness, and a positive emotional state for learning and growth—this visit gives us a chance to look at the emergence of these core developmental tasks. With these insights we have a chance for long-lasting positive intervention. It is through parent-infant exchanges that these vital forces for growth are activated. As stated by Greenspan[35] in a reflection on the importance of these early interactions in infancy:

> The self now exists in relation to others. It is aware of shared pleasures and joys and even of loss and despair, as when the caregiver doesn't return the infant's overtures . . . the consciousness that (now) embraces the human world—the sense of shared personhood as critical to the development of an individual's feeling part of the human community—flowers out of these early and enduring interchanges. (p. 53.)

The clinician has the chance to observe, support, and even participate in this most vital process—not a bad job!

DATA GATHERING
What To Observe

Following are observations the clinician should make during the course of the health care visit:

■ Does the parent enjoy the baby?
■ Does the parent look and act happy?
■ Do the parent's and baby's personal appearance show the parent's ability to care for the basics?
■ Is undressing, holding, and waiting sprinkled with game playing, dialogues, and toy object play?
■ Does the infant visually scan and auditorially monitor the room with a bright, active search?
■ Does the infant monitor your approach and initiate an interaction on a smile cue alone?
■ Are the infant's hands open, active, meeting in the midline?
■ Is the infant beginning to do verbal exchanges with the parent?
■ How many "games" are played as the infant is undressed, weighed, examined, etc.?
■ Does the baby invite interaction? How does he show it; what's his style?

What To Ask

Following are questions the clinician should ask the parents during the visit:

■ Are you enjoying the baby?
■ What games do you play together?
■ Describe the baby's personality. Is she like you? Like her dad?
■ Has the baby's schedule changed? Describe it.
■ Has your schedule changed (e.g., returning to work)?
■ Can you predict the infant's behavior from day to day?
■ What things does the baby do to settle into sleep? What are your bedtime routines?
■ What can you do to help?
■ Can he amuse himself for a time?
■ Can he wait for feedings if you call or pick him up?

- Does he stop crying just with anticipation?
- How regular is his schedule?
- Does he awaken during the night or during naptime?
- What does he do to settle himself back down to sleep?
- Does he get excited before his bath?
- Has he discovered his hands, feet?
- Does he play with both hands together?
- Does he respond to sound and visual objects easily?
- Does he bat at things?
- Can he hold onto simple toys?

Examination

During the examination the clinician should ask herself the following questions:
- Is this baby fun to deal with?
- Does he coo (ahs, ows, i.e., open vowel sounds with the beginning of labial consonants), smile, laugh? Does he do this without a prompt?
- Are his hands active? When visually regarding things, does he swipe, reach, grasp at things? Does he delight in doing so?
- Are his reach attempts symmetrical?
- Have the primitive reflexes disappeared (e.g., tonic neck reflex, grasp reflex, Moro, and walk-in-place reflexes)?
- Can the child lift head and hands up when prone?
- Does he repeat a behavior that produced an interesting event (e.g., place a rattle in his hand and see if he understands that his own activity causes the interesting sound)?
- Does he look at and follow you across the room?
- Is the baby positioned so he can look around the room? Are his hands free?

Modeling of play interactions during the examination may be particularly important to parents. Point out the baby's smiles as social elicitations. Develop a verbal or tactile game with the infant to see the response. Point out the infant's signs of overload or avoidance during the course of the physical examination or even with undressing. Does the child look away, dampen her expression, arch the back, change color to pale or mottled, or get fussy or frantic in movement? Consciously stop, pull back, and point out the infant's behavioral recovery. When is the baby ready to deal with you again?

Does the parent respond specifically to the infant's style and behavioral cues? Observations during weighing and measuring and after the immunizations may reveal the parent's response to various minor stresses.

ANTICIPATORY GUIDANCE

The clinician can offer parents advice and assurance about a variety of issues that arise at this age:
- Some active infants may jettison themselves out of infant seats at this time of increased activity. Therefore the old seat should be retired. The crib should also be lowered at this time.

- The importance of the child's own active exploration of the world, particularly her own actions, should be emphasized.
- The infant is still too young for joggers, bike seats, or vigorous throwing-around games. The baby may be ready for a backpack for walking, not jogging, with an adult if the infant's head control is good.
- Parents should be cautioned about overstimulation in toys, social interactions, and stressful events. Excess fatigue because of the loss of ability to handle environmental disturbances is a pitfall to be avoided. In considering any changes, think of ways to make the least number of alterations.
- The surge in activity often produces an increase in appetite and growth. It also means feedings may be more disrupted by wiggles and giggles.
- Emphasize the importance of holding and playing. Infants cannot be spoiled at this age. The baby should be near someone whenever awake.
- Siblings should receive cautious permission to interact with the baby under supervision. Help them learn what is too much.
- Breast-feeding turbulence is to be expected at this time. Explain its origin and options for management. A vulnerability to early weaning appears at this time.
- Babies at this age do not need to be fed at night, although their moms may wish to do so to maintain milk production.
- Sleep is marked by periodic awakenings. Parents should be encouraged to give the infant the opportunity to develop competency in this area, to not rush in with every noise, but to give the infant a chance to settle herself.
- Good sleep rituals begin at this age. The baby should be put to bed in a drowsy state without a bottle and with a quiet, calming song, poem, or pat.

REPRISE—CHAPTER OPENING CASE

Mrs. Martin needs to shift her parenting style so that she is more in tune with her child's growing competency and needs. She must learn to help him avoid too much stimulation at a time. She needs to understand what's behind her baby's eating behaviors so that she can manage things better. Finally, she needs help in enjoying her baby, either through her interaction with the health care provider or another professional.

REFERENCES

1. Parmelee AH, Wenner WH, Schulz HR: Infant sleep patterns: from birth to 16 weeks of age, *J Pediatr* 65:576, 1964.
2. Ferber R: *Solve your child's sleep problems,* New York, 1985, Simon and Schuster.
3. Ferber R, Kryger M: *Principles and practice of sleep medicine in the child,* Philadelphia, 1995, WB Saunders.

4. Anders T, Sadeh A, Appareddy V: Normal sleep in infants and children. In Ferber R, Kryger M, editors: *Principles and practice of sleep medicine in the child*, Philadelphia, 1995, WB Saunders.

5. Anders TF, Carskadon MA, Dement WC: Sleep and sleepiness in children and adolescents, *Pediatr Clin North Am* 27:29, 1980.

6. Hartman EL: *The functions of sleep*, New Haven, Conn, 1973, Yale University Press.

7. Zuckerman B, Blitzer EC: Sleep disorders. In Gabel S, editor: *Behavioral problems in pediatrics*, New York, 1981, Grune & Stratton, pp 257-272.

8. Anders TF, Halpern LF, Hua J: Sleeping through the night: a developmental perspective, *Pediatrics* 90:554, 1992.

9. Lozoff B: Culture and family: influences on childhood sleep practices and problems. In Ferber R, Kryger M, editors: *Principles and practices of sleep medicine in the child*, Philadelphia, 1995, WB Saunders.

10. Stein MT et al: Cosleeping (bedsharing) among infants and toddlers, *J Devel Behav Pediatr* 18(6):408, 1997.

11. Lozoff B, Wolf A, Davis N: Co-sleeping in urban families with young children in the United States, *Pediatrics* 74:171, 1984.

12. Brazelton TB et al: Early mother-infant reciprocity. In *Parent-infant interaction*, Ciba Foundation Symposium no 33, New York, 1975, Elsevier North-Holland, pp 137-154.

13. Madansky D, Edelbrock C: Cosleeping in a community sample of 2- and 3-year old children, *Pediatrics* 86:197, 1990.

14. Papousek H: Individual variability in learned response in human infants. In Robinson RJ, editor: *Brain and early behavior*, New York, 1969, Academic Press.

15. Ginsburg H, Opper S: *Piaget's theory of intellectual development*, Englewood Cliffs, NJ, 1969, Prentice-Hall.

16. Trotter S, Thoman E, editors: *Social responsiveness of infants*, Pediatric Round Table Series no 2, Skillman, NJ, 1978, Johnson & Johnson Baby Products Co.

17. Greenspan S: Clinical assessment of emotional milestones in infancy and early childhood, *Pediatr Clin North Am* 38(6):1371, 1991.

18. Dixon S et al: Early infant interaction with parents and strangers, *J Am Acad Child Psychiatry* 20:32, 1981.

19. Stern D: *The first relationship: infant and mother*, Cambridge, Mass, 1977, Harvard University Press.

20. Chance P: *Learning through play*, Pediatric Round Table Series no 3, Skillman, NJ, 1979, Johnson & Johnson Baby Products Co.

21. Gibson EJ: Ontogenesis of the perceived self. In Neisser U, editor: *The perceived self: ecological and interpersonal sources of self knowledge*, New York, 1993, Cambridge University Press.

22. Isabella RA: Origins of attachment: maternal interactive behavior across the first year, *Child Dev* 64:605, 1993.

23. Caudill W, Weinstein H: Maternal care and infant behavior in Japan and America, *Psychiatry* 32:12, 1969.

24. Dixon S et al: Mother-infant interaction among the Gusii of Kenya. In Field T et al, editors: *Culture and early interactions*, Hillsdale, NY, 1981, Lawrence Erlbaum.

25. Stern D: Mother and infant at play. In Lewis M, Rosenblum L, editors: *The effect of the infant on its caregiver*, New York, 1974, John Wiley & Sons, pp 187-213.

26. Cohn JF et al: Face to face interactions of postpartum depressed and nondepressed mother-infant pairs at two months, *Dev Psychol* 26:15, 1990.

27. Field T: Infants of depressed mothers, *Inf Behav Dev* 18:1, 1995.

28. Campbell SB, Cohn JF, Meyers T: Depression in first-time mothers: mother- infant interaction and depression chronicity, *Dev Psychol* 31:349, 1995.

29. Brazelton TB: *Touchpoints,* Reading, Mass, 1992, Addison Wesley.
30. Lipsitt L: The pleasures and annoyances of infants: approach and avoidance behavior of babies. In Lipsitt L, Reese HW, Bourne LE, editors: *Child development,* Glenview, Ill, 1978, Scott, Foresman, & Co.
31. Duhaime AC et al: Non-accidental head injury in infants: the "shaken baby syndrome," *N Engl J Med* 338:1822, 1998.
32. Tureki S: *The difficult child,* New York, 1989, Bantam.
33. Cohn JF, Tronick EZ: Three month old infants' reactions to simulated maternal depression, *Child Dev* 54:185, 1983.
34. Zuckerman B, Beardslee WR: Maternal depression: a concern for pediatricians, *Pediatrics* 79:110, 1987.
35. Greenspan S: *The growth of the mind and the endangered origins of intelligence,* Reading, Mass, 1997, Addison Wesley.

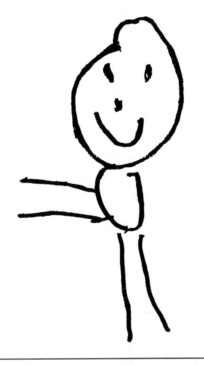

"A happy baby reaching out." By Jesse Naub, age 5.

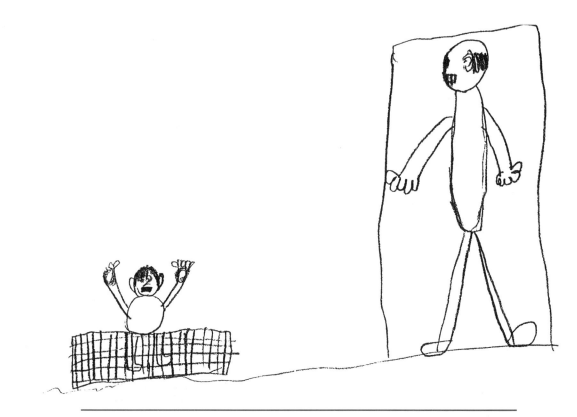

"Dad goes to the playpen to get the baby, who is reaching up to signal his wishes."

Six Months: Reaching Out

■ Suzanne D. Dixon
■ Michael J. Hennessy

KEY WORDS

Motor Development
Reach
Grasp
Ontogeny of Reach and Grasp
Self-Feeding
Motor Asymmetry
Sitting
Fine-Motor Skills
Handedness
Infant Stimulation Programs

> *Jason, brought in on time for his third set of immunizations, is a roly-poly, passive boy. His mother is concerned because he uses his left hand too much and puts everything in his mouth. She thinks she gives enough formula and cereal but wonders if he is still hungry. She wants to know when she can feed him foods like crackers and breakfast cereal bits. She says her brother is a "lefty" and always had trouble in school; she wants to know if Jason will have the same kind of trouble. On examination, Jason does reach first for your stethoscope with his left hand but will extend his right hand if the left is restrained. He grabs your pen more accurately with his left hand, shaping his hand before he touches the object. On the right side, his reach is less well directed and its form doesn't anticipate the pen's shape.*

Now that the baby has visually discovered his hands and has a simple grasp, the 5- to 6-month-old learns what to do with these new skills; sights can be explored in an active way. The texture, temperature, shape, and malleability of objects become new dimensions of the world that add interest and excitement to the child's life, as well as enhanced learning opportunities. The eyes, hands, and mouth work together. Reaching and grasping have a direct link to cognitive growth[1] because these behaviors allow for the active learning that is fuel for mental growth in infancy. The specific way that the skills of reach and grasp are refined during infancy and how these changes make interaction with the external world possible are the focus of this visit. Hand watching at this age and beyond will not only tell us about motor development but will allow us a window on cognitive development and social engagement with the environment. Knowledge of the workings of the hand allows the clinician to monitor not only motor skills, but also cognitive changes. This chapter is designed to build clinical skills in the monitoring of manipulative behaviors in early childhood.

BASIC PRINCIPLES OF MOTOR DEVELOPMENT

The pattern of acquisition of skills in this area illustrates several observations about **motor development** in general:

■ *Primitive* reflexes must disappear before *voluntary* behavior appears. For example, the grasp reflexes must be largely gone before voluntary grasp begins. Whether these reflexes are subsumed into voluntary patterns or disappear to set the stage for non–reflex-driven behavior is debated. However, the sequence of events is not. During a considerable overlap, grasp reflexes still influence hand behavior as volitional grasp emerges.[2]

■ Development follows a *proximal to distal* progression. This is evident in skill proceeding from the shoulder to the fingers. **Reach** precedes **grasp.** Control moves from the shoulder down to the fingers and from hip to ankle (see Chapter 12). The emergence of motor skills follows a relatively rigid sequence, although the timing and the style show variation from child to child and within some environmental supports or constraints.

■ *Pronation precedes supination.* Palm-down maneuvers, such as picking up objects, occur before palm-up maneuvers, such as putting objects in the mouth.

■ *Action and movement precede inhibition.* A child holds onto objects before being able to release them. Inhibition of a movement already started is harder than getting started. Once a reach is initiated, it is difficult for the child to stop. Once an early walker takes off, it is hard for the young child to readily stop.

■ Variation in motor development occurs in the *rate* of maturation of skills, with the timing at each stage being poorly predictive of the time at which the next stage will emerge.

■ The *exact* way a skill (e.g., grasping, forward progression) is completed each time varies. Every attempt is a new behavior in that sense. In fact, *lack* of variability in these behaviors, with rigid or stereotyped patterns of reach, is characteristic of a child with motor disabilities rather than of typically developing children.[2] The ability to modify motor actions in an ongoing process of learning and adaptation is a characteristic seen even in infancy.

■ The *sequence* of motor behaviors shows minimal variation.

The process of motor development is no longer conceived of as the inevitable rolling out of skills based upon neuromotor competencies. Rather, along with these evolving neuromotor competencies, changes in the biomechanical dimensions of the body and the child's internal motivation and drive to mastery create new movement possibilities. The environment provides challenges to adaptation, differing circumstances, and external motivators. Growth or change in one or more of these four areas (size, neural maturation, sparkle, or skills) creates an imbalance in the movement system. This prompts an imbalance that in turn leads to a minireorganization at a higher skill level. New skills emerge when system balance is restored across all these contributing systems. Old skills evolve into new skills as all these forces work together. One level blends into the next in an ever-changing, dynamic way. This view of a *dynamic systems approach* to motor development[4-7] allows us to see the vital interplay between child and environment in the emergence of motor skills. Support for active practice of skills with prompts to adapt to mildly challenging conditions means that caretaking can make a difference in this area, although this isn't the whole answer. Opportunities to exercise and use new skills are created by a supportive environment, which is quite different from practice that is repetitive, rote, and in some cases, passive. Children develop motor skills by using internal drive, maturing motor competencies, changing physical characteristics, and environmental prompts. Very large children and tiny children bring varying biomechanical factors to the situation. Adaptation is specific to the mix of these factors within each child.

THE REFLEXES

The grasp reflexes have been described in the classic work by Twitchell[3] and are presented in Table 10-1 and Fig. 10-1. The timing in the appearance of these reflexes testifies to neurological maturation and integrity. These have a predictable course that allows us to "date" central nervous system (CNS) maturation. From the child's vantage point, these reflexes help him start feeling the world (Fig. 10-2). They are like prepackaged software that gets the user (the infant) started.

TABLE 10-1 ■ Types of Grasp Reflexes

Reflex	Elicitation	Response	Emerges	Disappears
Mental	Touch chin	Hands close	Birth	At 6 wk
Palmar	Touch palm between thumb and index finger	Hands close	28 wk of gestation	2 mo
Traction	Stretch shoulder adductors and flexors	All joints of the arm flex	2-3 wk, peaks at 6 wk	Up to 5 mo
Instinctive grasp reaction orientation A	Light touch to radial side of the hand	Open and supinate hand	3-4½ mo	4-5 mo
Instinctive grasp reaction orientation B	Light touch to ulnar side of the hand	Open and pronate hand	5½-6 mo	6 (?) mo
Groping	Light touch to hand on the side	Hand will move toward stimulus	6-7 mo	7 mo (onset reliable volitional grasp)
Grasping	Light touch to the side of the hand	Hand will grasp object	6-7 mo	7 mo (onset reliable volitional grasp)

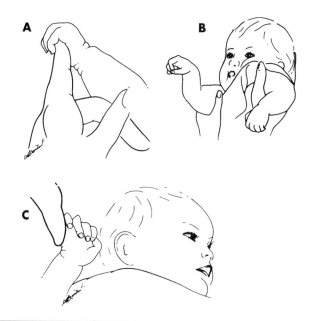

Fig. 10-1   Grasp reflexes. **A,** Reflex palmar grasp. **B,** Traction orientation grasp, type B, ulnar. **C,** Instinctive orientation grasp.

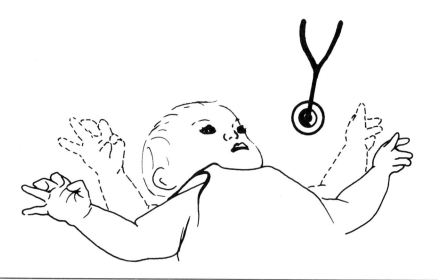

Fig. 10-2   Early infancy contains the earliest elements of reach and hand-arm and foot-leg activation with the presentation of interesting sights.

BOX 10-1	REACH

Arm and hand activation: 6 weeks to 2½ months
Closed hand reaching: 2 to 3 months
Hands open with reach: 4 months
Accurate reaching: 6 months
Anticipatory hand shape and movement: 9 months
Coordinated timing of hand closure with reach: 13 months

The asymmetrical tonic neck response, peaking at about 6 weeks of age, facilitates the infant's exploration of the hands. The infant is able to see what interesting things the hands are by turning the head to the outstretched hand even before having the strength and coordination to bring the hands before the eyes in the midline.

ONTOGENY OF REACH AND GRASP
Early Infancy

The behavior of the newborn contains precursors of reach and grasp in the form of the co-ordination of visual processing with hand activity, the presence of grasp reflexes, and some reaching behavior, particularly in the immediate neonatal period. The newborn in the quiet-alert state who visually fixates on a pleasant sight will begin to have mouthing movements, hands will open and close, and after considerable latency the infant will swipe toward the midline with hand and arm working as a unit. The feet and toes may also be activated in this process. The baby will reach up to touch the breast while nursing, a skill that goes away at a month or two. Infants as young as 4 weeks respond differently to objects that are in their range of reach than to those that are beyond that range[8]; they will swipe at reachable and touchable objects but not at those that are out of range. This shows a primitive visual-motor linkage. The infant may even show the ability to differentiate manual approach to two-dimensional versus three-dimensional objects with a curved swipe to the latter and a flat swipe to the former. The coordination of systems is present from the start, even though the accurate completion of the task and efficient control of hand movements may be months down the road (Box 10-1).

In this earliest form of reach, vision may initiate the reach but does not control it accurately: the infant cannot make ongoing corrections of efforts toward an object after starting a swipe toward it.[9] This lack of fully mature ability, plus the infant's one-handed swipe, makes success very unlikely at this stage. Additionally, a young infant will reach out in the dark for a pleasant sound, using mouth, hands, and feet, although success is unlikely here as well. In later infancy, reach becomes more dependent on vision and more adjustable based on visual input. Reaches in the dark without vision rarely occur at that time.[10]

The infant swipes with the whole hand and arm as a unit, with initiation of movement at the shoulder. The grasp will only occur if the hand touches something. This early type of volitional reach disappears at about 7 weeks of age. In a typical clinical setting, we rarely see it because we do not wait out the long latency period needed for this behavior to emerge, unbind the infant's arms, or provide the truncal support that is needed to see these skills. Moms may note that the baby reaches up to touch the breast and will comment on swipes at a mobile or toy while the infant is lying in a crib or in an infant seat. The **ontogeny of reach and grasp** is detailed in the following milestones:

■ *Mutual hand grasp* comes in at 2 to 3 months after a decrease in the tonic neck response. The infant really starts to explore the hands when this happens. Wrapping and propping so that the hands come together facilitate this process.

■ By 5 months of age, the automatic grasp responses to objects touching the hand have largely disappeared, although remnants may linger for years. *Volitional grasp* is prominent now and acts independently from reach (i.e., the hand moves separately from the shoulder). Increasing bulk and control of the shoulder musculature, as well as truncal strength and stability (i.e., sitting with slight or no support), enables reach to be more reliable at this age as well.

■ Fixed-extension postures at the shoulders or weakness of the shoulder girdle musculature, often present in the premature infant, may prevent the child from using reach and facilitating skill in this area. Applying external support with an increase in flexion at the shoulder (e.g., a rolled towel or small blanket behind the shoulders) often helps this group of youngsters develop these reaching abilities. For children with persistent truncal hypotonia, external supports may be needed to free up the hands for exploratory work.

■ By 3 to 6 months the hands should be loosely fisted at rest and *both hands activated* when the infant attempts to reach. Repeated failure to see one arm or hand move when the other extends is cause to consider perinatal stroke. Tightly fisted hands, with thumbs tucked inside, at this age are generally part of pathological hypertonia.

■ By 6 months the child should *reach across the midline* when the contralateral hand is restrained, although both hands are usually activated when a reach is started.

■ By 6 months the *thumb fully participates* in the grasp, although full thumb opposition may not be present until 2 to 3 months later.[11]

Grasp Development

Volitional grasp matures with increasing control, proceeding downward with decreasing shoulder movement, with more use of the wrist, and with increasing use of the fingers. The grasp is with the whole hand for medium objects, and a raking grasp is used for small objects at first. Then control of the grasp moves to the fingers as a unit, including the thumb, which is kept to the side of the hand, resulting in an "inferior pincer." When the tips of the fingers are used to deftly pick up a small object with the thumb across from the index finger ("opposed"), this is termed the pincer grasp. The pincer is used naturally only with visual coordination; we all revert to raking for objects in the dark, and blind children must be taught to use the pincer (Fig. 10-3).

Even before the pincer grasp is evident, the *index finger* takes the lead in grasping and exploring objects. Poking at things, particularly into holes at 8 to 9 months old, testifies to this maturation of specific finger skills and is usually coincident with the pincer grasp. It also means that electrical outlets, buttons, cracks, and other dangers become very attractive for this exploring first finger.

The grasp of medium-sized objects, such as small blocks, shows a similar progression from use of the whole hand and palm at 7 months to increasing use of the fingertips and finally to use of the index finger and thumb to stack the blocks "deftly and directly" (Fig. 10-3).[12]

The child shows increasing ability to anticipate the shape and weight of the object (Table 10-2 and Fig. 10-3). That is, as the child begins grasp or reach, near the age of 6 to 8 months, the hand position and the arc of movement of the arm and hand reflect the shape and distance away from the object sought, as shown in Fig. 10-4. As the baby begins to go after an object, the hand position, angle of arm movement, and postural adjustment show that the properties of the desired object are understood and that these concepts are transferred to the motor system. This system coordination, vision and reach, and the higher level of integration that it implies can be seen even in children who cannot successfully execute a reach or a grasp, such as a child with athetoid movements, weakness, hypertonicity, or an

TABLE 10-2 ■ Progression of Grasp*

Age (mo)	Term	Pattern Components
1	Nondirected swiping	Arms and legs activated, often beginning with startle; long latency; hands and mouth may open
3-4	Swiping	Moving arm up and down in attempt to contact objects
4	Corralling	Reaching out with entire arm and hand and sweeping arm toward body
4-5	Ulnar-palmar grasp of cube; rotates wrist	Fingers on top surface of object press it into center of palm, thumb adducted, wrist flexed
6-7	Radial-palmar grasp of cube	Fingers on far side of object press against opposed thumb and radial side of palm, wrist straight
6-7	Raking grasp of pellet	Raking object into palm with adducted, totally flexed thumb and fingers
7-8	Radial-digital grasp of cube	Object held with opposed thumb and fingertips; space visible between
7-9	Scissors grasp of pellet	Object held between ventral surfaces of thumb and index finger
9-10	Pincer grasp of pellet	Object held between distal pad of thumb and index finger
9-10	Voluntary release	Drops objects when desired

*Modified from Bayley N: *Bayley scales of infant development,* New York, Psychological Corp, 1969; Erhardt RP: *Developmental hand dysfunction: theory, assessment, treatment,* Laurel, Md, 1982, RAMSCO; Knobloch H, Stevens F, Malone A: *Manual of developmental diagnosis: the administration and interpretation of the revised Gesell and Amatrude developmental and neurologic examination,* New York, 1980, Harper and Row.

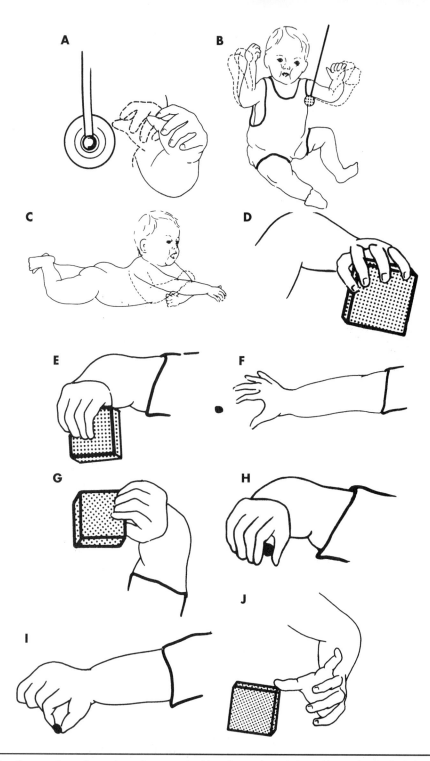

Fig. 10-3 Progression of reach and grasp. **A,** Nondirected, swiping, 1 month. **B,** Swiping, about 4 months. **C,** Corralling, about 4 months. **D,** Ulnar-palmar grasp of cube, 4 to 5 months. **E,** Radial-palmar grasp of cube, 6 to 7 months. **F,** Raking of pellet, 6 to 7 months. **G,** Radial-digital grasp of the cube, 7 to 8 months. **H,** Scissors grasp of pellet, 7 to 9 months. **I,** Pincer grasp of pellet, 9 to 10 months. **J,** Voluntary release, 9 to 10 months.

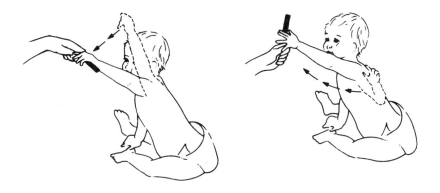

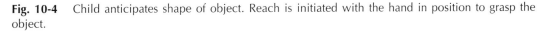

Fig. 10-4   Child anticipates shape of object. Reach is initiated with the hand in position to grasp the object.

arm in a cast or splint (see Fig. 10-4). Again, the clinician should look at the *quality* of the grasp attempt and the basis for it even when task accomplishment remains incomplete for reasons other than immaturity. Although difficulties with visual motor tasks will be more obvious as the child becomes capable of drawing tasks, difficulties may be evident at this age if the clinician watches these aspects of reach and grasp.

After 6 months of age, reach and grasp are separate. That is, the child can grasp a nearby object without a reach and can first reach for an object, grasping it only when it is near. This uncoupling is an example of the increasing efficiency of the motor system with maturation.

Between *5 and 7 months,* visually directed corrective movements can be seen in patterns of grasp. That is, the child watches the hand and amends its first moves to more closely accommodate the object's shape, distance, and texture. These ongoing corrections affect both the direction and velocity of movement.[13] Grasp is more specific, efficient, and smooth.

The volitional reach at this time is two handed and symmetrical, at least at its start. The child "misses" and "overshoots," occasionally getting the object batted into the opposite, available hand.

Between *7 and 11 months* of age, diminishing dependency on bimanual reach can be demonstrated and consistent single-hand reach becomes evident.[14] The transfer of objects is an outgrowth of these midline activities (Fig. 10-5).

The interest and vigor in the infant's investment in the manipulation of objects at this age make it both easy and exciting for parents and clinicians to begin to be "hand watchers." A dangling stethoscope, a red ball of yarn, or even a pencil can be used to watch the emergence of these hand and hand-eye skills throughout the first year (Box 10-2).

USE OF INSTRUMENTS

After a child learns how to use the hands well—reaching, grasping, transferring, manipulating—she learns to extend the functions of the hand through the use of objects. These instru-

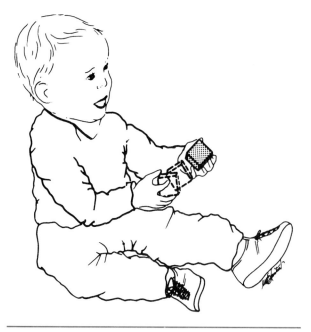

Fig. 10-5　Transfer of objects from one hand to the other.

BOX 10-2	GRASP

Regards toy: newborn
Activates with reachable toy: 1-4 weeks
Holds onto toy: 1-2 months
Hands open: 2½-3½ months
Grasp toy near hand, palm: 4-5 months
Two-hand grasp: 4-5 months
Rotates wrist: 5-7 months
Unilateral reaching: 6-7 months
Grasp two things in each hand: 7-8 months
Scoops (rakes) pellet: 6-8 months
Inferior pincer: 6-10 months
Pincer: 7-12 months

ments or tools allow her to reach farther, to act on things in new ways, and to do things that would be impossible through the use of hands alone. Although this seems like just a progression, it is conceptually an enormous step, allowing for much more elaborate exploration of objects. It is, at the child's level, the dawning of the age of technology. The progression of the *use of instruments* at this new age is shown in the following stages:

■ The first part of this progression is to discover that banging one thing against another makes an interesting sight and sound. Putting objects together in the midline and banging one object on the table with another demonstrate this first step.

■ The second stage is to see that an object extends reach, such as seeing that a stick can get a toy that otherwise would be out of reach. The instrument becomes a *hand extender,* doing the same thing as the hand, only farther afield.

■ The next stage is to see that a tool can do something *different than the hand.* This progression goes on through childhood with increasing agility with specialized tools that do more and more complex things, farther removed from the simple actions capable of the hand alone. For example, the child discovers that a spoon can scoop stuff that would otherwise squish between the fingers on the way to the mouth. Children start to use spoons at around 1 year, but are rarely adept at doing so until closer to 2. Forks do things very differently than hands and are generally used by age 3 to 4 years. Skill with a knife, requiring both hands doing very different but coordinated actions, will take years, into school age at 5 to 6 years. Scissors are used at 3 years.

■ Children can rotate their wrists while maintaining a grasp so they can open doors by turning the handle at 2 to 2½ years.

■ The child's hands become more adept at using these specialized tools, with more coordination between the hands and with increasingly separate use of the fingers being the parameters of complexity. Frustration, fatigue, and stress cause children to go backward in the demonstration of skills. For example, they may use their hands to eat or may tear something rather than cut it with scissors. In general, a slight gender difference arises in these visual-motor tasks, with girls being more skilled after age 2 to 3 years. Facility with preschool craft projects and some copying of letters or numbers may be slightly better among girls.

■ Drawing tasks and the coordinated use of pencils, markers, or crayons also put these visual motor skills to the test and are good to watch into school age (see Chapters 17 and 26).

ENVIRONMENTAL FACILITATORS AND DETRACTORS

Several factors may influence both the emergence and the demonstration of reach-and-grasp behaviors, including distraction, past experience with particular objects, temperament, and general state of the child (e.g., sick, tired, or hungry). Characteristics such as texture, shape, thickness, distance, and density of the object will also play a part because these factors will either prompt interest and adaptation or cause the child to withdraw from the task. Objects with varying shapes, colors, and characteristics that can be perceived as novel by the child have been shown to provoke the most manipulative behaviors by infants (Fig. 10-6).[15] As in other areas, *moderate novelty* elicits more activity on the child's part. An environment filled

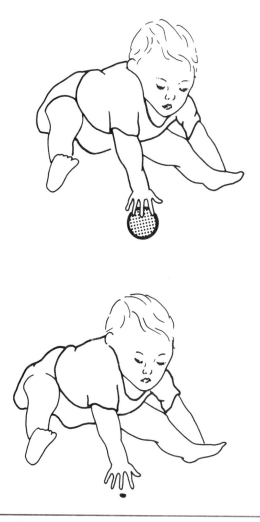

Fig. 10-6 Sitting steadily with hips abducted enables child to stretch to limits of play space and use vision effectively in going after objects of varying size and texture.

with a small variety of safe, reachable, graspable objects is fuel for development in this area. For some children who are more sensitive to all or some textures, this means a gradual, gentle approach to the consistent presentation of these objects.

Populations of preterm infants without significant perinatal complications may show specific delays in visual-motor activities even though other areas of development are normal.[16] The lack of self hand–monitoring in this population caused by shoulder girdle weakness and retraction may be at least part of the basis for this, although CNS dysfunction may also play a role. The clinician should pay particular attention to visual motor coordina-

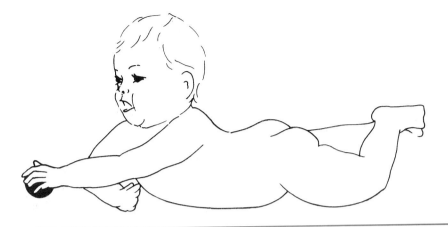

Fig. 10-7   Importance of the truncal stability of the prone posture is seen in situations when child is unwilling or unable to assume this posture. Reach and grasp are facilitated in prone position.

tion in this population. Assisting the infant in ways that bring the hands into the visual field may preclude any secondary deficits.

New "Back to Sleep" recommendations mean that day or awake tummy time is essential. These positions are illustrated in Fig. 10-7. This may mean specific supports for infants who have truncal weakness, instability, or hypertonicity, or for those who just resist this posture after weeks of being cared for in the supine position.

MOUTHING BEHAVIOR

The preponderance of young children's mouthing of and at objects should be expected because it is an integral part of the infant's early exploration of objects as part of the reach and grasp sequence. The child at 3 to 5 months and beyond goes after things with hands and mouth together, sucking at things that look interesting and bringing everything to the mouth when able. No evidence has shown unsatisfied oral gratification as the basis for these behaviors. As reaching and grasping skills mature, children learn to explore their world with increasing hand-to-mouth activity. Luckily, this produces a lot of drool to coat toys with antibody-laden saliva. Within limits of cleanliness and safety, it should be praised and encouraged. The child is extending reaching behavior into mouthing, another way to explore. With cognitive growth, the child learns more specific and complex ways to explore particular objects and mouthing drops out in typically developing children.

Feeding provides the optimal exercise for these emerging fine motor skills (Figs. 10-8 through 10-10), but hunger or lack of food is not the usual reason for mouthing. Foods with varying textures and sizes are a great way to get a child interested in **self-feeding**, as well as in learning more about the world. As soon as a child can sit with stability and is eating solids, self-feeding should become another laboratory for cognitive growth, as well as the increasing mode of feeding. If this period of maximal interest in hand activities and hand-to-

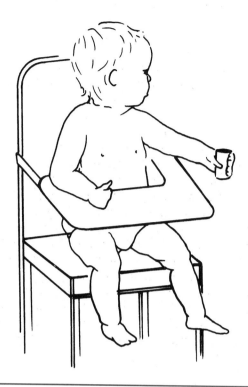

Fig. 10-8   Self-feeding is best initiated when sitting is steady, reach is unilateral, and grasp is at least scissor. The multiple sensory inputs in this situation and opportunities for exploration make it an exciting (although messy) part of the day.

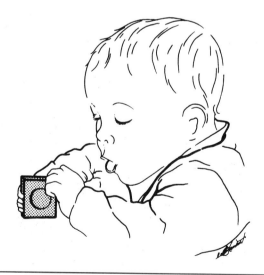

Fig. 10-9   Hands and mouth work together to explore the world, independent of hunger and adequacy of the feeding situation; this is to be encouraged.

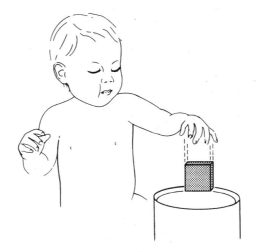

Fig. 10-10   Active experimentation with objects serves the important cognitive work of play. Simple objects allow basic principles to be clear to young child.

mouth behavior passes without such an opportunity, a long-term diminution of hand-to-mouth behaviors may result.

ASYMMETRIES

Children with **motor asymmetry** of reach or grasp in the first 3 to 4 months of life are likely to have a peripheral nerve deficit (e.g., Erb's palsy) or some bone or joint impairment or injury (e.g., fractured humerus). Central lesions (e.g., perinatal stroke) will manifest between 3 and 6 months with increasing asymmetry of spontaneous arm and hand movement, an asymmetrical residual Moro reflex, exclusive use of one hand, or asymmetries in movement when the child is upset. Differences in the maturation of reach and grasp between one side of the body and the other also may signal a central lesion. These may be observed in free play and exaggerated when the child is crying. Failure to use both hands to pull a cloth off the face also adds to evidence of central dysfunction in this age range. Asymmetries of this type should always be evaluated. By 6 months both hands should be used in this maneuver, perhaps with one predominating or leading as part of the early emergence of **handedness.** The lead hand can usually be identified by careful observation, but clear hand dominance before 18 months is not typical and calls for additional evaluation.

OBSERVATIONS

A few simple things in the office allow the clinician to be a good hand watcher with minimal effort. For a child in an alert state and comfortably supported, these observations are easy to set up (Box 10-3).

BOX 10-3	REACH AND GRASP BEHAVIOR SEQUENCE: USE OF SIMPLE OBJECTS IN ASSESSMENT

Raisin Behavior

5 months: regards, mouthing, activation
6 months: rake
7 months: inferior pincer
9 months: pincer

Pencil Behavior

2 months: follows with eyes horizontally
3 months: activates hands, follows vertically
4 months: bimanual reach, opens hands if touching
7 months: anticipates shape with hand opening at the start of reach
8 months: unilateral grasp
9 months: reaches across midline
12 months: makes marks on paper
18-24 months: imitates stroke on paper
30 months: imitates circle
3-5 years: mature hold on pencil

Stethoscope Behavior

2 months: regard across midline, follows vertically
3 months: bimanual swipes; brings to mouth if caught
5-6 months: reliable reach, hands open on contact
6-7 months: reach across midline if restrained
9-10 months: unilateral reach, with mirroring movements
13 months: unilateral reach with contralateral opening/closing

Block (1×1×1 inch) Behavior While Sitting

3-4 months: waves at block on the table, holds onto one if placed in the hand
4-5 months: brings both hands to block
5-6 months: brings block to mouth
6-7 months: picks up with one hand; holds onto one in each hand
7-8 months: bangs block on table
9-10 months: bangs two blocks together
10-13 months: stacks two blocks
15 months: stacks 3 blocks
18 months: stacks 4 blocks
24 months: stacks 7 blocks
36 months: stacks 10 blocks

HANDEDNESS

A child gradually comes to use one hand more frequently than the other; this hand is termed *dominant*. There are many ways to define dominance. A practical definition for the pediatric clinician, though somewhat arbitrary, is that the dominant hand is the hand used consistently to hold a spoon, stack blocks, hold a crayon, or throw a ball. It *may or may not* be the strongest hand.

Handedness is the most commonly observed manifestation of lateralization in the CNS. Although not commonly observed in clinical settings, subtle signs of lateralization may appear in very young infants.[17,18] In the child between 1 and 3 years of age, the dominant hand becomes more and more apparent. Dominance appearing in the first 18 months most often indicates an impaired peripheral or central control of the other hand (see above).[19] Normally, clear and consistent handedness is not fully established until 4 to 6 years of age,[20] with most children being right-handed. Mixed or indeterminate dominance is seen in a higher proportion of children than adults, suggesting a continuum of increasing lateralization with age. This process is related to differential function maturation of the cerebral hemispheres.[21] About 15% to 18% of children will still not have established clear dominance of one hand by school entry.

Left-hand dominance is believed to represent the consequence of less distinct cerebral lateralization, particularly in children and adults who write overhand with the left hand. The whole body participates in this laterality of function (e.g., eye, leg, arm, ear), but we focus on hand function because of its central importance in fine-motor functioning.

A strong genetic predisposition to dominance exists.[22] Only 2% of children of right-handed parents are left handed, whereas 42% of children with left-handed parents are left handed.[18] Higher level cerebral functions are better in left-handed individuals with left-handed relatives than in those without such a familial pattern.[23]

The left-handed child of a right-hand dominant family pedigree warrants *careful* evaluation. A detailed neurological examination should be performed at school entry or earlier to look for subtle signs of asymmetry of tone and reflexes, the perseverance of mirroring activities, and small amounts of tremulousness and overshooting. Although the majority of these children may demonstrate normal neurodevelopmental skills, in a few, left-hand dominance may be an early or subtle clue to a mild central motor disability. Hand preference should be placed in the global assessment of an individual child's health and development, not as a pathological indicator by itself.

Preterm infants and children with learning disabilities have a higher than expected rate of left-handedness, suggesting that this may be a subtle manifestation of CNS maturational dysfunction. The observation of an increased frequency among twins, regardless of zygosity and chorion type, may also reflect this process or may be related to some other unknown factor.

A WORD ON SITTING

Increasing truncal strength and stability enable the child to sit upright with decreasing amounts of support for increasing amounts of time. As **sitting** evolves, the spine increasingly straightens and the hands are used less and less for balance and support. When the hands are forward for balance and support, the position is called the *tripod sit* (5 to 7 months); this gradually emerges to an independent, stable sitting position, first on a regular surface (6 to 8 months) and then on an irregular or soft one (6 to 9 months). As soon as sitting is established, the hands are freed to manipulate objects, with gravity as a help rather than the hindrance it was when the baby was confined to the back. So object manipulation takes off when sitting is established.

For children with truncal weakness or with hypotronic or hypertonic postures, the delay in the ability to sit means that the learning opportunities provided by object manipulation are curtailed. Devices and activities that give the child support while sitting are worth pursuing so that these play opportunities are available to the motorically disabled child. Secondary cognitive difficulties might be avoided.

When sitting is well established, the child begins to map three-dimensional space. The child turns to follow and then get a toy going behind herself (8 to 9 months), provided that pivoting is stable; turning to get an object behind with only a sound cue happens at 8 to 9 months as does throwing toys from a high chair to see where they go and, of course, who will retrieve them. Increasing gross motor competency sets the stage for new learning opportunities.

SUMMARY

The emergence of voluntary reach and grasp is the time to look at motor competency, visual-motor coordination, and the appropriateness of the environment in exploring the object world.

DATA GATHERING
What To Observe

Age-appropriate milestones as delineated in Table 10-3 can provide an assessment scale, along with the following:

■ At 1 to 2 months, does the child move hands and mouth to go after object?
■ At 2 to 3 months, does the infant increase motor activity (wiggle) when looking at a novel object nearby?
■ Does the baby hold the hands together?
■ At 4 months, does the child bring hands to the midline?
■ At 6 months, does the child rattle the paper on the examination table or grab the feet?
■ At 7 months, does the child explore and manipulate toys, such as hitting them on the table, banging two blocks together?
■ At 10 to 11 months, does the child hold a toy out to show you?
■ How does the child use the hands and mouth in exploration?
■ Does the child use both hands and arms equally? Are the movements smooth?

During examinations from birth through the third year, the examiner should present objects toward which the child can reach. Five objects are suggested (see Box 10-3): (1) dangling stethoscope; (2) 1-in. cubed blocks with up to six available, beginning at 2 months; (3) a raisin or round cereal bit, beginning at 5 months; (4) a cup and spoon, at 9 months to 1 year; (5) unsharpened pencil, beginning at 4 months.

TABLE 10-3 ■ Reach Progression

Action	Age
Visual object pursuit	Birth
Arm/body activation (long latency)	2 wk-2 mo
Sustained hand regard	2-4 mo
Arm swipes, bilateral	2-3 mo
Alternating glances	2½-4 mo
Unilateral arm activity	3 mo
Reliable reach to midline	4 mo
Reach for object disappearing beyond visual field	4-5 mo
Unilateral reach	4-7 mo
Hand to hand transfer	5½-6 mo
Finger poke	8-10 mo
Plays midline games	8-12 mo
Visual anticipation of object shape	9-10 mo
Throwing objects	9-18 mo

The raisin offers the child the opportunity to demonstrate fine-motor activity with increasing use of the fingers. The pincer grasp should be seen at 8 months. The use of both hands equally during the course of this play should be seen. An unsharpened pencil or stick can be presented in the midline horizontally and then vertically to induce reach. The 4-month-old should have a bimanual reach and close the grasp if contact is made. The 6-month-old should anticipate the shape at the beginning of shoulder movement by shaping her hand to an accommodating posture. After 1 year the child will readily transfer the pencil and will begin to direct it downward to write. By 5 years of age, if not earlier, a mature "writing" grasp of the pencil may be the single best predictor of adequate **fine motor skills** for school achievement. Motor tone, the child's posture, and strength and control in the trunk, shoulders, and extremities should be noted throughout the course of the examination. The disappearance of the reflex grasp should be noted to follow the course outlined in Table 10-1.

The dangling stethoscope should elicit increasingly smooth tracking with activation of mouth, hands, arms, and lower extremities in the newborn period. Swiping should begin at 3 to 4 months of age. The reach should be reliable by 5 to 6 months of age, with both arms participating and the hands opening on contact. With one arm restrained, the child should reach across the midline. By 9 to 10 months of age the reach should be quite unilateral, although mirroring will be common. Reaching across the midline may not be seen reliably until the second year of life. Movements should be increasingly smooth with increasing use of the elbow and wrist.

A small block should be placed before the child on a surface while the child is sitting on the caretaker's lap. The grasp efforts should proceed as shown in Table 10-2 and Box 10-2. This activity can be done during the history taking. In the second year and beyond, this activity can move along the continuum of stacking blocks and building imagined structures.

Observe delays or abnormal patterns of the infant's fine-motor behavior. Persistence of primitive reflexes will interfere with the emergence of purposeful fine-motor skills.

In addition to observing laterality, observe what the other hand is doing. For example, at 7 months, are the hands equal in skill? At 10 to 11 months, is the other hand mirroring the active hand? At 12 to 13 months, is the other hand passive but fisted during a manipulation? At 4 to 6 years, is the other hand passive during a manipulation?

What To Ask

The pediatric clinician should inquire about the infant's achieving developmental milestones for reach and grasp as indicated in Tables 10-1 and 10-2 and Box 10-3. These are minimal competencies, not average. Failure to achieve these calls for further evaluation. The following are questions to ask parents during office visit:

- At 1 to 3 months, does the baby look at his hands?
- At 4 months, does the baby swipe at objects within visual space?
- At 5 months, can the baby reach for and hold onto toys?
- At 6 months, can the baby transfer an object from one hand to the other?
- At 7 to 9 months, does the baby feed crackers to himself?
- At 9 to 11 months, can the baby pick up a pea, raisin, or a cereal bit between the thumb and forefinger?
- Are there any imbalances, weaknesses, or asymmetries that caregivers notice?

ANTICIPATORY GUIDANCE

Play Activities. The child should be provided with a variety of safe materials to see, touch, and mouth. Parents can facilitate this through positioning the child in a variety of ways in different surroundings with a few simple, safe things for which to reach. The office should model this with safe, washable toys. With the advisory now to place children supine for sleep, it is even more important to provide prone time while awake to encourage object manipulation.

Feeding. When solid foods are introduced after 6 months, the child should be free to explore them with hands. When pincer grasp appears, the child will participate in self-feeding and effectively reach for and consume small, soft pieces of cooked vegetables, dry cereal, rice, pasta, and cheese. Failure to start allowing participation and to give over some control in this area spells the beginning of feeding difficulties.

Every room in the house should have some evidence of the child's work—a play place, the child's own magazines to tear up, a container of simple objects, and safe places to explore.

Asymmetry of reach or grasp should be taken very seriously because it may signal underlying neurological difficulty. Although subtle differences may be evident, persistent or worsening differences must be investigated. Parents should provide ample opportunities for the child to use the "less mature" hand. However, if these differences persist for 1 to 2 months, further evaluation is indicated. A short reevaluation time is needed.

A premature infant or any child with altered tone or strength should be placed with forward shoulder support to allow for good visual monitoring of hand activity. Prone positioning is particularly important in these groups even though it may take the child awhile to accept this position. Chest support will help. When the child is seated, a towel under the thighs flexes the hips, thereby relaxing the trunk and facilitating hand movement.

STIMULATION PROGRAMS

Parents should be cautioned about **infant stimulation programs** that promise gains in development. No program can provide a curriculum that is any better than the baby's own drive to use newly emerging hand-eye skills in productive ways. These programs may perpetuate a feeling among some parents that they must teach their children developmental skills. This is the wrong perspective. Their role as primary teachers for their child is one of facilitating the child's own efforts through careful observation and of developing a safe environment for the child's own free exploration. Many "developmentally appropriate" toys are available for purchase, but they do not possess magical qualities in themselves. Good toys are simple, safe, brightly colored (e.g., blocks and balls), and provide a variety of textures and actions. They also leave room for the child's imagination.

Excessive concern about stimulation equipment and programs should alert the clinician that these parents may be anxious about their child, feel incompetent as play companions and teachers to their child, cannot appreciate their own child's play needs, or have a distorted view as to what fuels a child's own development. The clinician should take these questions seriously and address the underlying parental issues. Motor competencies depend on the child's motivation (which can be supported through positive, but not overwhelming, response) and an opportunity for exploration of objects with hands (a setup parents can provide).

REFERENCES

1. Bushnell EW, Boudreau JP: Motor development and the mind: The potential role of motor abilities as a determinant of aspects of perceptual development, *Child Dev* 64:1005, 1993.
2. Touwen BCL: The neurological development of prehension: a developmental neurologist's view, *Int J Psychophysiol* 19:115, 1995.
3. Twitchell TE: The automatic grasping responses of infants, *Neuropsychologia* 3:247, 1955.
4. Thelen E et al: The transition to reaching: mapping intention and intrinsic dynamics, *Child Dev* 64:1058, 1993.
5. Thelen E, Corbetta D, Spencer J: The development of reaching during the first year: the role of movement speed, *J Exp Psychol Hum Percept Perform* 22:1059, 1996.
6. Thelen E, Smith LB: *A dynamic systems approach to the development of cognition and action,* Cambridge, Mass, 1994, MIT Press.
7. vonHofsten C: Motor development as the development of systems, *Dev Psychol* 25:950, 1989.

8. Bower TGR: Object perceptions in infants, *Perception* 1:15, 1972.
9. Bower TGR: *A Primer of infant development,* San Francisco, 1977, WH Freeman.
10. Clifton RK et al: Multimodal perception in the control of infant reaching, *J Exp Psychol Hum Percept Perform* 20:876, 1994.
11. Lantz C, Melen K, Forsberg H: Early infant grasping involves radial fingers, *Dev Med Child Neurol* 38:668, 1996.
12. Bayley N: *Bayley scales of infant development,* New York, 1993, Psychological Corp.
13. Matthew A, Cook M: The control of reaching movements by young infants, *Child Dev* 61:1238, 1990.
14. Goldfield EC, Michel GF: Spaciotemporal linkage in infant interlimb coordination, *Dev Psychobiol* 19:259, 1986.
15. Gramza AE: Response to the manipulability of a play dyad, *Psychol Rep* 38:1107, 1976.
16. Vohr BR, Garcia-Coll CT: Neurodevelopmental and school performance of very low-birth-weight infants: a seven-year longitudinal study, *Pediatrics* 76:345, 1985.
17. Caplan PJ, Kinsborne M: Baby drops the rattle: asymmetry of duration of grasp in infants, *Child Dev* 47:532, 1976.
18. Michel GF, Hawkins DA: Postural and lateral asymmetries in the ontogeny of handedness during infancy, *Dev Psychobiol* 19:247, 1986.
19. Erhardt RP: *Developmental hand dysfunction: theory, assessment and treatment,* Baltimore, 1982, RAMSCO.
20. Mandell RJ, Nelson DL, Ceumak SA: Differential laterality of hand function in right-handed and left-handed boys, *Am J Occup Ther* 38:114, 1984.
21. Wang PL: Interaction between handedness and cerebral functional dominance, *Int J Neurosci* 11:35, 1980.
22. Chamberlain HD: The inheritance of left-handedness, *J Hered* 19:557, 1928.
23. VanStrien JW, Bouma A: Sex and familial sinistrality differences in cognitive abilities, *Brain Cogn* 27:137, 1995.

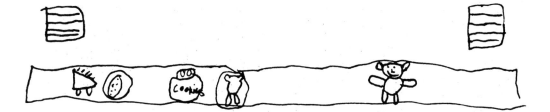

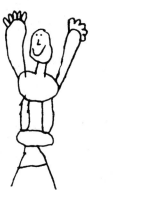

"Reaching Out." By boy, age 7.

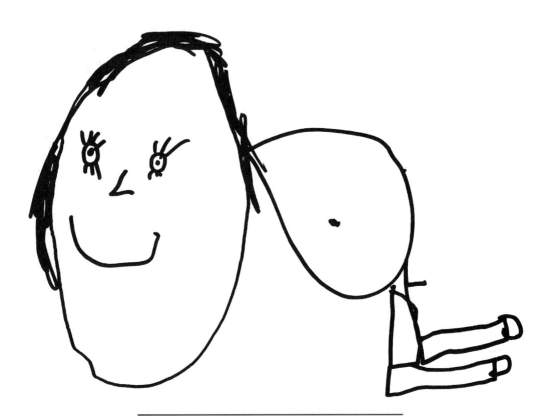

"My brother crawling." By Anne Atkinson, age 5½.

EIGHT TO NINE MONTHS: EXPLORATION AND DISCOVERY

■ Suzanne D. Dixon

KEY WORDS

Stranger Anxiety
Secure Base
Attachment
The Strange Situation
Separation
Divorce
Transitional Objects
Night Wakening
Safety
Food

> Katy, 8 months old, comes in for suture removal from her forehead. She had fallen out of her highchair during a struggle to lock her in. She screams and digs into her mother at your approach. Her mother says Katy just started these "tantrums" and is worried that this injury has made her fearful. She says that even Katy's grandmother cannot take her without protest anymore, and Katy is waking up crying at night. She believes all this "bad behavior" was caused by the laceration. Mother says she will just step out quietly while you remove the sutures because Katy cries even more when she is in the room. Besides, she is really tired, having been up three to four times a night with Katy, who has just started awakening again.

The landmark of social development described by Rene Spitz as "stranger anxiety" is reached after the midpoint of the first year.[1] This change from the all-trusting, happy-to-be-with-anyone baby to the screaming, fearful child does not appear to be a developmental advancement when first encountered, but it really is. This confusing behavior calls for some explanation, requires awareness by all who care for and make decisions about children, and testifies to the big gains in cognitive development that occur at this age. Play at this age is particularly interesting and important, offering a window to look at these new cognitive gains. The environment should be reviewed too because the baby's new skills bring the potential for getting into more trouble. We will explore safety from this developmental perspective.

STRANGER RESPONSES

The child has been sensitive to the differences between parents and strangers since the earliest weeks of life (see Chapter 9) and has shown real preference for the company and games of parents and other predictable adults. This continuum of development makes a quantum change in the second half of the first year. Real fear of being touched or picked up when approached by a stranger occurs at about 6 months, eliciting more discomfort than just seeing a stranger. However, a more apparent and overtly negative reaction known as **stranger anxiety** begins to appear at about 8 months and continues in its fullest form until about 18 to 24 months. This encompasses the period during which the child can envision and miss regular care providers (a cognitive skill we call object permanence for people), but does not have the linguistical and social skills to quickly negotiate a relationship with new people, the strangers. Although kids much older than 2 are still appropriately wary and worried about strangers, the degree and intensity of stress are much less than during this time frame approaching the first birthday. Also, other cognitive abilities allow the child to notice very quickly and become acutely distressed by the appearance, sound, and touch of unfamiliar people. Well-established routines of interaction and care are now in place, and the child becomes exquisitely sensitive to any differences from these expectations. Usually, the more dissonance, the greater the initial distress in a new circumstance.

The child needs reliable features of the environment as she starts to venture out to explore new territory, a scary proposition. The child can now change position in space and investigate things that were not possible to get to before. Familiar care providers are treated as safe sources of comfort in the midst of these little journeys; they serve as a **secure base** from which to explore.[2,3] The presence of the familiar care provider allows the child to take risks in moving away—creeping, crawling, rolling, or scooting—and later walking. When the child gets too far away or perceives a threat or danger, he counts on being rescued by care providers or on having them available to return to. If separated from them, and particularly if left in the presence of strangers, the child becomes, justifiably from her perspective, very upset. This reliance on care providers is evidence of attachment to them as well as of the child's new cognitive skills in visualizing them and wishing they were present when they are absent. Cross-cultural work provides evidence of this process as universal in healthy human development. The intensity and form of the behaviors may vary around the world, but this pattern between child and care provider has been observed everywhere it has been studied.[4,5]

DEFINITION OF ATTACHMENT

Attachment is the enduring emotional bond that humans feel toward special people in their lives. It encompasses trust that the other will be attentive and responsive to our needs and emotional state. It leads to behaviors that keep us close to the attachment figure. Absence from that person creates distress to some degree, and reunion brings relief from that distress. The work of the first year is to develop an attachment to one's care providers. This forms a model for other attachments throughout life. It is a requisite for healthy emotional development.[2,6-8]

We can observe behaviors that testify to that essential work of infancy if we have a structure to make the right observations. We can adapt some work from experimental psychology to help us in the usual clinical settings.[9]

THE STRANGE SITUATION

A predictable response in a young child who has experienced responsive care allows child development specialists to measure attachment using an experimental paradigm called **"The Strange Situation."** This procedure (abbreviated) is outlined in Box 11-1.

The child's distress with the mom leaving and the child's response to the stranger and to the mom on her return are used to characterize the nature of the child's attachment to the mom. Although this setup for distress may seem stressful, it replicates everyday events in a child's life, many of them in medical settings (although we would like to avoid them if possible). By making us aware of the range of possible responses to this situation, this work can assist us in identifying kids who are poorly attached and are at risk for long-term emotional and developmental problems.[10] In clinical settings we can make parallel observations without any extra time or special procedures, as seen in the opening case of this chapter. We can also ask focused questions about a child's behavior at home, on outings, or in other situations that involve separation.

- A *securely attached* child of 8 to 24 months looks wary at the approach of the stranger and will turn or move away with approach or touch. The child will protest, may or may not cry, and will try to follow the parent out. Upon the mom's return, the child will go to her for comfort, perhaps after a brief "punishment" of ignoring her. Crying is immediately reduced when the parent returns.
- An *avoidant* child seems unresponsive to the mom and demonstrates little distress when she leaves. The child reacts to the stranger the same as to the parent, and at reunion she avoids the parent or is very slow to approach. The child may resist being picked up and does not cling. Although this may be caused by cultural or temperamental differences,

BOX 11-1	THE STRANGE SITUATION

The mom* is seated and child plays in a room of toys.
A stranger enters the room and talks to the mom.
The mom leaves.
The stranger attempts to comfort or play with the child.
The mom returns and greets and comforts the baby.
The stranger leaves.

*Any familiar care provider may be in this role. The word *mom* is used because most experimental work has been done with moms. Work done specifically with involved fathers shows similar behaviors.

this pattern suggests to the clinician that more attention should be placed on monitoring the child's environment and emotional growth.

■ A *resistantly attached* child clings to the parent and doesn't explore the room at all. The child becomes very angry on separation and shows it on reunification with hitting, pushing, and failure to be comforted easily when picked up. This is worrisome and calls for more investigation of the child's environment.

■ *Disorganized* attachment is evident in a baby who looks flat throughout the procedure, showing little response to the mom's leaving or returning, often failing to cry, or crying at odd times. Gaze avoidance with the mom may be seen. Little or no toy exploration is seen. This is a serious observation, suggesting a significant lack of attachment in this child's life. This corresponds to infantile or anaclitic depression[1,11] and has long-term implications.[12]

Experimental work in this country and around the world has substantiated these observations as universally present.[13,14] The first type, securely attached, appears to signal the optimal response in all settings. The others display some form of attenuation of attachment, although other factors may play into this. Clinical use of these types of observations requires that these confounders be taken into consideration when evaluating a child's response. The following are factors that influence attachment behavior and color observations:

■ *Temperament* (see Chapter 2). An intense child may show a dramatic response to separation, whereas a mellow child may use more subtle behaviors to show distress. A positive approach child may be more intrigued by the stranger, whereas the child who usually withdraws from something new will be more quiet and clingy in this situation.[15,16]

■ *Cultural issues.* Although the strange situation test has been used around the world with similar results—the secure pattern being the most frequently seen response[5,17]—cultural values influence behavior in varying circumstances. For example, in Germany, the modal response tends to be the "avoidant" pattern. Parents in that culture value early independence and discourage clinging, so this might be expected.[14] Japanese infants more frequently reveal a "resistant" pattern, but they are rarely out of the mother's sight, and she fosters a dependent pattern of care in line with cultural values (see Chapter 2).

■ *Degree of familiarity.* A situation or care provider that is very different in style, appearance, or voice from a familiar one is likely to elicit more distress than if the circumstances are only moderately discrepant from the usual. A child at home will probably be less distressed than one experiencing separation away from home.

■ *Fatigue, illness, injury, pain.* We're all at low tide to cope with stress under these circumstances, and so are children. The most valid observations are made when the child feels well, is rested, and is comfortable.

Factors That Alter Attachment Behavior

The following are core influences on attachment behavior:

■ *Responsive care provision* is the most critical. Sensitivity to the child's needs and emotional states is important. This is played out in the course of everyday care. Social and emotional attunement, not just time put in, is the critical element. This means appropriate and prompt response, consistency, and tender and careful holding. An avoidant response may be seen when the care is too intrusive, too controlling, or overstimulating. A resistant pattern may follow from care that is inconsistent, negative, or rejecting.

■ The parent has an *internal working model* of responsive care, and behavior follows from that model. This may mean that the parent has experienced a strong attachment in her own childhood and emulates that early care. Parents who did not receive such optimal care can create a healthy internal model. It is most important in these cases that the parent has come to some understanding and resolution of her own care and has the insight to see beyond it. A new model of care can be constructed from others, from interactions with people outside the family. Mentors, friends, and other respected individuals can contribute to this model. Interventions for families at risk are probably most effective when they set up these models through relationships. When parents continue to harbor anger, resentment, or ambivalence, the "ghosts from the nursery"[18] will haunt their care of their own children. Inconsistencies in responsiveness and a fluctuating emotional climate will make it more difficult for the infant to attach to them. Therefore a parent's childhood history is important in understanding the milieu surrounding the baby's emotional growth.

■ *Altered mental state* will affect care. Parents with major mental illnesses, such as severe depression, bipolar disorder, or schizophrenia, cannot be attuned to the baby and the baby's needs. Depression, particularly, may be the final common pathway for many adverse circumstances to have a negative impact on child health and development (see Chapter 7). Substance abuse fits in here because the fluctuating mental status and availability that are part of the drug use pattern do not support good attachment. Because many women who use drugs self-medicate their depression, and those on stimulants may experience a serious depression when they come off drugs, drug use often makes a family at risk for poor attachment between parent and child. A baby's well-being has to be at the center of the family's care and focus. Conditions that marginalize the baby's care are not conducive to good attachment. Rote care, awkward handling, expressions of resentment toward the child, and little physical contact may be seen in clinical settings.

■ *Family and social stressors* play a role. A family with financial stresses, joblessness, unwanted moves, dissolved or troubled marriages, or a variety of other pressures may not be consistently available to the infant.[5,9,19] Further, a lot of changes in care or less than optimal care because of cost or parental absence creates stress. It is no surprise that resistant and avoidant attachment patterns are seen much more commonly in families struggling with such circumstances.[16,20] These conditions dramatically alter the interface between the child and the parent. This recalls Bronfenbrenner's social ecology model of development (see Chapter 2).

Dr. Geary noted that Logan, previously a roly-poly and jolly baby, seemed quiet and subdued at the 9-month-old checkup. He was sitting quietly in his mom's lap but didn't turn to her at all. Because it was 10:00 A.M., Dr. Geary asked how Lisa, Logan's mom, had gotten off work. She said she'd been laid off. As a single mom, she had no family support. She said she was looking for work. Logan's weight was down a little, and he looked pale.

A knowledgeable clinician will take into account other factors when observing directly or asking about a child's reaction to separation, strangers, and reunion.[9] The quality of the reaction to strangers is influenced by the infant's developmental age (remember, this tracks with cognitive development), temperament, presence of illness or fatigue, the stranger's demeanor, and the presence or absence of familiar figures. Conditions that heighten the fear response are unfamiliar surroundings (e.g., an examining room), active approach by the stranger (e.g., moving in quickly to examine the child), and close proximity to the stranger, especially with eye-to-eye contact. In addition, response to the stranger is more dramatic when the mother is present but not in physical contact with the infant (e.g., mother in chair, and child on examining table).

Factors that lessen the fearful behavior include a position close to or in contact with the mother or father, familiarization time in a new setting, and a stranger who approaches with toys and whose behavior is responsive to the infant's cues. Children who are exposed to many adults during infancy usually have less dramatic responses to strangers. Strangers who are similar to the parents in their responses to the child will elicit less anxiety than those who are different, no matter how "good" (i.e., sensitive) they are with children in general. Other children elicit less anxiety than adults do in children more than 1 year of age, although the erratic behavior of a toddler may frighten, as well as delight, an infant.

Individual infant temperament modifies the response. Some children sail through this period with a mild behavior change over a short period. Other children have predictable and dramatic fear responses that continue full-blown until the end of the second year. Dramatic negative responses are not the result of bad experiences in the past or of lack of love in the regular environment. These infants are likely to be shy, sensitive, and somewhat slow to warm up as part of their individual makeups. Transitions in people and events may require additional time and support in these children.

Cross-cultural investigations suggested that infants of all groups studied had the onset and the first peak of stranger anxiety at about 8 months of age.[7,14] However, in cultures where infants are regularly exposed to many caregivers, the response was less intense, was more easily overcome with a familiarization time, and lasted for a shorter period into the second year. In all cultures studied, even those described as "polymatric" (many mothers), the strongest protests came with separation from birth mothers. In the United States, infants attach to their parents, even those working outside the home full-time, if the parents' care is responsive and if time spent with the parents early in the infant's life has helped a relationship to start.

SEPARATION LINKS

The signs and rituals of leave-taking by a valued adult are associated with leave-taking in the infant's mind, so separation can be anticipated and anxiety builds before the actual **separation.**[7] This anticipatory response sometimes explains behaviors in infants. Clingy, irritable, whiny behavior is not caused by fear of the new provider, but comes from anxiety generated by the idea of separation from the primary care provider, who is responsive to the child's emotional and social needs.

> *Jared crawled toward his mom and screamed in what sounded like pain as she picked up her purse. Whenever she did so, he sensed that her departure was imminent. She picked him up for a good-bye hug and wondered if his long-time baby sitter wasn't taking good care of him any more. When she returned, he seemed very happy and came to her eagerly for comfort. He grabbed her purse and threw it down.*

Jared's protests don't come from an anticipation of unresponsive care. They are a testimony to his attachment to his mom. He has linked the purse to her leaving. Jared is anxious because of separation from a person on whom he has relied to orchestrate his life. This behavior is evidence of an attachment that is based on his emotional needs being met by his mom. Eventually it is the appearance of these same leave-taking and returning rituals that will help build the skills to anticipate return. The more clear and consistent the pattern, the easier it will be for him to become less anxious with these brief separations.

> *Jared's mom learned to take her wallet in her briefcase and leave her empty purse with Jared, putting it on the shelf before she left the house. "Mommy will be right back. See, I've left my purse. I'll get it when I come home." Jared liked to bring the purse into his room when the sitter put him down for his nap. He also was very clear that he needed his "blanky" right with him for sleep and when he went on an outing.*

Transitional Objects

Bowlby and Winnicott[6,21] have pointed out that a young child's attachment to a cuddly object, which they called the **transitional object,** is part of the developmental process of forming relationships and becoming independent. These first treasured possessions are frequently capable of filling the role of an important, though subsidiary, attachment when the primary attachment person is not there. The object is a substitute that is sought, especially when the child is hungry, tired, or distressed, just as the parent is sought. These props stand in for the absent parent.

Transitional objects are effectively used by children to shut out environmental stimuli and to calm themselves when upset. The selection of a special object may occur as early as 7 to 8 months but usually occurs between 1 and 2 years of age. Two thirds of children in the United States have a transitional object; other cultural groups have a lower rate,[22] perhaps because the cultural drive for and value of independence is less than in this country. This object may take many forms—a blanket, doll, toy, or piece of the child's or parent's clothing. Although most children discard the transitional object as they approach 3 or 4 years of age, when the separation process is farther along and peer pressure mounts, some children retain these attachments into their school years without evidence of psychopathology.[23]

Some parents may perceive the ever-present cuddly object as a weakness rather than a strength. Embarrassment may develop if they view it as a negative reflection on their parenting or on the child's ability to cope. Parents and the child may also receive pressure from extended family or child care providers to "give up that thing." The child's clinician can help parents appreciate their child's resourcefulness and emerging independence. Having a duplicate for washing or replacement is wise because these treasured items get heavy usage.[24]

Comfort Habits

Most children rock on occasion (usually when falling asleep), do some head banging, or later twirl hair, pull at their ears, or rub their faces. These comfort habits, along with the use of "loveys," are healthy ways to settle down, to cope with stress, or to fill in quiet time. These are positive steps in learning ways to solve life's little problems. The use of these comfort habits are healthy most of the time, but may be a concern if any of the following are true:

- The child prefers the lovey to people and spends more time alone with the lovey than with people.
- The child will not stop to acknowledge or respond to a parent when using the lovey or comfort routine.
- The child often leaves an activity to go to his lovey.
- The child hurts herself with the lovey or other comfort habit.

If any of these are the case, a further evaluation of development and the environment should take place.[24]

Coming and Going

As new motor competencies are discovered and practiced, the child can move away from a parent by crawling and eventually walking. This can be alarming; previously, proximity to the parent was predictable. Mahler et al[25] called this new emotional state "hatching." This refers to the realization by the child of being separate from mother, that the mother can leave or that the child can leave her and that proximity is not a guarantee during exploratory maneuvers. The drive for mastery and discovery is tempered by the realization that approaching new things or people in the environment increases one's distance from the familiar providers. An internal security is needed to go forward on these adventures. A child who is anxious will not explore as widely, as often, or as confidently. The child needs to "hatch" in order to grow developmentally. This implies that the relationship with the parent is secure and is like a reliable place to which the child can return physically and psychologically.

Another peak of stranger anxiety often occurs at 18 to 20 months of age. This is usually before the development of real language competency. The toddler relies heavily on the nonverbal communication patterns established with the parents. Strangers are not immediately a part of this individualized communication network. The emotional state of this second peak of stranger anxiety has been called *rapprochement*.[25] It is observed when the previously secure toddler intermittently checks in with a parent, either running back to a secure base or visually making contact across a room. This allows reassurance and refueling for more adventures. This resurgence of stranger anxiety at 18 months diminishes gradually as the child's mastery of communication skills allows communication with anyone.

Michael ran out of the examining room and down the hall. He stopped as the clerk at the desk greeted him. He quickly ran back and buried his head in mom's lap.

By 2 to 3 years of age, the child begins to show decreased distress and increased friendliness with strangers. This process of socialization and independence is gradual. As the preschool child explores new people and objects, he continues initially to draw closer to mother or father and plays less when encountering strangers. Children who are well attached to their primary caregivers use them as bases to venture out in ever-widening circles of exploration; children who are poorly attached do not venture out as readily, or when they do, they don't look back to check, to share a discovery, or to point to something of interest, an act of shared social attention. Children who remain extremely shy and clingy beyond age 3 or those who are not becoming more and more willing to explore when they are given familiarization and supports are worrisome. They are developmentally delayed, very insecure in their attachment to care providers, or so temperamentally withdrawn that it is an impediment to ordinary childhood experiences.

Separation Stressors

The opportunity to interact with adults outside the immediate family offers the infant new perspectives and the chance to learn about other people and self through these social interactions. The child's world is richer because of what others can bring to it. Friends, relatives, and other children add vitality to a child's life. The child learns that other adults can be trusted and enjoyed. This is not to displace the parents from their central position, but to expand the child's horizons.[20]

Alternative caregivers (grandparents, baby-sitters, etc.) can be introduced in a way that supports the child's efforts at social expansion without unduly stressing the child. A time of familiarization with the new caretaker, maintaining regular routines and place (if possible), and the initiation of leave-taking routines all make brief separations easier. The most important element, however, is an unambivalent attitude in parents. Parents must be comfortable with separation before the child can be because the child takes cues from them. Separations that are unplanned, prolonged, or accompanied by exposure to a caregiver who cannot meet the child's needs for consistency and contingency should be avoided at any age, but particularly from about 6 to 18 months, when these are the dominant developmental issues. Family vacations, visitation schedules, change of placement, business needs, and career decisions must take these needs into account in balancing family priorities.

> *Mark and Sharon wanted to go on a long holiday with Sharon's folks. Alissa, 10 months old, was an active child, and her grandparents weren't excited to have her on the month-long trip. Alissa's parents decided to forego the trip, go on a long weekend vacation by themselves, and then spend a week at a camp that had a kid's program and child care for Alissa.*

Divorce is hard on kids at any age, but it is particularly stressful at this time. Separation from the noncustodial spouse will be a stressor, and the changes in the emotional climate, financial pressures, moves, and changes in routine are very problematic to kids. *The more things change, the harder it is on kids.* Shared physical custody of the young child is particularly difficult at this time because it requires too much change in every aspect of life—bed, play space, feeding, etc. The child doesn't have the cognitive and linguistical skills to understand explanations of the situation and has no sense of time to understand when Daddy or Mommy are coming back. The family should look for other solutions to keep both parents involved without requiring that the baby absorb the great separation stress precipitated by change.

Shifts in foster placement and adoption are to be avoided at this time for similar reasons. A child's attachment to familiar people is the foundation of a sense of self. To blow that apart at this critical time will be detrimental even if the placement overall is better. Wait until age 2 to make these shifts if unable to do so before 6 months. Clinicians may have to be advocates for young children with social service agencies and the courts regarding shifts in care during this critical interval.

Chronically or repeatedly hospitalized children are at risk for poor attachments because their world changes from shift to shift and they do not have a chance to develop relationships with their parents because of the many demands and constraints of such a situation (see Chapter 25). One can identify a child with no real attachment to anyone in the hospital setting, one who is in serious trouble emotionally, by seeing who on the ward goes to anyone, who is carried around by everyone, and who rarely cries or turns to anyone special for comfort. This child is detached, a shallow and dangerous emotional state in which the child guards against any investment in anyone. The "pet" of the ward may be a child who is very damaged emotionally. The child not only is in trouble now, but will also have difficulties in the future with social relationships, personality problems, and perhaps delinquency. Healing must include the development of a relationship with a primary attachment figure, in the hospital or somewhere else. This is a behavioral emergency.

Daily Situations

Separations, strangers, and mild stresses are a part of life; they are opportunities for growth through widening social experience, the development of coping strategies, and the reenergization of parents. The clinician can identify the child's perspective by participating in discussion of family management decisions that involve separations. The clinician thus serves as the child's advocate by promoting the expansion of the social experiences and lessening any detrimental impact of prolonged separation.

On a daily basis for most families, leave-takings should be brief, affectionate, and accompanied by a clear statement of return, even for the child who does not understand words or time. These patterns should be clearly established in infancy and maintained over early childhood. Parents should never sneak out, lie about a return time, or promise gifts at each leave-taking. Trust is violated, and brief separations are seen as either a punishment or an extraordinary event.

Brief separations are a regular part of family life and are healthy for all concerned. The primary care clinician is in a position to observe these behaviors over time. The following behaviors should alarm the clinician regarding the response to strangers and separation:

- A child who shows no differential response to strangers by 1 year of age
- A child who is extremely fearful and clingy in all circumstances and doesn't change by age 2
- A child who becomes so upset with a brief separation that she repeatedly refuses to eat or stop crying
- A child who doesn't notice or become upset with the parent or care provider's departure
- A child who never checks back with the parent when exploring a new environment

The child's current caretaking environment and medical, developmental, and social history should be explored if such responses are present.[10] Prolonged or traumatic separations fuel excessive anxiety in response to the appearance of a stranger. Poor attachment to primary caregivers leads to the indiscriminate response. Parental anxiety during separation experiences heightens the child's own response. Children with developmental delays have a delayed onset of stranger awareness in line with their cognitive level. Those with disorders in the autistic spectrum will have both delayed and atypical responses to separations. A special look at the attachment process of kids in foster care, blended families, and atypical circumstances is certainly warranted.

BABIES WHO MAKE NOISE IN THE NIGHT

Night wakening that wakes up others often returns at this age. Some believe the basis for this is the ability to miss the parents because the child can now envision them when he wakens (i.e., object permanence). The child cries out to call them. Also, the ability to pull to stand means that the child can really wake up completely by trying out these new skills. If the child is worried or aggravated about being unable to get down or just wants to share the adventure, he will cry out for attention and reassurance. To parents, this feels like a big step backward; a solid night's sleep is gone. The distress is genuine, but what to do? Answer: go back to the basics:

- Form a simple, but consistent bedtime ritual that involves putting the child to bed while he is still awake.
- Be sure the child has a "lovey" for cuddling.

- When the child awakens and calls out, wait a minute or two to provide the opportunity for the child to get back to sleep on his own.
- If the cries are frantic, go in silently and tuck the child back in, using the same procedures that were done originally.
- Avoid taking the child out of bed unless you want to do that all night long.
- Reassurance delivered in a quiet, nonplayful way with brevity will help the child learn how to settle himself down and go back to sleep.

Other children resist going to bed at this stage, although that is usually more common with toddlers and beyond. The same solid bedtime ritual should help quiet things down.

Sleep means a separation, particularly as we set things up in this country. If you're a kid, you are in your own bed, away from others, in the dark, and alone until you wake up. Going to sleep means saying good-bye for a while. This, like other separations, creates a little stress for a child, so it's no wonder that sleep concerns are so common. For parents too, putting the baby to bed is a separation, and they may not come to the task without ambivalence. For this reason, when the clinician counsels families about sleep problems, the underlying issues are how everyone feels about separation, what they can tolerate, and what they really want. Family inconsistency and failure to follow advice usually come down to an attachment-separation issue, which should be addressed before dealing with the specifics of sleep problems. The following groups are likely to have trouble:

- Parents of a small, sick, or prematurely born baby, who are still concerned about losing the child even if the child is not physically ill. Often the parents themselves are not aware of this underlying worry (see Chapters 5 and 6).
- A family who has lost a previous child
- A divorced, separating, or single parent
- A working couple who are away from the baby all day
- A family with a history of loss issues, particularly recent ones (e.g., a move, a death in the family, loss of a job)

Night wakening is perceived as a bid for closeness and help rather than a manifestation of developmental change in these cases. These parents cannot let the child solve this issue on his own. The motivations and emotional needs of the parents must be addressed openly if night wakening is frequent and problematic. Temperamental issues in the child and particular cultural or family issues may also be the source of barriers to achieve the stated sleep goals.

The clinical management strategy is to allay anxiety while supporting the child's own efforts to go back to sleep. Too vigorous an intervention just further awakens the child, making settling down all the more difficult. No evidence shows that bringing a child into the parents' bed is either uncommon or leads to disturbance.[26] Some families choose a family bed and cosleeping.[27,28] Breast feeding may be enhanced in that circumstance.[29] This will not harm the child as long as the following are true:

- The child's bids for independence are met in other ways.
- The child doesn't become exposed to sexual activity that may seem violent.
- The adults aren't under such strong influence of drugs or alcohol that the baby is forgotten.
- Cigarette smoke is not in the environment.

EXPLORING AND SAFETY

> *Becky Jones, a 9-month-old obese child, was brought to the emergency room by her frantic mother. The child had a small scald burn to her left forearm and a large "goose egg" on her forehead, but appeared alert as she whimpered in her mother's arms. Mrs. Jones said her daughter had pulled over the coffee pot, spilling coffee on herself. Mrs. Jones said she didn't even know that Becky could go that far or move as fast as she did. She really had not been crawling until recently. Becky sat quietly at her mother's feet, playing with some papers from the desk while her mother got out some tissues to soothe her tears.*

With each new developmental competency, a child has the chance of getting into trouble in entirely new and surprising ways. The clinician can put into place the general concept that **safety** has to be linked to each new developmental gain. If the parents can see the world from their child's perspective at each new juncture of enhanced competence, they can anticipate how to make the environment safe while offering the child the chance to explore and learn to use new skills. This is a broader perspective than merely a list of safety issues or a checklist given at each visit.

This general dictum aside, at 8 to 9 months, dramatic changes in the child call for safety inspections in a lot of new ways. This is an ideal time to put the parental mind-set in place. The emergence of mobility in one form or another and the more adept use of fingers and hands mean more fun, learning, and safety issues.

When the baby can creep, crawl, roll, or scoot on her bottom, the child can change places in space. Now the sphere of safety widens to wherever the child can move. A whole room has to be made safe, and some spaces have to be blocked off because they contain too many things that can get the child into trouble. The goal here is not to discuss every safety issue, but to put forward a strategy of looking at safety issues that are triggered by developmental change. Then, whenever new skills emerge, a parenting pattern can be set up. For example, when the child can climb, what about the surface under play equipment? When the child rides the bus to school, what safety measures are needed? Box 11-2 shows some of the maneuvers that are appropriate for the newly mobile child who can now change location.

Because children are more adept with their hands working together at this age and in using the index finger and the pincer grasp, what they can grab and what they pull toward them must be considered. Exploring discoveries with the mouth is to be expected, so that also should be considered. Box 11-3 shows some of the things to keep in mind about the child who now has enhanced manipulative skills.

Parents should be told to get on their hands and knees and go around the house to see the world as the baby sees it. The lurking dangers, as well as the temptations, are more obvious with that activity than merely by going through a checklist.

It is also a good metaphor for seeing things from the child's perspective as one tries to anticipate or solve child-rearing problems. Many times it is the clinician who has to evoke

| BOX 11-2 | SAFETY FIRST FOR BABY ON MOVE |

Cupboard doors should have safety stoppers.

Household cleaning products should be put up out of baby's reach.

All stairways should be blocked by attached gates.

Outside doors should be closed tightly, perhaps with plastic sealers, or for older children, high hooks.

The crib mattress should be at the lowest level.

The diaper changing area should be safe in the event of falls. This may mean a pad on the floor or a low bed.

Baby walkers should not be used at all.

The car seat should be adjusted for size and never ignored. Watch for the child's wriggling out of it.

The garage and the bathroom should be off limits unless an adult, focused on the child, is present at all times.

Sharp corners of tables and cabinets should have protectors on them.

| BOX 11-3 | SAFETY FIRST FOR ACTIVE HANDS |

All electrical outlets should be plugged or covered.

Electrical cords should not hang down.

Protective caps should be put on faucets to prevent kids from turning them on.

All breakables should be put away.

Residents' and visitors' purses should be placed out of the child's reach.

All medicines must have safety caps that are kept on.

All siblings' toys with small pieces should be put away.

Pets and babies are a mix ready for trouble.

All houseplants should be checked for poisonous components and removed if present. If safe ones are kept, be ready for pruning that you didn't count on and roughage (i.e., dirt) for the baby that you didn't plan.

Cat and dog food should be kept out of the child's reach.

Anything tiny should be kept off the floor.

Sandboxes, beaches, and playgrounds should be inspected for tiny undesirables, such as cigarette butts, coins, and buttons.

the child's view of things for the parent to see the way through to problem solving. Starting in the first year, on their knees to check out safety issues, parents get a good start on seeing things from the child's viewpoint. It is a handy exercise for the clinician to suggest. A developmental matrix of safety is in Table 11-1.

FEEDING AND EATING AS EXPLORATION AND SEPARATION

No better classroom exists for learning about the world and exerting just a taste of independence than eating. With each new developmental gain, the child can explore **food** in new ways and take greater and greater charge of what goes into his mouth. This is a messy process. Parents have to be able to tolerate this and be ready to hand over control to the child. This is hard if the parents are anxious about the child, have a need to control, or don't like the mess and uncertainty that self-feeding involves. At 8 months, with the development of the pincer grasp and improved eye-hand coordination, the child should be allowed finger foods that he can handle and be allowed to explore the feel and texture of food. If the child is not given that opportunity, eating will be less interesting later or will turn into a battleground between parent and child. And it's a battle that parents never win. If there are struggles around food, there are likely to be struggles around a lot of things in the interaction between parent and child.[30]

Rayna was an obese, placid child who moved around very little during the 9-month visit. At every whimper her mother took out a bottle and gave it to her, cradling her and covering her head while feeding.

Rayna was found to be anemic and was drinking about 48 to 52 ounces of milk per day. Her mother reported that Rayna didn't want to feed herself and was "too little" to drink from a cup.

Rayna's mother is still treating her like a newborn, not responding to her developmental gains. Anemia and obesity are only part of the problem here—a "developmental arrest" in feeding interaction overall exists. The clinician should show mom what Rayna can and should be doing with feeding at this age and should explore why mom needs to keep this baby as a newborn. A mere prescription for feeding is unlikely to work here. Table 11-2 presents the developmental course of feeding.

With each change in the child, the feeding-eating situation should change.[31] If the child can't do age appropriate–self feeding, the clinician should explore whether the baby has developmental delays, oral-motor difficulties, unusual taste and touch sensitivities, or other difficulties. If these are not the case, the interaction between parent and child should be explored. Sometimes this means having the mom bring in food and try to feed the baby in the office. Although this may seem time-consuming at first, it can be efficient in identifying the source of the problem, as well as difficulties in the parent-child interaction overall.[32]

TABLE 11-1 ■ Age-Appropriate Safety Guidelines

Age	Child's Activities	Dangers, Risks	Questions and Suggestions for Parents
0-6 mo	Swimming reflex	Drowning, water intoxication, stress	Counsel on early swimming lessons.
	Immobile	Fire, smoke dangers	Place smoke alarm near infant's sleeping quarters.
	Rolling over	Falls, rolling off table	Use appropriate bathing facilities, restraints, safe changing area, padded floor.
	Attempts to sit up	Flipping out of infant seat (3 mo)	Keep child restrained in infant seat; remove infant seat at 3 mo.
	Sucking and mouthing objects	Ingestion, aspiration, strangulation from pacifier string or other objects	Keep toys clean; avoid letting child mouth keys.
	Motor excitement	Slipping in bath	Lower temperature of hot water heater (<120° F).
	Reaching for objects	Burns, cuts	
7-12 mo	Crawl, pull to stand, cruising	Burns; falls down stairs, into toilet bowl, or into tub	Block stairs; eliminate walker.
	Increased curiosity	Ingestions (medicines, plants, chemicals, household cleaning agents)	Have poison control phone numbers and ipecac available; lock cabinets.
	Pincer grasp	Aspiration of small objects, such as marbles and toy parts, pills, seeds, plants	Keep older children's toys (with button eyes, removable parts) and other small objects out of reach.
	Puts everything in mouth	Electric cord bites	Keep cords out of reach.
	Goes after hidden objects	Aspiration, strangulation (cords)	Look under tables, chairs, beds for dangers.
	Pulls objects down	Hot liquid burns, objects on tables	Put heavy or hot objects out of reach.
1-2 yr*	Walking, running	Traffic accidents	Does the child have access to the street?

*Highest accident rates of all groups.

TABLE 11-1 ■ Age-Appropriate Safety Guidelines—cont'd

Age	Child's Activities	Dangers, Risks	Questions and Suggestions for Parents
1-2 yr— cont'd	Loves to be chased (18-24 mo)	Runs away, into streets	Block doors, walkways; use automatic gate locks.
	Climbing (tables, desks, counters)	Ingestions, falls, burns	How are medications stored? Put chairs away from counters.
	Goes after hidden objects	Ingestions, electrocution	Are medications in purse? Are outlets covered?
	Increased independence and curiosity	Ingestions, burns, drownings	Is access to pool blocked?
2-3 yr*	Expanding world (backyard, garage, friend's house)	Ingestions	Is there access to garage, backyard, safe play equipment?
	Imitative behavior	Climbs, follows older children, ingests pills	Keep medications locked up and out of reach.
	"Swim" classes	Drowning, drinking pool water with hyponatremia	Avoid. Be sure of full parent participation. Do not expect child to be drown proof.
	Introduction to adult foods (nuts, popcorn, chewing gum)	Aspiration	Avoid access to nuts, popcorn, and chewing gum at this age.
	Resists constraints (e.g., car seats)	Car accidents	Possess, install correctly, and *use* car seat.
	False maturity leading toward less parental supervision (2-yr-olds)	All accidents	Keep under *constant* observation.
3-5 yr	Improved motor development: reaches high 'safe' places	Ingestions, burns, falls	Supervise play.
	Tricycles, big wheels	Spoke injuries, traffic accidents	Provide safe places to play
	Expanded world (school, neighborhood)	Car accidents, falls	Has traffic safety been taught?
	Continued drive to discover world	Burns (matches)	Discuss fire safety.

Continued

TABLE 11-1 ■ Age-Appropriate Safety Guidelines—cont'd

Age	Child's Activities	Dangers, Risks	Questions and Suggestions for Parents
3-5 yr— cont'd	Role playing, superhero imitations	Burns, ingestions, falls	Keep play areas safe; regularly supervise; discuss role models.
	Resists constraints (e.g., car seats)	Car accidents	Possess, install correctly, and *use* car seat.
6-14 yr	Independence, spends time away from home	Bike, skateboard, and car accidents; drownings	Child should: wear helmets; skateboard off streets, hills; use inline skates with wrist, elbow, and knee pads and helmets; swim in groups under supervision; take swimming and water classes.
	Unsupervised activities	Burns (fireworks and matches), alcohol and drug exploration or overdose	Talk to the kid.
15-17 yr		Car accidents; drug and alcohol use	Make sure child takes driver education. Discuss peer-proofing and other drug education programs. Apply reasonable curfews. All parties should be supervised.

PLAY AS AN ASSESSMENT

Children will demonstrate the cutting edge of their developmental competency in their **play** if we give them just a few props and a lot of support with few stressors. The 9-month visit, because it falls at a time of great developmental change and before real mobility and stranger anxiety make the child take flight at every encounter, is the perfect time to really look at how the child plays. Referrals for additional evaluations and enrollment in early intervention programs can all be completed before the first birthday if concerns are found at this assessment.

Formal assessments are done by only a few primary care clinicians. Most are left to specialists, special programs, or clinics. However, the concept of "developmental surveillance" (see Chapter 1), to which the clinician should be committed, demands specific observations that inform the situation with a given child. Some evaluation formats (see Appendix) are useful to back up parental concerns or ones evoked by general observations in the clinic.

TABLE 11-2 ■ Behavioral and Developmental Abilities Related to Feeding

Newborn–2 mo	Primitive reflexes (rooting, sucking, swallowing) facilitate feeding and quickly become organized into a while pattern of behavior; hunger cry initiates feeding interaction; minimal vocal, visual, or motor activity during feeding
2–4 mo	More alert and interactive during feeding; explosive cough to protect self from aspiration; beginning ability to wait for food; associates mother's smell, voice, and cradling with feeding; hand-to-mouth behavior quiets infant, increases interest in mouthing activities
4–6 mo	Readiness for solids; excellent head and trunk control; reaching for objects; raking grasp; increased hand-to-mouth facility; loss of extrusion reflex of the tongue; may purposefully spit out food as part of food exploration; adaptation to introduction of solids may be affected by infant's temperament
6–8 mo	Sits alone with a steady head during sitting feedings; chewing mechanism developed; holds bottle; vocal eagerness during meal preparation; much more motor activity during feeding
8–10 mo	Finger-food readiness; thumb-forefinger grasp (i.e., inferior pincer); grasps spoon but cannot use it effectively; feeds self crackers, etc.; enjoys new textures, tastes; emerging independence
10–12 mo	Increasing determination to feed self; neat pincer grasp; drops food off high chair onto floor to see where it goes; holds cup but frequently spills it; more verbal and motor behavior during feeding
12–15 mo	Demands to feed self without help; decreased appetite and nutritional requirements; improved cup use (both hands); uses spoon, fills poorly, spills, turns at mouth; can use spoon as extension of the hand; messy play
15–18 mo	Eats rapidly, short feeding sessions; wants to be motorically active (too busy to eat); fairly good use of spoon and cup; enhanced ability to wait for food; plays with or throws food to elicit response from parent
18–24 mo	Feeds self, using combination of utensils and fingers; verbalizes "eat, all gone," asks for food; negativism emerges, says no when really wanting offered food; wants control of feeding situation
2–3 yr	Uses fork; ritualistic, repetitive at mealtimes; food jags, all one food at a time; dawdles; likes to help set and clear table; may begin to help self to refrigerator contents
3–4 yr	Spills little; uses utensils well; washes hands with minimal help; likes food preparation; reasonable table manners while eating out
4–5 yr	Serves self; choosy about food; resists some textures; begins to request foods seen on television ads (especially junk food); makes menu suggestions; likes to assist in washing dishes; helps in food preparation

Continued

TABLE 11-2 ■ Behavioral and Developmental Abilities Related to Feeding—cont'd

5-6 yr	Uses knife; assists in preparing and packing own box lunch; can be responsible for setting and clearing table; aids younger siblings' requests for food or drink
6-8 yr	Does dishes independently and willingly; increases pressure to buy junk food; interested in, often critical of, and attempts to negotiate about daily menu; manages money for school meal ticket
8-10 yr	Enjoys planning and preparing simple family meals; wants supplemental spending money to buy snacks when away from home; more reticent about trying new foods; resists kitchen chores

TABLE 11-3 ■ Stethoscope Play Continuum

Action	Age
Regards in the midline	Birth-1 month
Follows to at least 90 degrees	2-6 weeks
Swipes at it	2-4 months
Reaches for it	4-5 months
Brings it to the mouth	5-8 months
Reaches across the midline	6-8 months
Pivots to get it while seated	8-11 months
Unilateral reach	9-11 months
Examines parts of it	12-15 months
Imitates use	15-19 months
Pretends with others	2 years
Knows where the heart is and maybe what it does	3-5 years

However, certain "essential" play activities inform the observer quite readily of where the child is on the developmental continuum, from newborn through adolescence:

- Block play (1" cubes)
- Response to the stethoscope
- Marker drawing on paper

With these few things and the structure to characterize the child's response, you can get a fairly accurate estimate of development with minimal time expenditure. For children with unknown developmental status, block play is a good place to start. Blocks can be brought out at the beginning of the visit, while you are talking to mom or dad before any

TABLE 11-4 ■ Block Play	
Action	**Age**
Regards the block at 8-10 inches	Birth-1 mo
Follows the block to at least 45 degrees while supine	Birth-2 mo
Mouth, hands, and feet activate, go after the block	1-3 mo
Swipes at the block	2-4 mo
Holds the block placed in the hand	3-5 mo
Holds 2 blocks	5-7 mo
Bangs 2 blocks together	7-8 mo
Releases the block to put it in a cup	11 mo
Builds tower of two	15 mo
Builds tower of six	20 mo
Builds tower of eight	25 mo
Builds bridge of three	30 mo
Builds stairs of six	35 mo
Counts one block	36 mo
Knows four different colors of the blocks	3½ yr
Counts five blocks	4-4½ yr
Can add two sets of blocks (i.e., 2 + 3 = 5)	5-7 yr
Can calculate take away to ten blocks	7-8 yr

procedures. You will get real data before the conversation is finished. Then you can decide whether you or another professional should spend more time on an evaluation with more formal tools and structure. Tables 11-3 and 11-4 lay out these structures. The drawing progression is presented in Chapter 24.

DATA GATHERING
Observation

On entering the examination room at the beginning of the office visit when the infant is 7 to 9 months old, you may observe either a wary expression on the child's face or a sobering infant. Observe the child's *social distance*—the limits of proximity that the child allows before showing signs of distress. This "extra data" is obtained without special effort, merely the systematic observation of the child as you begin your encounter. Within the visit, pay attention to the following kinds of observations:

- The parent's response to the child's distress will reveal the interactive style of the mother or father.
- Are the child's needs for comfort easily met (e.g., during the physical examination, when the child is being weighed, or at the time of an immunization)?
- Be aware of the signs of infantile depression in children who have experienced prolonged or particularly stressful situations (see case of Logan earlier in this chapter).

History Taking

Several issues can be addressed while taking the child and family's history by asking questions such as the following:

Stranger Anxiety
- How does the baby respond to seeing new people?
- Has the baby begun to be a bit wary of people seen infrequently?
- If the baby cries vigorously at these encounters, how do you respond?

Transitional Objects
- Does the child have a "lovey," a special toy or object?
- Ask if the parent notes any pattern to the child's associated behaviors when she wants the object (e.g., fatigue, hunger, stress).
- How do you feel about the use of the object?

Other Care Providers
- At this office visit or earlier, the parents' activities outside the home should be discussed in terms of their impact on the child.
- Is the child left with a regular care provider?
- What is the leave-taking routine?
- Is the baby's response different now than before?
- What helps the baby with these transitions?
- Do you plan any changes in the future?

Observation

Sitting down on the floor or with the child on some surface will get you ready to look at how the baby explores the world. At 8 months of age, in a *free play session,* we would expect the child to do the following:

- Sit without support
- Reach around the side to get a toy
- Reach for objects with both hands
- Anticipate the shape of an object with the shaping of the hand while reaching
- Transfer objects from hand to hand
- Stand while holding on (i.e., weight bearing)

- Move in some way—scooting, creeping, crawling
- Use a pincer grasp for small objects
- String phonemes together, such as "mamamama," "dadadada"
- May do pat-a-cake or wave bye-bye
- Hold a cube in each hand
- Bang cubes together
- Go after the stethoscope with one hand at a time, may imitate the dangling
- Be unable to let go of cube to put in a cup or a hand
- Look wary at first approach
- Cry when parent leaves or moves away
- Require help to sit and stand
- Try to put the ball and the cube together

ANTICIPATORY GUIDANCE

The cognitive basis for emerging stranger anxiety should be clearly explained. This puts it in a positive, normative framework; it doesn't mean the child has been abused or poorly cared for. The clinician can offer guidance for dealing with separation issues:

- Children should never be forced to show affection for a new person if they are distressed. This protest behavior must be seen as developmentally based and protective. Give children a chance to see the stranger in a familiar context for a period of time.
- Leave-taking rituals should be well established by this time. The routine helps children to cope with separations. This includes sleep; bedtime rituals are vital.
- When moving from room to room, parents should keep voice contact with children and reappear regularly.
- Baby-sitters should be introduced while the child is in the parent's arms, should approach slowly, and should give the child a chance to know them.
- Parents should never sneak away or go out after the child is asleep, if possible. The child's protest should be expected and tolerated rather than the parent violating the child's basic trust.
- Discuss separation issues as parents plan trips, vacations, and other separations. Discuss what can be done to support the child at times of necessary separations.
- Tell the family to avoid changes in the child's placement or custody between 6 and 18 months if at all possible.
- Avoid hospitalizations, if possible, during this time. The parent should always stay with the child at this age, even if they "cry more."
- If a child needs a medical procedure, encourage the parent to stay with the child. The child may cry *more*, but the stress of the situation will be *less*. Decreased crying is not necessarily the desired endpoint.
- Suggest the sharing of the infant's care with other adults if no other adults are regularly in the family. The child needs to be introduced to friendly strangers as opportunities for growth.
- Advise the parents to hold the child close after a separation until *the child* signals readiness to play or move away. This may mean that dinner preparation, laundry, or the mail should wait after a day at work.

- Discuss the night wakenings often seen at this age. Discuss management through allowing the child opportunity to get back to sleep.
- Suggest establishing falling-asleep rituals that can be replicated by the child when he awakens in the night. Tell the parents they should not put a child fully to sleep by holding unless they are prepared to do so all night long.
- Suggest support in choosing a transitional object for the child or family who is having trouble with separations.
- Beware of the chronically ill child who "likes everybody" in the hospital or the foster child who goes too easily to your arms. These children may have a serious derangement in attachment and may need extensive remedial work.

ACKNOWLEDGMENT

Previous versions of this work benefitted from the contributions of Pamela Kaiser, PNP, PhD.

REFERENCES

1. Spitz RA: The smiling response, *Genet Psychol Monogr* 34:57, 1946.
2. Ainsworth MDS: *Infancy in Uganda: infant care and the growth of attachment,* Baltimore, 1967, Johns Hopkins Press.
3. Bretherton I: The origin of the attachment theory: John Bowlby and Mary Ainsworth, *Dev Psych* 28:759, 1992.
4. Goin-DeCarie T: *The infant's reaction to strangers,* New York, 1974, International Universities Press.
5. vanIJzendoorn MT, Kroonenberg PM: Cross-cultural patterns of attachment: a meta-analysis of the strange situation, *Child Dev* 59:147, 1988.
6. Bowlby J: *Attachment,* vol 1, New York, 1969, Basic Books.
7. Bowlby J: *Separation: anxiety and anger,* New York, 1969, Basic Books.
8. Kagan J, Kearsley RB, Zelano P: *Infancy: its place in human development,* Cambridge, Mass, 1978, Harvard University Press.
9. Pederson DR, Moran G: Expressions of the attachment relationship outside of the strange situation, *Child Dev* 67:915, 1996.
10. Stein MT, Call J: Extraordinary changes in behavior in an infant after a brief separation, *J Devel Behav Pediatr* 19:424, 1998.
11. Main M, Solomon J: Procedures for identifying infants as disorganized or disoriented during the Ainsworth strange situation. In Greenberg M et al, editors: *Attachment in the preschool years,* Chicago, 1990, Chicago University Press.
12. Sroufe LA, Egeland B, Kreulzer T: The fate of early experience following developmental change: longitudinal approaches to individual adaptation in childhood, *Child Dev* 61:1363, 1990.
13. Isabella RA: Origins of attachment: maternal interactive behavior across the first year, *Child Dev* 64:605, 1993.
14. Grossman KE, Grossman K: The wider concept of attachment in cross cultural research, *Early Hum Dev* 33:31, 1990.
15. Waters E: The reliability and stability of individual differences in infant-mother attachment, *Child Dev* 49:483, 1978.
16. Vaughn B et al: Individual differences in infant-mother attachment at twelve and eighteen months: stability and change in families under stress, *Child Dev* 50:971, 1979.

17. vanIJzendoorn MH et al: The relative effects of maternal and child problems on the quality of attachment and clinical samples, *Child Dev* 63:840, 1992.
18. Fraiberg S: *The magic years,* New York, 1959, Charles Scribner's Sons.
19. Owen MT, Cox MJ: Marital conflict and the development of infant-parent attachment relationships, *J Fam Psych* 11:152, 1997.
20. Rutter M: Separation experiences: a new look at an old topic, *J Pediatr* 95:147, 1995.
21. Winnicott DW: Transitional objects and transitional phenomena. In Winnecott DW: *Collected papers: through pediatrics and psychoanalysis,* London, 1958, Tavistock Publications.
22. Lozoff B, Paludetto R, Lotz S: Transitional object use in the United States, Japan and Italy. Paper presented to the Ambulatory Pediatric Association, Carmel, Calif, May, 1985.
23. Sherman M et al: Treasured objects in school aged children, *Pediatrics* 68:379, 1981.
24. Leach P: *Your growing child,* ed 2, New York, 1989, Alfred A. Knopf.
25. Mahler M, Pine F, Bergman A: *The psychological birth of the human infant: symbiosis and individuation,* New York, 1975, Basic Books.
26. Lozoff B, Wolf A, Davis N: Cosleeping in urban families with young children in the United States, *Pediatrics* 74:171, 1984.
27. Stein MT, Colarusso, CA, McKenna J: Cosleeping (bedsharing) among infants and toddlers, *J Dev Behav Pediatr* 18:408, 1997.
28. Madansky D, Edelbrock C: Cosleeping in a community of 2-3 year old children, *Pediatrics* 86:198, 1990.
29. McKenna J, Mosko S, Richard C: Bedsharing promotes breastfeeding, *Pediatrics* 100:214, 1997.
30. Stein MT: Common issues in feeding. In Levine MD, Carey WB, Crocker A, editors. *Developmental-behavioral pediatrics,* ed 3, Philadelphia, 1997, WB Saunders, pp 392-396.
31. Telzrow R: Developmental considerations in infant feeding. In Howard RB, Herbold MH: *Nutrition in clinical care,* New York, 1982, McGraw-Hill Book.
32. Barnard K: *Nursing child assessment feeding scales (NCAST),* Seattle, 1978, University of Washington.

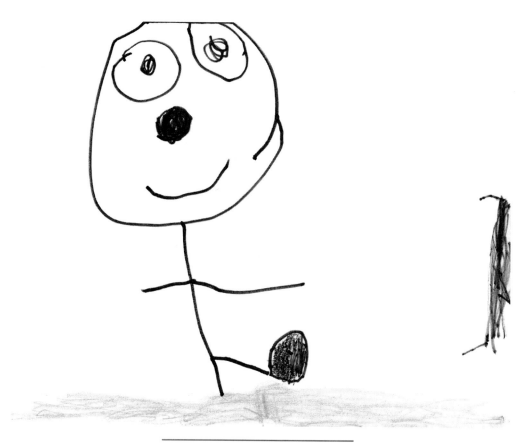

"A boy kicks a ball at a goal!" By Eric Stroiman, age 4½.

ONE YEAR: ONE GIANT STEP FORWARD

■ **Suzanne D. Dixon**
■ **Michael J. Hennessy**

KEY WORDS
Walking
Gross-Motor Processes
Gait Cycle
Running
Skill Appearance and Competency
Sleep Position and Motor Milestones
Infant Walkers
Sports
Shoes
Temperamental Characteristics

> *Jared's mom looks very glum as she comes in for his 1-year-old visit. She says that her mother-in-law wants Jared's legs checked and wants her to get advice about shoes. Mom admits that they're all concerned about Jared's not walking yet. His older brother walked at 9 months.*

The developmental milestone that parents focus on most prominently is the age at which the child starts **walking.**[1] Independent gait is greeted by parents as a source of pride and assurance of normality; any delay in its appearance may trigger worry and dire prognostication. Clinicians are also more likely to note and record this developmental landmark than any other.[2] Everyone, including the child, feels better when the baby walks, as if a big hurdle has been successfully overcome.

The child's perspective on the world and on himself changes dramatically when he can alter location, so he's a different child after walking. The visit of a 1-year-old offers the opportunity to look at the development of ambulation and **gross-motor processes** in general that emerge both before and after the start of walking. The goal is to see this area of development in the broader context of the whole child and in its importance to the family. The manner of emergence of this milestone provides great insight into a child and family from more than the motor vantage point. This view of the processes in and around motor development gives the clinician an expanded perspective on these readily observed and reliably noted milestones.

Some of the earliest perspectives on the regularities of early childhood development came from the observations of gross-motor milestones made by Gesell,[3] McGraw,[4] and others. This sequence came out of careful longitudinal and cross-sectional observations of normal children. The pediatric perspective on development in general has been strongly based on these schemes of motor milestones following from a neuromaturational model (see Chapter 2). Although we now know that not every aspect of gross-motor development can be accounted for by this model, the regularity and the readily observable nature of these motor achievements form a core of basic developmental appraisal, as shown in Figs. 12-1 and 12-2. Physical milestones in infancy are presented in Table 12-1. These are easy to observe, readily reported by parents, and easier than most to remember.[1] Through a chronicle of regular achievement of these skills, clinicians are assured of the child's neurological adequacy.

MOTOR SKILLS: GENERAL PRINCIPLES

Walking must be seen in the context of other gross-motor accomplishments. These all share, in addition to their regular sequence, certain characteristics[5]:

■ These skills are built on *neuromotor tone,* the base which determines behaviors, skills, and patterns. Hypotonic children, from whatever cause, will have delays in postural maturation and skill acquisition. Hypertonic children, with prominence of extensor postures, will have predictable "pseudoaccelerations" (e.g., rolling over, weight bearing on legs, and pull-to-stand) and delays (e.g., sitting).

■ *Volitional behavior is preceded by reflex behavior.* For example, the newborn reflex patterns of reciprocal kicking and automatic stepping clearly foreshadow the movements of walking seen near the end of the first year. These early patterns disappear at approximately 2 months of age to later reappear in the progressive emergence of independent gait. This sequence is thought to result from increasing suppression of the primitive reflexes by maturing cortical centers, leading to their reorganization into volitional movement patterns. Concomitant with increased strength and improved balance, the child learns to control the reflex pattern and use it to move.

■ Alternatively, it has been suggested that a *more continuous movement pattern evolution* characterizes motor development, avoiding this adaptation of the primitive reflex model.[6,7] A delay in the disappearance of early infant reflexes is associated with a comparable delay in the emergence of voluntary motor skills and can be anticipated by the clinician, although the mechanism of association is unclear. The sequence is clear, even if the description of the linkage is not. For example, the parachute reflexes, first the upper and then the lower, appear at about 9 months. Independent walking starts about 4 months after these appear, which suggests some orderly adaptation to the inevitable stumbles that early walkers experience.[8] Whether reflexes dissolve or are subsumed in more complex volitional patterns is not known. However, the regular unfolding and then disappearance of reflex behavior followed by the emergence of skilled movement offer the clinician an opportunity to point out to parents the integrity and internally regulated nature of the child's maturation.

■ *Maturation entails an increasing efficiency in the energy expenditure that is required to move through space.* The child becomes an increasingly efficient movement machine.[9,10] The bio-

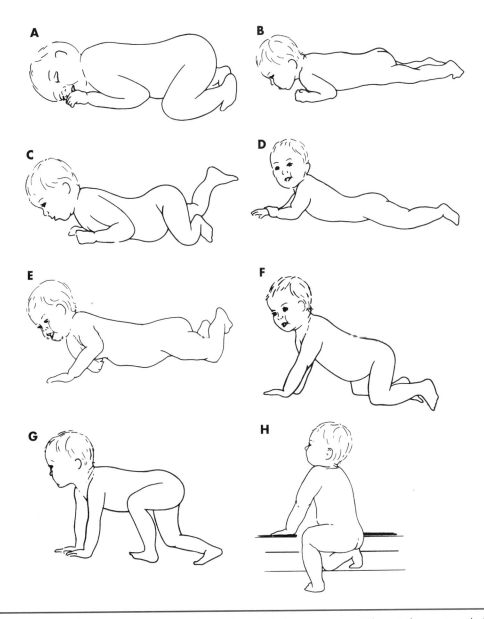

Fig. 12-1   Progression of prone posture. **A,** Newborn in flexed posture. **B,** Infant at about 1 month, head up briefly; some extension at hips and knees. **C,** Infant about 1 to 2 months old, head up to about 45 degrees, active legs. **D,** Infant about 3 to 4 months, up easily on forearms, head steady and able to be turned with minimal bobbing. **E,** Infant about 5 to 9 months up on hands; may use arm to pull self forward; may push with thighs and knees, creeping. **F,** Infant 7 to 11 months, crawling; reciprocal movement of legs and legs with hands. **G,** Crawling on feet. **H,** Child 8 to 18 months of age, climbs stairs.

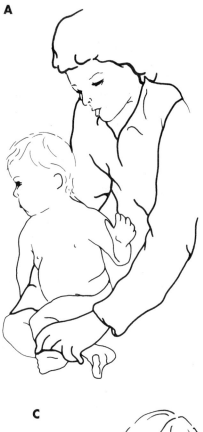

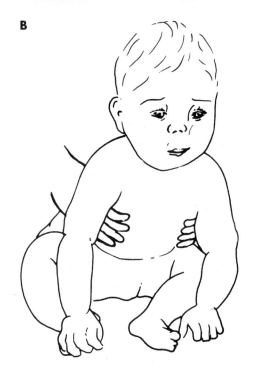

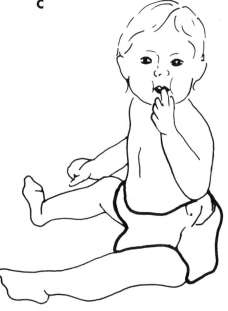

Fig. 12-2   Sitting progression: With each time period, steadiness and control of head increases; back becomes straighter from upper portion down; arms are held naturally further back, with external rotation at the shoulder. **A,** Age 1 to 2 months, sits with truncal support, head and shoulders steady, lower back still rounded. **B,** Age 4 to 7 months, sits in a pivot position with slight truncal support; all energy directed at maintaining postures. **C,** Age 5 to 9 months, independent sitting, back straight, able to pivot without losing balance.

TABLE 12-1 ■ Physical Milestones in Infancy

Behavior*	Age Range (mo)	Average Age (mo)
Raises self by arms while lying face down	0.7-5	2.1
Sits with support	1-5	2.3
Sits alone momentarily	4-8	5.3
Sits alone 10-30 seconds or more	5-8	6.0
Rolls from back to stomach	4-10	6.4
Sits alone quite steadily for long periods	5-9	6.6
Stands up holding onto furniture	6-12	8.6
Walks while adult holds hands	7-12	9.6
Sits down after standing	7-14	9.6
Stands alone	9-16	11.0
Walks alone	9-17	11.7
Walks sideways	10-20	14.1
Walks backward	11-20	14.6
Walks up stairs with help	12-23	16.1
Stands on left foot alone	15-30	22.7
Jumps off floor with both feet	17-30+	23.4
Stands on right foot alone	16-30+	23.5
Jumps from the last stair step to floor	19-30+	24.8
Walks up stairs alone with both feet on each step	18-30+	25.1
Walks a few steps on tiptoes	16-30+	25.7
Walks down stairs alone with both feet on each step	19-30+	25.8
Jumps from the second stair step to the floor	21-30+	28.1
Walks up stairs, alternating forward foot	23-30+	30+

*5th to 95th percentile.
From Bayley Scales of Infant Development, Motor Scale Record, The Psychological Corp, 1969, 1994. Used by permission.

mechanical parameters assure that with maturation and practice, forward movement is achieved with less change in the center of gravity, less overall joint movement, and refinement of muscle movement. This means more efficient movement.

■ *The progression of control is from more proximal joint movement to recruitment of more distal movement.* This usually means a refinement, a fine tuning of movement because the more

BOX 12-1	WORRY MARKERS*

No rolling prone to supine by 7 months
No rolling supine to prone by 9 months
No unsupported sitting by 10 months
No independent steps by 18 months
No running by 2 years
No jumping by 2½-3 years
No pedaling of tricycle or big wheel by 4 years
No bike riding by age 10

*These time frames should alert the clinician to problems that clearly call for more evaluation.

distal joint can make adjustments with less movement and more accuracy, as seen in the development of reach (see Chapter 10). Control of reach moves from the shoulder to the wrist; control of gait is transferred in part to the knee and ankle with maturation.

■ *The child increases in both speed and accuracy of movement with time.* These last characteristics (gains in efficiency, accuracy, and speed) are demonstrated in the specific developmental course of gait. Overshooting or undershooting, bilateral reach, and less well-directed movements are characteristics of immature movement.

MOTOR MILESTONES: THE TIME COURSE

The incredible importance placed on walking is curious. The age of independent ambulation, unless it is delayed beyond 18 months, predicts other areas of development very poorly. Accelerated motor development in general does not testify to superior mental skills; late motor development, except in the extreme, does not indicate mental deficiency. Delayed walking in children with perinatal difficulties is associated with an increased incidence of broader developmental delay, but without this history of risk, the age of walking has poor prognostic value.[11] (See Box 12-1.)

WALKING: A CHANGE IN PERSPECTIVES

New motor competencies dramatically change the child's view of herself and the world. Placement in space is now under the child's own control. The child now can choose (within limits) *what* to explore, not just *how* to investigate the objects within vision or reach. These skills allow the child to perceive, learn, and experience in entirely new ways by movement through space, such as choosing to go away from or toward caregivers. That new option is both exciting and scary. Everything changes because of this new perspective. Selma Fraiberg[12] describes the overwhelming world and self-view changes that a child experiences when he or she learns to walk.

In the last quarter of the first year, the baby is no longer an observer of a passing scene. He is in it. Travel changes one's perspective. A chair, for example, is an object of one dimension when

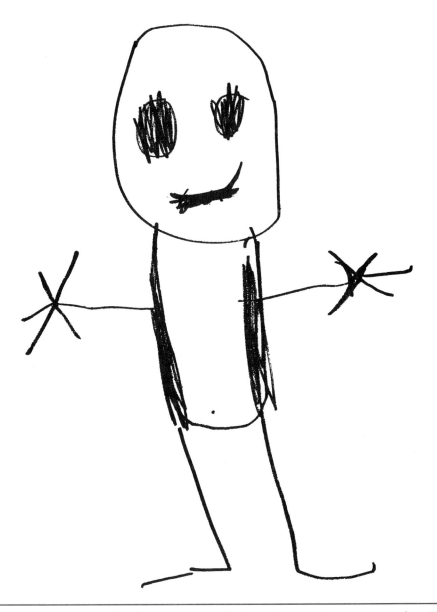

"Getting up on your own two feet" gives a sense of independence and an urge to explore. Belly buttons start to appear in drawings of 3½- to 5-year-olds. By Colin Hennessy, age 3½.

viewed by a 6-month-old baby propped up on a sofa. . . It's when you start to get around under your own steam that you discover what a chair really is.

The first time the baby stands unsupported and the first wobbly independent steps are milestones in personality development, as well as in motor development. To stand unsupported, to take that first step is a brave and lonely thing to do.[12]

All development is fueled by the ability to change position in space and to move away from a completely dependent vantage point. Or, as pointed out again by Fraiberg:

> The discovery of independent locomotion and the discovery of a new self usher in a new phase in personality development. The toddler is quite giddy with his new achievements. He behaves as if he had invented this new mode of locomotion and he is quite in love with himself for being so clever. From dawn to dusk he marches around in an ecstatic, drunken dance, which ends only when he collapses with fatigue.[12]

A motorically slow or disabled child suffers secondary disabilities because of limitations on visual, perceptual, and tactile experiences compared with walking, moving peers. The child also misses the energizing sense of competency that follows from motor gains. Seen in this context, therapies, surgical procedures, and external supports and braces for these children should be considered or evaluated from the perspective of their impact on these areas of development. Just normalization of position or posture is not enough if real mobility is not clearly improved.

THE ONTOGENY OF GAIT

Adult human ambulation is remarkably consistent and regular in terms of angles of displacement of the joints involved; the mathematical relationships between cadence, stride length, and velocity; and the timing of these events through the **gait cycle.**[10] Fig. 12-3 illustrates the gait cycle of events that occurs from heel strike to the next heel strike. These biomechanical events have specific durations, timing of muscle groups, and shifts of weight that mature over time, as shown in Table 12-2. The observation of gait throughout these phases allows a more accurate characterization of gait in both normal and abnormal conditions. The observation, "He walks funny," can be given more specificity if we understand what the parts of the gait cycle are and what to expect developmentally.

TYPICAL NORMAL WALK CYCLE

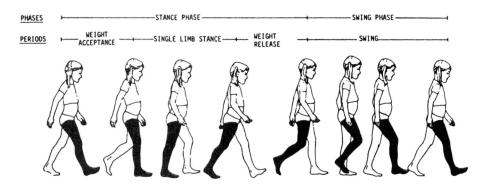

Fig. 12-3 Phases of the normal gait in childhood. (From Hennessy M, Dixon S, Simon S: *Child Dev* 55:844-853, 1984.)

TABLE 12-2 ■ Gross-Motor Development: 3-15 Years	
Age (Yr)	**Gross-Motor Development**
3	Stands on one foot; walks upstairs alternating feet
4	Pedals tricycle; runs smoothly; throws ball overhand
5	Walks downstairs alternating feet; skips; marches with rhythm; catches bounced ball
6	Hops; jumps
7	Pedals bicycle
8	Has good body balance
9	Engages in vigorous bodily activities, especially in team sports
10	Balances on one foot 15 seconds; catches fly ball
12	Motor awkwardness secondary to uneven bone and muscle growth
15	Gradual correction of motor awkwardness

Modified from Sahler OJZ, McAnarney ER: *The child from three to eighteen,* St Louis, 1981, Mosby.

All these gait parameters are moving toward maximal displacement in space with a minimum of energy expenditure. The body's center of gravity moves forward in nearly a straight line in a mature gait, the path of least energy expenditure. Extremity movements work together toward that end. Each of these parameters has its own developmental course as demonstrated by high-speed film analysis coupled with floor force plate and analysis of electromyographic (EMG) data. These highly technical studies have allowed a more complete and technically refined description of gait; they specify what the clinician can learn by careful additional observation.[10,13,14] These techniques are also useful in populations where gait is abnormal and surgical correction is contemplated. The following are characteristics of walking in a young child[9,10,14-17] (Figs. 12-4 to 12-6):

- The toddler's stance is *broad based;* as the child matures, the stance will narrow in absolute measure and in proportion to leg length. The narrower the base, the more mature the gait.
- Child's *knees and hips are flexed* even while standing and remain so as the toddler waddles one leg forward with a twist of the trunk; a changing hip position and a locked knee will emerge with development.
- Child's belly and bottom stick out because of the increased lordotic curve of the lower back. This provides balance in the immature walker. As the hips straighten (i.e., flexion), the child will tuck in the tummy and straighten the back.
- Ankle movement is minimal at first with flat-footed foot placement; as child matures, the ankle will dorsiflex and plantar flex. The child will develop a consistent heel strike after 30 months and a reliable lift-off with the forefoot and toes.
- When the child is first walking, the arms are abducted (out to his sides) and flexed at the elbow. They move little throughout the gait cycle, providing balance only. The arms first

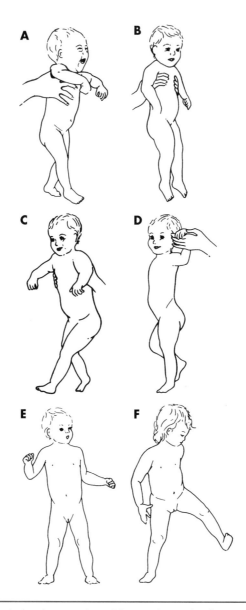

Fig. 12-4 Progression of gait development in toddlers and preschoolers. **A,** Reflex walk of the newborn, which usually disappears at 3 to 4 weeks of age. **B,** Before 3 months, infant bears little weight on legs. **C,** After 7 months, infant will walk with much truncal support. Excessive hip flexion with a forwardly displaced center of gravity means child is not ready for walking. **D,** Near 1 year of age, child's center of gravity is over hips and child can walk with help. **E,** During toddler years, positions of child's arm and feet testify to the level of maturity of gait. **F,** It is not until 3 to 5 years of age that child can balance steadily on one foot with all reciprocal truncal, hip, and arm adjustments that are required.

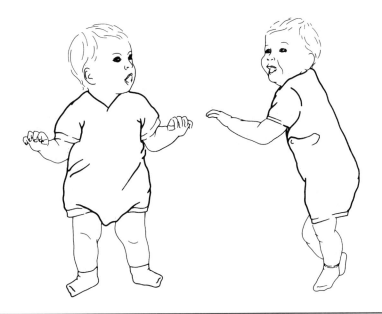

Fig. 12-5 Toddler's gait. Wide based, flexion at hip and knees, abducted feet, arms up and fixed.

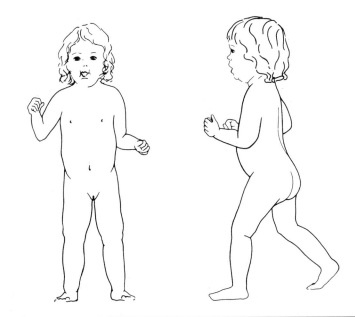

Fig. 12-6 Gait of the older toddler. Arms still used as part of balance. Feet turned out. Relative lordosis with trunk over hips.

come down, the hands go from fisted or splayed to relaxed, and then reciprocal arm movements are added.

- Feet go out nearly sideways. With maturation they turn more toward straight ahead.
- The center of gravity in a youngster just starting to walk shifts markedly up and down and side to side, an observation you can note if you just watch the umbilicus move throughout the gait cycle. This movement stabilizes throughout the gait cycle, and truncal rotation decreases.
- Angles of displacement at all joints decrease with time. Less overshooting or excess movement occurs.
- Acceleration forces are stronger than deceleration, so forward momentum is hard to check at first. Stopping is much harder than starting for the young child. Only later can stopping be combined with a pivot.
- Step length and walking speed increase, and cadence decreases with time, gradually approaching a fixed mathematical relationship. Older children take fewer steps to walk at a given speed largely because of an increase in step length. This, in turn, is related to leg length.

By 5 years of age, gait has matured to nearly adult patterns clinically and biomechanically (Fig. 12-7). The EMG patterns show adult patterns of muscle firing by this age as well.[18] Although increasing refinements emerge slowly and allow for more complex movements to develop, the mature biomechanical aspects of gait are established by school age.

Running emerges about 6 months after independent walking is well established. This involves a reduction of stance time (time with weight on both feet) to less than 50% of the gait cycle. Children don't increase their stride length when they run as toddlers; they just take more steps to go at a running speed. They keep the knees at a fixed flexion and don't use their feet to give a lift-off. Hip movement is as inefficient with running as it is for walking in the younger ages. All of the run parameters gradually shift to more mature forms across the preschool years.[19] Children will learn how to increase stride length, will add a "flight" phase when they lift off the ground briefly, and will learn to use reciprocal arm movement to propel themselves forward.

PREWALKING

The biomechanical precursors of gait are the reciprocal hip and leg movements of the kicking and crawling child, not standing or pull-to-stand.[6,7] These early spontaneous movements have the biomechanical characteristics, interrelationships, coordination, and rhythm of gait. However, not every child will crawl, and this does not reflect either motor or cognitive development. In fact, crawling may be the most overrated motor milestone in the first year. But all typical children will demonstrate ongoing reciprocal movement of the lower extremities that becomes smoother and more rhythmical and efficient from 9 to 12 months of age (Fig. 12-8). Spontaneous "swimming" movements are seen during bathing at about 9 months. These spontaneous movements are important to monitor (e.g., when a child is supine on an examining table) during the first year rather than merely checking off specific skill acquisitions, a process that can be misleading. These are the precursors of gait. Practice walking has not been

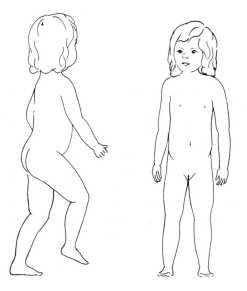

Fig. 12-7 Gait of the preschooler. Biomechanically, nearly at adult patterns. Heel strike present. Neck, shoulder, hips, and knees nearly vertical.

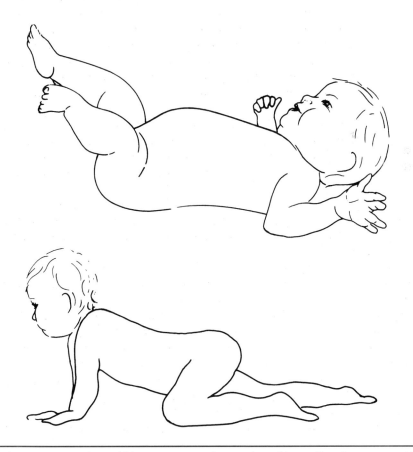

Fig. 12-8 Spontaneous reciprocal hip movements take a variety of forms. Practice opportunities are provided in prone.

shown to accelerate or decelerate the emergence of walking. Freedom to move in the prone position and enticements to explore in space by whatever means form the basis of gait.

GETTING STARTED AND REFINING SKILLS

Most children will cruise by 12 months, walking while holding on to objects at shoulder height, as shown in Fig. 12-9. Some children may resist any attempts at steps if their hands are held up because this eliminates the usefulness of arm position and truncal rotation, which provide stability. Cruising *on one's own* provides opportunity for real practice and the development of firm prototypes of movement that can be applied to varying demands, such as walking on a carpet versus walking on grass and going up the stairs or down an incline versus walking on a flat plane. The child is experimenting with new approaches to motor activity rather than simply repeating fixed actions. It is not rote repetition of a single activity

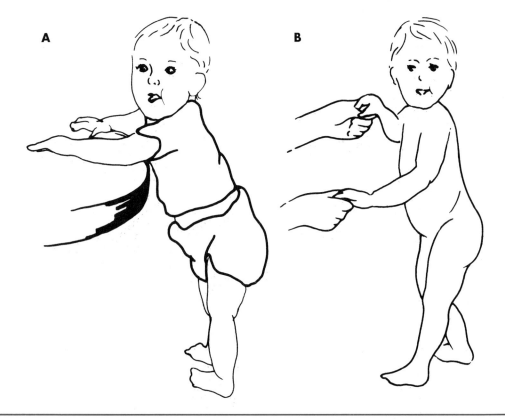

Fig. 12-9   Getting upright, cruising. **A,** Cruising on one's own provides opportunities to practice and explore. Most children do this by 12 months. **B,** Walking with help. Many families enjoy this activity. No evidence shows that this harms the child or accelerates walking. Some children resist holding on with both hands.

in a single circumstance many times over, but the accumulation of experiences that demands ongoing accommodation. For example, an adult could not claim competency in skiing after going down only one hill no matter how expertly that hill had been skied. Learning the skill (in the child's case, walking; for the adult, skiing) includes actively assimilated experiences in many circumstances and conditions. Passive practice or repetitive exercise of motor skills in isolation has no effect on skill acquisition, although range of motion at the joints may be maintained in a disabled child. *Self-initiated* actions, active movement, and exploration of the possibilities of movement are the necessary components of motor development.

Infant exercise programs for children without disabilities do not enhance motor development except as they energize the child and family through the enjoyment of movement and time spent together. Therapy programs that rely on *passive* movement may keep disabled children's joints flexible, but they do not ensure or augment skill acquisition. *No* evidence shows that repeated practice of motor movements (i.e., patterning) has any effect on the development of the handicapped or learning-impaired child.[20] Therapies should be designed to liberate the child from constraints based on tone, strength, or the preservation of premature reflexes to allow for active exploration and self-initiated movement.

ENVIRONMENT: INFLUENCING FACTORS

In spite of our own expectations, most children are *not* walking on their first birthday. The mean age for walking is about 60 weeks, with a 2 standard deviation range of 9 to 17 months.[21] The misconception that a child will walk by age 1 leads parents to feel worried and disappointed if the first steps haven't appeared by the first birthday. The clinician should mention the real norms if the child isn't walking, whether or not the parents bring up the issue. Many cultural groups will seek remedies for perceived weakness, bone problems, or foot irregularities in the child who is not walking by the first birthday.

 Mrs. Rodriguez asked Dr. Martin for vitamins to build up her Jorge's blood. "He's already 1, and his legs are weak and turned (bowed)."

The range of perception of achievement with **skill appearance** (i.e., doing the activity in any way or form), as well as **competency** (i.e., being able to do it without seeming to choose to exercise that skill, doing it regularly and automatically), is quite marked and is related to temperamental, familial, ethnic, and, to some degree, experiential factors.

Although regularity in the sequence of gross-motor development offers support for a prominent neuromaturational component in this area of development, a clear role is played by environmental factors as well. Neuromaturational readiness, physical factors such as leg length and strength, motivation of the child, and opportunities to hone and practice skills all play into this. Motor skills develop through an integration of previously acquired and practiced skills. This *dynamical systems* view is in contrast to the previous notion of motor skills developing nearly automatically with environmental supports having no role at all.

Expectations and timing of these events may vary by culture and family.[22] Familial patterns of walking may be related to the temporal aspects of nerve myelinization, to an inherited behavioral style, or to degree of emphasis on gross-motor activities. Basic neuromotor precocity and these individual factors may be the basis for the observed early acceleration of motor development in several groups, including African, Mexican, East Indian, and Middle Eastern children, when compared with that of white Americans.[13] Subgroup differences exist for the average age of achievement of motor milestones. A basic motor competency appears to be present at birth in these groups, which propels the infants forward at a faster rate and also leads to different patterns of handling that build on this early competency.[23]

Mr. Jackson, a black American, proudly held his 7-month-old son Miles's hands and walked him across the examining room to Dr. Strain. The baby bubbled with delight, squealing with every move.

Mrs. Williamson, a white American, held her daughter Melissa with strong support in a sit, her pale skin and feathery hair making her seem younger and more fragile than her 9 months. She delicately moved a toy back and forth without a sound, watching it and all the people in the room with an intensity that was almost alarming.

Severe experiential deprivation is necessary before any significant delay in motor development is noted. Dennis' study[24] of Hopi Indian infants placed on cradle boards demonstrated no alteration in the maturity or timing of walking, and more recent studies confirmed these classic findings.[25] These Native-American children, in spite of some early confinement (usually when sleeping), had ample opportunity for free movement and developed normally.[26] Specific training of motor skills (e.g., climbing) appears to have no effect on the time of emergence of those competencies.[4]

The new advisory on infant **sleep position**[27] has resulted in a slight shift in the timing of some **motor milestones,** such as rolling prone to supine, creeping and crawling, and pull-to-stand. Walking age shows no difference based upon sleep position. Importantly, those infants placed on their backs to sleep also had more awake time in that position, so it is unclear what contributes to this shift of less than a month in these motor landmarks. Experience may play a role in the development of these skills.[28] Tummy time while awake, back to sleep at night is a good practice to recommend.

The use of **infant walkers** in particular seems to have no effect on the appearance of independent walking.[29,30] Safety may be impaired in all children using these devices, so they should *not* be recommended. Extensor postures may be solidified in children with lower extremity hypertonia, undermining rather than facilitating walking in these youngsters.

Peripheral nerve myelinization and cerebellar growth increase rapidly from 6 to 12 months, and these changes appear to coincide with the movement changes that occur during that time. These processes in the central nervous system (CNS) set up basic readiness. Physical growth factors such as height and leg length may influence patterns of motor development[13] through biomechanical relationships that are necessary to get walking going. Obese children may have later gross-motor skill acquisition because of these biomechanical factors; they just have more mass to move.

> Brady, a 15-month-old of 28 pounds, was not yet walking and actually moved very little in the course of play. He was quite content in a playpen. However, he moved quickly in a crawl when he tried to grab the cat while he was on the floor.

A maturational readiness seems to be within a child, so motor skills emerge within a supportive but noninstructive environment. The environment alone can take little credit or blame for gross-motor achievements, but it acts with other factors synergistically. Or, as stated by Wolff,[31] "Neither intrinsic developmental timetables nor experience is a sufficient condition for motor skill acquisition. At every stage motor development depends not only on experience and quality of the stimuli, but also on brain mechanisms that assimilate and organize information from the environment and from action in progress."

An internal consistency within a child allows some anticipation of gross-motor skills. For example, a late sitter is likely to be a late walker. The style with which a child approaches motor skill development is also consistent.[32] Some children charge ahead to pull-to-stand, cruise, and walk with lots of energy and lots of falls. Others will take a more contemplative approach, studying the task well, winding up slowly, and feeling assured of each step before trying the next. The clinician will learn more about a child by monitoring *how* she achieves gross-motor skills than by focusing exclusively on the timing of these behaviors.

GAIT ABNORMALITIES

Although awkward at first, the gait of the young child should follow the sequence described previously and should show symmetry. A parent's saying something is wrong with her child's walking should be cause for careful evaluation. Some specific concerns are laid out in Box 12-2.

BOX 12-2   OBSERVATIONS THAT TRIGGER WORRY ABOUT WALKING

A "limp"
Gait asymmetry including asymmetry of the arms
Persistent toe walking or appearance of toe walking after 2 years
A decline in performance, ability, coordination, or endurance
A persistent waddling gait
Refusal to walk or bear weight
Persistent forward falling

> *In response to the question, "Do you have any other concerns?" asked at the end of a health supervision visit, the mother of a 12-month-old exclaimed, "Her left foot looks odd!" Developmental history revealed normal motor, language, and social skills in a child who took a few unaided steps 1 week before the visit. Physical examination was normal. The left foot was moderately inverted when standing; it was thought to be secondary to a mild positional deformity. The mother was reassured.*
>
> *At the 15-month visit, she reminded her pediatrician that "the left foot looks odd!" Examination revealed a normal foot and leg when examined passively but inversion of the foot when standing and walking. To the pediatrician's surprise, the left calf circumference was 0.5 cm smaller than the right side, and the left foot-exerting muscles were weak. Strength, tone, sensation, and deep tendon reflexes (DTRs) were otherwise normal and symmetrical. A magnetic resonance image of the spine demonstrated a congenital syringomyelia. Surgical exploration, drainage, and shunting prevented further neurological deterioration.*

A SPECIAL WORD ABOUT PREEMIES

The predictably altered motor tone of the preemie and enhancement of extension postures in this group of infants results in greater risk for an altered course of motor development. Even correcting for gestational age, preemies walk later and also seem to lack some of the coordination and efficiency that is age appropriate.[33] These factors in themselves do not predict other areas of development, although all children born prematurely are at risk for developmental concerns.

ALTERED PERCEPTUAL DEVELOPMENT: CHANGES IN MOTOR TIMETABLE

The impact of perceptual input on gross-motor development is illustrated through the motor development of congenitally blind infants[34] These infants demonstrate all the postural readiness (e.g., excellent truncal tone) and static skill acquisitions (e.g., stepping in place with support) at the same time as sighted children. However, they are predictably delayed in any movement through space, such as crawling, walking, and climbing. These skills do not begin to emerge until the child can reach toward sound cues alone, a landmark met by *all* children between 10 and 15 months. Some blind children will not crawl at all, won't walk until they are 2 or older, and may even begin sitting or standing late, although they may have the ability to maintain those postures. Until these children are able to use perceptual input other than vision to map their environment and to be able to understand the consistency of three-dimensional space, they are unwilling to risk moving about. In addition, the fueling that walking typically receives by way of visual input does not sustain the efforts of blind children through all the falls and uncertainties of early movement. It is a lot of work to walk, and the rewards must be there. Enhanced feelings of independence, greater perceptual input, and the attainment of goals (e.g., getting a toy) make the effort worthwhile. Perceptually handicapped children lack these incentives even if they have neuromaturational readiness. This emphasizes the role of internal motivation in the process of gross-motor development; it is not purely a neuromaturational process.

When To Worry

Motor milestones are not usually missed in clinical observation, but one needs a clear backstop about when to be worried after the average age of achievement has passed. Motor delays accompanied by alterations in motor tone generally, hypotonia, or hypertonia are more worrisome than the delay in one or more landmarks alone with normal tone and reflexes. Postures or positions not seen in the normal sequence should elicit concern, such as a frogleg position in supine. Late integration of primitive reflexes with delays in several areas is of more concern regarding slowed CNS maturation. Finally, some milestones should be weighted more than others. Unsupported sitting is a strong indicator of general developmental progress because it involves balanced truncal tone, good hip flexion and abduction, and excellent head control. In contrast, creeping and crawling are poor indicators because some children never do these activities and the timing and form are highly variable. With these general considerations in mind, some clinical precision points may be considered (see Box 12-2).

Later Motor Development

Although we often place the greatest emphasis on gross-motor development in the first 2 years of life, this sequence continues beyond walking.[35] These competencies are based on an increasing ability to *balance* on one side and to *lateralize* more and on other varying motor activities (Box 12-3). Children should be able to ride a big wheel adeptly at 4 years of age and should be able to ride a bike at 7. Skateboarding and in-line skating, activities we can neither condone nor stop, can usually be done by 7 to 8 years, although perhaps not safely. Observations of jumping, hopping, ball catching, and throwing, as well as specific questions about the handling of stairs and the type of vehicular travel that a child can handle will usually give you all the data you need on gross-motor competencies. Therapeutic implications and considerations are based on these increasing skills. For example, a big wheeler *may* be able to walk with crutches; certainly a biker can learn to do so if needed. A child who cannot hop will have difficulty using crutches because both skills require lateralization at about the same level. (See Table 12-2.)

LEARNING COMPLEX MOTOR SKILLS

Motor skills do not stand alone. Cognitive competencies have an impact on how a child learns new motor skills. It is not until midlatency or even adolescence that a youngster can use preknowledge of outcome to improve motor performance; younger children must experience the outcome of their motor activities to alter them, and they need considerable practice before they can do that. The ability to sequence concepts parallels the ability to sequence motor behaviors; only the older grade schooler or high school student can do this reliably if the sequence is longer than 2 to 3 movements. This has implications for the coaching of

BOX 12-3	LATER GROSS-MOTOR SKILL PROGRESSION

2-3 Years
Both feet on each stair, up and down
Full arm swing
True run begins
Jumps down a step
Jumps up stiffly
Hops 1-3 times
Throws ball with forearm extension only
Catches ball with fixed, outstretched arms
Pushes riding toy with feet, no steering

3-4 Years
Alternates feet up stairs
Walks in a straight line
Jumps, using arms
Broad jump, about one foot
Hops 4-6 times, arms and body helping
Catches ball against chest
Pedals and steers tricycle

4-5 Years
Alternates feet down stairs
Smooth run
Gallops and does one-foot skip
Hops 7-9 times on one foot smoothly
Throws ball with shift of body
Catches ball with hands
Rides tricycle very well

5-6 Years
Gallops and skips smoothly
Jumps up 1 foot
Broad jumps 3 feet
Mature throwing with shifts of weight
Adjusts body, arms, hands to catch
Rides bicycle

Modified from Berk LE: *Infants, children and adolescents,* ed 3, Boston, 1999, Allyn and Bacon.

sports. Children can refine movements only through practice and through suggestions made while the child is engaged in the activity. Lengthy discussions of sports skills may not be useful for young grade-school children. Sports activities, both individual and group, should be accompanied by individual and direct feedback to each child during the action. Complex group play often can only be understood when there is a "run-through" (probably several), with each child's experiencing the way all members should act together. Coaching from the sidelines is helpful only when closely associated with the child's own action.

A WORD ABOUT SHOES

The role of **shoes** is to protect the child from sharp, rough, hot, or cold surfaces. They do not shape the foot or assist in gait development. Barefoot walking best develops the lower leg, foot, and particularly the arch, so avoiding shoes when it is safe to do so is best. In typically developing children, high tops, wedges, inserts, and other expensive foot devices are not needed. Shoes should be changed frequently to accommodate rapidly growing feet. Those made of soft material that allows flexing and monitoring of fit are best. Orthotics for children should be reserved for those with clear neuromuscular problems and should be used only with the advice of a physician trained to evaluate and monitor these conditions.

THE DRIVE TO WALK

The drive to mastery that energizes all of development is never more obvious than in the child just learning to walk. The revelation that one's placement in space can be changed while visually monitoring and even holding onto an object is so overwhelming for a child that all else pales by comparison. Routine things such as feeding, diaper changes, and sleeping are terrible interferences with this new activity. A child's new interest in motor activities may even invade sleep time with wakefulness and restlessness. The child may pull to stand and cruise around the bed with every night wakening. Difficulties, as well as regressions, in other areas of functioning should be anticipated at the time of learning to walk. The child may be less interested in learning new words or engaging in sustained toy play. The expression of joy in accomplishment and a tangible excitement should be apparent in every child even if accompanied by looks of panic and wariness.

PARENTS' ROLE

The sparkle of joy testifies to the walking child's own sense of internal reward for a growing sense of competency. This sparkle is generalizable to other areas in which a child achieves mastery. An internal reward system is fueled as the child learns walking for walking's sake. An external reward system cannot have the energy or longevity of the internal one. The parents' role in this instance is to encourage, assure safety in exploration, prevent overtiredness, and enjoy (Fig. 12-10). It is not to exercise, instruct, or overwhelm the child with excessive praise. A parent's praise is welcome, if not overwhelming, but it isn't the key motivating factor.

Walking changes a child's perspective of self and of those around him or her. A sense of independence and ability to separate from parents is enhanced by this accomplishment. The child can play by roaming the environment with clear planning and direction and is no longer as dependent on caregivers to supply toys and orchestrate the day. The child can get into more trouble and can have more fun. The ability to ambulate independently heralds a whole new era. The child will soon discover temper tantrums, the word *no,* and running away. The infant becomes a toddler.

DATA GATHERING
What To Observe

Following are actions the clinician should observe to track the development of motor skills:
- At every encounter during the first 5 years, the child should be allowed free movement so that the clinician can observe the child's motor competencies. Place the child both supine and prone on the examining table to observe increasing head control, truncal stability, arm support, movement at the hip, and the smoothness and rhythmicity of the movement. Symmetry in movement is a vital observation.
- A line on the floor provides guidance for the child's directed walking. An area of some reasonable length (e.g., a hallway) must be provided for free-walking assessment. A child won't be able to follow a line exactly until age 2 or older.

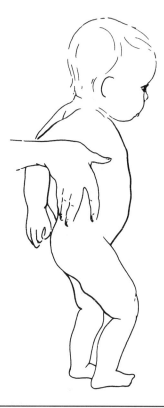

Fig. 12-10   Parenting support should be gentle, well-placed, but not compelling.

- Observe the amount of support the child requires to do other things, such as reach for a stethoscope. Note a decreasing need for support with sitting and increasing weight bearing on the lower extremities across the first year.
- Observation of the child walking with help and then alone should begin when the child is 9 months of age and continue until school age or beyond if there is a question. The walking base, the foot position, truncal rotation, and movement at the knee should be observed and should change along the lines presented above. The hand and arm position should change over time. The child's stopping and pivoting should improve. The rising to stand, stooping, and recovering will become smoother with time.
- The style, interest, and excitement of the child with motor activities should be noted at every encounter.
- At 3 years of age, knee and ankle motion should be good, and a heel strike should be present.

Climbing

A simple two-step climbing device kept in the examining room against the examining table can provide observations of increasing motor competencies. This apparatus will allow demonstration of lower extremity movement, proximal muscle strength, and coordination in climbing. Walking up and down stairs should follow age expectations (see Box 12-3).

Parent's Handling

A parent's handling of the child can give clues to both the child's competencies and the child's motor abilities. A parent who carefully supports the infant's head at all times when the child is 3 months or older may rightfully anticipate that this infant's head control is poor. Children around the world will be ready for upright packaging with or without attachment (e.g., backpacks, wrapping on the hip or back, cradle boarding) by 3 to 4 months. If a child is being carried like a neonate, something is wrong, either in the child's development or in the parent's ability to alter caretaking based upon the child's competencies.

Parents who cannot allow a 4-year-old to climb up on an examining table may anticipate that the child will be unsuccessful or awkward. Excessive "coaching" of a child during the motor assessment may also be a clue that the parent has a worry about function in this area.

What To Ask

Parents will usually find reporting of gross-motor skills the easiest of all areas of development. In addition to asking what the child can do, ask *how* the child approaches the task (i.e., with caution at one extreme or with abandon and impulsively at the other). The manner or style in which these skills are performed may reflect the emerging personality, family expectations, or difficulty with motor coordination.

The parents' response about the child's accomplishments may provide data about any underlying anxiety or specific worries. By beginning questions at a lower level of functioning than anticipated, the clinician can find the floor of the child's performance and convey the importance of individual expectations in motor development.

Children readily practice newly emerging skills in motor development, as well as in other areas of development. The relatively invariant order of motor-skill acquisition allows the clinician taking the history of a child whose development is generally normal to simply ask what kind of new movements or activities the child is doing. The internally regulated and self-fueling nature of this area of development is highlighted in this approach.

A child whose motor development is not synchronous with other areas of development, or is delayed beyond levels of normal variation (see Box 12-1) needs a more detailed history. Disorders of movement vs. disorders of tone and posture can be specified through history, coupled with a careful examination. Perinatal difficulties must alert the clinician to the need for a careful evaluation of gross-motor competencies, particularly if walking is delayed beyond 18 months.

Examination

Most of the gross-motor examination is best moved to the end of the assessment because those activities usually energize kids, who are then difficult to calm down. Doing activities that require child involvement while you are filling out forms is an efficient management of time. Following are other things to keep in mind about the examination:

- The clinician should assess passive motor tone of all extremities throughout the first 3 years. Move all four extremities as part of a playful game.
- Both slow and rapid motions should be applied to the limbs to elicit any lowered threshold to a stretch reflex.
- Deep tendon reflexes should be monitored.
- Asymmetries of tone or reflexes, or movement, provided the child's head is in midline, should receive very careful follow-up. Persistence of these signs may require further neurological evaluation.
- Early evidence of spastic cerebral palsy is tight heel cords with limited dorsiflexion of the foot or a "catch" in the Achilles tendon.
- Scissoring of the lower extremities when the child is held upright reflects adductor spasm.
- A limp requires complete neurological and orthopedic assessment by an experienced specialist.
- Head and truncal tone should be assessed through the pull-to-sit and prone positions, as well as the position of the child being held over the hand. In addition, the child's head and body control when being held upright, at the shoulder, or under the arms in front of the examiner should be assessed during the first year. Truncal tone is often reflected in how the child responds to handling and holding by the examiner. It's a perfect excuse to hold and handle the baby as part of every assessment until that is too troublesome, often at 15 to 18 months.
- Placing the baby both prone and supine offers the chance to assess increasing shoulder girdle tone and strength, as well as control of the lower body.
- Alternating hip movements appear at 5 months of age, but significantly increase in some form after 9 months.
- Weight bearing on the feet is observed in children from the age of 5 months to walking.
- Persistent standing on tiptoe is abnormal after 9 months.
- Walking with help should be attempted after 9 months but may not be present until after the first birthday.
- Climbing up stairs is seen from 8 to 18 months. After the age of 2 years, children will attempt to do this with feet only, two feet on the step. Only after 2 to 3 years of age do children alternate feet on steps. Gait should be observed during the second through the sixth years and beyond if indicated. As the toddler begins to walk independently, gait is typically wide based, accompanied by waddling hips and intermittent toe walking. With each observation, the base should narrow, the arms come down, and reciprocal movement should be added. Waddling at the hip should decrease, knees should move a bit more, ankle movement should increase, and a heel strike should be present at the age of 3 years. By the age of 5 years, a sticker placed below the umbilicus should move very little except forward as the child walks. Forward movement, either walking or crawling, should be smooth and rhythmical by and large. Any asymmetry in the gait is always cause for concern.
- Children can stoop about 6 months after independent walking. They bounce to music at 15 to 18 months of age. Getting up to sit or stand should be by a smooth roll to the side by 15 months.

- A soft, foam ball provides an easy way to assess catching skills (see Box 12-3). This game can be done at the end of the exam or as part of the weight-measure procedure of the nurse.
- Children who are consistently 3 to 6 months behind on motor-skill acquisition need a second look. Muscle tone, deep tendon reflexes, and the persistence of primitive reflexes and postures should be evaluated carefully. Cerebral palsy, hypotonias, and muscular and metabolic diseases must be considered. Through a careful history and assessment over a period of time, the primary care provider may determine whether the delays are global or are confined to the motor area. Further evaluation and intervention can become more focused with this in mind.

Anticipatory Guidance

- The clinician can support the parents' feelings of assurance and pride in their child's motor accomplishments and can highlight the individual **temperamental characteristics** of the child that affect all areas of development, including the style of motor achievements. Careful assessment should appropriately diffuse anxiety about individual patterns of development and confirm the child's integrity.
- Parents support development of gross-motor skills by providing opportunities for free exploration of the environment within safe limits. Excessive practice (adult perspective) and even overwhelming praise squelch the child's own innate drive for mastery and competency.
- A safe play area and encouragement of daily gross-motor activities for girls and boys in nonrestrictive, nonfussy clothes support development.
- Babies should be placed on their backs for sleep, which is in line with the sudden infant death syndrome (SIDS) prevention program. However, it is vital that babies get ample time in prone position *while awake* to get experience with pushing up, rolling over, and pulling to stand.
- Playing on the floor, wrestling sessions, and ball playing are good activities for both sexes if they are done in a relaxed, social manner. Baby gymnastics, swimming classes, and therapy programs are fine if they are done with those principles in mind; the activities themselves do not magically enhance development.
- Swimming lessons in particular may be dangerous for young infants,[36] and it is unrealistic for children to reliably sequence and coordinate the motor activities of swimming before the age of 4 years. Primitive reflexes are the basis for most behaviors in the water at younger ages.
- Beginning walkers are very energy inefficient. They require about 1200 kcal/day to sustain their new activities. This has to be delivered in six small meals because toddlers usually cannot sit still long enough for larger meals. Clinicians can anticipate these changes in feeding for parents. Children younger than 4 years should never be allowed to eat and walk at the same time because of the danger of aspiration.
- In spite of its name, the infant walker may *not* enhance a child's ability to walk.[29] Head injuries are common in young children in walkers. Children with lower extremity extensor hypertonicity do very well in walkers. However, that posture only exaggerates the

children's own abnormal preponderance of extensor tone. These children need to be on the floor, moving freely, and practicing reciprocal hip and knee movement. Every child can push a walker out doors, down stairs, and out into streets. Walkers contain children poorly and thwart prewalking progression. Individual therapy programs may include walkers for specific children, to stabilize the trunk. Other than in that context, it is better to actively discourage their use.

■ Programs based on the concept that *all* learning is facilitated through an integration of motor activities have no basis in science and have had no demonstration of effectiveness. These programs prescribe a rigid series of motor activities to be done by the parent so that patterns, either accelerated or remedial, can be established in the child. These activities consume up to 8 hours per day of "therapy" by the parent. Failures are attributed to non-compliance. These programs, under several names throughout the country,[37,38] victimize parents of handicapped children who are looking for anything to improve their child's outcome. No evidence shows that this "patterning" is important for development at all, certainly no evidence that learning to crawl has anything to do with learning to read. Secondary gain from increased parental attention, social interaction, and fun may have some benefit for some children in some circumstances, but the formal activities of these programs are incidental to these processes. Clinicians should be informed of what programs are operative in their communities and examine them carefully. Parents should be offered the clinician's professional input.

REFERENCES

1. Majnemer A, Rosenblatt B: Reliability of parental recall of developmental milestones, *Pediatr Neurol* 10:304, 1994.
2. Glascoe, F, Altemeier WA, MacLean WE: The importance of parents' concerns about their child's development, *Arch Dis Child* 143:955, 1989.
3. Gesell A, Thompson H: *The psychology of early growth,* New York, 1938, Macmillan.
4. McGraw M: *The neuromuscular maturation of the human infant,* New York, 1945, Hafner Press.
5. Wyke B: The neurological basis of movement: a developmental overview. In Holt K, editor: *Movement and child development,* London, 1975, Heinemann Medical Books.
6. Thelan E: Motor development: a new synthesis, *Am Psychol* 50:79-91, 1985.
7. Thelen E, Bradshaw G, Ward JA: Spontaneous kicking in month old infants: manifestation of a human central locomotor program, *Behav Neural Biol* 32:45, 1981.
8. Jaffe M et al: Relationship between the parachute reactions and standing and walking in normal infants, *Pediatr Neurol* 11:38, 1994.
9. Burnett CN, Johnson EW: Development of gait in children: parts I and II, *Dev Med Child Neurol* 13:196, 1971.
10. Sutherland DH et al: *The development of mature walking,* Oxford, 1988, Blackwell Scientific.
11. Chaplais JZ, MacFarlane IA: A review of four hundred and four late walkers, *Arch Dis Child* 59:512, 1984.
12. Fraiberg SH: *The magic years,* New York, 1959, Charles Scribner's Sons.
13. Hennessy M, Dixon S, Simon S: The development of gait: a study in African children ages one to five, *Child Dev* 55:844, 1984.
14. Freis S, Klemms A, Muller K: Gait analysis by measuring ground reaction forces in children: changes to an adaptive gait pattern between the ages of one to five years, *Dev Med Child Neurol* 39:228, 1997.

15. Preis S, Klenn S, Müller K: Gait analysis by measuring ground reaction forces in children: changes to adaptive gait patterns between the ages of one to five years, *Dev Med Child Neurol* 39:228-233, 1997.

16. Clark JE, Phillips SJ: A longitudinal study of intralimb coordination in the first year of walking: a dynamical systems analysis, *Child Dev* 64:1143, 1993.

17. Clark JE, Whitall J, Phillips SJ: Human interlimb coordination: the first six months of independent walking, *Dev Psychobiol* 21:445, 1988.

18. Berger W, Quinlern J, Dietz V: Afferent and efferent control of stance and gait developmental changes in children, *Electroencephalogr Clin Neurophysiol* 66:244, 1987.

19. Whitall J, Getchell N: From walking to running: applying a dynamical systems approach to the development of locomotor skills, *Child Dev* 66:1541, 1995.

20. American Academy of Pediatrics: The Doman-Delcato treatment of neurologically handicapped children, *Pediatrics* 70:810, 1982.

21. Bayley N: *Bayley scales of infant development,* New York, 1969, Psychological Corp.

22. Hopkins B, Westra T: Maternal expectations of their infants' development: some cultural differences, *Dev Med Child Neurol* 31:384, 1989.

23. Dixon S et al: Perinatal circumstances and newborn outcome among the Gusii of Kenya: assessment of risk, *Infant Behav Dev* 5:11-32, 1982.

24. Dennis W: Does culture appreciably affect patterns of infant behavior? *J Soc Psychol* 12:305, 1940.

25. Harriman AE, Lukosius PA: On why Wayne Dennis found Hopi infants retarded in age at onset of walking, *Percept Mot Skills* 55:79, 1982.

26. Chisholm JS: *Navajo infancy,* New York, 1983, Aldine.

27. American Academy of Pediatrics, Task Force on Infant Positioning and SIDS: Positioning and sudden infant death syndrome (SIDS): update, *Pediatrics* 98:1216, 1996.

28. Davis BE et al: Effects of sleep position on infant motor development, *Pediatrics* 102:1135, 1998.

29. Crouchman M: The effect of baby walkers on early locomotor development, *Dev Med Child Neurol* 28:757, 1986.

30. Ridenour MV: Infant walkers: developmental tool or inherent danger? *Percept Mot Skills* 55:1201, 1982.

31. Wolff P: Theoretical issues in the development of motor skills. In Lewis M, Taft L, editors: *Developmental disabilities: theory, assessment and intervention,* New York, 1981, Spectrum Publications.

32. Brazelton TB: *Toddlers and parents: a declaration of independence,* New York, 1974, Delacorte Press.

33. deGroot L, deGroot CJ, Hopkins B: An instrument to measure independent walking: are there differences between preterm and full term infants? *J Child Neurol* 12:304, 1994.

34. Adelson E, Fraiberg S: Gross motor development of infants blind from birth, *Child Dev* 45:114, 1974.

35. Sahler OJN, McAnarney ER: *The child from three to eighteen,* St Louis, 1981, Mosby.

36. Bennett HJ, Wagner T, Fields A.: Acute hyponatremia and seizures in an infant after a swimming lesson, *Pediatrics* 72:125, 1983.

37. American Academy of Pediatrics, Committee on Pediatric Aspects of Physical Fitness, Recreation and Sports: Swimming instructions for infants, *Pediatrics* 65:847, 1980.

38. Holm V: A western version of the Doman-Delcato treatment of patterning for developmental disabilities, *West J Med* 139:553, 1984.

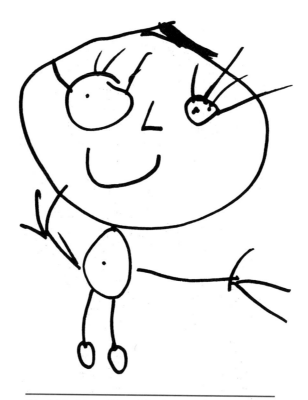

"A girl-baby walking." By Anne Atkinson, age 5.

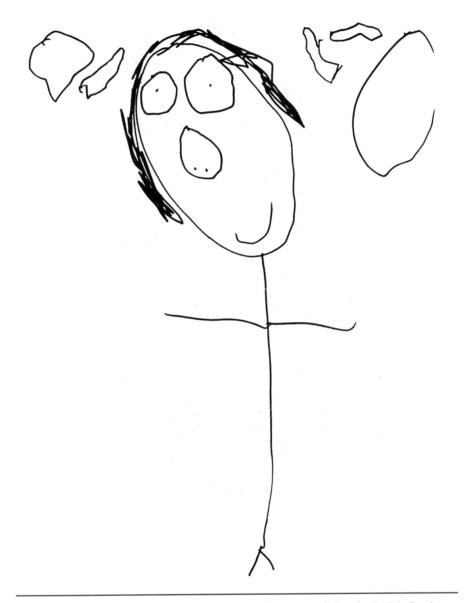

A 4-year-old boy shows himself walking under the sun and clouds. By Eric Stroiman.

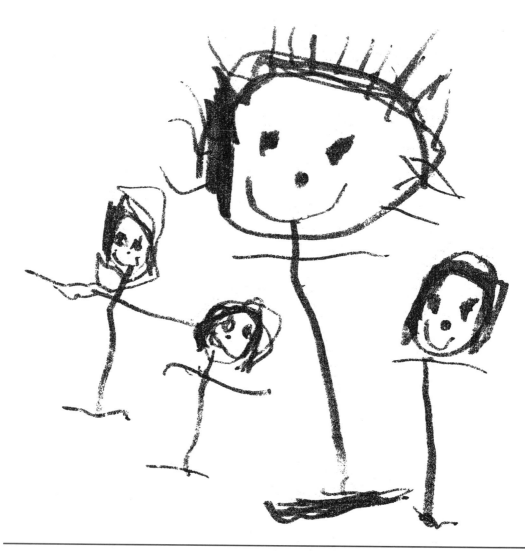

This picture shows the preschooler's perspective on the world, a healthy self-importance. This girl shows herself as the largest and central figure. Mom and Dad are shown close and well aligned, although smaller and looking a bit frazzled. Her older sister is off to the side, next to Dad. A sense of independence and a need to be in charge are balanced by a need to stay close and safe with the family. By Louise Dixon, age 3 ½ (original in brown marker).

CHAPTER 13

15 to 18 Months: Asserting Independence and Pushing the Limits

■ Martin T. Stein

KEY WORDS

Autonomy
Attachment
Discipline
Regressions
Self-Feeding
Rapprochement
Transitional Object
Behavior Modification

The mother of an 18-month-old girl asks if she should be concerned about her daughter's preference for a bottle—during the day and at bedtime. A standard response might be, "A child this age no longer needs her bottle. It's bad for her teeth and may encourage ear infections. My advice is to take it away and let her drink from a cup. She's a big girl now. She needs to grow up!"

An alternative approach would encourage a response based on a developmental history. Recognizing that maintaining a preference for the bottle represents holding onto an earlier, more dependent stage of development, an exploration of other milestones that reflect her autonomy might be useful. Focused questions to the mother, as well as office observations, reveal that this toddler feeds herself independently with a spoon and drinks from a cup, soothes herself to sleep each night with minimal fussing, and responds to her parents' verbal constraints at times of conflict. She enjoys the care of a regular baby-sitter and does not cry when her parents occasionally leave her at night. In the office, she plays by herself with toys. Periodically, she checks in with her mother and then returns to the toy box. She seems happy and able to move back and forth between the security of her mother and the autonomous, self-initiated play.

> *The child's development demonstrates a strong attachment to her mother while she is simultaneously becoming more independent in social and motor skills. Although the use of a bottle may be viewed as a residual symbol of infancy, perhaps this remarkably healthy girl needs a temporary "crutch" in the form of a bottle in order to negotiate the more demanding achievements of the second year.*

The discrepancy between what a parent tells you about behavior and development and what you observe in the office setting is perhaps most striking when the child is 18 months old. Although a parent may describe a child who now feeds him or herself, has the capability to express needs, can follow simple directions, and is a "delightful child," the clinician frequently observes someone quite different. In the office the same child may be suspicious of the clinician's kind and gentle approach, cling firmly to the parent, scream at any touch, and resist initial social interchange with a toy or an examining tool. How can this behavior be understood in a way that provides some insight into each child's development for the clinician and for the parents?

The behavior of an 18-month-old does contain many contradictions. The child seeks to be more independent in all areas but needs additional nurturance to refuel the push toward **autonomy.** Children need parents for additional security but at the same time seem to be always assertive in pulling away. The resistance and the negativism of this age try the patience of parents. Simultaneously, these forces supply the energy the child needs to act independently.

The toddler appears to have an innate resource of energy to master new skills in an even more complex world. Unfortunately, attention span, cooperation with playmates, motor dexterity, and, perhaps most significantly, tolerance for frustrating events are limited. Although drive for mastery of the environment appears to be built in (some parents describe the toddler's efforts as driven, striving, or searching), the child's psychological tasks inevitably apply limits and precipitate conflicts as the child reaches out for more independence. Frustration is a fact of life for a child struggling to do more things, explore more places, and push at the limits of behavior and the restraints of the real world.

The 18-month-old has developed a strong emotional tie with the parents; events in the outside world are measured against that link. At this age, the child frequently checks back with a parent as if to say, "Is it safe? Can I continue to play . . . to move forward?" Parents are a secure base from which to explore.[1] This behavior can be seen in day-care centers and playgrounds when the toddler is brave and independent and then suddenly searches and runs to a secure area when the social environment changes or becomes threatening. For some toddlers, even the benevolent approach of a physician or nurse threatens a fragile internal stability; in the office, the child runs quickly to the parent, seeking a sanctum and security. The same child might have appeared more secure with the clinician during the first half of the second year, but by 18 months a "rapprochement"[2] with the parent and outer world produces what, on the surface, appear to be more infantile behaviors (clinging to a parent, crying at a stranger, or refusing the approach of a playmate). It is as if the maturation of the central nervous system (CNS) has produced greater awareness of the external world (e.g., other children, other adults, toys, furniture), and this awareness now comes into conflict with a previously secure, parentally modulated environment. Cognitive skills have matured enough that a child can imagine a threat.[3] Communication is appreciated as important in handling the world, but an 18-month-old cannot effectively communicate with strangers. The toddler is lost without parental translation and interpretation.

Helping parents through this period is easier when the clinician's observations and expectations of behaviors are based on these developmental phenomena. The patterns of interaction that are established at this time have great longevity. Parents must see the struggles for mastery and independence as both inevitable and a positive sign of the child's emotional and social growth. This will sustain them through the "first adolescence."

Three aspects of behavior and development often surface at this age either in the questions parents bring to the office visit or in what a clinician observes in the office setting: (1) discipline and temper tantrums; (2) toilet training; and (3) changes in feeding patterns. All of these can be seen within the context of this drive for independence.

DISCIPLINE

The newly discovered capacity to walk, run, and climb opens up new pathways of exploration for the toddler. Not only can the child get to things, he or she now can manipulate objects into new forms that follow from imagination. Fine-motor and visual-perceptual skills allow the toddler to shape, invent, and explore objects; these manipulations give definition and form to the child's world. Simultaneously, receptive language function is developing rapidly; the child now *understands* many words, follows simple directions, and can even point to some parts of the body when a parent sounds its name.

These new skills emerge rapidly and must be incorporated into a psychological framework that previously was dependent on caretakers' passive manipulation of the child's environment. The sudden awareness that through language, motor, and perceptual skills the child can shape and pattern the world brings about inner conflict for most children. These conflicts can be seen when a tower of neatly stacked blocks falls; when a playmate, benign and cooperative at one moment, commits the awful sin of touching a child's toys momentarily; or when a parent removes a child from one enjoyable activity and moves him or her to another place (e.g., from playing with toys to the dreaded high chair). The toddler now can make a choice about a toy, a playmate, or a meal. Infringement on those choices produces inner disharmony that may lead to anger and aggression. The young toddler does not possess the psychical structure to delay gratification, to suppress or displace angry feelings, or to manage these difficult situations through verbal communication. The child cannot wait, see things from another's point of view, anticipate compound effects of actions, or cope effectively.

Seeking alternative responses consistent with developmental capacities, the child pouts, cries, becomes morose, or has a temper tantrum. Behavior outbursts by the 18-month-old can be viewed as developmentally predictable (Fig. 13-1). The frequency and intensity with which an individual child manifests these behaviors is dependent on many factors, such as (1) the degree of attachment to parents, (2) the toddler's individual temperament and way of adapting to new and stressful situations, and (3) the parents' style of responding to various behaviors in the child.

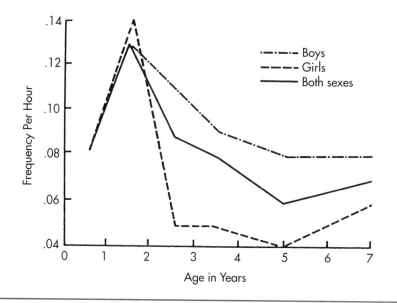

Fig. 13-1   Frequency of anger outbursts, with peak between 18 months and 2 years. (Modified from Goodenough FL: *Anger in young children,* St. Paul, 1931, University of Minnesota Press. Cited in Helms DB, Turner JS: *Exploring child behavior: basic principles,* Philadelphia, 1978, WB Saunders.)

Emotional **attachment** to parents is a major goal of the first year of life, whereas in the second year, children need to be encouraged to broaden the focus of that attachment and become more independent. (In fact, some observers of human development have suggested that the guiding psychological goal throughout life after the first birthday is to detach from one's parents!) Parents can be encouraged to allow self-play, mistakes, mishaps, and consequent frustrations in their child. If a parent is too protective and limits the development of independent skills by providing an overly protective environment, infantile attachment behaviors become more secure and lock the child into an earlier phase of development. New situations—without mommy or daddy or when frustration is inevitable—become intolerable. When a toddler is allowed, even encouraged, to experience modulated amounts of frustration during the course of play, the child learns to manage angry feelings, feelings that may be directed toward parents, play objects, or a playmate. These kinds of experiences assist the child in the gradual journey to becoming more independent from parents.

A toddler's *temperament* is reflected in the style of response to conflict with self, others, and the environment. Toddlers vary significantly in the energy released when a frustrating experience arises. A youngster with a high level of adaptability to change and a positive approach to new stimuli will probably move quickly from a conflictual situation to one that is harmonious. At the opposite end of the spectrum is a child with intense expressions of mood and negative withdrawal responses to new situations. This child may be easily frustrated at seemingly minor conflict. The intensity and duration of crying, screaming, and level of consolability will, in part, relate to these innate aspects of temperament. Although most children are somewhere between these temperamental extremes, a clinical appreciation for them can be helpful in assessing a particular child and the parents' responses to that child.[4]

Finally, *parental styles of responding* to a toddler's tantrums affect the resolution of the episode, as well as the nature of future tantrums. Children are sponges of adult attitudes and actions at this age. They learn how to handle their own anger, aggression, and frustration as they observe parents and other caretakers. Often those parents who seem able to manage toddler tantrums are less threatened by their child's aggressive moments and emerging independence. They do not get drawn into the struggle themselves. They recognize, often unconsciously, the strengths of this autonomous act and can freely assist the child in handling feelings. Other parents may feel challenged or threatened by the child's bids for independence and respond only with anger. Styles of parenting the child at this age often reflect a parent's own sense of self-effectiveness and own experiences from childhood. The toddler can call forth feelings and responses that many parents did not even know were within them.

Discipline at this age means teaching, guiding behavior, and showing the child how to cooperate. It is not simply the parents' response to a tantrum. When viewed constructively, discipline can be seen as a process of teaching the toddler to place limits or boundaries on behavior within family and cultural limits, to learn to "use words" to express anger, to feel comfortable with feelings of anger, and to learn to cope with the inevitable frustrations of normal life. It may be useful to compare tantrums with a blown fuse. The tantrum serves a purpose in itself; it releases tension as it provides an exit for bound-up energy that momentarily finds no other outlet. Occasional toddler tantrums viewed in this manner can be accepted, understood, and allowed to occur by the understanding parent. In the healthy toddler, occasional tantrums usually cannot be stopped and should even be seen as helpful.

From another perspective, "discipline solidifies the boundaries, as well as the core of the ego."[5] It offers the child a way to manage conflictual feelings and unacceptable behaviors. Because the fragile ego is developing a sense of self (see Chapter 17) at this time, conflicts directed at parents, peers, siblings, and toys are necessary. These conflicts collectively define the child's emerging ego; simultaneously, the child needs an adult to define acceptable limits of behavior. Pushing and testing those limits may be the only way to be sure of their firmness. The push-pull process of a toddler's development is now seen in terms of both the child's behaviors and the parental responses to those behaviors.

TOILET TRAINING

Five milestones must be reached before a toddler is ready to master bowel and bladder control. They are a result of neurological maturation, an increased attention span, an attachment to a caretaker whom they want to please, and the emerging ability to sequence events (Box 13-1).

These milestones of development reflect mastery of the motor, social, and language skills that usually come together after the second birthday; for some, it may be a few months earlier; for others, developmental readiness may not be apparent until 3 or more years of age (Table 13-1). From the child's viewpoint, toilet training that is too early or too rapid has no advantages. It may be detrimental if it creates expectations the child cannot handle. When viewed from the standpoint of the child's needs, toilet training demands a level of complex,

BOX 13-1	DEVELOPMENTAL PREREQUISITES FOR BOWEL AND BLADDER CONTROL

Maturation of the central and peripheral nervous systems to the degree that voluntary control of the anal and urethral sphincters is possible, ability to sense and signal the urge to go

Ability to sit on a potty seat quietly for a moderate period of time with the conscious intent to have a bowel movement or to urinate

Desire to gain satisfaction from the successful completion of defecation and urination, to recognize the pleasure in the supervising parent and within oneself through growth in competency as a form of positive reinforcement

Ability to understand the sequence of requirements of the task

Drive to imitate greater than drive to oppose parents

multistepped, voluntary control that could not be obtained previously. Motor, social, and receptive language skills come together to make this a big event in a child's life. It is an opportunity for growth and increased feelings of self-esteem.

At her second birthday, Janelle's parents initiated potty training, but Janelle refused their efforts. She balked at sitting on a brightly painted potty seat. When her father read a book to her, she would sit on the seat but would neither urinate nor defecate. She popped up and ran out of the bathroom as soon as the story was finished. When Janelle's pediatrician inquired about the parents' attempts, they said that they were not sure she made a connection between sitting on the potty seat and a bowel movement. At 30 months of age, Janelle seemed to enjoy sitting on "my potty" and defecating with ease. At this time, her facial expression demonstrated pleasure when her parents congratulated Janelle on her new skill.

As a form of anticipatory guidance, it is helpful to discuss toilet training at the visit when the child is 18 months old for three reasons: (1) to prevent parents from rushing into training before the child is ready, (2) to bring out the developmental significance of training as a way to assist parents in understanding and responding to the broader developmental events at this age, and (3) to help parents begin to set the stage for this process later on. Clues that a child is physically and emotionally ready for potty training may be observed some time between 18 months and 2 years of age in most children. Following are examples of such clues:

■ The child will demonstrate having made the connection between the feeling (muscular contractions) of urination or defecation and what is produced. This connection is communicated to the parent as the child points or looks at the urine or bowel movement.

■ The child has increased periods of daytime dryness (i.e., increased bladder capacity and sphincter control), tells the parent after having a bowel movement or urinating, and can sit quietly for a period.

TABLE 13-1 ■ Guide to Toilet Training Readiness: A Developmental Approach

Child's Behavior/Competencies	Parental Response
Complex, multistep behavior; completing household tasks; completing tasks in sequence	Narrate the process while the child is watching parent or siblings at toilet.
Undresses self	Allow child to undress self; loose, easily removed clothes are preferred; praise the child while mentioning that he or she will soon use a potty seat.
Shows interest in a potty seat Demonstrates ability to understand requirements of various tasks	Keep potty seat in a regular place in the bathroom; let the child know he or she can sit on it and what it is used for; some children can learn about the seat initially by sitting on it with diaper on.
Points to, looks at, or announces BM* in diaper	Put diaper/BM in seat; dispose of it later; acknowledge the production.
Increasing periods of daytime dryness	Use training pants during the day.
Ability to sit quietly on potty seat for a moderate period	Praise the child for knowing about the seat and discuss its use; encourage sitting on the seat.
Shows satisfaction in having BM	Praise moderately by showing pleasure in completion of task
Asks to use potty seat or uses it in self-directed manner	Encourage use of potty seat after a meal (gastro-colic reflex) or (for some children) at a time when the child usually has a BM.
Desire to please by imitating parents	Praise the child by pointing out that "my big girl is now ready to use her potty seat."
Partial voluntary control of anal and urethral sphincters, demonstrated by having a BM or urinating at a planned time on the potty seat	Show pleasure in task completion while expecting setbacks, both at times of stress and spontaneously.
Interest in successful use of potty seat	Try training pants; encourage child to remove training pants by self.

* BM, bowel movement

■ The child shows interest in the toilet, shows imitative behavior in other areas (e.g., dressing, household tasks), is interested in compulsively putting things away, and is not violently negative.

At this time, parents can be encouraged to introduce a potty seat, explain its function to the child, and make it available. Parents must take the child into the bathroom and discuss and demonstrate the process. Having the child sit on a potty chair (initially with the diaper attached) is a first step in getting acquainted with the chair. The parents should be positive toward the behavior and the product (feces). The child will see the bowel movement as a part of self; parents should not regard it as "yucky." Parents can be encouraged to show their pleasure at a successful movement, but overenthusiasm is not warranted because this exaggerates the importance of using the potty chair, adding stress to the child and inviting negative behavior. Conversely, parents whose 2-year-old does not seem interested in a potty chair should be encouraged to wait a few months. It is often helpful to point out to parents that just as some normal children do not walk until after 15 months, some toddlers require more time to attain consistent voluntary sphincter control and to be willing to exercise it. It is not a measure of intelligence on the child's part or of adequacy of child rearing on the parents' part.

The initiation and continuation of toilet training is dependent on the child's personal health and environmental events. External events such as intercurrent illness, birth of a new sibling, a family vacation, or absence of a parent for a prolonged period can be expected to delay or cause a setback in the mastery of toilet training. When some of these events are predictable, potty training may be delayed by the parents. **Regressions** without any explanations also should be expected. The child's self-respect should be preserved in these circumstances. Parents should be informed that other less predictable changes in family function may delay mastery of this new skill. Boys generally train 2 months later than girls. Firstborn children train 1.7 months later than children born later. In most families, the whole process will take months.

FEEDING AND SELF-DETERMINATION

As fine-motor skills and visual-motor coordination advance, the 18-month-old enjoys the use of a cup and spoon. Self-feeding represents a significant form of mastery in the use of an instrument to extend and expand the abilities of the hand and in the honing of visual-motor skills (Box 13-2). It is also another psychological separation from dependency on parents. It is helpful to point out to parents that, although messy and seemingly disorganized, allowing a child the freedom to feed him or herself assists development and mastery at several levels.

As with any new skill, learning may progress at different rates for children of various temperaments, and setbacks (or regressions) may occur after intercurrent events in the family. As with most new experiences that require mastery, feeding is particularly vulnerable to individual differences and fluctuations. Particular attractions or dislikes for certain foods

BOX 13-2	DEVELOPMENTAL SKILLS ENHANCED BY SELF-FEEDING

Fine-motor skills
Hand-to-eye coordination
Independent actions yielding an enjoyable response
Learning to choose from and enjoy different food textures and colors

are common at this time. Prolonged periods of refusing one food group are common (i.e., food jags). Excessive intake of juice at this age can satisfy a toddler's appetite, discourage the intake of more caloric-dense foods, and lead to failure to thrive. However, as long as the child's physical growth has not been compromised, parents need reassurance that fluctuations in diet are normal and self-limited. Demonstrating the child's rate of growth on a standard growth curve is often reassuring to the parent who perceives the toddler as "starving herself." Food refusal provides an opportunity to explain to parents the importance of self-directed feeding in terms of emotional independence.

> *Robbie was known to his pediatrician as an engaging and socially interactive infant. At his 18-month-old health supervision visit, his clinician observed that he was walking around the room with a bottle of juice. Even block play did not distract him from a firm grasp of the bottle. Robbie's mother listed only a single concern on the pre-visit Q card (see Appendix)—his refusal to eat most foods. She tried to make meals that he might like and spoke to other parents about their children's food interest. Nothing seemed to help.*
>
> *Robbie's physical exam and developmental assessment were normal. In fact, he had engaged several areas of mastery of independent skill, including falling to sleep by himself, playing with toys for an extended time period, and a few early signs of readiness for toilet training. However, his growth chart revealed a decrease in the velocity of weight gain, most likely a result of inadequate caloric intake caused by excessive juice intake. Robbie's clinician not only made use of the encounter to counsel about the need for calorie-rich foods and significantly less juice, but saw an opportunity to point out to his mother that exchanging the bottle for a cup would also give a boost to Robbie's development. The cup, similar to self-feeding, becomes a symbol of growth and self-reliance.*

The more the clinician can do to assist the parent of a toddler in understanding these new skills as a reflection of mastery and "separation" from infantile dependency on the parent, the better equipped the parent will be for "letting go"[5] through continued guidance and surveillance without squelching further growth. A parent has never won a feeding battle with a child. Ingenuity and patience are required to set up feeding as a source of good nutrition, physical and psychological.

The "push-pull" process that characterizes this stage of development can be viewed as one of daily increments of psychological growth achieved by mastery of more complicated skills. These skills require adequate maturation of the toddler's nervous system and the parents' ability to simultaneously stimulate and pull back, that is, to encourage self-feeding, potty seat recognition, and creative play while letting the child master these objects and events independently. To be sure, it is a delicate balance that requires parental skill that will vary in different families. The child's clinician can point out the developmental necessity of this balance. It can be demonstrated during the physical examination with toys or examining instruments or when observing the child's play during the interview with the parent.

DATA GATHERING
Observations

Watching the 18-month-old child, both at independent play and while in interaction with the parent, provides insight into the developmental goals of this age. As the history is recorded, helpful observations include the following:

- Does the child play independently, making use of toys in the examining room?
- Fine-motor dexterity and visual-motor skills can be observed through play. Does the child play spontaneously with toys in the office, make a tower out of four cubes, scribble spontaneously, try to remove clothes by him or herself?
- Does the child have a transitional object? Was it brought to the office? If so, how is it used by the child?
- Does the parent allow the child to move around the examining room independently, to experiment with the available toys?
- How does the parent modulate the child's play, verbally and nonverbally?
- When you walk into the room, what is the child doing? Does the activity change in your presence?
- What is the intensity and duration with which the child clings to the parent? How does the parent respond?
- What is the content and style of the parent's verbal interactions with the child?
- Assess the child's response to your examination.

History

To discover the point on the developmental pathway from dependency to autonomy for a particular toddler, the clinician may ask a parent to describe a typical morning at home with the child. Motor, language, and social milestones are documented. Feeding styles, behaviors, disciplinary responses, and play content are often discussed spontaneously by looking in detail at one time interval. If not, focused questions can be directed to the parent(s), with the goal of assessing psychological independence:

- Does the child play alone for short periods? What kind of toys are of interest? Does the home have safe places for exploration? Is there a place for the child in every room?
- Does the child experience temper tantrums? What appears to set them off? When do these occur? How intense are they? What are your usual responses? How do they make you feel?
- Do you and your spouse agree on expectations for and management of the child's behavior?
- Does the child have a favorite thing to carry around or take to bed? How do you feel about it? Do you always make it available?
- When the child is doing something that is off limits, how do you respond? What do you say? What do you do?
- Many parents of toddlers find it hard to say *no* so many times each day. How do you manage to change behaviors without always saying *no*?
- Have you thought about toilet training? If so, what ideas do you have about when and how to accomplish it?

Examination

Approach the child cautiously. If when you enter the examining room, the toddler is on the floor or at a table playing with toys, you might bend down to the child's level. Sitting on the floor and engaging the child with a ball or other toy may yield a temporary alliance and permit effective interaction with the child. A simple, brief comment about the toy the child is playing with or a color (or pattern) on clothes may be helpful.

Frequently at this age the toddler may react with alarm at your entrance into the examining room, usually seeking out the mother and either clinging to her or sitting quietly on her lap. Reassure the parent that this is a normal and expected behavior at this age. In fact, it represents an emotionally close attachment between the child and parent.

The physical examination is usually performed optimally with the child in the parent's lap. Stranger awareness is lessened in this more secure position. Physical abnormalities can be assessed accurately while the parent holds the child. In the same manner, assessment of language, motor, and social skill can be successful when the child is sitting on the parent's lap. The extent of the stranger-awareness response will determine how much developmental information can be observed; other data can be obtained from the parent's history.

Because the move toward independence is in progress at this stage, coupled with the unfamiliar examining room where the assessment is done, development at the age of 18 months can appear more delayed than it is. Explaining this to parents is helpful. They should not feel embarrassment when their toddler screams and clings to mother at the clinician's approach. A comment such as, "Maggie certainly knows who is important in her life!" will go a long way to ease any tension the mother may experience.

Anticipatory Guidance

The pediatric perspective for parent education at this examination should focus on (1) the anticipation of either behavioral or developmental problems based on the clinician's data base during the interview and physical examination and (2) assisting parents with the next developmental stage by pointing to new milestones and anticipated behaviors.

The child's temperament, behavioral responses to new situations, progress in self-directed feeding, and independent play will guide the discussion of anticipatory guidance. Not every visit at 18 months will require the discussion offered in these guidelines. For some parents, reassurance that development is on track will suffice. However, insight into broader meanings of new skills is appreciated by all parents.

Behavioral and developmental education for parents of an 18-month-old may include the following topics:

Concept of Rapprochement[2]

Without using the term *rapprochement*, which may be confusing or misleading to some parents, an explanation of the child's anticipated behavior is helpful. It refers to the frequently observed and normal change from independent play and exploratory activity to a period of clinging to the parent in the presence of other children and adults. It is usually seen between 18 and 24 months and may last for a week to several months. It is age appropriate, transient, and, for some children, a developmental necessity before achieving greater independence in play, language, and motor skills.

Self-Feeding as an Expression of Control and Independence

The clinician can help parents see mealtime as important in the child's growing expression of control and independence.

- Talk about feeding time in terms of the *child's* needs, not only the need for nutrients, but also for self-directed mastery over an important part of the environment.
- Point out that appetites are often erratic at this age, but that toddlers do not starve themselves.
- Let parents know that the appetite control mechanism in the hypothalamus is well developed and that given the availability of nutritious foods, the 18-month-old will choose adequate nutrients over time.
- Discourage forced feeding or battles over food intake. Redirect the discussion to help the parents view feeding in developmental terms, as an expression of learning to be satisfied through a self-directed task.
- Let parents know that messy feeding behaviors are both expected and appropriate at this age.
- Praise parents for allowing the toddler to exercise new visual-motor skills that provide the hand-eye coordination to use a cup and spoon successfully. Socially accepted eating patterns are nurtured over time by a positive approach to these social situations.
- Explain that foods the family eats should be the bulk of the toddler diet.
- Tell parents that the child's throwing food and screaming mean the child is done eating and should be put down.

Transitional Object[6]

About two thirds of toddlers will have an inanimate **transitional object** that is used for comforting, especially when they are falling asleep and at times of stress. Some parents need the reassurance that these old, threadbare blankets, dolls, or toys are a reasonable way to find the security required at certain moments in each day. Their use may persist until the third or fourth birthday and occasionally later. Developmental assessments at 10 years old, comparing children who used a transitional object with those who did not possess an obvious one, showed no significant differences in behavioral or educational outcomes.[7] Some youngsters seem to need an object. Parents may appreciate the theoretical insight about the meaning of the object as described by Winnicott et al.[6]

Toilet Training Readiness

This examination (usually the last health supervision visit before the second birthday) is an ideal time to anticipate the parents' expectations, knowledge, and plans for the initiation of toilet training. Readiness skills have been discussed earlier. Ask the parents, "What are your ideas or plans for toilet training?" Providing developmentally appropriate information at this time in terms of motor, social, and receptive language skills goes a long way in preventing either a too rigid or too lenient program for the child. Table 13-1 provides guidelines for the early stages of the process. It is helpful to teach parents that learning to use a potty seat is an important milestone in the toddler's ability to take control of the environment while gaining a sense of mastery and feeling good about oneself. The focus should be on the *child's* control, not the parents'.

Anticipating Disciplinary Problems

To assist parents in understanding the expected development of negative behavior in the form of emotional outbursts is a significant task for the child's clinician at this time.[8] It should be explained and interpreted in terms of the toddler's striving for psychological independence while the ability to manage anger and frustrations is limited by both language and attachment to parents. It is the child's bid to have a say in what is going on, to have his or her perspective appreciated.

> *The mother of an 18-month-old who has been brought to your office for a health supervision visit is surprised to discover a poster and brochure in your waiting room that encourages alternatives to spanking. Just as you do as a part of each patient's visit at this age, you mention the poster and ask the mother what she thinks about it. "What's so bad about spanking? We spanked our two older kids when they needed it. When the kids get wild or don't mind, a quick swat on the behind lets them know what's right. I don't do it a lot, but all kids need a spanking sometimes," she responds.*

This situation is both an opportunity and a challenge for the clinician. Several different responses are possible:

A. "You should never spank your child. It is an act of violence that gives your child the wrong message. I'm sure you don't want to teach him that physical violence is a way to solve conflicts. Such behavior will encourage physical responses when he gets angry as an older child or teenager."

B. "There are other ways to manage your child when he is angry or out of control. I'd like to show you some of these methods, especially what we call distraction and time-out. I'd also like to talk about preventing tantrums by showing you the value of praising your child when he does things well or when he behaves well."

C. "You seem to have learned that spanking gets a quick response." Pause, wait for a response.

Or,

"Can you give me an example of your child's behavior that is usually followed by spanking?" Pause, wait for a response.

Or,

"What do you hope to accomplish when you spank your child?" Pause, wait for a response.

Or,

"Many parents who use spanking as a form of discipline tell me that they were spanked by their parents. Can you tell me about your family and how you were disciplined?"

The first response is authoritative and leaves no room for negotiation. The parents' method of discipline has been sent to the jury and given a guilty verdict, complete with a huge dose of guilt. The second response is a reasoned lecture to the parent about alternatives to spanking that provide punishment without spanking. A statement about positive reinforcement as a method to prevent conflict and tantrums is tacked on. However, the clinician has closed the door on negotiation through discussion.

The third response attempts to engage the parent in a dialogue about personal experiences, perceptions, and feelings about spanking. This approach provides an opportunity to explore moments when the parent was effective in discipline; it gives the clinician an opportunity to help the parent generalize from those to other situations. Through open-ended or focused questions, the clinician demonstrates respect for the parent's personal history. These simple questions, followed by a pause (the hallmark of active listening), give the parent an opportunity to explore a potentially difficult issue with the child's clinician. Beyond that, it brings about an opportunity for the development of mutual trust, a necessary ingredient for successful education.[9]

For many families, an open and frank discussion about spanking as a form of punishment will require direct, focused questions by the child's clinician. The American Academy of Pediatrics recognizes that corporal punishment in the form of spanking carries significant risks to a child's psychological and physical development. The many effective alternative responses to tantrums and misbehaviors have led most child advocates and clinicians to conclude that spanking is an unnecessary form of punishment. Following a consensus conference of participating pediatric clinicians and social scientists, at which the available research on corporal punishment was received,[10] a policy statement was published to encourage clinicians in their guidance for parents to seek alternative methods for dealing with undesired behaviors (Box 13-3).

Some parents find it difficult to accept or understand the push-pull nature of toddler behavior even when provided with an explanation of the behavior as a requirement for psychological independence. These parents may have experienced a rigid or strict form of child rearing from their own parents; some may have been physically abused as children; and others may have a rigid personality structure with a limited capacity to tolerate conflict. Parents may also be struggling with issues of autonomy themselves. Whatever their background, these parents need special guidance in behavior management.

Parents must see how easy it is to be drawn into conflict and that this is always a no-win situation. They must see how the child's needs for control are undercut by a power struggle on the one hand and lack of control on the other. For some families, cultural imperatives act as a strong influence in shaping parents' approach to discipline. Secure limits that are consistently and kindly presented are what the child needs. It may be helpful to provide parents with guidelines to assist them in clarifying their perception of the child's problem and a strategy for intervention. Box 13-4 gives critical questions for effective interactions by parents.

Communication Skills

Teaching parents that the toddler often has a receptive vocabulary that is at least ten times greater than the expressive vocabulary may encourage some parents to talk to their

BOX 13-3	AMERICAN ACADEMY OF PEDIATRICS: POLICY STATEMENT ON "GUIDANCE FOR EFFECTIVE DISCIPLINE"

Corporal punishment involves the physical application of some form of pain following undesirable behavior. Corporal punishment ranges from slapping the hand of a child about to touch a hot stove to identifiable child abuse, such as beatings, scaldings, and burns. Because of this range in the severity of punishment and the form of punishment, its use as a discipline strategy is controversial. While significant concerns have been raised about the negative effects of physical punishment and its potential escalation into abuse, a form of physical punishment, spanking, remains one of the most commonly used strategies to reduce undesired behaviors, with more than 90% of American families reporting having used spanking as a means of discipline at some time.[11] Spanking, as discussed here, refers to striking a child with an open hand on the buttocks or extremities with the intention of modifying behavior without causing physical injury. Other forms of physical punishment, such as striking a child with an object, striking a child on part of the body other than the buttocks or extremities, striking a child with such intensity that it results in marks lasting more than a few minutes, pulling a child's hair, jerking a child by the arm, shaking a child, and physical punishment delivered in anger with intention to cause pain, are unacceptable and may be dangerous to the health and well-being of the child. These types of physical punishment should never be used.

Despite its common acceptance, and even advocacy for its use, spanking is a less desirable strategy than time-out or removal of privileges for reducing undesired behavior in children. Although spanking may immediately reduce or stop an undesired behavior, its effectiveness decreases with subsequent use. The only way to maintain the initial effect of spanking is to systematically increase the intensity with which it is delivered, which can quickly escalate into abuse. Thus, at best, spanking is only effective when used in selective infrequent situations.

A number of consequences of spanking lessen its desirability as a strategy to eliminate undesired behavior:

- For children younger than 18 months, spanking increases the chance of physical injury, and the child is unlikely to understand the connection between the behavior and the punishment.
- While spanking may result in a reaction of shock by the child and the cessation of the undesired behavior, repeated spanking may cause agitated and aggressive behavior by the child that may escalate to physical altercation between the parent and child.
- Spanking models aggressive behavior as a solution to conflict and has been associated with increased aggression in preschool and school age children.[12]
- Use of spanking and threats of spanking lead to altered parent-child relationships, making discipline substantially more difficult when physical punishment is no longer an option, such as with adolescents.
- Spanking is no more effective as a long-term strategy than other approaches,[13] and reliance on spanking as a discipline approach makes other discipline strategies less effective to use.[14] Time-out and positive reinforcement of other behaviors are more difficult to implement and take longer to work when spanking has previously been a primary method of discipline.

From American Academy of Pediatrics, Committee on Psychosocial Aspects of Child and Family Health: *Pediatrics* 101:723, 1998.

Continued

| BOX 13-3 | AMERICAN ACADEMY OF PEDIATRICS: POLICY STATEMENT ON "GUIDANCE FOR EFFECTIVE DISCIPLINE"—cont'd |

■ Long-term undesired and unintended consequences of spanking may occur for parents and children. Because spanking a child may provide the parents some relief from anger, the likelihood that the parent will spank the child in the future is increased.[15]

Parents who spank their children are more likely to use other unacceptable forms of corporal punishment.[16] The more children are spanked, the more anger they report feeling as adults, the more likely they are to spank their own children, the more likely they are to approve of hitting and to hit their spouses, and the higher their level of marital conflict as adults.[15] Spanking has been associated with higher rates of physical aggression in children, more substance abuse, and increased risk of crime and violence when used with older children and adolescents.

Because of the negative consequences of spanking and because it has been demonstrated to be no more effective than other approaches for dealing with undesired behavior in children, the American Academy of Pediatrics recommends that parents be encouraged and assisted in the development of alternative methods other than spanking for dealing with undesired behavior.

From American Academy of Pediatrics, Committee on Psychosocial Aspects of Child and Family Health: *Pediatrics* 101:723, 1998.

| BOX 13-4 | HELPING PARENTS TO ANTICIPATE DISCIPLINARY PROBLEMS[17] |

What am I trying to teach?
Why is this important to me?
How am I trying to teach it?
What is my child learning?
Anticipating problems, the clinician may use this and subsequent visits to explore various change strategies.

children more effectively. The use of simple, clear phrases and sentences that express parental emotions and directions can be encouraged. Clear directives that are brief, are unequivocal, and do not imply a choice when there is none are best (e.g., "It's time to go to bed" versus "Would you like to go to bed?").

Anticipating and Short-Circuiting Excessive Frustration

Many children at this age experience a tantrum when their immediate environment overheats (e.g., a supermarket, a large family gathering, dinner preparations causing a busy end of the day). The excessive sensory stimulation may be visual, auditory, tactile, or, as is often the case, a combination of sensory inputs. The time of the day may be a contributing factor (e.g., in the morning when parents are busy preparing for work or school, end of the day when parents and older siblings return home, or bedtime). Many parents are not aware of the temporal and situational patterns that tantrums follow. It may be helpful to suggest change indirectly by asking, "Do you think that changing some of these situations may help your child by decreasing moments of frustration?" Specific suggestions might include shopping at a different time (when the child is more rested or, if possible, without the child), providing an alternative activity during dinner preparations (e.g., having the child watch *Sesame Street* or some other child-oriented television program or videotape or arranging for an older sibling to play with the toddler).

Consistency in Discipline

Children at this age require consistency in all aspects of their life. Too many caretakers, too many different activities, and too many different people giving different cues confuse expectations and responses of the toddler. It is not surprising that parents often have inconsistent approaches to child rearing in general and to toddler discipline in particular because they are products of different families and often of conflicting parenting styles. In addition, the inconsistencies in behavior responses may be between a grandparent and parents or between the parents and day-care personnel. When inconsistency in discipline becomes apparent, the clinician should point out the advantages, indeed the necessity, of providing consistency. A conference with both parents is often required to explore and solve this problem. Basic philosophies, as well as very specific issues, must be discussed in a frank, open manner within a family. This process ideally starts in the first year; it becomes a clear necessity in the second.

The link between the action and the response of the parent has to be very close at this age for the child to get the linkage. Delayed responses will only confuse the child about what is expected. Repeated redirection will be needed because the child's memory skills are still very immature.

Behavior Modification

The reinforcement of positive behaviors and ignoring of minor negative behaviors form the core of **behavior modification.** Some parents encourage negative behavior unconsciously by either overreacting to minor outbursts of anger or by making frequent demeaning statements when behavior is contrary. Point out that this kind of attention only raises the child's interest in pursuing negative behaviors. Conversely, frequent praise for positive behaviors teaches the child that parental attention and appreciation is the reward for doing things well, such as drinking from a cup independently, using a potty seat, asking for a toy or milk, or making something with toys.[18]

Children under 2½ usually need specific help to move to an activity that is not forbidden. Give them the alternative and praise their participation in it. Yelling "No!" across the room only invites the toddler to tease by doing it again.

Dealing With Tantrums

When parents recognize that most tantrums in children at this age are a result of acute frustration, the simple method of *distracting the child from the situation* that appears to be associated with the frustration usually is effective. In fact, distraction as a way of life may be the method of survival for some families at this stage of development! Suggest that the child can be *physically removed from the conflictual or unsafe environment* and placed in a less conflictual or safer place. An alternative toy, a book, or an interactive game with a parent or other person usually serves to ameliorate the screaming child if given with a hug or loving touch. Body contact is important.

Other tantrums will require a *verbal dialogue* between parent and child. Removing the toddler from the conflictual environment and sitting with him or her in a quiet place are the first step. *Holding the child closely* while talking is settling and reassuring for some children. *Asking a question or making a statement that reflects the child's feelings* at the moment gives the child an opportunity to reflect on the emotional content of the behavior, a feeling or thought that may not be available unless it is articulated by a person the child trusts (Box 13-5). Examples of this form of communication are shown in Box 13-6.

Although the intensity of the tantrum, the child's temperament, and the parent's ability to confront emotional material will predict the effect of this method, it is a very powerful tool, not only as a method of response to negative behavior, but more significantly, as a potential foundation for parent-child communication about feelings.[19]

Time-Out Period for Excessive Tantrums

When a child with a severe tantrum does not respond to verbal communication or to being picked up, it may be helpful to give the toddler a time-out period. The removal of positive parental attention in the form of a time-out increases compliance with parental expectations by 25% to 80%.[20] An explanation is required ("you will stay there until you stop crying; mommy (or daddy) is in the kitchen, and you can come to me after you stop crying"). For some children this technique redirects out-of-control behavior, allows the anger to run its course, and provides a time for reinvestment with the parent as the tantrum terminates.[21] When time-out is used consistently for age-appropriate duration (approximately 1 minute for each year of age), not excessively, and with a planned strategy for escape behavior, it is more likely to be successful.

For some parents, reading one or two books on behavior during this period may be helpful (see Chapter 27). Other parents may benefit from parent-toddler play groups, a parent education group, or day care.

The child's clinician can be helpful as a guide to parents who are going through the experience of a toddler with tantrums. However, it is important to refrain from simply providing parents with a "recipe" for behavior change. Behavior modification techniques are helpful as part of an overall management plan that includes an understanding of the many variables contributing to the child's problems. Listening carefully to parents and children, observing parent-child interactional styles in the office, and communicating with them through active listening skills will often provide a sufficient foundation for the parent to understand both the nature and response to various negative behaviors. "Prescriptions" for behavior change can give the clinician a false sense of security. Teaching parents about their toddler rather than how to change their toddler's behavior has a bigger payoff in the long run. Having said this, some specific guidelines can often help parents in distress (Boxes 13-7 and 13-8).

A comprehensive approach to the assessment process includes consideration of the parent-child relationship, shaping and teaching desired behaviors, and reducing undesired behaviors; this model will guide the clinician in the determination of which aspects may require intervention.[22]

BOX 13-5	EXPRESSING EMOTIONS THROUGH IDEAS

Greenspan's model for child development emphasized the interaction between emerging emotional capacities and through processes at different ages. He has pointed out that the 18-month-old exhibits **specific behaviors to express emotions through ideas:**

Dependency and security—Caring for and holding a doll or stuffed toy

Pleasure—Showing smiles and excitement to accompany play; indicating fondness for certain food or a special toy

Curiosity—Hide-and-seek or exploring drawers or closets; search play with dolls or stuffed toys

Assertiveness—Making needs known verbally; putting doll or stuffed toy in charge of activities of other toys

Protest and anger—Using words such as *mad* to express anger; getting mad at an uncooperative toy

Setting self-limits—Punishing a doll or stuffed toy for being naughty; responding to parental "no"

In this model, "a tantrum is seen as the result of a frustration—an inability to master a task, to communicate a desire, to understand why things are as they are." Following a calming-down period, the parent can then reengage the child in the world of ideas and teach a valuable lesson: closeness between parent and child can occur even after a disruptive emotional experience. By teaching a child to label feelings, to learn to make use of pretend play and by using words to discipline, the child's emotional and cognitive skills are blended to encourage growth.

Greenspan offers the following example of managing a toddler temper tantrum:

"Jimmy enjoys taking care of his stuffed dog in pretend play, but has temper tantrums when frustrated. Today, his mother cannot find his green car just when he wants it. He manages to say, 'Car. Green,' and then when it doesn't instantly appear, he turns red in the face and starts kicking, stomping, and throwing things all over the place in a full-fledged tantrum. At moments of rage like this, your teaching about ideas obviously needs to wait until you have calmed the child down. So Jimmy's mother yells a little, threatens a little, and physically stops Jimmy from kicking until he quiets down. The two then sulk in mutual annoyance for a few minutes with Jimmy going off by himself and starting to play. At this point, his mother sits next to him, becomes a partner in his play, and then gives him a hug to show that everything is all right. While she is giving him a hug, she also says, 'Are you still angry?' This gives the child a chance to learn the word for the emotions he felt, as well as the idea that emotions can be labeled. Gradually, his mother explains about patience and how to look for things he cannot find right away. Later on, when he wants his green car again, his mother might be able to convince him to be patient and look further. She can show him, even in hide-and-seek fashion, how to look. 'Is Mr. Green Car in the closet? No, he's not here. Under the chair?' etc. This use of ideas will probably not work each time, but he may be willing to wait and look rather than throw a tantrum at least some of the time. Your ability to tolerate intense emotion and to reconnect with your child will encourage his use of ideas to express feelings."

Modified from Greenspan SI: *Psychopathology and adaptation in infancy and early childhood: principles of clinical diagnosis and preventive intervention*, New York, 1981, International Universities Press and Greenspan S, Greenspan NT: *First feelings: milestones in the emotional development of your baby and child*, New York, 1985, Penguin Books.

BOX 13-6	TANTRUMS: STATEMENTS THAT UNLOCK A CHILD'S FEELINGS

"Gee, you sure are upset right now!"
"Sometimes we get real angry and upset inside us when things aren't going well."
"Isn't it awful when you can't do something you really want to do?"
"You seem really mad at me now."

BOX 13-7	DISCIPLINE IN EARLY CHILDHOOD MANAGEMENT: CONCEPTS FOR CLINICIAN

Achieving a helping relationship—Parent should perceive the child's clinician as someone available to discuss behavioral outbursts and other negative behaviors.

Identifying problem areas—Through a screening checklist or focused questions, developmentally predictable behavioral problems should be queried.

Exploring genetic, historical, and social predisposing factors—Include questions on maternal depression, prenatal events, perinatal stress, the health of siblings, the vulnerable child syndrome, substance abuse, and the parents' own childhood memories.

Viewing parenthood as a developmental process—Recognize that parenting skills are established through maturation, knowledge, experience, and guidance. Development of effective parenting skills takes time.

Encouraging parents to take an active role in deciding how to manage the child's behavior—Explore methods previously used by the parents and provide support for their ways or suggest modifications that might be more effective.

Respecting different parenting styles—Cultural, social class, and past experience provide parents with variable responses to child behaviors. Variations in child rearing among families can be instructive for the clinician. A "best" way to manage a behavioral problem does not exist.

Providing appropriate models—Increase parental awareness that children imitate and identify with their parents' behavior. While modeling healthy adult behavior, the clinician can be a useful guide to the parent.

Consistency—Rules are essential for discipline. For toddlers, the number of rules should be limited and parents should enforce only the important ones. This should help with consistency.

Talking about discipline—Parents (and other child care providers) should discuss with each other expectations for the child's behavior and agree on management approaches. Discuss acceptable conduct as well as unacceptable behaviors.

Rewarding appropriate behavior—Praise, encouragement, and rewards increase a child's happiness, security, and self-esteem.

Punishment to discourage some behaviors—Consistency is important. Design to motivate socially approved behaviors and to be specific for a particular offense. Explanation must accompany punishment. Carry out as soon as possible following inappropriate behavior. Administer in context of a warm parent-child relationship.

Modified from Smith EE, VanTassel E: *Pediatr Clin North Am* 29 (1):167, 1982.

BOX 13-8	DISCIPLINE IN EARLY CHILDHOOD MANAGEMENT: CONCEPTS FOR PARENTS

Provide exemplary models.

Frequently discuss with each other behavioral expectations and agree on uniform approaches to management.

Limit number of rules and appropriate behavior with your child at a calm time.

Expect your child to need several trials to learn appropriate behaviors.

Compliment your child frequently concerning correct behavior.

Establish and maintain schedules and routines.

Give your child choices when appropriate.

Anticipate and avoid unnecessary conflict situations.

Use punishment sparingly, but consistently.

Individualize punishment for particular offenses and provide simple explanations as to why you are punishing.

Be mindful of individual and marital needs apart from your child.

Modified from Smith EE, VanTassel E: *Pediatr Clin North Am* 29 (1):175, 1982.

Anticipating Parental Distress

The rapid changes in the development of a toddler may be overwhelming for single (especially adolescent) mothers, the socially isolated family, families experiencing economic stress, and the family undergoing a significant life event (e.g., divorce, illness, or an unplanned move).

Young children are barometers of the family's emotional life. Although regressions in recently acquired milestones are common for all children at this stage, they are predictable among children in families experiencing increased stress. Developmental regressions in toddlers include refusal to use the potty seat, throwing food when in the high chair, screaming with seemingly mild frustrations, and increased periods of night awakening. Although these behaviors are transient setbacks in development, they are particularly frustrating to the parent in distress. The child's demands may be just too much for the parent to handle. He or she may not be able to see beyond the behavior. Some parents internalize the child's behavior and seem to see it as a failure in parenting ("She was so good at eating by herself and using the potty seat a few weeks ago. What have I done to cause these new behaviors?"). Along with guilt, these parents experience anger and fatigue as the toddler's infantile responses become more difficult to manage in the presence of acute or chronic family distress. An astute clinician will either anticipate or recognize the accompanying anxiety or depression in the parent (or its effect on the child), explore the severity or chronicity of the problems, and, when appropriate, offer assistance in the form of a referral to a parent group or a counseling resource.

In concluding the office visit, the clinician will find that a summary statement about the child's current stage of development is beneficial when it is then followed by what the parents might anticipate. At 18 months, the emphasis should be on the following:

■ Language skills as they develop, with the emerging use of two- and three-word phrases and mimicking as a way to communicate and reflect on experiences

- The importance of play, with self-initiated play in a safe environment that provides the arena to use new motor skills followed by parallel play with other toddlers
- Behavioral changes that allow increasing levels of tolerance for frustrating events, such as limit setting during play time, bedtime behaviors, feeding behaviors, and toilet training

REFERENCES

1. Ainsworth MDS: Infant-mother attachment, *Am Psychol* 34:932, 1979.
2. Mahler M, Pine F, Bergman A: *The psychological birth of the human infant,* New York, 1975, Basic Books.
3. Kagan J: *The nature of the child,* New York, 1984, Basic Books, pp 43-48.
4. Carey WB: Clinical use of temperament data in pediatrics. In Porter R, Collins GM, editors: *Temperament in infants and young children,* Ciba Foundation Symposium no 89, London, 1982, Pitman Books.
5. Brazelton TB, Gatson RL, Howard RB: Developmental feeding issues. In Howard RB, Winter HS, editors: *Nutrition and feeding of infants and toddlers,* Boston, 1984, Little, Brown & Co.
6. Winnicott DW: Transitional objects and transitional phenomena. In Winnicott DW: *Collected papers,* London, 1958, Tavistock Publishing, pp 229-242.
7. Sherman M et al: Treasured objects in school aged children, *Pediatrics* 68:379, 1981.
8. American Academy of Pediatrics, Committee on Psychosocial Aspects of Child and Family Health: Policy statement on guidance for effective discipline, *Pediatrics* 101:723, 1998.
9. Wissow LS, Roter D: Toward effective discussion of discipline and corporal punishment during primary care visits: findings from studies of doctor-patient interaction, *Pediatrics* 94:587, 1994.
10. American Academy of Pediatrics: The short- and long-term consequences of corporal punishment, Part 2, *Pediatrics* 98:803, 1996.
11. McCormick KF: Attitudes of primary care physicians toward corporal punishment, *JAMA* 267:3161, 1992.
12. Eron LD: Research and public policy, *Pediatrics* 98:821, 1996.
13. Roberts MW, Powers SW: Adjusting chair time-out enforcement procedures for oppositional children, *Behav Ther* 21:257, 1990.
14. Wilson DR, Lyman RD: Time-out in the treatment of childhood behavior problems: implementation and research issues, *Child Family Behav Ther* 4:5, 1982.
15. Straus MA: Spanking and the making of a violent society, *Pediatrics* 98:837, 1996.
16. Graziano AM, Hamblen JL, Plante WA: Subabusive violence in child rearing in middle-class American families, *Pediatrics* 98:845, 1996.
17. Vaughan VC, Litt IF: *Child and adolescent development: clinical implications,* Philadelphia, 1990, WB Saunders, p 204.
18. Showalter JE: The modification of behavior modification, *Pediatrics* 59:130, 1977.
19. Gordon T: *P.E.T.: parent effectiveness training,* New York, 1975, Plume Books.
20. Scarboro ME, Forehand R: Effects of two types of response-contingent time-outs on compliance and oppositional behavior of children, *J Exp Child Psychol* 19:252, 1975.
21. Drabman RS, Jarvie B: Counseling parents of children with behavior problems: the use of extinction and time-out techniques, *Pediatrics* 59:78, 1977.
22. Howard BJ: Advising parents on discipline: what works, *Pediatrics* 98:809, 1996.

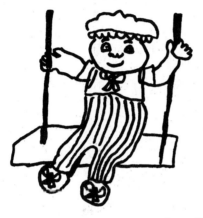

"A baby in the park."

"A baby learning to talk." By Ryan Hennessy.

CHAPTER 14

TWO YEARS: LANGUAGE EMERGES

■ **Suzanne D. Dixon**

KEY WORDS

Symbolic Function
Language Development
Language Difficulties
Language Delays
Gestures
Bilingualism
Hearing
Speech Difficulties

Jared, age 2, comes in for an ear check after an episode of otitis media. His tympanic membranes now appear nearly normal. Upon questioning, his mother says that he has about 10 to 20 single words and hasn't put together any words except "gimme." The fourth child of this family, born 8 years after his next older sibling, Jared had a mildly difficult birth, but recovered well. He has had four episodes of otitis media since birth. His mom says that he doesn't talk more because all of his sibs do everything for him. "There's no need for him to say anything, or even point, for that matter," she says. She feels he's "younger" than the other kids were at his age, but she says that she's to blame; she really enjoys her baby. Jared doesn't say anything in the office.

The second birthday falls in a period when a whole new set of capabilities emerge. These include the core concept of one thing standing for another, called **symbolic function.** Another closely aligned concept is the ability to understand rules and systems that generalize from one situation to another. Language comes out of and further fuels these basic cognitive processes. Major reorganization of brain systems at this time coincides with this behavioral shift. **Language development** and growth in cognitive abilities together allow the child to interact with the world in new ways, and they represent a big transition in development, from infancy to childhood. A new plateau is reached—the era of the talkative, questioning, active 2-year-old.

COGNITIVE ABILITIES

The clinical appraisal of language has now been shown to be even more critical than in previous eras of pediatric practice. Language assessment should become a prominent part of child health surveillance for some important reasons. For example, work in developmental psychology has defined more of the links between language and cognitive abilities.[1] A look at language is a look at the mental structures that may be critical to the skills needed in school years and beyond. For example, although a child who has early **language difficulties** may not have continuing **language delays** per se by the entry of school, the child may have verbally-based learning disabilities, difficulties in the speed and accuracy in verbal processing, and social adjustment problems. Early identification and remediation through the provision of appropriate services may prevent school failure and its emotional sequelae.

Secondly, the chief complaint of language delay may identify youngsters with atypical development, such as the autism spectrum of disorders, a class of disabilities that may be on the rise. For these youngsters, early remediation through jump-starting language before the age of 7 gives them a substantially better outlook than the potential for children without useful language by that age. These youngsters are hard to spot early if one does not have a strong vigilance about language development.

Child health care providers rarely miss disabilities in the motor sphere, but those involving cognition and language are often missed or dismissed in spite of the fact that they are among the most common of developmental disorders.[2] This won't happen if the clinical milieu is set up to regularly evaluate language and if the clinician has a strong sense of how language develops, including the limits of variability. A proactive evaluation process built upon a strong understanding of language development allows the child health care provider to do good developmental surveillance in this area.

LANGUAGE DEVELOPMENT COURSE

Language, of course, begins long before the second birthday, and continues beyond it. The specific patterns of early childhood language development have been summarized by many workers.[1,3-7] The following represents a synthesis of these works, and Table 14-1 lays out the sequence.

Prenatal and Infancy

Language development begins before birth as the infant perceives the sounds of the womb, quiets to their steady rhythm, and begins to synchronize movements to mother's voice and body sounds. Increasing evidence suggests that the fetus responds to environmental sounds long before birth and begins to develop some memory of these. Specific pieces of music may result in the fetus' turning toward the source and showing heart rate changes suggestive of alerting (see Chapter 4).

Responsiveness to specific sounds and interactional synchrony between infant movement and parental voices and rhythm are well developed at birth.[8] Discrimination of even similar sounds (e.g., pa, ba) is present in the first weeks of life, although this ability may be lost later in the first year if a specific sound is not present in that child's language. This

TABLE 14-1 ■ Clinical Evaluation of Language Skills

Age	Receptive Skills	Expressive Skills	Specific Indication for Referral
0-1 mo	Recognizes sound with startle; turns to sound and looks for source; quiets motor activity to sound; "prefers" human speech with high inflection	Differentiated crying; body language of positive and negative response	No response to pleasing sound when alert; neonatal sepsis; meningitis; neonatal asphyxia; prematurity; congenital infection; familial deafness; renal abnormalities; aminoglycoside therapy
2-4 mo	Prolonged attention to sounds; responds to familiar voice; watches the speaking mouth; enjoys rattle; attempts to repeat pleasing sounds with objects; shifts gaze back and forth between sounds	"Ed, ih, uh" (hind mouth vowels); cooing, blows bubbles; enjoys using tongue and lips; reciprocal cooing; play dialogues; loudness varies	No response to pleasing sounds; does not attend to voices
5-7 mo	Seeks out speaker; localizes sounds; understands own name, familiar words; associates word with activity (e.g., bath, car)	Initiates sounds; pitch varies; babbles with labial consonants ("ba, ma, ga"); uses sounds to get attention, express feeling; sounds directed at object	Decrease or absence of vocalizations
8-12 mo	Begins word comprehension; responds to simple commands—"point to your nose," "say bye-bye"; knows names of family members; responds to a few words, those associated with specific objects	First words, five to six— "mama, dada"; inflected vocal play; repeats sounds and words made by others; "oo, ee" (foremouth vowels); intentional gestures	No babbling with consonant sounds; no response to music
13-20 mo	Single step element commands; identifies familiar objects	Points to objects with vocalization; vocabulary of 10-50 words; pivot and open class words, rate, and content varies	No comprehension of words; does not understand simple requests
18-24 mo	Recognizes many nouns; understands simple questions	Telegraphic speech; vocabulary of 50-75 words; 20-word sentences, phrases; stuttering common	Vowel sounds, but no consonants; no words

Continued

TABLE 14-1 ■ Clinical Evaluation of Language Skills—cont'd

Age	Receptive Skills	Expressive Skills	Specific Indication for Referral
24-36 mo	Understands prepositions; can follow story with pictures	Identifies body parts; vocabulary of 200 words; dependent on phrases, three-word sentences; uses words for expressive needs; pronouns; early grammar	No words; does not follow simple directions; no sentences
30-36 mo	Understands some syntax (difference between car hit train and train hit car); understands opposites; understands action in pictures	Sentences of four or five words, three elements; tells stories; uses "what" and "where" questions; uses negation; uses progressive and past tense, all regular form; uses plurals, regular form	Speech largely unintelligible to stranger; dropout of initial consonants; no sentences
3-4 yr	Understands three-element commands	Talks about what she is doing; uses "I" with grammar by her own rules; vocabulary of 40-1500 words; speech intelligible to strangers; "why" questions; commands; uses past and present tense; passive speech in spontaneous speech; nursery rhymes; says colors, numbers 1-4, full name, sex; articulation of "m, n, p, h, and w"; four-word sentences	Speech not comprehended by strangers; still dependent on gestures; consistently holds hands over ears; speech without modulation

is true, for example, with the "r" and "l" sounds that are not differentiated in Japanese. A selective attention to one's own language, parents' voices and changes in tone, or prosody in the surrounding language has been seen in newborns. Infants do selectively quiet to the unique tones, rhythm, and timing of lullabies around the world. Children in the first year acquire a sense of what sounds are words, the units of language, and pay more attention to words that have been presented to them before. They are building a storehouse of words that will serve them in the second year when they begin to develop a vocabulary of their own.

TABLE 14-1 ■ Clinical Evaluation of Language Skills—cont'd

Age	Receptive Skills	Expressive Skills	Specific Indication for Referral
4-5 yr	Understands four-element commands; links past and present events; decreasing ability for second language acquisition	2700-word vocabulary; defines simple words; auxiliary verbs "has" and "had"; conversation mature with "how" and "why" questions in response to others; articulation of "b, k, g, and f"; five-word sentences; "normalizes" irregular verbs and nouns; increases in accessibility of forms	Stuttering; consistently avoids loud places
5-6 yr	Understands five-element commands; can follow a story without pictures; enjoys jokes and riddles; can comprehend two meanings of a single word	Correct use of all parts of speech; vocabulary 5000 words; articulation of "y, ng, and d"; six-word sentences; corrects own errors in speech; can use logic in recounting story plots	Word endings dropped; faulty sentence structure; abnormal rate, rhythm, or inflection
6-7 yr	Asks for motivation and explanation of events; understands time intervals (months, seasons); right and left differences	Articulation of "l, r, t, sh, ch, dr, cl, bl, gl, and cr"; has formal adult speech patterns	Poor voice quality, articulation
7-8 yr	Can use language alone to tell a story sequentially; reasons using language	Articulation of "v, th, j, s, z, tr, st, sl, sw, and sp"	
8-9 yr		Articulation of "th, sc, and sh"	

Expressive language also begins early; cooing, the production of vowel sounds without the formation of syllable units, begins in the first 2 months of life. Loudness of cooing begins to vary at about 1 month of age,[5] and pitch variation develops between 2 and 4 months of age. "Conversations" with 2-month-olds should thus show some variation in tone, as well as sound. Cooing sounds are heard from children who are completely deaf, although with decreased frequency and not in a conversational or interactive setting. Babbling, the production of sounds containing both vowels and consonants, is heard by 6 months of age and is heard in a similar manner among all language groups around the world.[9] Babbling requires a marked increase in fine-motor control of all the oral pharyngeal musculature. Babbling appears to exercise these speech organs and to allow the child to discover the ability to talk. The quantity and quality of babble are less in children who have reduced or no hearing or who are rarely interacted with verbally.

Imitation of adult speech, called jargon or jabber, with the phonetical and intonational parameters of the child's native language occurs regularly by the ninth month, earlier in some children. This always precedes the first words. Pointing at objects begins between 9 and 12 months and is a very important language milestone. It precedes the naming of objects and engaging in communication with the world through shared attention to objects.

By the age of 1 year, a child usually has two to eight "words," short utterances that are produced in a specific context or to identify a specific person, event, or object. The minimum competency would be one word other than "mama" and "dada" and following one-step commands and **gestures.**

Gestures

Often infants' gestures are part of emerging language abilities.[1,10,11] While pointing is the precursor to naming, some gestures may be the precursors to asking. These are called instrumental gestures. For example, a toddler's pointing and grunting at the cookie jar is a request for the contents. Symbolic gestures at 13 months are also highly correlated with later language ability (e.g., recognizing a telephone by lifting it toward the ear, categorizing a shoe by touching it to the foot, or labeling a toy car by moving it back and forth on the floor). These then expand to be even more elaborate pantomimes, demonstrating a connection between two events, imitating an event, and developing themes in play. These are analogous to short descriptions or stories. Children who can say or wave "bye bye" or do "pat-a-cake" with a verbal prompt are testifying to the emergent cognitive and language skills. Children with a rich gesture communication system in toddlerhood are likely to develop normal linguistical skills even if they are late bloomers in terms of language production itself. Children without such gestures are likely to have persistent language difficulties.[1] The clinician is well advised to ask about, observe, and engage in gesture games with the infant and toddler. These are not trivial.

The toddler both overextends (e.g., using the word "doggy" for all interesting animals) and overly restricts (e.g., using the word "doggy" only for the family dog) the meaning of these early utterances in the struggle to order and understand the world. The child is experimenting with the rules and structure of language and will gradually refine this so that "dogs" are the creatures we identify as such, and Fido will get his own proper name. Feedback is absorbed from listening to others' use of language rather than specific teaching about terms or words. The child may point and look for an affirmation of naming. From this feedback and rapt attention to the language around him, the toddler puts the linguistical puzzle together. A rich verbal environment facilitates this process.

The acquisition of new words during the period from about 12 to 18 months tends to be quite slow. These words tend to be simple, salient, and overgeneralized naming that allows the child's needs to be met and the primitive sharing of simple observations. These are called the nominative and instrumental functions. Things that a child can act on or things that change or move are usually the first named. The size of the average vocabulary of an 18-month-old is between 50 and 100 words, but this is extremely variable between children and may even fluctuate periodically within a given child, who may only use a word in a special context and not anywhere else. Words will appear and disappear in seemingly random fashion. The child may depend more on others' gestures and visual reinforcers in the context of the family's simplified, overemphasized speech to increase her own receptive language capacities. Families do expand and clarify these utterances through a process that may help to fuel further language development.[12] *Talking to children, responding to their utterances as if they had full communicative intent, and avoidance of overcorrecting word attempts will boost language skills.*

The apparent lag period in language progress is often followed by an explosion in either words or phrases. The second half of the second year and the beginning of the third are characterized by rapid increases in vocabulary and the use of verbs, adjectives, and even some adverbs. The most significant event in this period is the creation of original linkages of words that express a complete and original thought (e.g., "da da come," "dight hot," "now nigh dark"). These combinations imply, but may not explicitly have, a subject, verb, and perhaps an object or modifying word, although they are telegraphic or without connecting words over three fourths of the time.[3] They are in contrast to the simple naming of objects or expression of simple demands (e.g., "doggy," "wa-wa") that are characteristic of the "prelanguage" heard earlier. Some prelanguage may have sentence forms (e.g., "I wanna," "ah done"), but are always used all together in a single word and are called holophrases. True sentences show original linkages and associations, using the interchange of word combinations across differing circumstances. These generally emerge when vocabulary reaches a threshold of 50 words.

The processes of learning words, word order, and the semantic cues of language seem to reside in several areas of the brain, including the right and left parietotemporal and the frontal areas. As a word or phrase is learned and becomes part of the established language bank, the left temporal area becomes the site for this ongoing use of language. Word retrieval and the rapid recognition of words and utterances, nearly automatic, become available at a time of brain reorganization, at about 18 months to 2½ years old. The laying down of language subsumes bilateral brain systems, whereas the ongoing use of previously learned language is increasingly localized to the left temporal lobe, particularly the essential elements of grammar.[13] This geographical distribution has some flexibility. Children with early brain lesions of the left hemisphere will still acquire and use language, but with an altered time frame and facility. Other areas of the brain seem to pick up these functions in these circumstances.

SEMANTICS—THE WAY WORDS ARE PUT TOGETHER

The 2-year-old shows an understanding of the rules of language through the differential ordering of words to alter their meanings, such as "go car" versus "car go."[6] In addition, the toddler's confusion is obvious when requests are stated in the child's own telegraphic style.[3]

Talking "like a baby" to the child is likely to confuse her. The toddler anticipates that language will be interpreted by those around her and that correct grammatical form will be spoken. More than 90% of utterances in a 3-year-old are grammatically correct. New constructions (e.g., "I like it.") for the child of this age are sometimes learned in their entirety and applied in several contexts as an experiment. The 2- to 3-year-old child may use more than 300 words, nearly half the number that adults use in everyday conversation. The toddler may delight in just trying out this new skill, both in public and in private. The explosion of speech production comes from the awareness of the power of this newfound skill. The child can use dialogue to share experiences, negotiate, and pretend, delighting in drawing adults into conversations and relying on them for expansion, clarification, and refueling of the efforts. The creation of original utterances is part of an expanded interactional world of people and events.

Receptive language is always ahead of expressive language, so the child always understands more than she can say. This usually results in a mild to moderate degree of frustration, which is a source of energy for the child trying to expand linguistical skills. It can also lead to developmental stuttering, the verbal tumbling over words that won't come out fast enough to satisfy a busy preschooler's mind. This is very different than the stuttering that is a block in speech production, usually with an initial sound of a word, that emerges in late preschool and early school-age years. A little help with slowing down, best guesses about what the wanted word really is, and the avoidance of pressure or embarrassment will help the young child get mouth in line with mind in learning to speak.

Receptive language is usually more regular in its development because it is more closely linked with cognitive development than is expressive language. The latter, in turn, is more variable, being influenced by individual temperament, environmental prompts and constraints, and even the interpretive skills of the listener. Receptive language is much more predictive of long-term language abilities than expressive, although in most kids, they clearly track together.[1] *The clinician should be much more worried about the child who has difficulty understanding age-appropriate utterances that are presented without visual prompts than about a child who has little to say, but does follow verbal input at an age-appropriate level.*

For the clinician, the development of receptive language means caution should be used in discussions with a parent in front of a child because understanding will be far ahead of what the child says. Even if vocabulary is not available to the child, the prosody, general idea, and many words will be understood. Sensitive subjects and negative behaviors or situations should be discussed out of earshot of a child older than 3. Even some younger children may be able to understand such discussions.

CRIB SPEECH

Children in the preschool years practice speech in private, as well as with others. "Crib speech" serves linguistical, emotional, and cognitive purposes as it is used to sort out the day, the experiences, the struggles, and the misunderstandings. Crib speech offers a direct view of the child's mind at work, putting language and life in order.

> *Jason, almost 4, was in his room for a nap with a stuffed dog as his companion. His mom heard his conversation. "Go, go go gooooooing, ing ing ing, thing sing a song. We didn't go go sosobad. Stop hitting now wowwow. You go to sleep right now wowwow. Put jacket for the store in the store in the car in the car. I mean it. The red jacket. The red jacket, with Barney."*
>
> *Jason is very busy, working on suffixes, sound, rhyme, the "w" sound, prepositions, pronouns, compound adjectives, adverbs, and, it sounds like, some discipline issues about a car trip that may not have occurred because of some behavioral issues. He tells us a lot about his language development, his abilities, and how he uses it to manage his day.*

LANGUAGE MILESTONES

A clinician should be concerned about the child who fails to reach the minimum competencies shown in Table 14-2. With such a child, the clinician should take a more detailed look at language and evaluate neurological concerns, possible **hearing** problems, and other social-interactional issues.

The years between age 2 and 5 are characterized by a gradual expansion in sentence complexity. The length of a child's phrases and sentences increases dramatically during this time from an average of one or two elements at under 2 years of age up to three to five elements by age 4. Linguists use this measure, mean length of utterance (MLU), to evaluate language maturity. Clinicians can evaluate the longest thing a child says to get an approximation of this measure. It should increase at every visit between ages 2 and 5.

Rules are overapplied at this time, so "mistakes" are made that didn't appear before. "He has two feets," "The mices are teasing the cat," "The boy putted the cars away," are all examples. This is linguistical progress, not regression. The late preschooler is now conscious of rules governing language and is overly fastidious in their application. He will self-correct these irregularities over time without teaching; no didactic instruction is needed here.

Verb tenses are added in orderly sequence[3]; systems of negation and the form of questions also have their own specific developmental course. The "w" words appear in the 3-year-old's talk. The 2-year-old can communicate with family members easily; the 4-year-old should be intelligible to almost anyone who speaks the child's language 100% of the time. The regularity of these processes is quite striking.

After 5 years of age, all the basic components of language are in place, although these forms become more accessible and usable with time. A vocabulary of 800 to 14,000 words is common by age 6.[14] Poetry, puns, and jokes, all subtle turns on language, are enjoyed by early grade school. The study of grammar is appreciated with relish in the early school years, and foreign languages have particular interest for the child at this time. Foreign languages learned early create at least bilingual people and facilitate the later learning of language. Vocabulary increases should be a lifelong process, and sentence complexity increases into adult life. Table 14-1 shows the developmental progression.

TABLE 14-2 ■ Backstop Parameters that Call for Referral if Not Met

Age	Milestone
Newborn	Turns to a soft voice, especially the parents'
By 3 months	Cooing sounds. Looks alert, interactive, smiles
By 6 months	Coos and jabbers and does more every day Turns to a new sound and familiar voices, laughs
By 9 months	Babbles mamamama, bababab Knows name, turns when called
By 12 months	Points at objects Has one word in addition to "mama" and "dada" Follows one-step commands Gives or shows objects to the caretaker
By 18 months	Produces five or more words Comprehends more than 50 words
By 2 years	Produces more than 50 words Puts two words together Follows two-step commands Points at pictures in a book Names or attempts to name objects Uses "words" to request things
By 3 years	Talks in sentences most of the time Is understood by strangers at least half the time Says name, age, gender, and birthday month Names most objects in her daily life and at least three body parts Tells stories in three-sentence or phrase "paragraphs" Knows one color
By 4 years	Sustains a conversation Understood by a stranger Uses pronouns

WHY DO CHILDREN SPEAK?

The question "Why do children speak?" raises considerable controversy among psychologists and is not satisfactorily answered by any one school of thought. *Innate theorists,* or nativists, contend that children speak because a predetermined neurosensory capacity (i.e., language acquisition device [LAD]) kicks in at some point in development.[15,16] These theorists note the regularity in language development across all cultural and language groups and the production of sounds in deaf infants. However, this school cannot account for the experientially determined disturbances of language in a neglected and emotionally disturbed child or for the interactional variables from child to child that strongly influence language development. Experience is needed, in the nativist's point of view, to trigger this genetically determined capability. Other than that, this school sees the environment as relatively unimportant to the learning of language.

The *learning theorists* (see Chapter 2)[17] maintain that children speak because they imitate the speech around them and are rewarded in their efforts. Language emerges from the need to name objects, make demands, and comply with the verbal environment around them, based on the models and reinforcements provided them. Certainly, children in isolation do not learn language, and children learn the language and dialect to which they are exposed. However, these theorists do not account for the unsolicited and private babble and practice done by the infant and young child, even up through the school years, that serves no communicative intent. Predictable developmental "mistakes" in grammar and syntax made by children at certain periods have no parallel in adult speech. These detours cannot be accounted for by imitation. Indeed, they are temporarily unavailable to specific adult correction. In fact, adults rarely correct or negatively reinforce these language errors in their children.[12] Adults respond to the content and factual correctness, rather than the form of the child's speech.[6] In general, practicing speech with a child does *not* improve the quantity or quality of language, so direct imitation does not explain the bulk of language development. Or, as stated by Cazden,[4] "as 'foots' and 'goed' and 'holded' show, children use language they hear as examples of language to learn *from*, not samples of language to learn." Although a model for speech is necessary, children translate adult speech into their own grammar or rule system, implying a more complex processing problem than simple imitation.

The *interactionalist school* presents a synthesis of these perspectives, saying that children speak as an outgrowth of their interactions with parents and significant others.[1] These important people in a child's life respond to, elaborate on, and clarify early utterances, and these interactions fuel the child's growth in language. Basic cognitive processes must be present to allow children to use that input in the development of their own language skills. The neural basis of language must be present to take in the linguistical experience, order it, and reproduce it in original combinations. Children exposed to only mechanical speech (e.g., television) do not speak. Language is an outgrowth of adequate emotional development and serves the emergence of new cognitive skills. The social environment is organized to bring a child into it as a participating member, no matter what the cultural context.

In support of this position, observations of early language suggest that this interaction is vital. The amount and variety of babbling and imitative speech production at 9 to 18 months to some extent is a reflection of the amount of the mother's (or significant caretaker's) speech that the child has experienced. However, during that late infancy–early toddler period, subsequent growth in language competency is dependent on the amount and variety of *responsive* speech.[12,18] The size of a 2-year-old's vocabulary is directly dependent on how much the mother speaks to her. In other words, the development of language is built on early interactions with caregivers and is augmented later by the presence of a rich, conversational environment. *The presence of early dialogues with the child, building and expanding on the child's own utterances, and the later enriched verbal reinforcements around the child are directly related to early language acquisition.*

BOX 14-1 SUPPORTING LANGUAGE DEVELOPMENT IN YOUNG CHILDREN

Talk to the child. Beginning in infancy, talk to the baby, naming things in the environment, narrating the events of the day. A rich verbal environment supports language development all the way to college.

Speak slowly and in short phrases for the young child and give emphasis to particular words. Higher pitch gets a young child's attention.

Talk in regular language forms, including complex sentences, to provide good models to imitate. Children with more advanced language forms have families who speak to them in longer utterances. Use pronouns as appropriate; don't substitute proper names.

Respond to the child's speech as if it has meaning. Beginning at 2 months, respond to the baby's sounds with an echo or an enhancement. The baby will learn that her noises create a response.

Repeat what a child says often so that the child experiences being heard.

Respond to the meaning and not the form of the child's speech. Expand on what is said; don't correct the attempts. Help the child get ideas across.

Ask questions and wait for an answer. Language development is enhanced by giving kids a prompt and time to respond. Children who are expected to answer will have enhanced language competency.

Look at books together; name the pictures; talk about the images and the stories. Let the child start to tell the story his way when ready.

Never punish or shame a child for any language effort. Give a new model if needed, but don't overcorrect or drill.

Increase interest in language with exposure to music and rhymes.

Encourage gestures to communicate and to use in games. These will enhance, not detract from, the development of speech.

As clinicians, we can make use of all of these perspectives in conceptualizing language development. Children speak for the following reasons:

■ They have a basic neurosensory and cognitive readiness
■ Speech around them provides models
■ Speech is fun, both alone and, more importantly, with significant others

Deficits in any of these areas will be reflected in abnormal or delayed language development. The clinical perspective should be to look for basic neuromaturational competencies, a rich linguistical environment, and evidence that the child is loved, talked to responsively, and free of other sources of developmental energy drain. An appropriate and responsive environment can support the development of language. Box 14-1 gives ideas on how to provide that environment.

LANGUAGE AND COGNITION

Language development is intricately entangled with cognitive development. Much discussion and research have been devoted to the question of whether language is necessary for cognition (i.e., whether or not we need words and semantical structure to think) or whether language is merely an outcome or reflection of growth in mental capacity.[3,19] This chicken-and-egg question aside, the clinician will find that language assessment becomes increasingly enmeshed in other areas of functioning as a child grows because the usual evaluation of language, using standard instruments, is really one of cognitive growth and vice versa. Most often, language and cognitive development *are* linked in an individual child, but not necessarily so. Language development, particularly in a population of disabled children, is highly predictive of overall functioning, and language remains the best predictor of cognition. School systems are heavily biased to verbal skills, so it is not surprising that school performance and linguistical abilities are linked. Early language disorders are highly predictive of learning difficulties in school. Most studies show that greater than 40% of children with early language difficulties will have learning difficulties in school.[20]

Emotional and cognitive deficits may be secondary to primary language disorders, particularly in a society that places so much emphasis on verbal competency and formal schooling performance in its children. Conversely, emotional disorders may have language-delay symptoms.[10] In any case, the language-delayed child must be carefully and comprehensively assessed for these associated difficulties.

VARIATIONS IN LANGUAGE DEVELOPMENT

Receptive and expressive language in the normal population of children varies significantly.[1,21] In addition, style differences surface with some children adopting "frozen" phrases in their entirety (e.g., "I wuv you"), and others hesitantly building sentences from a large stock of available words (e.g., "Daddy botta Julia"). Some are late to develop expressive language, whereas some use words or phrases very early. Those late talkers who do catch up are more likely to have a rich gesture communication system and to have normal comprehension.[11]

Minority groups in the United States may be at a disadvantage in language evaluation and its close relative, cognitive assessment, as measured in the school setting and in standardized tests, for several reasons:

- Vocabulary differences
- Unfamiliarity with verbal interchange with adults in a test situation
- Temperament differences
- Systematical differences in grammatical structures that lead to misunderstandings and assumptions
- Inhibition based on fear of ridicule

A minority child in a majority setting may be inhibited from using advanced language structures. Compounding the problem is the tendency for even well-intentioned teachers to interact verbally with students who are verbal, take verbal initiatives, and respond with longer utterances.[4] The reluctant child from any group will get increasingly less verbal encouragement, practice, and reinforcement.

Socioeconomic class differences in language development may additionally reflect other differences in verbal environment.[19] Middle-class children experience a richer verbal environment, have received instructions in a complex verbal form, and are required from an early age to use verbal interchanges. Not unexpectedly, language in this group is often more advanced in early childhood.

MYTHS ABOUT LANGUAGE DEVELOPMENT

Parents and clinicians alike may explain away a child's language delay using one of several formulations that have no grounding in science. Adherence to these may lead to delay in diagnosis and treatment. Examples of these are the following:

■ *His brothers get him everything he wants, so he doesn't have to talk.* Although children lower in the birth order, when compared with firstborn children, show a slight delay in expressive language in terms of quantity of utterances, they should have no such delay at all in receptive language, gesture language, or crib speech. Also, the type and complexity, if not the quantity, of things said should follow developmental expectations for age. Children talk because of neuromaturational factors, not environmental need alone. Siblings can prompt language a bit and may provide vocabulary, both good and bad. Birth order effects do not account for significant delays or atypical language progress.

■ *He's a boy, so what do you expect?* The gender difference in language development is small, with girls ahead of boys in both quantitative speech and complexity after the first birthday. As a group, girls retain the advantage in verbal tasks throughout school. Again, this is a subtle difference of weeks to months. Significant delays cannot be explained by gender. Many detailed tests of early language have different norms for boys and girls to account for these small differences. If a screening test does show delay, further specialized evaluation should take gender into account.

■ *He's in a bilingual household, so we expect him to be delayed.* **Bilingualism** means a lot of different things, and research is not clear because of the nonexperimental nature of this situation. However, a few conclusions can be drawn from the work that has been done.[19] Children raised in bilingual households do have a slight delay in expressive language up to about 2 years of age while they put the components of language together. They mix the syntax and vocabulary of both languages, perhaps using both languages in a single utterance. However, a single object will have a single name in one or the other language until age 2. After that, children are able to switch appropriately from one language to another in context and have a *combined* vocabulary that meets the usual expectations. Bilingualism is not a good explanation for language delay after age 3 and even before if we look at the receptive skills and the ability to do early word combinations. Bilingual exposure facilitates language development rather than hampering it over the long term. If delays are present after age 3 in a bilingually exposed child, an underlying cognitive deficit or ongoing conflict surrounding the child is being played out in the use of one language or another.[22]

■ *He's lazy.* Young children have an internal drive to mastery (see Chapter 2) that means that they exercise newly developing skills as these emerge. They don't hold back unless they are fearful, stressed, intimidated, or ill, needing their internal resources elsewhere. If developmental energy is lacking, it is because the energy is needed for other purposes. If a child is performing below age level, it's because that is the best that the child can do at that time. To say the child is lazy reveals a basic lack of understanding of the nature of child development.

■ *He'll grow out of it.* This is usually the case experientially. All but a few children learn to speak. However, as we have seen, these children with early or continuing delays are at risk in early childhood because of what the lack of language prevents them from doing, for emotional difficulties, for behavioral problems, and over the longer term, for subtle or not so subtle language and learning difficulties.[23]

All these viewpoints do not explain a significant language delay or justify significant delays in further evaluation or referral. Beware of such unfounded explanatory models. Further clinical work should be done to investigate the nature of the delay and its etiology. Observation of these delays demands an ongoing appraisal of all aspects of development.

CLINICAL LANGUAGE ASSESSMENT

Some peculiarities regarding the appraisal of language in the usual clinical settings provide a bit of a challenge, such as the following:

■ Most standard language assessments depend upon expressive language, which in turn is the most variable aspect of language. Gesture language and receptive language are much better indicators of long-term language development, but these areas should be specifically evaluated. This requires a careful history, or better, a chronology because as these competencies emerge over time, we get a broader picture of the whole process.

■ Language, particularly but not exclusively expressive language, is an "acute phase reactant" that stagnates or even regresses in the face of any stressor, such as illness, separations from primary care providers, and family changes. Because these are the times and circumstances during which we often see children, it is even more imperative that a good record be taken at the regular health supervision visits, when stressors are at a minimum. Otherwise it may be unclear whether a language delay is primary or secondary, short or longer term.

■ The office visit itself is a stressor, so productive language is difficult to assess because children often do not speak for the clinician. Indeed, in some cultures and subcultures the very idea of interacting verbally with an unfamiliar adult is very foreign.[24]

■ Recall of language milestones, even with sophisticated observers, is notoriously faulty, whereas almost all families remember the exact moment a child walked alone, a gross-motor milestone. *Current* language production is the only reliable history. If you miss asking the question, the history taken later becomes so unreliable that it is nearly useless unless language is egregiously delayed.

■ Parents are so skilled at interpreting the child's intent and providing so many gesture contexts and visual prompts that they and you may overestimate the child's isolated receptive language abilities. Although you want parents to be that way, it can be problematical in assessment. Further, atypical use of language may be thought of as indicating precocity.

> *Mrs. King reported to Dr. May, when asked about language development, that her son of 28 months not only said sentences, but that they were several words long. This was a surprise because he had said no words and was not pointing at the 12 and 15 month visits. He had been an irritable, somber baby whose general development had been a bit slow. Saying "ah" and screaming were the only sounds Dr. May heard in the office. When being given his shot by the nurse, the boy was heard to echo very clearly, "Now this won't hurt a bit" and, "Hold still." Further investigation suggested that he had no spontaneous speech or gesture language and that his social interaction and toy play were atypical. A diagnosis of autism was confirmed upon referral.*

To do a good job with ongoing language assessment of children in a primary care setting, the whole interaction has to be set up with this as a goal. It takes no more time, but it does take a commitment, a focus, and a framework to evaluate the child's linguistical skills. The office staff should listen to the child's utterances at the beginning of the visit, during weighing and measurement procedures, and in interaction with the parent(s). Instructions that are part of the routine should be first given *without visual supports,* adding a gesture if it is needed. Keep your hands in your pockets or at your sides and look at the child while giving instructions. Give one-step instructions (e.g., Take off your shoes) and then lengthen instructions based on expectations or until you get confusion (e.g., Take off your shirt and get up on the table).

Beware of the interfering parent in this interaction with the child because it may be telling you something. The parent may already know that the child can't understand your requests, and that in itself is a clue that you are asking for something beyond the child's linguistical abilities. Children may signal their difficulty by ignoring you, looking at you very intently, changing the task, trying to guess what you want, or leaving the scene. Interactions with toys in the room, in the waiting room, and in the course of the examination provide a language sample on which to build an appraisal, although these usually represent minimal competency. The best assessment is still the direct recording of what a child is saying at that time, done at each health supervision visit.

When To Worry

One should not only track normal development, but also have a system to make referrals at a particular time (see Table 14-2). Minimal expectations should be met or a referral made. One needs this backstop because it is all too easy to focus on motor development, to explain the lack of language in the clinical setting, or to say, "We'll check it next time."

The best assessment is the report of the parent on the child's current language function, including receptive and expressive language and, for the youngest children, gesture language (Table 14-3).[2] Parents' expressing a concern about speech or language will be justified about *three quarters of the time,* so ignoring such a complaint is foolhardy. A further assessment is almost always needed. This can be done quickly with the checklist provided in Table 14-2 or with the language component of several parent questionnaires that should be part of every health supervision visit. Table 14-1 gives an expanded checklist. If these indicate the possible presence of a language delay or atypical use of language, the primary care clinician or a specialist should take a more detailed look. The MacArthur Communicative Inventory Infant and Toddler forms[21] provide this detailed look at child language up to age 30 months. A few more questions on social development will help to address the possibility of a disorder that falls in the autistic spectrum (see Appendix). Also, Table 14-3 presents primary care records that identify the emergence of real language delay.

TABLE 14-3 ■ Case Study in Emergence of True Language Delay*

Medical Chart	Comments
2 mo: Small child, doing well.	The continuing small size of this child may have contributed to the delay in recognition of the language problem. Our expectations of development are lowered in a proportionally small child in general.
4 mo: Petite. Happy.	
6 mo: Sitting. Pulling up. Cooing. Jabbering. Things in the mouth.	Cooing should have been present at the 2 mo and surely by the 4 mo visit. Babbling at this age is what we're looking for.
8 mo: Petite. Not too verbal.	A key observation. Expect lots of "talking" at this age.
12 mo: Pulls to stand, cruises, crawls. Da, da. No words, no pointing. Petite.	These phonemes are coming in late, should be strung together and one word present. The absence of pointing is suggestive of real delay. Motor development is normal.
15 mo: Walking well, running. Jabbers. No words. Will get hearing test. Growth at bottom curve. Mom small. Note: Hearing test OK.	Worry is setting in. The first step is always a hearing test.
18 mo: Understands a lot. Her own language. No words. Affectionate. Play OK. Does bye-bye, pat-a-cake. No pointing. Mom not concerned; was late talker.	Receptive language is considered, but without an assessment, we can't be sure that this child is using spoken language alone with the support of gestures. No words by this time is abnormal. Autism is considered, hence the comments on play, affective development, and imitation. However, these imitative games mentioned are first-year level imitation. As usual, imitative play and language track together, and both are delayed in this child. Family history is important, but not enough to ignore the problem at this point.

*Notes on development extracted from a primary care record: Child with no health concerns and five entries for minor illnesses, one otitis media only, not included here.   *Continued*

TABLE 14-3 ■ Case Study in Emergence of True Language Delay*—cont'd	
Medical Chart	**Comments**
2 yrs: Six words, no more for 4 mos. Understands things in family. Neuro OK. Speech sounds OK. Lots of gibberish. Growth at 5th, same. Denver OK except lang. Family doesn't want to pursue. Divorce, stress, money. Recheck 3 mos.	This vocabulary is very low, and at this level we wouldn't expect to see word combinations. Two-word links are what we should see. No change at this time of rapid growth in language is a big red flag. Concerns about global developmental delay and neurological conditions are addressed through specific assessments, although it would be unusual to discover something now with this much contact and continuity. Social turmoil is pulling attention away and cutting down access to services. Return interval signals worry.
3 yrs: 17 words, Mom's list, animal noises, names of family, one verb. Repeat hearing. Mom ready for referral. Tears. Grandma involved.	The level of expressive language is beginning second year and is not "instrumental" at all. The family is now ready to address this after failing earlier return as suggested. Mom's list testifies to her "buy-in" at this point. Audiology can now detect more subtle hearing loss that would be important to identify but would not explain this level of delay.

*Notes on development extracted from a primary care record: Child with no health concerns and five entries for minor illnesses, one otitis media only, not included here.

Differential Diagnosis

The primary care clinician should screen for other conditions for which language delay could be a symptom, such as the following:

- Hearing loss
- Global developmental delay
- Psychosocial deprivation
- Chronic illness
- Acute stressors
- Autism spectrum of disorders
- Elective mutism

      Although these categories are not mutually exclusive (i.e., most autistic children are delayed, and most neglected children have slowed development), they do provide direction for further assessment and intervention. About half the children with language delays have delays in other areas.[25] Further, even if the final diagnosis is in the category of specific language disorder, the job isn't over.[26] Even with therapeutic and educational intervention, this group is at risk for difficulties in school, both cognitive and social. Specialized intervention that puts language in place before age 7 is imperative here. If a child has no language before puberty, it is unlikely that language will emerge thereafter. Behavioral problems may be prominent in this group, particularly when communication difficulties raise frustration levels.

SPEECH DIFFICULTIES

The clear articulation of the sounds of speech is distinct from the content and form of those utterances, which is language (Table 14-4). The ability to reproduce the sounds of one's native language has its own developmental course. A child in the first year of life can distinguish all of the sounds that exist in his language (losing the ability to hear those sounds that are not in the native tongue by 9 months of age). However, the child may not be able to say all the complex blends of sounds until school age. Intelligibility for the unfamiliar adult (i.e., the clinician) should increase with the child's age, being about 50% of the time for the 2-year-old, 75% for the 3-year-old, and 100% for the 4-year-old. By 2 years of age, beginning consonants should not be omitted ("oy" for "boy"). By 3½ years the ending consonants should always be present ("did" should not sound like "di"). The "th" sound will not be present until age 3; the "r" and "l" sounds will be mixed until age 5.

If speech in general sounds babyish or immature for the child's age although the form and complexity are at age level, an articulation problem is probable. However, language and **speech difficulties** often overlap.

Some general irregularities of speech require referral or further evaluation, such as the following:
- A decrease in the amount of speech
- Lack of change in speech for 3 to 6 months in a child younger than 5 years old
- Explosive or constantly loud speech
- Hoarseness

TABLE 14-4 ■ Speech Disorders

Type	Description
Deficits of resonance	Disorders are characterized by abnormal oronasal sound balance. Deficits most commonly appear as hypernasality (e.g., in cleft palate) or hyponasality (e.g., in adenoid hypertrophy).
Voice	Problems appear as deviation in the quality, pitch, or volume of sound production. Such impairments have either psychological or physiological bases. Thyroid disease and laryngeal polyps from overuse are some considerations.
Fluency	Disorders reflect disruption in the natural flow of connected speech. The most common type of fluency disorder is stuttering.
Articulation	Disorders include a large group of problems often encountered by the physician. They are characterized by imprecise production of speech sounds. Most articulation "problems" are common at certain ages and are, in fact, normal. However, their persistence often requires intervention.

From Levine M, Brooks R, Shonkoff JP: *A pediatric approach to learning disorders,* New York, 1980, John Wiley & Sons.

- Awkward, unusual cadence or lack of prosody (emotionality) in speech
- Child's being embarrassed by speech

Some speech irregularities should draw the clinician's attention to oral motor function and, perhaps, motor function overall. Poor articulation of frontal consonants, giving the speech a garbled or swallowed character, may give a clue to hypotonia or mild cerebral palsy, particularly if accompanied by drooling or difficulty swallowing. An overly nasal quality to speech may suggest palatine dysfunction, perhaps a submucosal cleft palate. Hearing loss must be considered with any speech concern.

There is reason to investigate speech if the child is ashamed of it, is teased about it, or if it is noticeably less mature than that of other children the child's age. Additionally, if the child regularly experiences frustration in trying to get the meaning across, a formal evaluation is needed. Referral should be made to a speech and language specialist who is experienced in working with young children.

DATA GATHERING
What To Observe

An office visit offers an important opportunity for evaluation of language development. Observing the following will help in such an evaluation:
- What does the child say in amount, clarity, prosody, and length?
- How much of what the child says do you understand?
- How much does the parent interact with and speak to the child? What kinds of things are said? Is the child expected to answer?
- What does the child understand? Give one-, two-, and three-step commands to see what the child can do.
- What verbal output accompanies play in the waiting or examining rooms?

What To Ask

The following are examples of questions to ask the parents. Box 14-2 gives more examples.
- What can the child say now? Words? Phrases? Sentences?
- What is the longest thing the child says?
- How many words does the child know?
- Can the child follow one- (two-, three-) step commands? (Be sure you leave out gestures and verbal supports)
- Does the child know his name? Siblings? Age?

Ask the following of the child, using picture books, simple toys, and a toy telephone to help:
- What's that? (pointing to a picture)
- Which one is the _____? (in a book)
- Give me the _____ (from among the objects).
- What's your name, etc.? Start a conversation.
- After age 3, ask a child to describe an experience, such as a birthday, an outing.
- Present one- to three-step commands as part of the physical exam.

BOX 14-2	SAMPLE QUESTIONS FOR PARENTAL REPORTING OF SEQUENTIAL ITEMS

When did your infant smile at you when you talked or stroked his face?

When did your infant produce long vowel sounds, such as "eeeee" or "aaaa"?

When did your baby first give you the "raspberry"?

When did your child first babble, such as "ba ba, ma ma"?

When did your child say "dada" or "mama," but inappropriately?

When did your child begin to use "dada" and "mama" appropriately?

When did your child say a word other than "dada" and "mama"?

When did your child first point at objects?

When did your child begin to follow simple commands, such as "Give me

_____" or "Bring me _____," accompanied by a gesture?

When was your child able to follow simple commands without an accompanying gesture?

When did your child begin to speak jargon—to run unintelligible words together in an attempt to make a sentence?

How many body parts can your child point to when named? Which ones?

When did your child start to put two words together?

When did your child use three pronouns?

Modified from Capute AJ, Accardo P: *Clin Pediatr* 17:847, 1978.

Assessment

Use Table 14-2 to look at a child's language. If that raises a warning flag, look at Table 14-1 to see if you should be really concerned at this time. If so, the following are options for the next step:

■ Use the Early Language Milestone (ELM)[27] or other instrument to look at the issue in more detail. The MacArthur CDI, the REEL, CLAMS, and other assessments are available for a more detailed look.

■ Evaluate general development, oral-motor function, and emotional responsiveness to look for comorbid conditions.

■ Ask for more details of family history and medical risk factors for hearing loss or developmental delay.

■ Order a hearing test. Any language delay requires this.

REFERRALS

If data indicate the need for further examination and possibly treatment, consider the following specialists:

■ A speech and language pathologist familiar with young children should be involved early for evaluation and treatment.

■ For concerns about general development, a developmental specialist, pediatric neurologist, or child psychologist should see and evaluate the child. The DDST (II) is a helpful screening tool in these cases and can be used in a primary care setting.

- Any suggestion of a hearing loss requires the consultation of an ear, nose, and throat (ENT) physician, as well as a skilled audiologist. It's *never too early* for hearing augmentation if recovery by other means is not likely.
- Early intervention services, special education, or a language enhancement program should be consulted, depending upon the specifics and the services available.
- Loss of language skills, severe language difficulties, or the presence of seizures requires an electroencephalogram (EEG) with consideration of Landau-Kleffner syndrome.

ANTICIPATORY GUIDANCE

Offer parents the following guidelines regarding their children's language:
- Parents can support language development by talking *with* their children, engaging them in dialogues, asking questions, and encouraging them to narrate experiences. The linkage of tactile and verbal games and the reading of body language cues in the first year begin this process.
- The playful use of language in the second year through rhymes and jingles fuels interest in words.
- Expanding the child's expressions and speaking clearly and simply with correct words and grammar are also important.
- When talking about a present object or event, beginning the description with "look" or another orienting word allows the child to focus attention. Important words should be repeated.
- Narration of parental activities and caretaking events provides a rich verbal environment.
- Encourage the use of words rather than actions to express feelings and wishes.

READING TOGETHER

The reading of stories and other quiet listening activities in the third year are helpful. All of these should be consciously modeled by the clinician in the interaction with the child. Reading together supports language with its own developmental course. Parents who may find it awkward to know what to say to their young children may be supported in their efforts at verbal exchange through the specific use of books together. Offer parents the following types of advice:
- Beginning in the first year, parents may point to objects and identify them.
- Parental pointing progresses to the child's pointing and naming things in the early second year of life.
- Picture explanation with brief descriptions of the immediate action grows into short story telling by 2 to 3 years of age.
- Children who are 3 and 4 years old will expand the action beyond the picture, can follow stories, and anticipate events through the medium of books.
- Children older than 7 years regularly enjoy stories without pictures.
- Jokes and riddles for the 5- and 6-year-olds are often based on words with double meanings or vagaries of language. Enjoyment of these by parents and kids reinforces this new plateau of language development.

■ Poetry and other interesting uses of language can be introduced at this time, if not earlier. The physician should have a stock of simple jokes and puns in mind to highlight this new skill in a clinical setting.

SUMMARY

The language of the third year of life is a landmark of change for the child and the family. The child can now share observations of events, recall past events to himself and others, and communicate original thoughts and feelings to others. For most children, this is a liberating and exciting event. For parents, this often marks the undeniable end of infancy. Their child becomes more of an individual and an active participant in family life. Much of the work of exposing the child to objects and events, talking to him without obvious response, and learning about him through body language and nonverbal response now pays off as the child speaks. The joy, amazement, and amusement of toddler speech are tainted by the loss of the totally receptive infant. This step requires developmental work for the whole family. Language acquisition marks another step in individuation for the child and a separation for the family. It may also represent the single most significant developmental process in that it may be unmatched in its complexity and in the fact that it makes the child particularly human.

REFERENCES

1. Thal D, Bates E: Language and communication in early childhood, *Pediatr Ann* 18:299, 1989
2. Glascoe F: Can clinical judgment detect children with speech-language problems? *Pediatrics* 87:317, 1991.
3. Brown R: *A First language: the early stages,* Cambridge, Mass, 1973, Harvard University Press.
4. Cazden CB: *Language in early childhood education,* Washington, DC, 1981, National Association for the Education of Young Children.
5. de Villiers PA, de Villiers JG: *Early language,* Cambridge, Mass, 1979, Harvard University Press.
6. Garvey C: *Children's talk,* Cambridge, Mass, 1984, Harvard University Press.
7. Coplan J: Evaluation of the child with delayed speech or language, *Pediatr Ann* 14:203, 1985.
8. Condon W, Sander L: Neonate movement is synchronized with adult speech: interactional participation and language acquisition, *Science* 183:99, 1974.
9. Ferguson C: Baby talk in six languages, *Anthropology* 66:114, 1964.
10. Thal D, Reilly J, editors: Origins of language disorders, special edition of *Devel Neuropsychol* 13: 1997.
11. Thal D et al: Continuity of language abilities: an exploratory study of late- and early-talking toddlers. In Thal D, Reilly J, editors: *Devel Neuropsychol* 13:233, 1997.
12. Snow CE: Mothers' speech to children learning language, *Child Dev* 43:549, 1972.
13. Mills DL, Coffey-Corina S, Neville H: Language comprehension and cerebral specialization from 13-20 months. In Thal D, Reilly J, editors: special edition of *Devel Neuropsychol* 13:397, 1997.
14. Anglin J: Vocabulary development: a morphological analysis, *Monogr Soc Res Child Dev* 58:238, 1993.
15. Chomsky N: Formal discussion. In Bellugi U, Brown R, editors: The acquisition of language, *Monogr Soc Res Child Dev* 29(92):35, 1964.
16. Pinker S: *The language instinct,* New York, 1994, Morrow & Co.
17. Bandura A, editor: *Psychological modeling,* Chicago, 1971, Atherton, Aldine.

18. Ringler NM: The development of language and how adults talk to children, *Infant Ment Health J* 2:71, 1981.
19. Elliot J: *Child language,* New York, 1981, Cambridge University Press.
20. Aram DM, Hall NE: Longitudinal follow-up of children with preschool communication disorders: treatment implications, *School Psychol Rev* 18:487, 1989.
21. Fenson L et al: Variability in early communicative development, *Monogr Soc Res Child Dev* 59:242, 1994.
22. Grosjean F: *Life with two languages,* Cambridge, Mass, 1982, Harvard University Press.
23. Levine M, Brooks R, Shonkoff JP: *A pediatric approach to learning disorders,* New York, 1980, John Wiley & Sons.
24. Super C, Harkness S: Why African children are so hard to test. In Adler LL, editor: *Cross cultural research at issue,* New York, 1978, Ethos.
25. Kolvin I, Fundudis T: Speech and language disorders of childhood. In Apley J, Ounsted C, editors: *One child,* London, 1982, William Heinemann Medical Books—Spastics International Medical Publications.
26. Richardson S: The child with delayed speech, *Contemp Pediatr* 16:55, 1992.
27. Coplan J et al: Validation of an early language milestone scale in a high-risk population, *Pediatrics* 70:677, 1982.

ACKNOWLEDGMENTS

Earlier versions of this chapter benefited from the contributions of Elizabeth Bates, PhD, and Heidi Feldman, MD, PhD. They and colleagues, Donna Thal, PhD, Judy Reilly, PhD, and Doris Trauner, MD, continue to provide insights into the development of language, from which the chapter draws heavily.

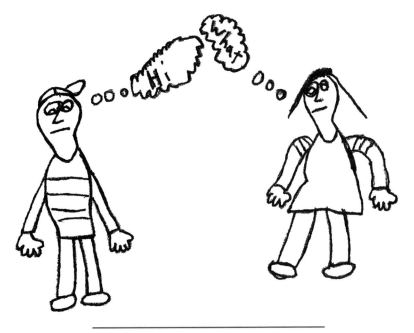

"Two kids talking." By Taylor Roberts, age 9.

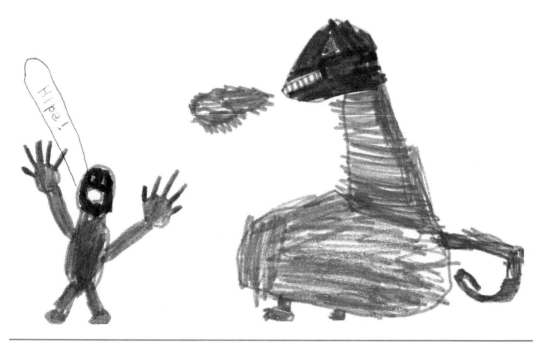

Neil, age 4½, shows his stress in the face of an imaginary dragon attack. His large hands and grounded feet suggest that he feels able to handle this terrifying situation. Aggressive themes are often in the drawings and play of 3- to 6-year-olds, and not uncommonly later.

THREE YEARS: EMERGENCE OF MAGIC

■ **Suzanne D. Dixon**

	KEY WORDS
	Imagination
	Fantasy
	Symbolic Function
	Imaginary Friends
	Lying
	Fears in Childhood
	Dreams and Nightmares
	Monster
	Night Terrors
	Stories, Fairy Tales
	Television

> *Mr. Jackson brings in his 3-year-old son because the boy does not tell the truth about drawing on the wall and spilling milk. He says Marc has an imaginary friend who is always sitting in his chair at home. Marc also seems to be afraid to take a walk after dinner with his dad, a thing he used to enjoy. Marc has nightmares at least twice per week, which he had never had before. His dad wonders if he is turning into a "wimp" and needs more discipline.*

Although the charm and fascination of a child's **imagination** are apparent to all caretakers, we rarely reflect on its developmental significance and function. The emergence of imagination is both a marker of cognitive growth and a tool of mental and emotional development. It is a vital probe into the inner life of a child, provided we have a framework on which to place a child's play, stories, fears, and actions. Imagination is in full flower at age 3, so it is the perfect time to evaluate what this aspect of the child can tell us about mental and emotional growth. The 3-year-old floats at a hazy border between reality and **fantasy.** If you let yourself be pulled into his world, you'll learn a lot and be ready to offer informed advice on many areas of preventive mental health. Selma Fraiberg's classic book, *The Magic Years,* should be required reading for all child health care providers in order for them to understand and appreciate this special part of young children.

SYMBOLIC FUNCTION: CORE OF BOTH LANGUAGE AND FANTASY

The young of all higher animals play—with actions, objects, and with others—but only human young engage in fantasy play. This uniquely human mental function, along with true language, relies on the child's ability to let one thing stand for something else. This is called **symbolic function.** An object can be treated as something else entirely, just as a sound or a group of sounds indicates an object, real or imagined. Although children do simple imitation, even delayed imitation, at a much earlier age, the late second to fifth years see the ready creation of unique play in scenarios, with roles, costumes, voices, and sequenced events. Play goes beyond simple linkages or imitations at this age; it now contains novel components and combinations. When real sentences are heard and language really takes off, we can be sure that increasingly complex pretend play will follow. Conversely, if all language is significantly delayed, the child's play will not reflect this ability to fantasize. These are linked mental functions.

Tools for Cognitive Growth

This new mental capacity, the ability to use fantasy, emerges in toddlerhood and is exercised frequently. That is why toddlers more readily fit into fantasy and pretend play. The child now uses mental actions to link and transform events, actions, sounds, and meanings. This is an active mental process that attests to a new level of ability to order experience and learn about the world. The ability to fantasize strengthens the ability to learn and in no way detracts from the skill of understanding "the real world." Quite the contrary, as stated by Fraiberg,[1] "A child's contact with the real world can be strengthened by periodic excursions into fantasy in a world where the deepest wishes can achieve imaginary gratification." (See Fig. 15-1.) The ability to use imagination and fantasy opens an entirely new world for a child. Previously this world was limited to direct experience; now the child can imagine possibilities, reasons, and sequences of events that go beyond the immediate.

 Jason looked at the pattern of the bathroom tiles and thought he saw a face. He wondered who was behind the wall. He refused to go to the bathroom by himself.

The child of this age can review, rework, and repetitively process the events of daily life through actions, language, and "mental movies." Events of the day may be overwhelming and incomprehensible. Through fantasy the child can recall them, process at his own rate, and set down memory.

 Brandon was heard talking to his stuffed animal in bed at night. "Now, just you stop this. I told you never to do it. Bad Barney. OK, you're all right now." Clearly he was reworking a little rough spot in his day.

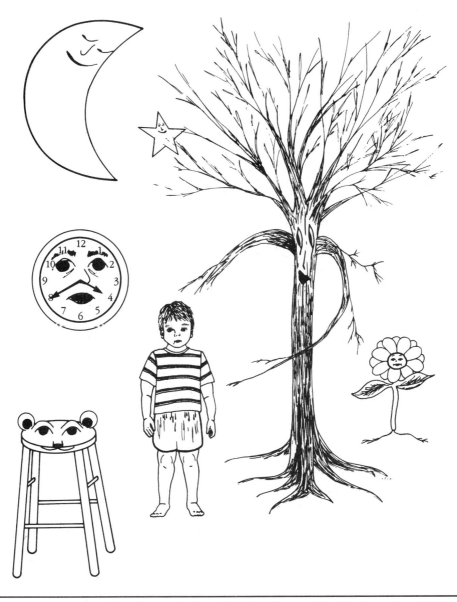

Fig. 15-1   The magical quality of a preschool-aged child is illustrated in this picture, in which inanimate objects are assigned human feelings and motives (animism).

In addition, the ability to fantasize enables the child to experiment mentally with new sensations, an enhancement or elaboration of cognitive structures. The child can try out activities and roles that may be beyond her capability in real life. With the help of playmates, these activities may be stretched even further, with new ideas, roles, plans, and actions.

 Justin and Kevin were playing firemen with pretend hoses, running around and putting out imagined fires. Kevin said, "Now the firemen go to space. There's a rocket fire." They then sat down and "blasted off."

Interactional play is now a regular event and results in more elaborate schemes than children usually come up with on their own. They often recall and experiment with rules, limits, or behavior. Fantasy can serve, as well as define, a new level of cognitive growth throughout the preschool years.

Tools for Emotional Growth

Fantasy also serves emotional growth in that it allows children to experiment with strong feelings, work through areas of tension, and assume aspects of identification of those around them. They can try out new roles for themselves in a safe, flexible way in imagined forms, such as roles of the opposite sex, of their parent, of a monster, or of an animal.[2]

 Every time Christopher talked to his doctor about visiting his newly remarried Dad on the weekend, he got into the posture of a dog and used his "growl voice."

Negative feelings can be expressed in ways that won't draw rejection or punishment, especially when those feelings are directed toward loved ones. Fantasy provides the ability to work through interactive difficulties with siblings, playmates, parents, and caregivers. These melodramas allow not just venting, but preservation of self-esteem and practice at resolution. The child has strength and power in fantasy life that cannot be achieved in real life. Aggressive themes may be evident in the play of the mildest mannered child. Costumes, puppet play, and doll play are forums and props for this developmental work.

Expressive language abilities lag behind the child's cognitive capacities (see Chapter 14), so these nonverbal forms of fantasy are particularly important for the child of 3. The child can both work through and communicate feelings, frustrations, anxieties, and wishes in safe ways.[3] Adults should pay close attention to play to understand what the child is about. Negotiation with words becomes more available after age 4.

Imaginary friends are very useful to young people. They are created by many children, but particularly by girls, firstborns, and only children. These magical creatures serve many functions, such as the missed presence of the parent, an idealized parent, a playmate, the willing slave of a toddler struggling with power and autonomy issues, or the victim in a power struggle. These friends can be the scapegoats for misdeeds, a comforter after discipline, or even a jolly companion for a long afternoon or a dark night. These valuable people come and go, depending upon the situation. Too careful a scrutiny of them or even too much attention to them by adults makes them disappear because they don't survive in the hard light of reality. They should be prized and respected as being the product of a creative, adaptive, and developing person. No evidence shows them to be harmful, indications of pathology or unmet needs, or cause for concern.

Tools for Social Growth

The emergence of fantasy allows a child to play with other children in new ways.[4] The assumption of imaginary roles, however brief and ever changing, allows longer and more elaborate play periods, as well as solitary and cooperative play with other children. One child can be caught up in another's imaginative structure, have fun, and learn from it.[5] Play with older children allows toddlers to function at a higher level.[6]

> *Sherrie, age 3, was playing house with her 5-year-old cousin. She was pouring the "tea" (water) into cups when her cousin told her to "be careful. Tea makes a big stain." Sherrie asked, "What's a stain?" "A big mark you can't get out even if your mom washes it." Sherrie was just settling in when her cousin announced that they now had to do the washing. Sherrie hadn't done that before. They turned over the step stool for a pretend basin. Sherrie is being pulled up by this interaction with her cousin into play that is much more complicated than what Sherrie would do on her own.*

Cooperative play means learning about give and take, negotiation skills, assertiveness, and demands for communication beyond the circle of family interpreters. Play with others, interactional play, should be the norm at this age, rather than parallel play, as was seen earlier. Increasing complexity and extended lengths of play should be evident from ages 2½ to 5 years. Ask at health encounters how long a child plays with other kids. The length of play should be longer each time you ask.

Parent interaction in play can increase the complexity and length of play episodes, provided the parent doesn't take over, push too hard, or ignore signs of disengagement (e.g., the child leaving, playing with something else). Parents, however, cannot provide an exciting enough play experience by themselves. Children in the third year need other children, such as relatives, neighbors, a play group, or a preschool group. Learning to get along with other children and to develop mutually regulated play interactions are the goals at this age rather than any structured learning. Parents should think of peer play at this age as a necessary enhancement for the child, not a substitute for their primary social experiences in the family. Introduction of a group experience is nearly mandatory at this age if it hasn't occurred before. Some children will need more time and support than others to embrace this expanded world. Mild stress with group play is inevitable and is a prompt for growth in social competency. Learning to get along, to initiate interaction, and to get your own position across to others is an important task at this age.

Lies, Thefts, and Other Misdemeanors

An active imagination is a healthy sign even if it generates "untruths." Children at this age do not *(indeed cannot)* intentionally lie or plan to deceive another. However, their reports of events, particularly under pressure, most often reflect how they perceive things to be, how they creatively process those impressions, how they wish things were, or how they think things should be to please. These perceptions are real even if the reported events are not. These stories are not formed out of moral lassitude.[7] They should be seen as "creative coping" with a situation that may be stressful for the child. Parents should reflect on the underlying issue rather than struggle with the content of the story. Untruths should not be supported, but it does no good to press a child to retract a story. Reflect on the obvious and give a specific action plan to correct it. The child will know that the story is not correct. Forcing an admission of **lying** will just cause the child stress and greater reliance on the safe fantasy.

Mrs. Curtis looked from the broken vase to her very guilty-looking 3½-year-old daughter. Mrs. Curtis said, "I'm very sad about this vase. You shouldn't be playing in here. Now let's clean it up. I hope you feel sorry for what happened."

Children also have very fluid concepts of property rights when it comes to things they want. They may "borrow" a sibling's toy or a playmate's tricycle if the object is attractive enough. They may then imagine that it is OK, that the owner said it was OK, or that they will give it right back. The guilt of a candy heist at the grocery store is easily covered over by fantasy. Clearly the rules of society and the rights of others must be taught to young children, so these behaviors shouldn't be ignored. Parents must give a message, in very concrete terms, about what is acceptable behavior and how to correct a wrong. Generalities, such as "behave" or "act nice" make no sense to a young child. Children this age cannot understand the event from the other child's perspective, nor can they understand the need for a broad social order (Box 15-1). They have a hard time generalizing from one situation to the next even if adults think the situations are similar. Direct confrontations don't usually work at this age.

Parental concerns or even events in the examining room are opportunities to give parents developmental perspective and to model age-appropriate responses to these "crimes."

FEARS IN CHILDHOOD

Every child, beginning in infancy, has fearful responses to some things, but at this age, fears are more complex. The child can imagine fearful things that *might* happen and can imagine other meanings to the things that have happened in the past or are occurring in the present. Current and future events can be feared not just for their immediate danger, but for what is

BOX 15-1	RESPONDING TO 'CRIMES' OF TODDLERS

Developmentally Appropriate

"I bet you wish that the crayon marks weren't on the wall. Let's clean it together."

"You and Jeremy must have had a fight. Tell him you are sorry for hitting, and let's go out to swing."

"Give Jason's truck back; it's his, not yours. Ask him before you play with it."

"My pack of gum is in your room. Put it back in my purse. Ask me if you want gum."

Developmentally Inappropriate

"That's Jason's truck. How would you feel if he took your things? Play nice."

"Did you take the gum in my purse? Tell me, did you? You can't just take things that belong to other people. How would it be if everyone did stuff like that?"

perceived as an anticipated or ongoing threat. The ability to fantasize can enlarge and modify these real or perceived dangers, as well as help the child to manage them better.

The **fears in childhood** have their own expected developmental course[8,9]; these are presented in Table 15-1.

Types of fears seem to be linked to cognitive development (i.e., bright children have precocious fears; delayed children have fears consistent with their mental age).[10] Although subject to both individual and circumstantial flavoring, the objects of fear are remarkably consistent across children. Some emerging fears appear regressed. For example, a fearless 5-year-old may become afraid of a monster in the closet after turning 6. No child can be protected from working through these fears. Children's fears, especially in early childhood, seem to cross cultural barriers,[11] although the intensity of the child's response and the *specific* circumstances that intensify fears vary from child to child and across groups.[10] The expression of fear is individual, ranging from fleeing or calling for help to shyness or irritability or even to increases in activity and aggression.

Elkind[12] suggests that as children are exposed to increasingly complex issues and adult developmental issues, we may anticipate that the situations and concerns that evoke fears may also grow in diversity and complexity. For example, fear of pollution, car accidents, or even interpersonal violence may be part of many children's lives (see Chapter 24).

Management of Fears

Fears cannot be avoided, and they shouldn't be because they serve to keep us safe, restrain our behavior, and help us draw what we need from the environment. Support for adaptive coping and protection from unreasonable fears are the goals here.

It's healthy for toddlers to be afraid of strangers, dogs, noisy environments, and separation from care providers. Stranger anxiety peaks from 8 to 18 months, and separation anxiety is expected. New adults should approach a toddler slowly after talking to the familiar adult and should be prepared to back off. Children should not be told to kiss every

TABLE 15-1 ■ Fears in Childhood

Age	Fears
0-7 mo	Change in stimulus level, loss of support; loud, sudden noises
8-18 mo	Separation, strangers, loud events, sudden movements toward, touching, physical restraints, large crowds, water, being bathed
2 yrs	Loud sounds, dark colors, large objects, large moving things, hats, mittens, changes in location of physical things, going down the drain or toilet, wind and rain, animals
2½ yrs	Movement, familiar objects moved, moving objects, unexpected events linked (e.g., Grandma in mom's hat)
3 yrs	Visual fears, masks, old people, people with scars, deformities, the dark, parents going out at night, animals, burglars
4 yrs	Auditory fears, the dark, wild animals, mother's departure, imaginary creatures, recalled past events, aggressive actions, threats
5 yrs	Decrease in fears; injury, falls, dogs
6 yrs	Fearful age; supernatural events, hidden people, being left or lost, small bodily injuries (e.g., splinters, small cuts), being left alone, death of loved ones, the elements, fire, thunder
7 yrs	Spaces (cellars), shadows, ideas suggested by television, movies, being late for school, missing answers in school
8-9 yrs	School failure, personal failure, ridicule by peers, disease, unanticipated events
10-11 yrs	Wild animals, high places, criminals, older kids, loss of possessions, parental anger, remote possibilities of catastrophe (e.g., earthquake), school failure, pollution
12-17 yrs	Physical changes in one's own body, isolation, sexual fears, loss of face, world events

Modified from Jersild AT, Holmes FB: *Child Dev Monogr* 20:358, 1935; and Ilg FL, Ames L, Baker SM: *Child behavior*, New York, 1981, Harper & Row.

stranger[1], pet every dog, or be scolded for crying with a stranger's approach. Repetitive leave-taking and return rituals help toddlers to cope with necessary separations.

Preschoolers' imaginary fears should be respected as sources of anxiety. Parents should acknowledge the fearful feeling without adding credence to the imaginary creature. Reassurance of support and safety and giving a child a sense of control of part of the situation will restore some equanimity. Drawings and pretend play with dolls or with others can be used to cope effectively. Attempting to argue kids out of fantasy is usually futile. Avoidance of overwhelming images or events will help keep the lid on fears. Giving children time to size up a situation before acting will also help.

School-age children need openings to expose their fears and worries and focused discussions on what might happen. At this age, information generally reduces fears, whereas it may overwhelm the preschooler. Unmentionable events become very fearful (see Chapter

24). Reassurance of the normalcy of fears is usually helpful. Good models also help to show children this age how to face fears. Parents can help by sharing some of their own worries and concerns and then talking through how they have coped or will cope. Kids like to rehearse mentally or talk through their plans about fearful things. Most days in a clinical practice offer opportunities to see children's fears and their coping styles (Box 15-2).

The interpersonal environment of children who chronically are excessively fearful should be examined to see if it lacks support for resolution of their fears or if it is too overwhelming for their ability to cope. Past events, separations, and abandonments leave the scars of chronic fearfulness that become generalized. Clinicians can model for parents ways of discovering their child's basic fears through a sensitive clinical interview. Then appropriate responses can be modeled commensurate with the child's developmental level. Children who are too shy to make age-appropriate relationships with others need a very careful look. Their linguistical skills, social awareness, or sense of security should be evaluated. *Extremely shy and fearful children are at high risk for emotional disorders and should be followed closely.*

A child's fears should never be dismissed as trivial. They offer clear testimony to a child's affective, cognitive, and social level. Fears are the other side of fantasy, and both are to be respected as sources of and testimony to mental growth. The fear is real even if the object of the fear is not.

DREAMS
Nightmares and Night Terrors: Things that Go Bump in the Night[13,14]

The emergence of symbolic function means that **dreams and nightmares**—nighttime fantasies—will also make their appearance. They are another piece of evidence of this new level of cognitive growth. In addition, they serve in the resolution of the dilemmas and tensions of daily life. They are a useful outlet for a young child, as well as for older kids and adults.

Nightmares and dreams are the product of rapid eye movement (REM) sleep, a mentally active part of the sleep cycle. Not every REM period has dreams; these are more likely to emerge in the early morning, particularly as the child grows. Children may waken from dreams and may or may not be able to tell you about content, depending on cognitive level and linguistical skills. They respond to comfort and reassurance. When the child remembers the dream or has specific nighttime fears (e.g., **monster** in the closet), a general reassurance is needed, not an exhaustive exploration of the room for a monster. This "buying in" of the parent just adds confusion (was that monster real?), anxiety (I guess there could be a monster in my closet), and inability to get help (my mom even has to get it out). Dream content is a jumble of things and events for mental sorting, so it is no wonder that they increase at the time of stress. Kids caught in a recurrent pattern of the same dream need help to look for the stressor, *not* exploration of the dream content itself. Firm, consistent bedtime rituals help all kids cope with nighttime fears and awakenings. Avoidance of overly intense images on television and videos will cut down on some nighttime fears.

Night terrors, on the other hand, are abrupt partial wakenings from deep sleep and are accompanied by dramatic physiological arousal with no wakefulness or responsiveness to comfort. Although very frightening to parents, they are not harmful and go away without

BOX 15-2 IMPENDING IV: MANAGING FEARFULNESS IN MEDICAL SITUATIONS

Situation

Marissa, age 18 months, needed an IV started because of croup. She clung to her mother throughout the whole assessment, really yelled as the nurse approached, and was whiny but consolable. On the table she struggled with the restraints and went into an hysterical pitch when her mom left to retrieve a purse left in the waiting room. Upon mom's return, she stopped screaming, but sobbed inconsolably. She barely flinched with the stick itself. In her room, in the tent, she slept. Her mom was in the bathroom on her awakening and she immediately screamed and grabbed her blanky.

Helps at this Age

Presence of mom, loved one
Avoiding eye contact with a stranger
Support of a lovey
Ability to protest
Maintenance of as much of a routine as possible

Situation

Jason, age 3½, saw the preparations for the IV. The nurse seemed to have pointed teeth like a lion, and her long fingernails were sharp. He thought he'd never get away if she pinched him. The IV looked like it could crush him, and the syringe looked the size of his dog at home. It might just go right through his arm into his heart—Clunk! Move your arm away!

He was really sorry he wrote on the walls this morning—this was a pretty bad punishment. He thought the nurse was really dumb to put the needle in one hand when that sore red part was on the other. He wished he had brought his Power Rangers—they'd get 'em. The nurse asked him what color cover he wanted on his IV.

Helps at this Age

Calm reassurance
Reassurance of lack of blame
Ability to use fantasy to cope
Limiting long explanations
Giving control where possible

Situation

Darryl, age 9, asked the nurse a million questions in the treatment room while they were getting set up: "How big is the needle? Will you die if a bubble gets in? Do you ever slip? How long will it take for the medicine to go in? Can the needle come out? What if you move?" He said he was sure he wouldn't cry. He wanted to hold still. In a small voice he said over and over, "don't cry, don't cry, hold still." His dad asked him if he wanted him to hold his hand. He said, "No thanks," and looked up at the ceiling.

Helps at this Age

Good, calm explanations
Questions answered concisely
Exact expectations laid out clearly
Giving of a time frame, a plan
Giving a little time for getting ready
Respect for apparent lack of need for support

intervention. Parents should keep kids safe while they thrash around but shouldn't expect either responsiveness or memory. These usually occur in the second sleep cycle (the 11 o'clock news phenomenon), increase at times of fatigue and stress, and run in families. Children appear flushed and wide eyed, but unresponsive to comfort. They will not remember the event later.

STORIES AND BOOKS

Stories, including **fairy tales,** are a delight to kids, but they are useful as well. They assist kids in working through their own fantasies, conflicts, and experimentation with roles. Bettelheim, in his classic work,[15] talks about the adaptive significance of fantasy stories. He encourages adults to read the stories right through without interpretation. He believes that kids should construct their own explanations of the book based on their own issues. A little less dogmatic approach would be to allow the child to discuss anything about a story with pauses, mild prompts for comment, and a brief response from the parent. This approach, along with urging the child to retell a familiar story, has been shown to be effective in improving reading and speaking skills in young children, even in the relatively short term.[16]

Book reading starts in the first year with familiarity, turning pages, and looking at and pointing to pictures and progresses as follows:

- Between age 1 and 2, children can talk about one picture at a time.
- At age 3 to 4, children learn how the pictures are connected in a story and then can tell the story with no book present.
- The ability to guess "what will happen next?" is really evident at age 5 to 6, about the same time that the child appreciates motivations in the book's characters.

Listening to how parents read to their child will not only tell you about the child, but also about the interaction between parents and child. Simple books in the exam room allow this observation to be made incidentally. Direct physician involvement with encouraging reading (e.g., Reach Out and Read—a program from Boston University School of Medicine) seems to be highly effective in getting it to happen at home. If children are read to at home, they will do better in school, have more complex vocabularies, and ask more complex questions.[17]

TELEVISION AND MOVIES

The average American watches 6 or more hours of **television** per day, and most children over age 2 watch at least 2 hours per day.[18] Because TV is such a pervasive part of children's lives, it is important to look at how and to what degree TV affects children.

The influence of TV on young children has been a matter of concern since the 1960s.[19,20] Although the research is ongoing, areas of ambiguity and problems related to issues of causality remain. These concerns include the form of television (i.e., how it delivers information), the content of the material, and what other parts of a child's life TV displaces. These concerns will be discussed in turn.

Television delivers *many different types of information,* some commercial, some pure fantasy, and some factual or documentary. A child under age 5 cannot distinguish between these categories and will remain confused about what's what on TV until at least age 7. As we have seen in this chapter, the preschooler lives with one foot in fantasyland at all times anyway, so TV is always "real" at that age. The preschooler cannot distinguish what is pretend and what is not. Further, the cognitive ability to know that one thing can stand for another (symbolic function) is just emerging and remains incompletely developed until age 7 or so. Children believe that all the characters act and feel as portrayed and that they somehow live in the TV setting between shows. They assume ongoing relationships and do not understand the concept of acting and rehearsing, even if all this is explained to them. By the time they are 3, children start to pick up story bits, particularly if emotionally tense. Bad dreams and daytime worries are the result at this age, even if there was no effect earlier. For all these developmental reasons, watching TV is a very different experience for a young child than for an older one or an adult.[17,18]

The mode of TV is to present material in short, fast-moving bits of imagery and talk to maintain attention. Children under 3 are fascinated by these images, but don't have the cognitive skills to understand them. Children need a lot more processing time to understand what's going on than do adults, and they do not benefit from close-ups, music, or lighting techniques to draw attention to salient features of the story; these techniques are confusing, and the story seems cut up. Flashbacks and multiple story threads make no sense to preschoolers. As in real life, kids need a lot of support to make transitions, and that is generally not available on most programs when transitions are made frequently and fast. Even kids in middle school will be challenged to follow the action in a fast-paced program. The *mode of TV* then means that kids miss a lot of what they see, often don't make connections, and are likely to focus on the most intense, not the most important, images and story components.

Because of these factors and the receptive nature of the media itself, watching TV *requires little mental work.* At a time when the central nervous system (CNS) is establishing important connections based upon active mental processing, time spent watching TV is time on idle, mentally.[21] It is also time taken away from more physical play, family and peer interaction, and other activities that are interactive. This is the displacement problem with TV. Further, the inactivity, combined with food advertising, sets up the link between TV, obesity, and physical inactivity.[22,23]

The *content of TV* is also of concern in three areas: stereotypes, values, and violence. Although much has been done in the past two decades to broaden the diversity in TV programming, stereotyped images still show women as dependent and less competent; the elderly as weak, foolish, and incompetent; and minorities as comic figures, similar to images from an earlier era.[24] Most families will find some of the situations, solutions, and relationships depicted on TV at odds with their own values. These will include sexual mores, attitudes towards drugs and alcohol, suggestive conversations and innuendos, attitude toward crime and law enforcement, etc. Without other models or alternative views on how to handle life problems, kids quickly pick up TV programs' solutions and assumptions. Consequences of actions are not depicted, and children are left to believe that certain actions have no negative outcomes. As discussed earlier, school-age kids handle fears and stress through adaptation of role models and through mentally practicing how they would handle various situations. TV images fall on fertile ground at this age for models and solutions.

The area most studied is the effect on children of exposure to *violence,* which more than 80% of TV programs contain. Although the subject has been studied much, the answers are not completely conclusive.[25,26] There is no question that children will show more aggressive behaviors after being shown aggressive acts on TV, and children who watch more TV are, as a group, more aggressive. Imitation of actions can be seen at age 14 months, so it's no surprise that older kids imitate what they see. This has been shown in multiple studies. Although many have commented that recent outbreaks of egregious violence perpetrated by youth are related to this near constant exposure to violence, science has not been able to prove a direct link as yet. At this time, most would agree that watching violent images is associated with acting more aggressively or, as stated in Cole and Cole[17] after a review of the literature, "The current consensus is that watching violence on television does in fact increase violent behavior in many viewers, whether or not they are otherwise 'predisposed' to it." (p. 451)

Is TV all bad? NO! Parental involvement can significantly improve the gain it can provide children.[24] And a lot of good shows are developed with the young child's needs and interests in mind, such as preacademic, social, and fantasy programs. Children are exposed to things, good and bad, that couldn't otherwise be available at home. Without TV, they would miss some of the "language of the culture." But it takes parental involvement, vigilance, interaction, and discussion to help children link what they see on TV with their lives, reflect, clarify, emphasize the main points, and place their own interpretations on the programs (Box 15-3). This means that the TV shouldn't be a baby-sitter, shouldn't be on during meals, and should be limited in time and in content.

Most of the discussion about TV also applies to videos and movies; although these aren't as pervasively present, parents are usually more involved in the choices, and the beginning of a rating system and published reviews are available to help concerned parents make choices. A word of caution, however—many videos labeled for kids, like TV cartoons, contain violence without consequences, pacing that exceeds children's ability to follow, and stereotypes.

BOX 15-3	PARENT MANAGEMENT OF TELEVISION AND VIDEOS

Spouses should discuss the TV plan for their child on the first birthday and review it on
   every birthday thereafter.
Never use TV as a reward.
Limit to 1-2 hours per day maximum.
Plan what to watch; don't "surf"!
Turn off TV when program ends.
No TV during meals.
Consider channel lockouts or V-chips.
Specifically suggest and set up another activity.
Discuss programs with kids, including advertising.
Check on the policy of the use of videos and spot check its practice in day care, preschool,
   or school.
Contact local networks and sponsors for accolades and complaints.
Watch **with** kids.

DATA GATHERING
What To Observe

The clinician should observe and make note of the following:
- The child's use of toys in the office: Suggest the use of puppets, small doll figures, blocks, small cars, blackboard. What does playing with toys reveal about the child's cognitive level?
- Ability to fill in empty times (e.g., time in the waiting room or during mother's interview) with imaginary events: Does the child approach and play with other kids?
- Interest in books
- General response to the office environment and any manifestations of fear, wariness. How does the child cope?
- Is the child wearing a costume, a special shirt, or carrying a toy that tells you about an interest in "pretend"?

What To Ask

The clinician should ask the following questions during the examination:
- How does the child use fantasy at home?
- What are the child's favorite toys? How are they used?
- Does the child have imaginary friends or enemies and an interest in costumes, role playing, or assignments?
- What types of books does the child like? How does he read them?
- Does the child discuss imaginary events, sequences, or creatures? What role do they serve?
- How much television does she watch? What programs? Are parents present?
- Does the child sing television jingles, talk about advertised products?
- Is the child assigning new functions to familiar objects (e.g., toothbrush becomes a spaceship, a banana is a gun)?
- Is the child having dreams or nightmares?
- What things make the child fearful?
- What is the parent's response to nightmares and fearful situations?
- Who does the child play with? What and how does she play?
- What about "untruths" and "unlawful borrowing"? How is it handled?

Assessment

The following factors should be assessed during the examination:
- Does the child move into puppet or doll play?
- Can the child accept and use your own fantasy suggestion (e.g., tongue blade becomes a car)?
- Will the child accept a nonsense word for a familiar object?
- What does the child do with some nondescript objects (e.g., several tongue blades, paper clips, paper cup)?
- Can the child do clay play with imagination?
- Is the child fearful? If so, how is fear handled?

Anticipatory Guidance

Following are some guidelines for clinicians to help guide parents of toddlers:

■ *Explain the importance of handling the TV monster.* Encourage limiting television to 2 hours per day *maximum.* Go through child-oriented programs *of value.* Parent's (or other adult's) viewing participation with children should be for at least half of the time child is watching TV. Reflection on show content should occur during and following the show. In other words, parents should make it a social and active event.

■ *Encourage play with toys that require at least two thirds of their use to be determined by the child* (e.g., blocks, balls, toy buildings, dolls, puppets, crayons and paper, and simple vehicles).

■ *Reflect to parents the usefulness of stories, imaginary friends, role playing, and "untruths."*

■ Reflect on the emergence of *dreams and nightmares* as markers of this new phase of cognitive and affective development. Welcome them as indicators of healthy mental development. Parents should respond to the child's reaction to the nightmare rather than to the content of it. Brief reassurance of the parent's protection should be central to this response. Parents should never dismiss or attempt to explain away this or other frightening experiences.

■ *Parents should read to the child every day.* Hand out books from the office and have a variety of books available.

■ Parents should *preview books* and perhaps develop good library habits or exchanges with friends beginning in the third year of life.

■ *Old clothes and simple costumes* are good props for this phase of development.

■ *Parents should never ignore a child's fears.* They tell of the child's inner life and developmental level. Listen patiently.

■ *Parents should not stress or elaborate on their own concern* about a situation that frightens the child. Assurance of parental protection and support is most important.

■ *Parents should never force the child to meet the object of fears.* The child should not be ridiculed or threatened for being afraid.

■ If a child appears *excessively fearful or nightmares are very frequent,* look at the child's daily experience for evidence of overstimulation and exposure to emotions or situations that are overwhelming.

REFERENCES

1. Fraiberg S: *The magic years,* New York, 1959, Scribner.
2. Winnicott D: *Playing and reality,* New York, 1971, Basic Books.
3. Murphy B: *The widening world of childhood,* New York, 1962, Basic Books.
4. Chance P: *Learning through play,* New Brunswick, NJ, 1979, Johnson & Johnson.
5. Bruner J: Children at play. In Lewin R, editor: *Child alive,* Garden City, NY, 1975, Anchor Press.
6. Goncu A: Development of inter-subjectivity in social pretend play, *Human Dev* 36:185, 1993.
7. Kohlberg L: Development of moral character and moral ideology. In Hoffman ML, Hoffman LW, editors: *Review of child development research,* vol 1, New York, 1974, Russell Sage Foundation.
8. Lewis M, Rosenblum M, editors: *The origins of fear,* New York, 1975, John Wiley & Sons.
9. Rutter M, editor: *Scientific foundation of developmental psychiatry,* Baltimore, 1981, University Park Press.

10. Mussen, PH, Conger JJ, Kagan J: *Essentials of child development and personality,* New York, 1980, Harper & Row.

11. Konner M: Aspects of the developmental ethology of foraging people. In Blurton-Jones N, editor: *Ethological studies of child behavior,* New York, 1972, University of Cambridge Press.

12. Elkind D: *The hurried child: growing up too fast too soon,* Reading, Mass, 1981, Addison-Wesley.

13. Ferber R, Kryger M: *Principles and practice of sleep in the child,* Philadelphia, 1995, WB Saunders.

14. Anders T, Eiben L: Pediatric sleep disorders: a review of the past 10 years, *J Am Acad Child Adolesc Psychiatry* 36(1):9, 1997.

15. Bettelheim B: *Uses of enchantment,* New York, 1976, Random House.

16. Whitehurst G et al: A picture book reading intervention in day care and home for children from low income families, *Dev Psychol* 30:679, 1994.

17. Cole M, Cole S: *The development of children,* ed 3, New York, 1996, WH Freeman and Co.

18. Comstock G, Paik H: *Television and the American child,* New York, 1991, Academic Press.

19. Lesser G: *Children and television,* New York, 1974, Random House.

20. Surgeon General's Scientific Advisory Committee on Television and Growing Up: *The impact of televised violence,* Washington, DC, 1972, US Government Printing Office.

21. Valkenburg PM, vanderVoort THA: Influence of TV on daydreaming and creative imagination: a review of the research, *Psych Bull* 116:316, 1994.

22. Taras HL et al: Television's influence on children's diet and physical activity, *J Dev Behav Pediatr* 10:176, 1989.

23. Taras HL et al: Children's television viewing habits and the family environment, *Am J Dis Child* 144:357, 1990.

24. Signorelli N: Television portrayals of women, and children's attitudes. In Berry GL, Asamen JK, editors: *Children and television,* Newbury Park, Calif, 1993, Sage.

25. Bryant J, Zillman D, editors: *Media effects: advances in theory and research,* Hillsdale, NJ, 1994, Lawrence Erlbaum.

26. Sege R, Dietz W: Television viewing and violence in children: the pediatrician as agent of change, *Pediatrics* 94:600, 1994.

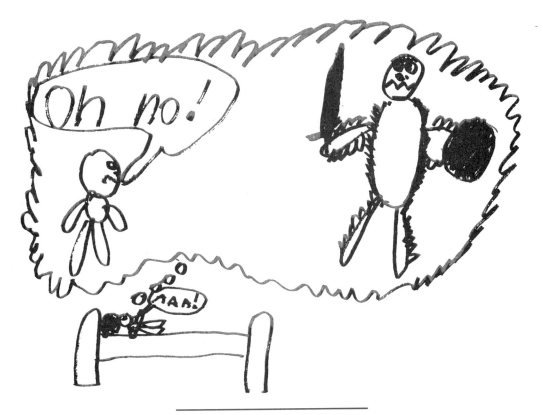

"A scary dream." By Ryan Hennessy.

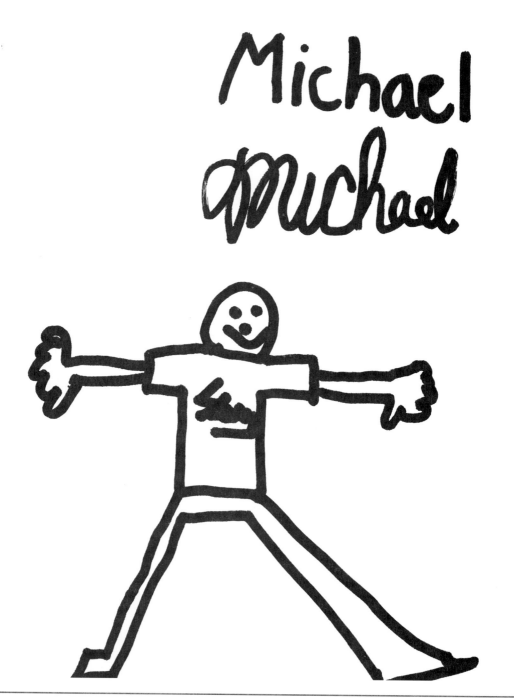

This boy demonstrates his positive self-image with his exuberant stance, large hands, and his care to make sure we know who he is and that he can even write his name in cursive. By Michael, age 6½.

CHAPTER 16

FOUR YEARS: CLEARER SENSE OF SELF

■ **Suzanne D. Dixon**

KEY WORDS

Self-Concept
Initiative and Guilt
Gender Identity
Gender Stability
Gender Role
Sexual Exploration
Ethnic Identity
Aggression
Moral Development

> Samuel's mom apologizes as you enter the exam room for a health supervision visit, saying that her son "looks like a mess" today but "he insisted on wearing these clothes." She also apologizes for her delay; the teacher had pulled her aside to say that she was worried that Samuel was being "too aggressive on the playground." Mom's concerned about that, as well as that his lying has become frequent. Samuel sits and looks out the window, his Power Ranger in hand, with a Batman T-shirt, a string of beads around his neck, and red fingernail polish. A baseball cap tops off his outfit.

The 4-year health supervision visit often brings into sharp focus the important process of the development of the self as an individual with definition beyond the immediate family. Exploration of the place, the roles, and the identity that one has is the proper work of this age. This is done through observing the modeling of significant others, trying out various persona in looks and actions, and experimenting with social roles in the family, the preschool, the neighborhood, and with peers. These are the child's laboratories in developing a real sense of self in many dimensions.

The child is beginning to be able to describe himself, whereas before he couldn't even understand the request "Tell me something about yourself." Now this query or a comment such as, "You look very strong to me," and the follow-up prompts result in a lot of rich information. Damon and Hart[1] have characterized how children from 4 years onward describe themselves along the physical, activity, social, and psychological dimensions. These

TABLE 16-1 ■ The Emergence of a Self-Concept: How Kids Describe Themselves in a Developmental Perspective

Level	Physical	Activity Based	Social	Psychological
Categorical identification (4-7 years) Basic descriptive features Concrete, often external	I have green eyes. I'm 5 years old.	I play soccer. I play on the computer.	I'm in Mrs. Smith's class. I'm Jake's friend.	I think about Power Rangers. I'm happy.
Comparative assessments (8-11 years) The line-up of self with peers Linear, often rigid and rule based	I'm stronger than most kids. I have the longest hair of anyone in my class.	I'm not very good at school. I'm good at math, but I'm not so good at reading. I'm the best kicker on the team.	I'm the second most popular girl in my class. I do well in school because I do more book reports than anyone.	I'm not as smart as most kids. I cry more than the other kids.
Interpersonal implications (12-15 years) Sense of self based upon relationships Personal characteristics as the basis and reasons for relationships Often lack of flexibility	I am soooo ugly; everyone makes fun of me. I have blonde hair, which is good because boys like blondes. No one sits near me because my pimples are so bad.	I play basketball, which is good because girls like athletes. I treat people well so I'll have friends when I need them. I like to join things so I can do things with people.	I can keep a secret, so people trust me. I'm very shy, so I don't have many friends. I can almost always get the rebound, so people pick me for their teams.	I understand people, so they come to me with their problems. I'm the kind of person who loves being with my friends. We can talk about anything.

Modified from Damon W, Hart D: *Self understanding in childhood and adolescence*, New York, 1988, Cambridge University Press. In Cole M, Cole S: *The development of children*, ed 3, 1996, New York, WH Freeman.

stage shifts testify to how the sense of self emerges over time, in the context of social interactions (Table 16-1). By asking a child to describe himself at health supervision visits through adolescence, first with concrete probes and later with more open-ended questions, we can monitor an increasingly refined **self-concept** along several dimensions. How a child sees himself along these dimensions helps us chronicle this stage-based emergence of a sense of self. A child should be able to define some aspect of himself that is positive and satisfying even if other dimensions are concerning for himself or others. Home, school, sports, and activities are the locations in which a child defines himself. We should ask about activities in these locations in order to tap into how a child sees himself.

The preschool child is faced with the task of gaining enhanced mastery over emotional, sexual, and aggressive impulses. He is learning not only who he is, but how he is expected to behave. More self-control, self-care, and self-regulation should be asked of him to support healthy development; the family must be ready to give more over to him at this age. If not, struggles, diminished self-esteem, and anger or sadness ensue.

This visit marks the time at which the clinician can really interact in an extended way with the child herself. The child in turn becomes an active and usually cooperative participant in the assessment process. She can converse about past and future events, ask and answer questions, and is often curious about herself. Data are easy to obtain; she'll usually reveal everything by word or action. This should be an efficient and quite entertaining encounter if you focus on what kind of person this child is becoming, how she defines herself, and how she gets along in the outside world. Interventions on behavioral regulation, sexual issues, and moral development as a foundation for discipline can be very effective at this age. These discussions can now be directed to the child, as well as to the family.

LANGUAGE AND MOTOR DEVELOPMENT: NEW SKILL LEVELS

Enhanced skills in the areas of language and motor development at this late preschool period give the child new ways to figure out who he is (Table 16-2). Language skills blossom during this period, which enable complex social interactions that go beyond the family. They also help the child get more specific information from all aspects of the environment. The child's vocabulary increases, and speech begins to contain all the elements of adult speech with regard to syntax and grammar. The "w" words—who, what, when, etc.—enable him to probe every event in detail. Conditional phrases, qualifiers, and subordinate clauses mean his narratives, arguments, and negotiations are much more complex. Although speech may be slightly imperfect in articulation (e.g., "r's" and "l's" may still be confused), the child is, for the most part, intelligible to strangers (e.g., the health care provider) virtually 100% of the time. He has a whole host of "facts" ready for recitation (Table 16-2). You should be able to have a real, although brief, conversation with a 4-year-old. The length, complexity, and content will vary by temperament and context. A child of 4 should be able to interface a bit with the outside world without the full interpretive skills of the parent.

Large-motor skills have now improved, so more elaborate play and outside activities are available to the 4-year-old (Box 16-1). Fine-motor skills have also matured, so work with pencils, scissors, and other tools produces more skilled craft creations. Competence in activities that demand greater accuracy or careful timing and sequencing, such as baseball, ballet, soccer, or football or a complex project with several steps, is still several years off, although

TABLE 16-2 ■ Language and Cognitive Skills in Preschoolers

Language Area	Ability Level
Vocabulary	Hundreds to thousands of words; parents can't even begin to count
Verbs	Uses suffixes and helper verbs (have, had) to indicate past, ongoing and future
Nouns	Uses plurals including some but not all irregulars ("mice" but also "feets")
Adjectives and adverbs	Lots
Intelligibility	100% to strangers
Articulation	A few errors ("r" and "l" confusion)
Prosody (emotional expressiveness)	Lots
Content	Asks questions using "w" words Uses clauses and phrases Understands conditionals; e.g., "If it rains tomorrow, we will. . ." Can give full name, gender and age of self and siblings, name of the teacher, and the name of at least one friend and can describe that friend Identify colors, maybe some letters and numbers. May write name or a few letters Can identify composition of object and function ("What's a car made of?"; "What does your heart do?") Can follow a story, anticipate events and ascribe feelings and motivation. ("What will happen next?" ; "How does he feel?") Copies a "+" Draws a person with two to five parts Sustained cooperative play

many sports activities are enjoyed and are to be encouraged. The components of these activities that are still to emerge are the following:

■ Understanding rule systems and applying them in context
■ Advanced motor planning (e.g., running and catching a ball on the run)
■ Sustained attention to the actions of others (e.g., anticipating the action on a playing field)
■ Memory skills (e.g., football plays; baseball instruction, "if this happens, do that")
■ Ability to conceive of the steps of a task leading to completion (e.g., basketball play setup)

    Although these activities may be introduced at this age, pressure to succeed at team sports should not be applied. These activities will look very different at this age than they will even 1 to 2 years later. Cooperative group games, excursions around town, and craft activities involving more than one step can be anticipated, learned, and enjoyed.

    Four-year-olds can assume more responsibility for washing and dressing themselves. They should pick their own clothes within the bounds of cleanliness, decency, and

| **BOX 16-1** | **MOTOR SKILLS IN PRESCHOOLERS** |

Walks up and down stairs, alternating feet
Skips on one foot
Can broad jump
Climbs up jungle gym
Throws overhand and catches a large ball
Stands on one foot for longer than 10 sec
Holds crayon well
Uses scissors
Can use a computer mouse
Uses table utensils well except knife
Pours reliably
Dresses self (mostly, most of the time)

specific outside rules (e.g., long pants for church). They should be able to do simple, regular household chores, although these should be one- to two-step (e.g., collect the wastebaskets and throw their contents in a bin) and very specific (e.g., "pick up the blocks," not "clean your room"). Practiced, prompted, and praised activities always take more time than the adult's doing the task, but these are ways to build a sense of responsibility on top of the child's new skills. This will build a sense of self that includes being a contributing member of a family.

SOCIAL AND EMOTIONAL DEVELOPMENT

Much of the developmental work of this period has to do with the acquisition of enhanced self-control over sexual, emotional, and aggressive impulses through identification with important adults and older children in the child's life. The internalization of norms and expectations for behavior is part of the development of the concept of self. Self-regulation is the working task here. The acceptance of the limits of behavior through identification with positive role models is the job.

Freud[2] emphasized the strong attachment that children, beginning at 3 to 5 years old, show for the parent of the opposite sex. This closeness is often associated with a certain amount of anxiety that motivates the child at about 6 years of age to redirect identification to the parent of the same sex. The successful negotiation of this "Oedipal phase" helps to instill the beliefs, morals, and behavioral manner of the parents, including the societally defined gender-specific behavior.

 Lisa told her mom she was going to marry daddy when she grew up. She then marched off in her mother's shoes.

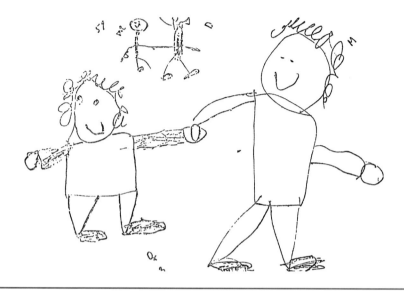

Between 4 and 6 years old a strong attachment often develops with a parent (or other important adult) of the opposite sex. In this drawing, a girl 5 years and 9 months old drew herself holding hands with her father (above), and drew her younger sister and mother in smaller images. Normal sibling rivalry was the focus of the family's attention.

Erik Erikson[3] emphasized the conflict between the feelings of **initiative and guilt** at this age. Taking the lead, standing up for oneself, and making needs clear is a big part of the work at this age.

> *Jared grabbed back the toy crane that Michael had just taken from him and said he had it first and wasn't finished. Then he asked Derek to play with him. They "did cars" in the corner.*

Learning to take social initiatives without ever feeling excessively guilty or imping-ing excessively on the rights and feelings of others is a sign of healthy emotional develop-ment during the preschool period. Conversely, the child who is always bullied, is taken ad-vantage of, or uses adults as mediators all the time needs some support to take more initiative in social interactions. All kids swing back and forth between the extremes, but the child who is overly shy or clingy all the time, or conversely, overly intrusive to others, needs help. The bully, one who only knows how to relate through aggression, domination, or dis-respect of others, also isn't on track with this developmental work. Children who have no friends at this age or who are always marginalized in the preschool or neighborhood are of concern. The other kids know whether a child is beyond the norms of aggression, guilt, or dependence on adults, even if they cannot report why that child is disliked. Other children are generally good barometers of appropriate social adjustment.

DEVELOPMENT OF GENDER CONCEPT

The part of self-concept that includes gender emerges in stages, beginning at birth but becoming prominent in the preschool period. One's *anatomical gender* obviously is determined at conception and during fetal life, and many components of sexual behavior, perceptual and cognitive structures, and aspects of emotional life are influenced by genetic and prenatal forces. When the gender of an infant becomes known, the interpersonal environment starts to add to that definition of self. Parents immediately begin a style of interaction that varies by gender in talking, in holding, in expectations, and in application of meanings to appearance and behavior. This *gender attribution* is difficult to change after it is ascribed in the first hours to days after birth.

 Doug Martin described his newborn son as "really strong." Eric Johnson told the doctor he was surprised how delicate his newborn daughter's hands were — "like my wife's."

Genital exploration begins in infancy, but a peak of interest occurs in the middle of the second year. By 2 years of age, a child knows that she is a girl and that genital touching is pleasurable. She has a **gender identity** that is nearly impossible to alter thereafter. Further, she is able to classify other people correctly by gender using hair or clothing. The continuity, immutability, and permanence of this attribute (**gender stability**), however, will take years to be clearly acquired, so it's not uncommon for a young preschooler to say that he will grow up to be a mommy or that the new baby girl will become a "big boy like me." The exploration of different identities with cross-gender dress-up, fantasy play, stories, and statements is the way children learn that gender is a stable part of one's self.[4] In preschool this is an appropriate, normal activity. Children under 3, and often older, define gender by external attitudes rather than by differences in genitals, although when asked, they reveal that they know that boys are, in the words of Mr. Rogers, "fancier on the outside," whereas girls are "fancier on the inside." Clothing, hair styles, and possessions may actually be more salient, hence the belief that gender may be as changeable as your costume.

The preschool years are ones in which a child acquires a sense of what expected, gender-specific behavior is. This is the beginning of the acquisition of the **gender role,** the external behavior that reflects the inner gender identity.[4] Play activities and toy preferences, language, body posture, and movement start to become differentiated subtly in the second year but become striking by age 4. Children are more rigid than adults in judging what is gender-appropriate play after age 5, no matter how liberal or how restrictive their environment has been, because they cling to rules and predictability to order their world. As they solidify an understanding of this aspect of themselves without the ability to blend categories of anything, they may go through almost hyper-male or hyper-female role playing. This stereotyped definition of gender role stays through grade school.

 When asked if the girls in his school played baseball, Samuel, age 6, replied that that was silly. "Girls don't play baseball; they do soccer."

Specific interest in the genitals of self, as well as of others, reaches another peak at this age, so **sexual exploration** is to be expected. Sexual interest then goes underground at about age 6 with the forces of socialization and with children's learning that sexualized interest or behavior, at least that done in public, draws disapproval. Children older than 6 who are still seductive or exhibitionistic, or do any sexual exploring publicly are atypical and require further investigation.

Interest in sexual issues bubbles just under the surface across grade school, however, as evidenced by the fascination with jokes, words, gestures, or stories that have to do with elimination or implied sexual function. These continue throughout grade school. Peeks at pornographic material, as well as renewed interest in sexual information, are common as middle school approaches. During adolescence, sexual interests are prominent as the child works toward an understanding of the sexual part of himself, his sexual orientation, and intimacy. (See Chapters 21-23.)

Boys' Play and Girls' Play

We can learn a lot from the play patterns of kids, so it's not lost time to ask about it at any age. From the preschool period on, play shows marked gender differences. Although scientists note these in the second and third year, and some studies even show infancy differences, it's really beyond age 3 that these play pattern differences are obvious. Boys play more physical games and hierarchical and one-upmanship games in which there is a winner and a loser; they are likely to play in larger groups. Their games usually involve a lot more action, even if played on a computer. Boys can be seen building the highest tower or the longest train. They like to say they run the fastest and gladly report successes in competitive play. They may be threatened if someone suggests an alternative activity.

Girls play in smaller groups and have games in which there is no winner or even an endpoint. They enjoy the process of play with a lot of inclusion in role playing. They are less overtly aggressive, although verbal aggression and some manipulation of people are regularly observed. Girls build enclosures; they change roles frequently so that everyone gets a turn at being the boss, the teacher, or the mom. They try to get lots of kids involved with their play and may make offers to get them to do so (e.g., "you can be the mom if we play house"). They like it when people have other ideas, but usually try to reshape the proposal, engaging in what is often a prolonged negotiation. Both sexes imitate household activities as they play house at age 3. The girls take over at age 4, and the boys run around with their own, more active games. Standoffs, space violations, and mutual raiding of play spaces continue to occur, however. After age 5, children with a clear sexual identity will choose same-sex playmates if they have a choice.

Sexualized Behavior

Young children often will engage in behavior that reflects their interest in these sexual matters; this should be expected. Parental responses should be in concert with a family's own values, but should include clear, nonhysterical feedback from which the child can learn the expected norms. Shaming a child, punishing without explanation, or refusing to discuss this area of behavior sets the stage for sexual problems later. Moral, social, and family rules may restrict specific behaviors; the clinician should be aware of what's abnormal for children at a given age, developmentally harmful, or indicative of inappropriate sexual experience or emotional deprivation. Box 16-2 lists some parameters to apply when confronted with questions about whether some sexualized behaviors are within the normal range.

Sexual behavior is likely to emerge and be obvious in the preschool period, whether it is flirtatious behavior with an adult or exploratory behavior with another child, so it's a good time to elicit parents' concerns and to encourage sex education at the level of the child's concerns. Areas of concern should be given developmental context.

BOX 16-2   SEXUAL BEHAVIOR IN CHILDHOOD—WHEN TO BE WORRIED

Masturbation begins in infancy and is nearly universal from toddlerhood on. There is no
   evidence that it is problematical unless one of the following is true:
   It is compulsive, taking a child away from other activities
   It is consistently done in public in spite of counsel to do otherwise
   It is done in groups
   It is done with objects
Exploring of other children's genitals, "playing doctor," is very common. This is worrisome
   if one of the following is true:
   It is forceful exposure or touching, not mutual
   The participants are more than 2 years apart in age
   Penetration is attempted
   Behavior is accompanied by aggressive themes or activities
Infrequent interest in pornography is common, but repeated, chronic interest is a concern
Simulated intercourse or penetration with objects is abnormal in childhood
Explicit sexual conversations with significantly older or younger children
Preoccupation with sexual themes in play or conversation
Sexual activities or exploration with animals
Violent sexual ideas, themes in play, or actions

"Sex education" begins in infancy with establishment of comfort with physical touching and emotional closeness. It becomes explicit in this preschool period when children begin to connect sex organs with reproduction and sensual pleasure, and it includes the development of the ability to set limits and not be forced to closeness on any level. Children should be given the freedom to ask questions about this area. Parents should provide accurate answers for the questions asked, following the child's lead. At this age, a full explanation of sexual intercourse is usually not needed or wanted. Parents who follow a child's lead usually provide the right level of information and set the stage for coming back for more when the child is ready.

> *Annie paraded around the living room in her mom's nighty while her dad read the paper. She said she was practicing her dancing.*

Sexual Exploration

Preschool children show a great deal of interest in the "private area" (roughly that part of the body covered by a bathing suit) of themselves and others. Games involving undressing or exploration of another child's body are common by age 4. "Toilet talk" becomes particularly interesting as the structure and function of these private areas are verbally explored. Sex play, sometimes played as "mother and father" or "doctor," is common in preschool children. Children of this age often attempt to engage in physical contact with other family members, such as touching their mother's breasts; both "exhibitionistic" and "voyeuristic" activities are common and normal. These behaviors should be seen in the positive sense that they testify to the child's work on the resolution of these important relationships. They do not predict continuance of these behaviors, but do demand explicit feedback about what the norms really are in the home and school.

> *Mrs. Allen found Jessica and her friend Kyle, both 4, under the blankets in Jessica's room. Jessica's panties were down and they both looked guilty. Jessica said they were playing house. Mrs. Allen explained that "clothes off is not good play." She redirected them to some play outside. A similar episode was never repeated.*

Such behavior in children can lead to conflict between parent and child and can also create strained relationships between parents with differing views on management. It is helpful for the pediatric clinician to be able to reassure parents that sexual play among preschool children is a natural consequence of growth in the child's cognitive, emotional, and social development. The parents' response will reflect their own views, but should incorporate this developmental framework. Parents can be told that children of this age are intensely interested in learning about themselves and their bodies and that this interest extends to other children and adults as well. In fact, this is the age at which children are most likely to notice differences between individuals, including differences in weight, race, and eye color, as well as sex organs. Again, observing and noting these differences helps the child obtain a clearer sense of herself as a unique individual with specific traits and characteristics.

At what point parents need to set limits on sexual exploration by preschool children is a matter for each family to decide, consistent with its own values and tolerance for such behavior. Parents may be told, however, that overreacting to sexual play in childhood may only temporarily suppress such behavior, actually heighten sexual curiosity, and create unnecessary anxiety in the child. On the other hand, parents who are overly permissive may expose their child to situations that are beyond his ability to handle. This, in turn, may be anxiety-provoking for the child. In general, parents should be helped to communicate to their children that an interest in the genital organs is healthy and natural, but that nudity and sex play are generally not acceptable in public, between children and adults, or when forced upon anyone. Parents should discuss the degree of nudity allowed in a family to ensure consistency. Parents also should tell children of this age that no other person (including friends and family) has permission to touch them on their "private area." Such conversations between parent and child should take place on numerous occasions before adolescence if the child is to incorporate such values as his own level of understanding matures.

ETHNIC IDENTITY

In the preschool years children become increasingly aware of the differences between people and the similarities and differences between themselves and others. With an interest in categorizing and labeling these observed differences, preschoolers come face to face with racial differences and **ethnic identity.** By the age of 4, children can sort dolls and pictures by ethnicity and, even at age 3, will be able to group people about half the time. Skin color is less salient than other features, such as dress, behavior, and speech. They then can label themselves on this dimension.[5,6] This is the age to discuss racial differences in appearance as these issues emerge, either by direct questions or through stares by children. Children exposed to a multiracial environment may notice ethnic differences earlier; those with less exposure may be less aware. But before school age, children clearly notice, label, and then begin to develop expectations based upon ethnic differences. If parents don't want those concepts guided entirely by outside (particularly media) forces, they have to take opportunities to discuss stereotypes, prejudice, and pejorative language directly. If racial issues are dismissed as not appropriate to talk about, children will develop their own ideas. These will be shaped by what they see and hear and will be in line with their cognitive imperatives to label, categorize, and make linkages. Children will not be kept "color-blind" by putting this issue underground.

AGGRESSIVE BEHAVIOR

Overly aggressive behavior may become a problem during preschool years because emotions, a sense of self, and identification with powerful figures are developmental themes. A child engages in problematical aggressive behavior when she shows a disregard for the feel-

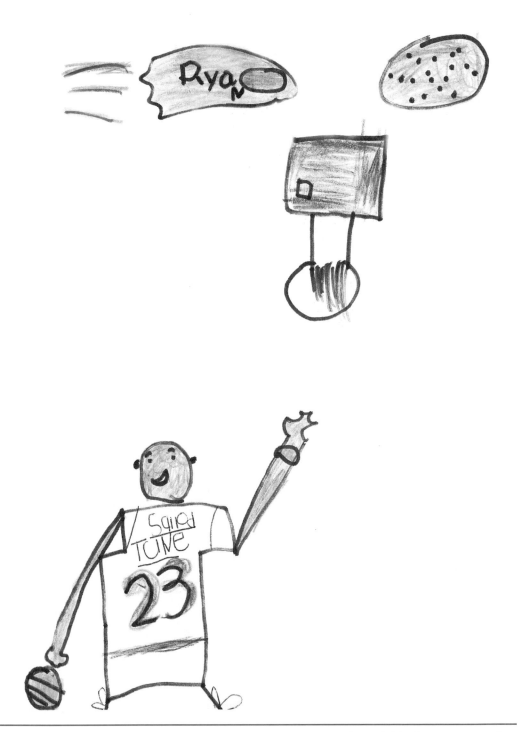

A black boy shows himself shooting baskets. The dark skin is unusual in a child's drawing, even when racial pride and ethnic identity are strong and positive.

ings, property, rights, or physical safety of other individuals. Aggressive behavior can be distinguished from assertive behavior, in which the child attempts to satisfy her own needs in a direct, energetic, perhaps even willful manner, while still respecting the basic rights of other children. In contemporary Western culture, we want our children to certainly be assertive (and a *little* aggressive), but not *really* aggressive.[7] The child must struggle to keep **aggression** under *her own control* while becoming appropriately assertive. The balance is hard to achieve and is probably a lifelong process; the struggle is prominent at this age. The expanded social world and enhanced interpersonal abilities bring this issue forward at this age.

Some theorists find that aggression is a biological instinct and believe that better child-rearing practices channel this aggressive instinct into socially acceptable behaviors.[8] Because our evolutionary past favors successful competition, we are prewired to be aggressive. Other theorists view the development of aggressive behavior as a response to frustration in the early life of a child and positive reinforcement for aggressive behavior that occurs in some families, and as a result of a child's following the model of powerful adults who exhibit aggressive behavior. The former theory of aggression as instinct is supported by the ubiquity of aggressive behavior in preschool children. Films taken of children in preschool settings indicate that all children engage in aggressive acts toward their peers many times each hour. Other evidence shows that girls will engage in frequent aggressive behaviors like boys do, provided they feel relatively assured of going undetected; girls may also be particularly verbally assaultive.[9]

These aggressive acts are rewarded in early childhood because most of the time the aggressor gets what he wants. On the other hand, theories that view aggression as a learned response are supported by studies that show that many problematically aggressive preschoolers come from homes in which the parent-child relationship is of a hostile, rejecting type or where interpersonal and environmental violence is often present. Such children may merely be imitating their parents' disciplinary behaviors or interpersonal style. A child's aggressive behaviors may be the only behaviors that draw parental attention, thereby imbedding them as a habit and style for the child. Television and movies model physical aggression as the way to solve problems, and aggressiveness may be increased by this exposure (see Chapter 15).

Developmental Course

The developmental course of aggression is that aggressive physical acts to get a desired object typically begin early in the second year. By the third year, these are surpassed in frequency by verbal aggression. *Hostile aggression,* an aggressive act designed to hurt another person without any object being involved, may become prominent in the fourth to sixth years and require support to resolve. Girls particularly exhibit *relational aggression* as they isolate, distance, or exclude another person. In preschool, children challenge many other children of different ages, sizes, and abilities. By grade school, they have learned to restrict the targets of aggressive challenges to kids with whom they have a chance of winning. These tussles are inevitable and provide an opportunity to learn about self, relationships, negotiation skills, and the limits of behavior. Unless conflicts are excessive, adults should stay out of the middle because children need to learn to self-regulate. Significant imbalance in this back and forth or an escalating pattern between peers or siblings may require some intervention, suggestions for alternatives, or exploration for the basis of the excessively combative interaction. Arguments and some fighting are inevitable, however.

Behavior that Calls for Closer Attention

Preschools in general understand these outbursts of aggression and usually help children learn to control themselves, use words to negotiate, and redirect their attention. If a preschool says that a child is overly aggressive to the point that staff members cannot handle her or don't see progress, this is a serious concern for the clinician to address. Being thrown out of preschool is highly suggestive of a serious behavioral problem that demands clinical attention.

To understand a particular child's aggressive behavior, the clinician can take an appropriate history from the parent. Following are things that trigger the need for an exploration of the chief complaint of aggressive behavior:
- The more serious the aggressive behavior is (i.e., bodily harm)
- The more frequently it occurs
- The more widespread the settings (home, school, and community)
- The more frequently that hostile aggression occurs rather than object competition aggression

Isolated instances of aggressive behavior, regardless of the degree of actual physical or property damage incurred, can be a part of a normative growth process. The child who appears chronically angry or anxious is more worrisome than a child whose aggressive act comes out of a positive, open approach to life in general. The angry child may not feel good about himself or his place in the family or society or trust that his needs will be met with consistency. Sad (depression) is very close to mad (anger) and bad (misbehavior) in early childhood. Chronic aggressors may be depressed or anxious youngsters. These issues call for further exploration, suggestions for support for a more positive self-image, or, occasionally, a referral to a mental health professional.

DISGUISED ANGER AND AGGRESSION

Following are examples of behaviors that are really disguised aggression:
- Fecal soiling in a child who has previously demonstrated normal bowel control
- Fecal smearing
- Intentional self-destructive, self-injurious behavior
- Intended destruction of objects
- Willful harm to animals

Jeremy came into the classroom while everyone else was outside. He opened several kids' lunches and stepped on their sandwiches.

Biting behavior beyond age 2½ calls for further exploration. It indicates a delay in language, lots of anger, or levels of frustration beyond the norm. These behaviors must usually be interpreted as angry, aggressive acts. The "accident prone" child may likewise be demonstrating aggressive behavior toward self. Girls who are labeled "sneaky" may be covertly aggressive, and this label should not be disregarded. Children labeled by other children as *bullies* usually need at least short-term intervention. Children's drawings with teeth, strong force lines, and lots of forceful coloring-in should be looked at carefully and cautiously to see if aggression is predominant in feeling and thought (see Chapter 26).

BEGINNINGS OF MORAL DEVELOPMENT

Through a gradual process of identification of parents, the foundation for **moral development** is laid down. The 4-year-old shows increasing reasoning ability and can apply this to some moral issues, but the child is still "flawed" in judgment because of thought processes. She can understand rules but still bends them to accommodate immediate circumstances, especially under pressure. The primary goal is to obtain approval and reward (and avoid negative outcomes), so behavior is still shaped by a close link between behavior and consequences. The 4-year-old can understand the idea of promises but can't always keep them herself when time or new circumstances intervene. The child can recognize the difference between truth and fantasy but doesn't always tell the whole and complete truth.

 Justin told his mom that he didn't break his brother's truck, in spite of clear physical evidence and the lack of another, plausible suspect. He said he was trying to fix it.

"Inaccurate talk" is a better term than "lies" at this age. Premeditated plans to deceive will be a possibility after age 6 to 7 years. At age 4, the child can recognize the rights of others ("It's Johnny's turn now."), but not always respect those rights because his own needs are paramount. Property rights often are a little vague, particularly if the property is attractive. The child may really believe that he's "just borrowing" a toy. He cannot cognitively take the part of the other "dispossessed child," so an appeal to retrospective empathy really has no meaning at this age.

Merrill said that her friend Kristin had said she could borrow her Barbie when it came home with Merrill from preschool. Kristin's mom called later, saying her daughter said Merrill stole it and that she was crying. Merrill and her mother drove over and returned it.

On the other hand, the 4-year-old demonstrates a good sense of justice ("That's not fair; Jason never gets to be first.") and can show unselfish sympathy and concern for others when directly confronted with some unfairness or sadness on the face of another.

Moral judgments must be confined to the immediate instance, so lessons should be structured with the specific (e.g., "Give Sarah's book back. She did not say you could borrow it," *not* "Don't take other people's stuff."). The 4-year-old wants to please, wants approval, and may even become a bit self-righteous in this newfound awareness of the rules that govern conduct. The child likes consistency, clear expectations, and instances where the same judgment is applied to everyone. Direct, specific feedback on both correct and incorrect choices, as well as the experience of consequences closely linked to actions, are the forces that begin to infuse a moral code at this age. The child's moral sense is still linked to the specific consequences of her actions rather than any abstract moral code. She is building that sense over time through specific interactions and reactions.

DATA GATHERING
What To Observe

- What is the child wearing? Does this reflect some aspect of who he is trying to become and who he wants to be?
- In the waiting room, what does he do, play with, and say? The office staff can really help.
- What is his relationship with his mom or dad? Has it seemed to change since the last health supervision visit? What are signs of growing independence?
- Does he initiate an interaction with you? Does he carry on a conversation?
- Does his manner or appearance reflect a specific gender identity?
- What toys or activities does he bring with him? What do those tell you about his sense of self?
- What kind of picture does he draw? What does it reveal about him? How does he hold the crayon?
- Does he separate from the parent easily, such as for weighing or another nonstressful event?
- Can he dress and undress himself? Does the parent intervene, expecting a problem?
- Can he follow a three-step command and get up on the exam table without difficulty?
- Is there appropriate shyness about the examination of the genitals or even undressing?

What To Ask

Following are examples of questions to ask the child:
- How are you? Why did you come today? Comment upon appearance, clothing, or possessions that are evident.
- Do you have anything you want checked? Is there anything you want to ask me?
- How are things in school/daycare/home, good or not so good?
- What is your favorite thing to do there? What is bad that you have to do?
- Tell me your friend's name? What do you do together? What do you play?

These questions and conversation should be continued as you explore how this child sees herself in her world and who is important in her world. You are also listening for language, in line with the skills outlined in Table 16-2. Specific questions are seen in Table 16-3. You should be able to understand all of the child's speech. Parents should

TABLE 16-3 ■ Questions To Be Asked During Examination

Questions for Children	Objective
Does a dog live at your house? Is it a boy or girl dog? How can you tell?	Assess the child's awareness of sexual differences; if the clinical situation suggests any confusion in the child's own gender identity, clinician may follow up with questions such as, How can you tell if you are a boy/girl? What do you like about being a boy/girl? Is there anything you don't like about being a boy/girl?
What do you do when you want something and mommy/daddy says you can't have it?	Assess the child's perception of his own responses to parental limit setting: does the child admit to throwing tantrums that he later regrets (a good sign)? Does the child relate a number of different levels of responding to frustration (e.g., "sometimes I cry, but sometimes I just go to my room and play.").
How do you like your preschool/daycare center, etc.? (by name if possible)	Assess the child's reaction to and success in separation from family members.

Questions for Parents	Objective
What kinds of play activities does your child enjoy?	Parental reports can provide much information about the child's actual motor skills (e.g., can she ride a three-wheeler?) and social skills.
What does the child's pre-school teacher (babysitter, grandparent, etc.) say about him/her?	Obtain additional information about the child's personality and behavior while separated from parents, and at the same time assess parents' openness to feedback about their child from outside the home; some parents find difficulty in accepting any negative feedback about their child, while other parents seem surprised at favorable reports from outsiders about a child with whom they are experiencing difficulty.
What do you like most about your child? What would you say is his/her most trouble-some quality?	Determine the parents' capacity to identify and articulate the child's positive and negative qualities; inability to report some highly positive quality is unusual for parents and should be a sign for further evaluation by the clinician.
How often does he/she misbehave? What kinds of things does he/she do? What do you usually do when this happens?	Assessment of discipline practices at this age is absolutely essential; the clinician should be alert to the presence of inappropriately high or low behavioral expectations during this period; disciplinary techniques may be inconsistently applied, too harsh, or otherwise ineffective.
Do you take him/her out to dinner at a friend's house or a restaurant?	Assesses the parents' comfort with their efforts to help the child meet social expectations outside the home; regardless of the parents' standard of behavior, parents should have a degree of confidence in their child's behavior by age 4 or 5.

Continued

TABLE 16-3 ■ Questions To Be Asked During Examination—cont'd

Questions for Parents	Objective
How does he/she act when he/she is angry? What does he/she usually do when another child grabs something away from him/her?	Allows the parents to discuss concerns regarding the child's aggressive behavior or lack of aggressive behavior.
How does he/she show you that he/she knows he/she is a boy/girl?	Allows the parent to discuss the child's gender identity formation and their own degree of comfort with it.
Has your child expressed an interest in his/her body by asking questions, or examining him/herself or other people?	Allows the parent to discuss evidence of sexual curiosity in the child, while defining this as a normative process.
Does your child behave differently around his/her father/mother than he does around you? In what way are his/her relationships different with each of his/her parents?	Provides opportunity for the parents to discuss the Oedipal phenomenon at its various stages, while allowing the clinician to assess and comment on the age appropriateness of this behavior.

allow and enjoy this conversation; excessive intrusion at this age means something is of concern.

Parental issues also should be elicited. Some exploration of these should be done with the child present, but all sensitive or negative concerns should be discussed without the child. The child can be asked to draw with the supervision of office staff, or a return appointment can be set up. Any sign of serious shame or embarrassment calls for a change in the venue of the discussion. Children should not be shamed or embarrassed, although their own views of difficulties should be elicited.

Dr. Gann said to Mark, "Your mom tells me you've had to stay in from the playground many times. Tell me how that happens. What starts those problems?"

Ask parents for several details about the child's life, such as the following:
- Child's favorite type of play
- Child's favorite toys
- Child's preferred playmates

These all give clues to the child's sense of himself.

- Ask how the child contributes to the household with chores, duties.
- Ask about how much self-care she does.

ANTICIPATORY GUIDANCE

The following guidelines can help the clinician guide parents of 4-year-olds:

- Assess the appropriateness of the child's preschool setting. Does she need more or less structure, more or less self-control? What are her relationships with the other children? Does she have friends and engage in cooperative, sustained play?
- Discuss the normalcy of sexual exploration at this level. Elicit questions and concerns.
- Discuss with the family appropriate limit setting, management, and the importance of consistency in family expectations.
- Discuss toys and play vis à vis a broad range of interests but with expectations of sex-specific activities. Stress the importance of role playing.
- Explain the importance of reviewing television and movies that children watch and of limiting exposure to violent and/or sexual themes and sex stereotyping.
- Explain the importance of peer play and help a family orchestrate playmates if this does not occur naturally. A child this age should bring kids home (or participate in parent-initiated get-togethers), or the parents should find out why the child does not.
- Explain the basis for outbursts against the same-sex parent and "over" attachment to the opposite sex parent. Physical closeness should continue with parents' being alert to the need to limit overly sexualized behaviors.
- Children should have regular responsibilities around the house.
- Self-care should be nearly complete, although checks and prompts on cleanliness, as well as finishing touches, will still be needed.
- Discuss stories with social or moral themes. Begin to build a sense of systems, rules, and norms.
- Discuss sex education for the preschooler. This usually includes providing names for all genital parts and explaining that touching of genitals should be done only in private and that breasts are for feeding babies. Parents should answer the child's questions but not overload her with too much information at one time.
- Children need to be counseled about their own private parts, that they are for no one to touch except parents and health care providers. Children should be empowered to resist all touches that feel bad. Parents should give them permission to discuss these. All reports of bad touches should be taken seriously.
- Caution parents about the differences between "inaccurate talk" and "lies" and the difficulty with respecting the property rights of others at this age.
- Overly aggressive behavior should be discouraged but *not* answered with aggression because that gives a mixed message and has been shown *not* to be successful. Encourage parents to model appropriate problem solving.
- Differences between people (because of individual, ethnic, or disabled characteristics) should be discussed openly, neutrally, and positively. Children's curiosity about these issues should be respected.

■ Discuss the importance of family rituals and traditions in giving children a sense of self.
■ Children enjoy going through baby books and seeing old pictures of themselves as they struggle with a sense of self. Going over a baby book and displaying baby pictures are good ideas. Telling the birth story or a special anecdote helps define one's point.

ACKNOWLEDGMENT

This chapter benefits from the earlier contributions of Nicholas Putnam, M.D.

REFERENCES

1. Damon W, Hart D: *Self understanding in childhood and adolescence,* New York, 1988, Cambridge University Press.
2. Freud S: *New introductory lectures on psychoanalysis,* New York, 1965, WW Norton.
3. Erikson E: *Childhood and society,* ed 2, New York, 1963, WW Norton.
4. Dixon S: Gender identity: early orientation to atypical behavior. In Rudolph A, Hoffman J, Rudolph C, editors: *Rudolph's pediatrics,* ed 20, Stamford, Conn, 1996, Appleton and Lange.
5. Bigler R, Liben L: A cognitive-development approach to racial stereotyping and reconstructive memory in Euro-American children, *Child Dev* 64:1507, 1993.
6. Hirschfield LA: Do children have a theory about race? *Cognition* 54:209-252, 1995.
7. Pomerantz E et al: Meeting goals and confronting conflict, *Child Dev* 66:723-728, 1995.
8. Lorenz K: *On aggression,* New York, 1963, Harcourt.
9. Crick N, Grotpeter N: Relational aggression, gender and social psychological adjustment, *Child Dev* 66:710, 1995.

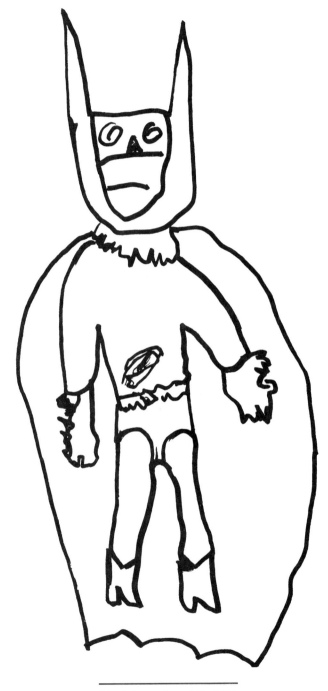

"A picture of me." By T.W.

ALE+PS

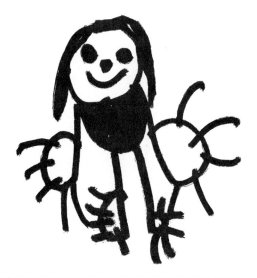

A girl 3 years and 10 months old shows her advanced school readiness skills in language, social, and motor areas. This drawing would receive a mental age of 5 years, 6 months. Advanced artistic skills may reflect advanced cognitive skills generally or may be the beginning of a special talent in artistic endeavors.

FIVE YEARS: ENTERING SCHOOL

■ Philip R. Nader

KEY WORDS
Entering School
Readiness
Individual Variation
Kindergarten Entry
Type of School

FOCUS OF DEVELOPMENTAL WORK

It has been suggested that as play is the work of the preschooler, school is the work of the child. Contemplating a child's **entering school** holds realistic promises and realistic perils for both the child and the family. To many parents, the transition to school represents evidence of effective child rearing up to this time. How that transition is negotiated and when and what the child and family experience and learn in the early school years often has long-lasting effects on several areas of psychological well-being. These include future achievement or lack of achievement, personal sense of worth, ability to contribute to others, and satisfaction with life. Box 17-1 lists the developmental tasks facing the child at school entry. Rutter[1] points out the profound and enduring influence of the school environment on the child. Getting off to a good start is of critical importance.

THEORETICAL FRAMEWORK

A variety of theoretical models of development have relevance for the pediatrician approaching the evaluation of school **readiness.** Conceptual models of Freud, Erikson, Piaget and Inhelder, and Gesell and Ilg[2-5] (see Chapter 2) illustrate many of the critical developmental tasks on which interaction of the individual with the environment is about to unfold. The conceptual framework of cognitive social learning theory[6] is also of value in understanding the reciprocal interactions that shape an individual's sense of competence (see Chapter 2).

This comprehensive theory of learning is useful to those involved with the education and socialization of young children. Bandura[6] points out the important influences of modeled and observed behavior on learning. The formulation also stresses the importance that mastery of a given task gives to the child's developing sense of competence as an individual. Bandura's theory takes into account the mutual influences of the individual, the physical and

367

BOX 17-1	DEVELOPMENTAL TASKS FACING CHILDREN AT SCHOOL ENTRY

Separation
Increasing individualization
Integration of cognitive skills required to learn to read
Ability to form relationships with other children and adults
Ability to participate in group activities and follow rules and directions
Gradual formation of a sense of self or identity, both inside and outside the family environment

psychosocial environment, and the task or behavior to be learned. All of these factors are important in learning.

The skilled and experienced pediatrician approaches evaluation of the child's school readiness with a healthy caution because **individual variation** in "normal" behavior and cognitive function at this age is great. *Readiness at a given age does not necessarily imply either accelerated or retarded development.* The purpose of a readiness evaluation should not be placed in the context of prediction of disease or dysfunction, but in the context of attempting to optimize the chances of a successful early school experience. The limitation of existing tools for assessment and the potential power of a medical pronouncement support the need for proceeding with caution in the evaluation of school readiness.

The time before school entry is an opportunity for the pediatrician to systematically review a 5-year data base that should be available to critically assess the potential fit or lack of fit between child, family, and school factors. It is unlikely that moderate to severe developmental problems, disabilities, or illnesses will have gone undetected up to this time. Naturally the pediatrician will already have been involved in the care plans and management of schooling or special education interventions for children with such difficulties. The Individuals with Disabilities Act mandates an equal educational opportunity for the disabled from birth through the twenty-second birthday.[7]

It is the more subtle developmental and behavioral variations that present problems for detection of potential inimical influences on schooling. Two children may be very similar in their temperamental characteristics, social behavior, ability to attend, ability to screen out distractions, visual-motor abilities, and language development. Yet how they do in school may be quite different, depending on parental views and expectations and the style and expectations that the school environment places on them. Therefore determining the attitudes, values, and expectations of the parents first is important. It is also wise to ascertain those that seem to be prevalent in the community as expressed in the educational philosophy of the school.[1] For example, parents may describe an "active, inquisitive, independent, and creative" 5-year-old who is later described by a teacher as "restless, stubborn, resistant, and rebellious." Parental desires and expectations for performance should be determined, and comparison of these hopes with the child's school experiences can sometimes be helpful in forming more realistic expectations of the child. Problems result when underexpectations and overexpectations are placed on the child's school performance.[8]

BOX 17-2	CRITICAL AREAS DESERVING SPECIAL ATTENTION

Presence or absence of potential biological insults to the nervous system
Indicators of language dysfunction
Indicators of problems in attention and impulsivity
Successful socialization or separation experience from the parent or parents

Despite the wide variation in the term "normal," several critical areas within the child deserve special attention at this time. These developmental requisites provide some touchstones in the evaluation process (Box 17-2).

BIOLOGICAL FACTORS

We know that prematurity, maternal illness, poor nutrition, and adverse perinatal events can potentially affect brain maturation and subsequent developmental outcome. We are becoming increasingly aware of the more subtle effects of these factors on learning abilities and specific areas of cognitive function, such as memory and attention.[9] These arise from a number of intrauterine, perinatal, and early life experiences. It is increasingly recognized that early biological factors, such as low birth weight, are further influenced by potentially modifiable environmental influences, such as poverty, maternal education, and home environment.[10] Minor surgical procedures, hospitalizations, self-limited illnesses, and other medical or biological events were previously thought to have little bearing on issues of education and future learning. Now it appears that such events may have a significant influence on *specific* cognitive abilities, emotional factors, or motor competencies.[11] The impact of recurrent ear infections on subtle hearing deficits (either transient or permanent) with subsequent impact on cognitive function is receiving greater recognition. Recurrent otitis media seems to have its greatest effect on early language development among children living in homes with the least amount of language stimulation.[12]

LANGUAGE

The presence of a delay in language development has been shown to be the best single predictor of later learning problems. Particular attention should be given to a child who has a history of early language delay, even if the current language competency falls within the expected range. We should also be alert to how the child's language develops. Were there problems in fluency, comprehension, and the naming of objects? Expected language milestones are shown in Table 17-1 and discussed in greater detail in Chapter 14. These language developmental milestones may also reflect other cognitive functional areas that are important to the tasks of new learning that will be expected in school. It is now recognized that in children with dyslexia (a difficulty in reading associated with normal intelligence, motivation, and education) the neurobiological defect is in a specific component of language develop-

TABLE 17-1 ■ Selected Language Guideposts

Skill	Age 2 yr	Age 3 yr	Age 4 yr	Age 5 yr
Comprehension	Follows simple commands; identifies body parts; points to common objects	Understands spatial relationships (in, on, under); knows functions of common objects	Follows two-part commands; understands concepts of same and different	Recalls parts of a story; understands number concepts (3, 4, 5, 6); follows three-part commands
Expression	Labels common objects; uses two- or three-word sentences; uses minimal jargon	Uses three- to four-word sentences; uses regular plurals; uses pronouns (I, me, you); can count three objects; can tell age, sex, and full name	Speaks four- to five-word sentences; can tell story; uses past tense; names one color; can count four objects	Speaks sentences of five words; uses future tense; names four colors; can count ten or more objects
Speech	Intelligible to strangers 25% of the time	Intelligible to strangers 75% of the time	Normal dysfluency (stuttering)	Dysfluencies resolved

ment. These children, who constitute up to 10% of a school population, have a deficit in their ability to break down the smallest segment of speech in a word. This deficit in phonological awareness can be detected during a pediatric evaluation.[13]

Most developmental tests overemphasize verbal skills in estimating intellectual competency. However, when performance in school is considered, these verbal skills and the cognitive function that underlie them may be of central importance. Bilingual or non–English-speaking families present special difficulties in assessment of children's language development. The pediatrician should be wary of ascribing learning and language problems entirely to bilingualism.[14] It is often noted that true language delay is present in both English and the natal language. By school age, confusion in the use of the two languages should be gone and the child should not have language dysfunction because of bilingualism.

ATTENTION PROBLEMS

At or before the age of 3 to 4 years a cluster of behaviors that has been associated with a high risk of school learning problems is identifiable; these behaviors are a high degree of activity, lack of ability to sustain attention, and impulsive behavior with little ability to delay gratification. The progressive improvement in a child's ability to focus and to differentiate between what is important to a task and what is not is often a key factor in how well the child can master early learning skills in the standard school environment (see Chapter 18). The child who can sustain attention only when information is given in a certain mode or when all distractions are eliminated will have difficulty when faced with the complexities of the usual classroom.[15]

SOCIALIZATION AND SEPARATION

It is increasingly rare for a child not to have had some experiences outside the home or away from parents before entering school. The pediatrician can obtain direct (from preschool teacher) and indirect (from parent) information on how the child functions in separating from a parent and on how the child gets along with new adults and other children in a preschool environment. For some kindergarten children, riding a bus to school is a new experience that may challenge social skills and modify the response to separation. Nursery school teachers' written observations, when blindly rated on such characteristics as peer relationships, teacher-pupil relationships, independence, participation in group activities, leadership characteristics, task orientation, attention span and persistence, self-confidence, and immaturity, were found to be relatively good predictors of school achievement and behavior in later elementary school (grades 2 to 6), as reported by Chamberlin and Nader.[16]

Parental and child factors appear as the child faces school entry. Not only is the child required to successfully negotiate a partial separation from the parents, but the parents themselves must be able to separate from the child. A child with a shy or timid temperament may be challenged when separated from a parent at the start of school. The best predictor of a successful separation and entry into school is a previous successful experience. Parental views on their child's vulnerability (see Chapter 3) and the pattern of child rearing up to this time will have an impact on this process. As in other areas of medicine, a focused history will help the clinician identify problems on which to work and strengths to reinforce.

> *Stephanie had a difficult time separating from either parent when she started preschool at 3½ years old. After 3 weeks of refusal to separate and prolonged crying when either parent left her at preschool, she was withdrawn from the class and cared for at home by her grandmother. At 4½ years old, she had the same experience. Stephanie was described by her parents as shy and fearful of new experiences.*
>
> *Recognizing that difficulty with separation experiences might affect kindergarten entry, Stephanie's pediatrician counseled her mother about the benefit of arranging multiple brief separations—with other child care persons, while playing at the park, and at a friend's home—and said that an early visit to the school, before the start date, might make Stephanie more comfortable with the new teacher and classroom. The pediatrician also suggested a children's book about starting school that might allay Stephanie's fears.*

DATA GATHERING

The assessment before **kindergarten entry** should include a complete update and review of the child's medical history and the family's medical and social history. Previous day-care or preschool experience should be reviewed. Rocky past experiences may suggest additional considerations. Data should also be obtained on preschool resources, expectations, requirements, and educational programs and philosophy. The examination and formal assessment procedure should include a general physical examination with a growth assessment if one has not been recently completed. It should include a neurological screening and recent evidence of visual and auditory acuity. Finally, some paper-and-pencil tasks or assessment tools should be administered. At this age the child should be reasonably comfortable with the examination as long as the parent is present, should be able to answer simple, concrete questions, and should comply with requests. The child should be an active part of the assessment process.

What To Observe

The clinician should observe the child carefully during the examination and during even brief separations from her parents to make assessments regarding development. Table 17-2 outlines factors to be evaluated.

What To Ask

Table 17-3 presents questions that should be asked during the examination. Questions can be directed to the child and the parent as the clinician engages both during the encounter.

TABLE 17-2 ■ Observations To Be Included in Examination

Observation	Assessment
Is the child quiet and reserved, outgoing, verbal, inquisitive, at ease, or frightened? Does the child initiate questions or comments?	Child's social interaction during interview and examination. How does the child handle interactions with adults, parents, and non–family members?
Is the child active, passive, slow to warm?	Child's temperament and behavior in examination situation
Can child be completely understood? Is language appropriate for age? Are sentences clear, compound, and complex? Is articulation clear? Does the child modulate speech well?	Child's language and verbal skills. Can use items from Denver Developmental Screening test, Early Language Milestone Scale (see Appendix and Table 17-1)
Does child show excessive dependence or independence? Observe separation effect(s) if occasion arises. What does the parent allow the child to do?	Parent-child interactions
Can child follow 1- to 3-step instructions and assist with examination by holding still, looking at a specific point, cooperating on the neurological examination? Is child easily distracted by environmental stimuli?	Ability to attend and cooperate
Does child show evidence of ability to solve hypothetical problems, ask questions, draw interesting pictures?	Curiosity, creativity, problem-solving ability

Examination and Assessment

Obtaining a careful history and observing and talking with the child will give the physician a good data base; next the clinician should examine the child. Drawing, paper and pencil tasks, and games of developmental assessment can often be done first unless a pressing reason exists to perform selected portions of the physical examination immediately.

Pediatricians will find it valuable to build into their repertoire a battery of tasks they believe they can administer in a reproducible, standardized way. The Denver II developmental screening test (see appendix), Draw-a-Person (see Chapter 26), Pediatric Examination of Educational Readiness (PEER), drawing of geometrical figures, and other tests can be used. Office personnel can administer some or all of these tests, and the physician can review the data. Children at risk for learning disabilities can and should be identified at school entry. Box 17-3 has specific questions about letter identification, verbal memory, and letter-sound associations.

Table 17-4 shows age-appropriate abilities. Familiarity with these behaviors, drawn from the most popular tests for young children, will assist the pediatrician in the assessment process.

TABLE 17-3 ■ Questions To Be Asked During Examination*

Question	Objective
Tell me about _____. What words would you use to describe _____?	Determine parents' views of child; what characteristics they mention first; it is better to have parents describe behavior rather than make judgments about it ("he gets along well with other children").
What happens when _____ is with friends or playmates? Who in the family is ___ like? How do you expect _____ to do in school? Why?	Follow-up of this line of questioning can open up areas of parental concern, expectations, and their own experiences with the education system.
To the child: Do you have any friends? What do you do with your friends? How are you the same/different than your friends? Who in the family are you like? Your mother, father, or who? How do you expect to do in school? Why?	
Tell me what you know about the school where _____ will be starting.	Should bring out real or imagined view of today's school; whether or not there has been a visit to the school or discussion of the school with neighbors may indicate degree of parental investment or interest.
Describe how he uses crayons, pencils, scissors.	One child may laboriously use scissors to cut out a doll, whereas another will be engaged in a task, use the scissors, lay them down, and proceed with the next task.
What does he like to do? Dislike? To the child: What do you like to do?	This may help in determining leisure time use, amount of television viewing, interest in reading or being read to
If _____ does _____, what do you do?	Helping parent to focus on behavior will give information on discipline methods, parental ability to cope, guide, direct, and support child.

*Some questions are for both child and parent. They can be used when clinician is interviewing them together or separately.

Observation of how the child approaches various tasks, including those to facilitate the physical examination, can be revealing:

■ Can the child follow auditory directions with no visual clues? (e.g., "Take off your shoes, get up on the exam table, and sit back.")
■ Can these be one-, two-, or three-step directions?

BOX 17-3	TESTS USEFUL IN IDENTIFYING CHILDREN AT RISK FOR DYSLEXIA

Letter identification (naming letters of the alphabet)
Letter-sound association (e.g., identifying words that begin with the same letter from a list: doll, dog, boat)
Phonological awareness (e.g., identifying the word that would remain if a particular sound was removed: if the /k/ sound was taken away from "cat")
Verbal memory (e.g., recalling a sentence or story that was just told)
Rapid naming (rapidly naming a continuous series of familiar objects, digits, letters, or colors)
Expressive vocabulary or word retrieval (e.g., naming single pictured objects)

From Shaywitz SE: *N Engl J Med* 338:307, 1998.

TABLE 17-4 ■ Appropriate Abilities at Preschool and Kindergarten Entry Ages

Years	Abilities
3	Picks longer of two lines Can point to chin and teeth on request Cuts with scissors Makes 3-cube pyramid in about 15 seconds Copies a circle Jumps with both feet together
4	Goes upstairs and downstairs one foot per step Copies cross (+) Washes hands Can tell "how many" when shown two circles Completes "A hat goes on your head, shoes on your . . ." Can button
5	Dresses self (except tying shoelaces) Copies square Can count six objects Can answer: "Why do we have houses, books, clocks, eyes, ears?" Can tell: "What is a chair made of? A dress?" Knows (or can be taught): address, phone number, where mother and father work Finger counting (how it is done, pointing to or not) and finger identification Digit span—should be able to repeat four digits forward
6	Tells how a crayon and a pencil are the same and different Can tell differences between common objects: dog and bird, milk and water Can complete "A lemon is sour, sugar is . . ." Can tell what a forest is made of

From Hoekelman R, Blatman S, Brunell PA: *Principles of pediatrics,* New York, 1978, McGraw-Hill Book.

- How attentive to the task is the child? (e.g., can the child complete a drawing?)
- How facile is the child with pencil tasks? (e.g., holding a pencil with a mature grasp; steady lines that are connected; clear hand dominance)
- Is the task easy or slow and pressured? (e.g., What does the child's face look like while doing the tasks?)

The value of performing a so-called amplified neurological examination to detect soft neurological signs is not necessary for an individual patient during a routine school entry evaluation. For the child in whom problems with attention or learning are suspected from historical data, a brief neuromaturational assessment is helpful. An evaluation for digit span (recall of four numbers at 5 years old), memory of serial commands (at least four directions), and right-left discrimination may reveal problems with attention, listening skills, impulsivity, and organization. The testing of various higher central nervous system (CNS) functions in sensory, coordination, motor, and spatial areas is better assessed from observation of behavior. More static, permanent CNS dysfunctions should be assessed with enough of a standard neurological examination to ensure the absence of mild neurological deficits (e.g., mild cerebral palsy and the clumsy child).[17]

Many pediatricians find it valuable to ask the 5-year-old: "Draw a picture of your family doing something." Neuromaturational skills (e.g., visual-motor integration and fine-motor coordination) and psychosocial characteristics of the child and family will be revealed in these drawings (see Chapter 26).

No child should enter school without the benefit of formal vision and hearing acuity tests. Many schools have such screening programs in place for entrants. Updating routine immunizations and other health screening tests (e.g., tuberculosis and lead tests in high-risk communities) are now requirements in the United States for a child to enter and remain in school. A screening urinalysis is recommended only once during childhood, usually at the 5-year-old examination.[18]

STANDARDIZED EVALUATIONS FOR SCHOOL READINESS

Because of increasing pressure on schools to ensure academic success of their students, some schools have instituted testing to determine so-called readiness for formal schooling. Such tests are often unstandardized and untested with regard to reliability and predictive validity.[19] The decision to enter school is always based on legal age of entitlement. No child should be deprived of this right, although the learning environment should be adapted to individual needs. A distinction must be made between tests of academic readiness, which evaluate the child's ability to perform basic learning skills, and developmental screening tests, which attempt to evaluate a child's level of gross-motor, fine-motor, language, and personal-social development in comparison with the performance of age-mates. What one has learned at home does not ensure the ability to profit from a specific educational environment. Conversely, lack of academic skills does not predict school failure.

Most pediatricians are familiar with the items from the Denver II (formerly Denver Developmental Screening Test) and with the task of copying geometrical figures, which en-

TABLE 17-5 ■ Neuromotor Accomplishments

Age (yr)	Gross Motor Skills	Fine Motor Skills
2	Runs well Kicks ball Goes upstairs and downstairs (one step at a time)	Builds tower of six cubes Imitates vertical crayon stroke Turns book pages singly
3	Goes upstairs (alternating feet) Jumps from bottom step Pedals tricycle Stands on one foot momentarily	Copies circle Copies cross (+)
4	Hops on one foot Goes downstairs (alternating feet) Stands on one foot (5 sec) Throws ball overhand	Copies square Draws person with two to four parts Uses scissors
5	Stands on one foot (10 sec) May be able to skip	Copies triangle Draws person with body Prints some letters

From Levine MD et al: *Developmental and behavioral pediatrics*, Philadelphia, 1992, WB Saunders, p 40.

compasses the ability to copy a circle (3 years), a cross (4 years), a square (5 years), a triangle (6 years), and a diamond (7 years). The forms should be presented to the child to copy, and the clinician should not routinely demonstrate drawing the form. Table 17-5 presents a summary of expected neuromotor accomplishments. Special attention to these tasks should be given with children who were born prematurely or those who had a difficult perinatal course (see Chapter 6).

The PEER is a combined neurodevelopmental, behavioral, and health assessment designed primarily for children 4 to 6 years of age. It requires a substantial amount of time plus familiarization with test administration before it can be used. Thus it could not be considered a frontline, quick-screening instrument. However, it may be a useful tool for the clinician to use with a child if questions arise about the child's abilities in one or more areas. It can be ordered from Educator's Publishing Service, Inc., 31 Smith Street, Cambridge, MA 02138-1089.

ANTICIPATORY GUIDANCE

The greatest danger in assessment of school readiness is a tendency to overinterpret findings. The pediatrician should avoid dogmatical pronouncements of prognosis. Strive to describe the child in the most accurate way possible. The child's particular strengths should be brought into focus so that the parents and the school may build on them. Clearly identify areas of concern. For most, it will not be possible to predict the outcomes. Concentrated efforts at support can evolve, and occasionally remediation will be indicated. Examples of summaries follow:

> *Johnny, age 5 years, is an only child. He has no serious health or medical problems; he displays the behavior, skills, and knowledge of most 5- to 6-year-old children. His ability to handle paper and pencil tasks is more like that of a 4-year-old. The parents, college graduates, describe him as fun loving, able to concentrate on things, and having several good friends. He had a good preschool experience and preferred large-motor activities, sandbox, cars, and trucks to drawing and puzzles. The physician's knowledge of the school's kindergarten program is that attempts are made to take children at the speed they can work, and formal prereading skills are introduced after the first month of school.*
>
> *Jennifer, age 5 years, is the third of five children and the only girl. She has a history of recurrent ear infections, but her hearing at this time has been tested as normal. She is slightly overweight for height. She tends to be shy, apprehensive in new situations, and quiet in large groups. However, her neurological examination and developmental assessments show her to perform at or above age level. She learns most readily with visually presented materials. Her parents describe her as "serious." She has two close friends. Jefferson School's small class size should be ideally suited to bring out the skills of this lovely girl and to encourage gross-motor activities.*

The pediatricians in these situations can be optimistic and encourage the parents to be regularly involved in visits at open houses and to listen to the child's descriptions of the school experience. Ongoing monitoring of each child's progress and fit with the school is indicated.

Parents may ask the pediatrician for advice on what **type of school**—public, private, parochial, or specialized—to select if they have a choice. The pediatrician will ask the parents for a little more information before venturing a suggestion:

- Are the parents concerned about ethnic or minority mixing?
- Are they under any misconceptions regarding the quality of education that can be obtained?
- What are the traditions and social expectations of the family?
- What was the parents' experience with the schooling they received?
- What is the profile of the children in a given school?
- Will this child fit in, be able to make friends, and succeed?

In general, quality education is available in most schools and is often highly dependent on the teacher. Recent research[20] indicates that continued positive effects of preschool and Head Start experiences, especially for low-income children, are dependent on the quality of the subsequent school experience. Therefore a parental visit to a prospective school should be advised. This is desirable even if no choice is anticipated because all children do better if parents are visible and involved from the start.[21] A classroom environment that is able to adapt to the needs of a wide variety of development levels would be the most ideal. Public schools, for the most part, have access to a greater range of specialized services for children with special needs than do private or parochial schools. In some public school systems, a cluster of schools focuses on a specific area of interest (e.g., science, math, drama, music, history) that may be more suitable to a particular child. Parents can also be encouraged to inquire about classroom size, which may vary within schools and between school districts. Smaller class size may enhance learning among children with learning disabilities, inattention, or behavioral problems.

Frequently parents may ask if the pediatrician thinks their child should be kept out of school, kept at home for another year. Parents who perceive their child as excessively shy and slow to warm up in new situations, clingy, or less advanced than others in motor or language skills may raise this issue. A child should almost never be kept out of school. Socialization, learning, and school readiness activities are often exactly what is needed and should not be delayed. Preliminary data now suggest that old-for-grade students (even those who have not been retained) have increased rates of behavioral problems, especially as adolescents.[22] Such questions about delaying school entry can serve as a springboard into exploring reasons for the parents' concerns. If it turns out during evaluation that serious, previously undetected developmental problems are present, appropriate diagnostic and remedial efforts should be instituted. However, these efforts often involve school-based resources and special programs. When in doubt, the pediatrician should encourage attending school, even with a modified program, rather than continuing day care or remaining at home. Close contact with the kindergarten teacher is mandatory, especially if the patient entering school is a boy, very close to barely making the 5-year-old age cutoff, and is small (at or below the 25th percentile for height).

When the child experiences difficulty or when adjustment or advance in learning does not occur, further evaluation and referral are indicated. Psychoeducational testing aimed at formal evaluation of cognition, attention, and behavioral factors that could impede progress may be necessary. Waiting 1 year for the child to "mature" only serves to delay necessary remediation. If the educational expectations are found to be excessive and the child is within range of normal abilities for age, adjustment of the learning environment is required rather than the child's being labeled as deviant. Repeating kindergarten as a remedial step without formal evaluation and program restructuring is not indicated and is invariably nonproductive.

The pediatrician's door should always be open to a discussion of how the child is doing in school. With the increased mobility of today's society, the pediatrician should be aware that children who have moved frequently are more likely to have emotional and behavioral problems and are more likely to repeat a grade than are students who have never moved.[23] If the response to a query of how a child is doing in school is less than a superlative from a parent, it deserves further exploration. Carrying out the preschool assessment sets the stage for ongoing monitoring of family and school behavior and achievement. In this way the pediatrician can be alert to early signs of a lack of fit between what the child brings to the situation and what the parents and school expect. Also, the pediatrician can share in the joy and excitement of a young school-aged child's successful social and intellectual growth.

REFERENCES

1. Rutter M: *Fifteen thousand hours,* Cambridge, Mass, 1979, Harvard University Press.
2. Freud S: *New introductory lessons in psychoanalysis,* New York, 1965, WW Norton & Co.
3. Erikson EH: *Identity and the life cycle,* New York, 1959, International Universities Press.
4. Piaget J, Inhelder B: *The psychology of the child,* New York, 1968, Basic Books.
5. Gesell A, Ilg F: *The child from five to ten,* New York, 1946, Harper Brothers.
6. Bandura A: *Cognitive social learning theory,* Englewood Cliffs, NJ, 1977, Prentice Hall.
7. Individuals with Disabilities Act, Pub L No 101-476, 104 Stat 1146 (1990).
8. Wright G, Nader P: Schools as milieux. In Levine MD et al, editors: *Developmental and behavioral pediatrics,* Philadelphia, 1992, WB Saunders.
9. Wender EH, Solanto MV: Attention deficit/hyperactivity disorder. In Hoekelman RA, editor: *Pediatric primary care,* ed 3, St Louis, 1997, Mosby, p 675.
10. McCormick MC, Workman-Daniels K, Brooks-Gunn J: The behavioral and emotional well-being of school-age children of different birth weights, *Pediatrics* 97:18, 1996.
11. Klein PS, Forbes GB, Nader PR: Effects of starvation in infancy (pyloric stenosis) on subsequent learning abilities, *J Pediatr* 87:8, 1975.
12. Teele DW, Klein JO, Rosner BA: Otitis media with effusion during the first three years of life and development of speech and language, *Pediatrics* 74:282, 1984.
13. Shaywitz SE: Dyslexia, *N Engl J Med* 338:307, 1998.
14. McNamara J: Cognitive basis of language learning in infants, *Psychol Rev* 79:1, 1972.
15. Levine MD: Middle childhood. In Levine MD et al, editors: *Developmental and behavioral pediatrics,* Philadelphia, 1992, WB Saunders.
16. Chamberlin RW, Nader PR: Relationship between nursery school behavior patterns and late school functioning, *Am J Orthopsychiatry* 41:597, 1971.
17. Taft LT, Barowsky EI: The clumsy child, *Pediatr Rev* 10:247, 1989.
18. American Academy of Pediatrics: Recommendations for preventive pediatric health care, *Pediatrics* 96:373, 1995.
19. American Academy of Pediatrics: The inappropriate use of school "readiness" tests, *Pediatrics* 95:437, 1995.
20. Lee VE et al: Are Head Start effects sustained? A longitudinal follow-up comparison of disadvantaged children attending Head Start, no preschool and other preschool programs, *Child Dev* 65 (spec issue 2):684, 1994.
21. Comer JP: The Yale-New Haven primary prevention project: a follow-up study, *J Am Acad Child Psychiatry* 24:154, 1985.
22. Byrd RS, Weitzman M, Auinger MS: Increased behavior problems associated with delayed school entry and delayed school progress, *Pediatrics* 100:654, 1997.
23. Simpson GA, Fowler MG: Geographic mobility and children's emotional/behavioral adjustment and school functioning, *Pediatrics* 93:303, 1994.

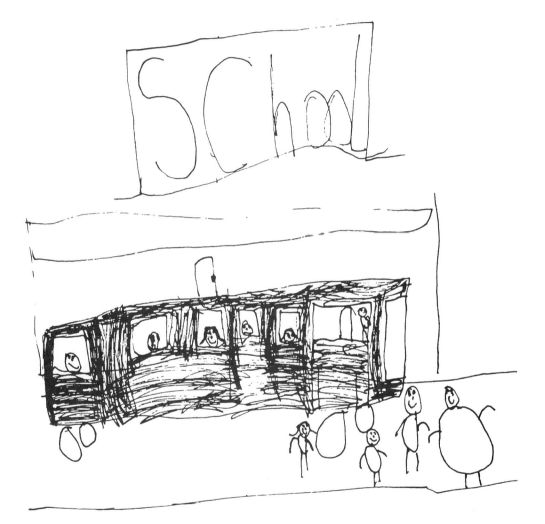

"A girl and a boy get on the bus. Their parents are watching."

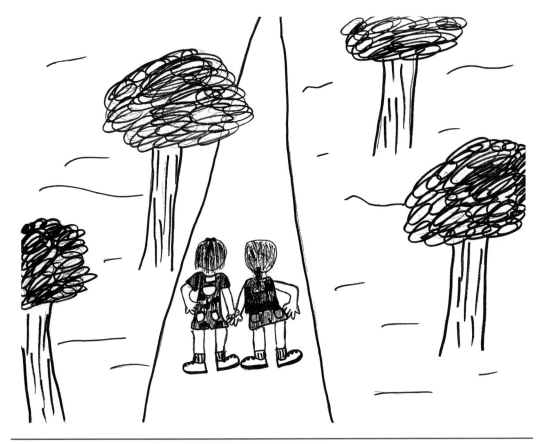

"Friends Forever" A precocious ten year old shows herself walking with a friend. Clear distance perspective usually emerges at an older age. By Kaitlin Thomas, age 10

CHAPTER 18

SIX TO SEVEN YEARS: READING, RELATIONSHIPS, AND RULES

■ Martin T. Stein

KEY WORDS

Concrete Operations
Attention Deficit
Learning Disabilities
School Refusal
Truancy
Separation Anxiety

 Bryan, age 6 years, was referred at his school's request to see if "something couldn't be done" about his activity level. His first grade teacher thought him much more active than the other boys in her class because he frequently spoke out of turn, moved about the classroom during less structured class periods, and invaded his peers' work space and private conversations. He was an only child whose parents both worked. He was adored by all four grandparents, who lived nearby and provided much of his daily care. His parents had encouraged his outgoing personality and excellent verbal skills and were quite tolerant of his high energy level during their times alone with him. His pediatrician found him to be physically healthy with no neurological abnormalities and with a history of excellent language and motor development. He was rather presumptuous in his stance toward the pediatrician, asking the doctor what kind of car he owned and how much the examination would cost. His mother had difficulty concealing her amusement at this inquiry by Bryan. Psychometric evaluation by the school psychologist documented Bryan's academic achievement at above grade level in all academic areas.

The pediatrician convinced Bryan's parents to work closely with his teacher in making clear to Bryan their support of classroom behavioral expectations. His parents began to follow through with the teacher's rewards and consequences for unacceptable behavior at school. Improvement in impulse control was not dramatic, but by second grade his teacher commented that Bryan was a "challenging, but gratifying student to have in class."

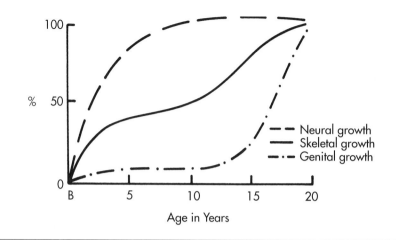

Fig. 18-1   Organ growth curves drawn to a common scale by computing values at successive ages in terms of growth. (Modified from Harris JA et al: *The measurement of man,* Minneapolis, 1930, University of Minnesota Press.)

The 6-year-old child stands on a threshold of exciting new cognitive and social experiences. With regular school attendance actually required for the first time, this age marks the beginning of a lifetime of obligations and adherence to schedules and routines imposed outside of the familiar family environment. This time of transition may present a crisis to the child or her family while at the same time providing an opportunity for rapid cognitive, social, and emotional growth.

The accelerated physical growth of the preschooler begins to slow as children enter the years of middle childhood. By age 5 years the brain has attained approximately 90% of its adult weight, and over the next 2 years the final myelinization of the central nervous system (CNS) will be completed (Fig. 18-1). The nearly mature CNS coincides with qualitative advances in cognitive capacities. Simultaneously, the child may participate in activities requiring the integration of fine and gross motor skills, such as dance, sports, and, in the classroom, handwriting and arts and crafts projects.

COGNITIVE DEVELOPMENT

The 6-year-old begins to show less evidence of the cognitive stage described by Piaget[1] as "preoperational" thinking—thinking marked by so-called magical qualities. The sensitive observer will find most first graders questioning many of their previous assumptions about the world. The typical 6-year-old does not take fantasy for granted and may question magical events. Nevertheless, she may have difficulty in performing mental operations that involve simultaneous changes in more than one variable. Instead, she may continue to focus on one aspect of a situation, a phenomenon known as *centration.* For example, the child may believe that a tall, narrow bottle of soda contains more soda than a short, wide bottle with an equal volume merely because the former is taller. Likewise a child may be able to make her way from home to school with great accuracy, but may be unable to mentally reverse the directions to appropriately plan the trip home. She may be able to participate in a multifaceted game, but will have difficulty learning it from verbal directions alone or explaining the rules with clarity. She may resent a sibling whose birthday "comes before hers" without consolation from the sense that soon thereafter the situation will be reversed.

Piaget[1] was able to demonstrate preoperational thinking and the transition to **concrete operations** with simple techniques, using readily available materials. For example, an adult can form a ball of clay for a child and ask him to form a similar ball with "as much clay" as the first ball. When the child agrees that both balls have exactly the same amount of clay, the tester can flatten one of the pieces, roll it into a narrow cylinder, or break it into two or more chunks. If the child is asked which of the original two balls now has the most clay, his answer and reasoning may reveal his capacity to conserve mass cognitively despite the physical manipulations that were carried out before his eyes. However, the child of about 6 years or less also may give an answer that demonstrates he does not conserve mass cognitively. The child may state that the original ball of clay now contains more clay because it is longer than the other ball or less clay because it is flatter. The child who retains the concept of mass despite these changes in appearance has achieved, in part, a new level of reasoning called "concrete operations" (Fig. 18-2).

The age at which children demonstrate these changes in cognition varies considerably, often beginning around age 6 years and gradually evolving over the next 4 to 5 years.[2] By age 5 years, most children demonstrate that they understand the concept of the conservation of length. Many younger children will maintain that a long string and a shorter wooden stick are the same length if they are arranged so that the ends of the string coincide with the ends of the stick. Conservation of mass and weight are accomplished mentally by most children 1 year or more later, and conservation of volume is achieved much later, when children reach the last 2 years of grade school.

Six-year-olds continue to demonstrate many of the preconceptual qualities of thinking typical of preschoolers (see Chapter 17). First graders may still believe the sun and moon were made artificially and move because man or God makes them move. They may feel sorry for a car that is heavily loaded with passengers as if the car had feelings. In fact, even adults may think in egocentric, magical ways, depending on many factors, including the context of the cognitive task. The ways in which children think and attain knowledge as they develop into middle childhood are apparently less rigidly tied to specific Piagetian cognitive stages as was once thought.[3]

As children move through the early years of grade school, they do manifest more of the qualities of thinking that Piaget described as "concrete operational thought." This stage is marked by the ability to consider multiple variables concerning objects or situations simultaneously, perform mental operations relating to concrete objects (e.g., adding or subtracting objects, creating maps), understand serial relationships (e.g., ordering pictures, number concepts), and appreciate classification systems. Classification tasks, common in modern schoolwork, require the identification of a common factor in groups and subgroups.

Although the thinking process of the 6- to 7-year-old is qualitatively different from the thinking of older school-age children, the typical first and second grade child should manifest those qualities that make possible productive classroom participation and learning.

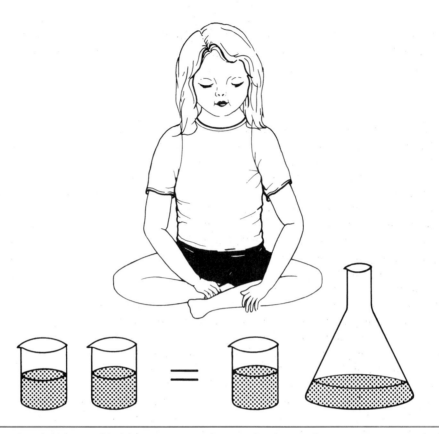

Fig. 18-2 This child is proudly able to appreciate that equal volumes of water are maintained when the shape of the container is changed, a demonstration of conservation of mass in a child who has entered the stage of concrete operations.

In first grade, academic demands are made in addition to the behavioral, social, and emotional demands of kindergarten. Academic failure in the first grade results when children cannot demonstrate in school that they have the capacity to perform the primary decoding tasks of reading, solving simple addition and subtraction problems, and writing simple sentences with properly spelled words.[4] Although these skills are generally taught to all children at about the same age, normal children vary substantially in the age at which they achieve the capacity to read, spell, and work with numbers. A modest delay in the development of these abilities, even if the delay is maturational and not otherwise significant, can create serious psychological and behavioral difficulties for a child whose self-image is tarnished by the experience of academic failure at an early age.

Academic difficulties in the first and second grade may diminish the child's self-esteem, color her future attitude toward school, and result in considerable anxiety in parents. It is important that the pediatrician begin to help the parents understand the source of their

BOX 18-1	ACADEMIC UNDERACHIEVEMENT AND BEHAVIORAL PROBLEMS: CLUES TO ETIOLOGY AND INTERVENTION

Neurologically based problem with sustained attention
Learning disability that limits effective mental manipulations necessary for learning
Psychological disorder that may be a primary cause of school failure or a secondary manifestation of a learning disability or chronic inattention
Disorganized home environment that may be the result of marital discord, poverty, a major life-event change, substance abuse, or child/spousal abuse

child's academic difficulty and collaborate with the child, her parents, and the school in designing a program to address the child's specific needs.

A useful model to evaluate academic success in first grade curriculum assumes that children have both the cognitive power and the cognitive style to deal effectively with the classroom environment.[5] The child with insufficient cognitive power may be generally dull, with mild or borderline mental retardation that does not become apparent until the child is faced with the academic demands of first or second grade; or selective cognitive deficits (i.e., learning disabilities) may appear in a child who otherwise shows normal intelligence. The child with even a mild form of mental retardation may have a history of delayed attainment of early milestones in language development. Another child with a selective learning disability may seem bright, with a good fund of general knowledge and normal developmental milestones, but has difficulty with specific academic tasks during the first grade in a way that is quite unexpected by parents and teachers, who perceive the child as normal in intelligence and in demonstrating good work habits.

The child who has difficulty learning in the first 2 or 3 years of school is a challenge to pediatric clinicians because of the similarity of behavioral symptoms and academic outcomes for a wide variety of developmental, neurological, and psychological conditions. The challenge is more apparent when a clinician appreciates that these many variables may be variations on a normal spectrum of behavior or may reflect problems that are inherent in the child or her environment. Inattention and distractibility in the classroom, poor organization skills, frequent daydreaming during learning exercises, and awkward social skills are often found in many first and second grade children who are not achieving academic progress. Among children with these behaviors, with or without poor school performance, the clinician should consider four broad categories that can provide useful clues to etiology and intervention (Box 18-1).

PROBLEMS WITH SUSTAINED ATTENTION AND LEARNING

Perhaps the most common disorder of cognitive style in the differential diagnosis of academic failure is **attention deficit** hyperactivity disorder (ADHD). A child with a primary attention disorder is presumed to suffer from intrinsic inefficiencies in maintaining selective attention.

- The process of attention in a learning situation has different components that may reach maturation at different chronological ages in an individual child. These functions of attention include planning and reflection, vigilance and awareness of salient information, resistance to distraction, a sustained mental effort, and an ongoing monitoring capability to detect errors and make corrections.[6]

- A history of early temperamental difficulties (e.g., withdrawing from novel situations, being slow to adapt, having intense emotional responses or negative moods [see Chapter 2]), perinatal stress events, sleep disorder, and inattention in multiple settings and situations is found in some but by no means all children with an attention disorder.

- Minor neurological abnormalities (so-called soft neurological signs) may be apparent on physical examination. These nonlocalizing neurological findings include motor impersistence, synkinesis (moving a body part without intention when focusing on another body movement), right-left confusion, and poor short-term memory.

- Inattention, associated with poor listening skills, impaired memory, impulsivity, and disorganization, will often surface in an office setting when a child with a significant attention problem is asked to repeat a series of digits, follow a serial command, or demonstrate right-left discrimination.[7]

Although a deficit of attention is the central problem in children with ADHD, many of these children are overactive (hyperactivity) and demonstrate problems with impulse control. The diagnosis is made largely on the basis of history, including teacher and parent reports and, in selected cases, psychometric testing, rather than physical examination. Teachers, who have the advantage of classroom observations, identify far more children as inattentive and overactive than do parents or clinicians.[8,9] To succeed in the classroom, the first grader must be capable of focused and sustained attention for periods of 25 minutes to 1 hour. Good students in standard settings are not easily distracted, are selective in what they attend to, and must be able to shift the focus of attention rapidly. Parents and teachers are not surprised when a child who lacks these qualities earns low marks in the first grade, often after experiencing a difficult time in kindergarten. Such a child may be seen as so unhappy, so distractible, or so preoccupied that academic failure can be predicted early in the school year.

As a guide to clinical assessment, the core symptoms of inattention, hyperactivity, and impulsivity have been described with specific clusters of behaviors (Box 18-2).

The ADHD diagnostic classification requires the presence of a specified number of symptoms for at least 6 months beginning before the age of 7 years and present in at least two or more settings, including at school, home, and play. When these criteria are applied, approximately 5% to 8% of school-age children seen in a primary care pediatric setting will have ADHD. Similar to most pediatric disorders of behavior, an accurate diagnosis of ADHD is complicated by the fact that many of the core behaviors can be seen in the course of typical child development.

Recently, the American Academy of Pediatrics published a diagnostic classification of behaviors seen in primary care medical settings; the classification emphasizes the broad spectrum of normal and abnormal behaviors seen in infants, children, and adolescents.[10] *The Classification of Child and Adolescent Mental Diagnoses in Primary Care: Diagnostic and Statistical*

BOX 18-2	DIAGNOSTIC CRITERIA FOR ATTENTION DEFICIT HYPERACTIVITY DISORDER

Three categories of ADHD

Attention Deficit Hyperactivity Disorder, Combined Type: This subtype should be used if six (or more) symptoms of inattention and six (or more) symptoms of hyperactivity-impulsivity have persisted for at least 6 months. Most children and adolescents with the disorder have Combined Type.

Attention Deficit Hyperactivity Disorder, Predominantly Inattentive Type: This subtype should be used if six (or more) symptoms of inattention (but fewer than six symptoms of hyperactivity-impulsivity) have persisted for at least 6 months.

Attention Deficit Hyperactivity Disorder, Predominantly Hyperactive-Impulsive Type: This subtype should be used if six (or more) symptoms of hyperactivity-impulsivity (but fewer than six symptoms of inattention) have persisted for at least 6 months. Inattention may often still be a significant clinical feature in such cases.

Inattention

Often fails to give close attention to details or makes careless mistakes in schoolwork, work, or other activities

Often has difficulty sustaining attention in tasks or play activities

Often does not seem to listen when spoken to directly

Often does not follow through on instructions, and fails to finish schoolwork, chores, or duties in the workplace (not because of oppositional behavior or failure to understand instructions)

Often has difficulty organizing tasks and activities

Often avoids, dislikes, or is reluctant to engage in tasks that require sustained mental effort (such as schoolwork or homework)

Often loses things necessary for tasks or activities (e.g., toys, school assignments, pencils, books, or tools)

Often distracted easily by extraneous stimuli

Often forgetful in daily activities

Hyperactivity

Often fidgets with hands or feet or squirms in seat

Often leaves seat in classroom or in other situations in which remaining seated is expected

Often runs about or climbs excessively in situations in which it is inappropriate in adolescents (may be limited to subjective feelings of restlessness)

Often has difficulty playing or engaging in leisure activities quietly

Often "on the go" or acts as if "driven by a motor"

Often talks excessively

From American Psychiatric Association: *Diagnostic and statistical manual of mental disorders,* ed 4, Washington, DC, 1994, American Psychiatric Association.   *Continued*

BOX 18-2	DIAGNOSTIC CRITERIA FOR ATTENTION DEFICIT HYPERACTIVITY DISORDER—cont'd

Three categories of ADHD—cont'd

Impulsivity
   Often blurts out answers before questions have been completed
   Often has difficulty awaiting turn
   Often interrupts or intrudes on others (e.g., butts into conversations or games)

Some hyperactive-impulsive or inattentive symptoms that caused impairment were present before age 7 years.
Some impairment from the symptoms is present in **two or more settings** (e.g., at school [or work] and at home).
Clear evidence must exist of clinically significant impairment in social, academic, or occupational functioning.

Manual for Primary Care (DSM-PC), Child and Adolescent Version can assist clinicians in the process of sorting out a typical developmental variation from a disorder that meets specific diagnostic criteria. For ADHD in particular, the *DSM-PC* should be helpful in separating typical overactivity, inattentiveness, and impulsivity from such behaviors in children who need further evaluation and treatment.

The diagnosis of an attention deficit disorder should be made with careful deliberation, including an assessment of a child's behavior from both a parent and a teacher. It is important that parents understand that this diagnosis is largely descriptive of the child's behavior and does not reveal the etiology of the problem, dictate treatment, or predict the individual child's prognosis. Children with early-onset, severe ADHD do carry a significant risk for serious maladjustment in adolescence and beyond.[11]

Although longitudinal outcome studies of children with ADHD are limited, those with less pervasive attention problems may eventually do quite well. Feedback to the parents should emphasize specific problem behaviors that have been identified and should focus on possible strategies that might mitigate these problems and enhance adjustment to school. The use of stimulant medication may improve the inattentiveness, hyperactivity, and impulsivity of children who have this disorder, often making them more ready to learn. Medication will not improve academic achievement directly. Improved progress will be achieved through clear behavioral management (perhaps including medication) and a focused educational intervention, using all avenues of learning available to the child.

Stimulant medication will not by itself turn a student's D's into A's and will not correct a specific learning disability. An unjustified shift to a medical versus an educational diagnosis may lead to unduly high expectations from the medication and the lack of a directed, specific educational program. Whereas a stimulant medication is often the most effective intervention for a child with ADHD, it should not be used without equal attention to the learning environment, individual learning style, and the psychosocial assessment of the child and family.

The evaluation and management of children with chronic inattention involves ongoing contact with the school, as well as referral to educational and mental health specialists when indicated. This is equally true when stimulant medications are prescribed. The pediatrician must therefore develop an alliance with the child, parents, and teacher so that a long-term collaboration is possible. An environment that supports the child's efforts to maintain focus on tasks and be successful can be created only by this collaborative effort.

LEARNING DISABILITIES

A learning disability refers to a consistent difficulty in learning basic academic skills related to reading, spelling, and mathematics. **Learning disabilities** are presumed to be neurologically based, a reflection of the "hard-wiring" network of the CNS. They are seen in 3% to 15% of school-age children with a wide variation of aptitudes, from those children with average intelligence to those with superior intellectual abilities. In fact, a learning disability is often suspected when the difference between aptitude and achievement is wide. Most learning disabilities do not come to the attention of parents, educators, or clinicians until a child is challenged with cognitive work that requires the acquisition and use of reading, spelling, or arithmetic skills.

A clinically useful perspective on learning disabilities is achieved with the recognition that we learn primarily by visual or auditory inputs of information. Assuming that a child has adequate visual acuity and hearing capacity, most learning disabilities can be conceptualized as a developmental variation in the processing pathways of the CNS.[6] Visual-dependent learning problems may cause a delay in learning to read and manipulate numbers. The recognition and comprehension of the symbolic language represented by words or numbers is altered in a manner that may affect the development of reading skills (dyslexia) or mathematical abilities (dyscalculia). Children with auditory-dependent learning problems find it difficult to comprehend spoken language when presented with new information. These disabilities result in either a visual or auditory processing disorder that may have significant impact on the quality and quantity of learning. The variety of specific learning disabilities that become apparent during early elementary years are defined in Table 18-1.

Although the diagnosis of a learning disability is usually based on more data than the physician can obtain during the interview with the family and examination of the child,[12] procedures can be accomplished in a primary care setting that provide critical clues to a learning disability. It is essential to obtain the results of educational testing from the school or other source or to ask that such tests be performed if necessary. Schools are required by federal law to respond to a parent's request to assess learning or behavioral problems that affect school function. Difficulties with cognitive style are usually not apparent in the pediatrician's office, an environment that differs from a classroom environment in many important ways. Specifically, most children with ADHD do not display inattention and hyperactivity in a medical office setting[9] unless visual, auditory, or motor domains associated with learning are assessed by neurodevelopmental tests. Data on the child's learning patterns and output (grades), attention span, and social and behavioral adjustment can be obtained by contacting

TABLE 18-1 ■ Definitions of Learning Disabilities

Term	Description
Visual perception deficit	The inability to differentiate between similar looking letters, numbers, shapes, objects, symbols; may habitually skip over lines in text
Auditory discrimination deficit	The inability to distinguish similar sounds ("pig" and "big") or confusing the sequence of heard or spoken sounds ("ephelant")
Dyslexia	Difficulty sounding out letters and confusing words that sound similar resulting in problems acquiring basic reading skills
Dysgraphia	Difficulty expressing thoughts on paper and with writing associated with unreadable penmanship and problems in gripping and manipulating a pencil
Dyscalculia	Problems with perception of shapes and confusion of arithmetic symbols leading to poor comprehension of simple mathematical functions
Dysnomia	Inability to recall names or words for common objects.

teachers directly with the parent's permission. Teachers are often eager to have an opportunity to discuss with a clinician the children whom they find most challenging. A number of standardized teacher report forms are also available if the pediatrician wishes to obtain a more formal profile of the child's behavior in school.[13,14]

The case of Bryan provides an example of how a child's temperament and experiences in the family can result in disruptive behavior in school. ADHD is only one of a number of disruptive behavior disorders occurring in childhood. In Bryan's case, it would not be appropriate to label his difficulties in school as a disorder because they resulted from typical variations in the personalities of child, parents (and grandparents), and teacher. Specific learning disabilities most often become apparent during first grade, although other specific subtypes of academic difficulty may emerge initially in fourth or fifth grade (see Chapter 19), and still others become apparent for the first time in junior high school (see Chapter 20). It is essential that physicians routinely inquire about the progress of 6-year-olds in the first grade. Any concerns raised should not be dismissed as "adjustment" problems or entirely maturational in origin (i.e., "he will grow out of it"). This will provide a data base that may reveal the sequence in which academic problems develop and prove the need for appropriate remediation before the establishment of a cycle of failures. Children with a primary learning disability can show academic difficulties without attentional, behavioral, or emotional problems if evaluated early enough. However, without diagnosis and intervention, such children may subsequently develop low self-esteem and have disturbances in emotions and conduct as a result of academic frustration. These secondary effects of academic failure will make accurate diagnosis much more difficult later. Because the best medicine is preventive medicine, it is important that learning disabilities be recognized early so that specific remedial measures may be undertaken to lessen the occurrence of secondary problems with emotions and conduct.

PSYCHOSOCIAL PROBLEMS THAT AFFECT LEARNING

A child's emotional life, family environment, school, and community are other important factors to consider when problems with learning occur in the first and second grades. Among children with mental health problems (e.g., depression, anxiety, oppositional behavior, or conduct disorder), 30% to 80% have problems with academic achievement and classroom behavior. A low self-esteem and poor self-image in these children affect learning, especially in those with an associated learning disability. Chronic family dysfunction or, in the vulnerable child, even a temporary life-event change in the family may cause or exacerbate school failure. Separation, divorce, an illness (in the child or in a family member), substance abuse, and child abuse or neglect are seen in many young school-age children with learning problems. Finally, the child's extended environment in the school and community can affect learning. A curriculum that does not fit the learning needs of a child, an unmotivated or overwhelmed teacher, a teacher (or parent) whose expectations for academic success are discordant with a child's abilities, or a community where violence is pervasive or where school achievement is not a major goal may have the same effect on learning as a neurologically based learning disability or disorder of attention. Dworkin[15] has pointed out the following.

> School processes are more important determinants of students' performance than such features as whether schools are public or private, class size, the age and spaciousness of the school building, and student-teacher ratio. Rather, the school's academic emphasis, expectations for attainment, amount of homework, teachers' actions during lessons, use of group instruction, and use of rewards and praise are major influences on students' performance. Aspects of the school's social environment (such as the amount of praise offered to children) may be particularly important for children from disadvantaged homes in which less emphasis is placed on academic attainment and standards for classroom behavior.

SCHOOL AVOIDANCE

All clinicians who work with children sooner or later will evaluate a child who refuses to attend school.[16,17] Unexcused absences from school follow a bimodal pattern of incidence, with peaks in the early primary grades in about 5% of children, particularly first grade, and a second peak again in junior high school in 2% of youth. The clinician should carefully and systematically determine the reason the child is not attending school before developing an approach to the problem. Some children are kept home from school by parents, although most unexcused absences from school are attributable to **school refusal** by the child.

> Most first graders who refuse to attend school do not roam the community **(truancy),** but spend the school day at home. These children may have a variety of physical complaints, including stomachaches, headaches, dizziness, and fatigue, which often subside as the day progresses (Fig. 18-3). Although a few of these children may be suffering from an actual phobia[18] of school itself or of some particular aspect of the school experience, such as travel on the bus, most first graders who refuse to attend school appear to be suffering from **separation anxiety.** When examined in the pediatrician's office, these children usually appear healthy and have a normal physical examination, although some initially appear pale, sad, and emotionally depressed.

SICK

"I cannot go to school today,"
Said little Peggy Ann McKay.
"I have the measles and the mumps,
A gash, a rash and purple bumps.
My mouth is wet, my throat is dry,
I'm going blind in my right eye.
My tonsils are as big as rocks,
I've counted sixteen chicken pox
And there's one more—that's seventeen,
And don't you think my face looks green?
My leg is cut, my eyes are blue—
It might be instamatic flu.
I cough and sneeze and gasp and choke,
I'm sure that my left leg is broke—
My hip hurts when I move my chin,
My belly button's caving in,
My back is wrenched, my ankle's sprained,
My 'pendix pains each time it rains.
My nose is cold, my toes are numb,
I have a sliver in my thumb.
My neck is stiff, my spine is weak,
I hardly whisper when I speak.
My tongue is filling up my mouth,
I think my hair is falling out.
My elbow's bent, my spine ain't straight,
My temperature is one-o-eight.
My brain is shrunk, I cannot hear,
There is a hole inside my ear.
I have a hangnail, and my heart is—what?
What's that? What's that you say?
You say today is . . . Saturday?
G'bye, I'm going out to play!"

Fig. 18-3 *Sick.* From Silverstein S: *Where the sidewalk ends*, New York, 1974, Harper & Row.

These children are experiencing stress in response to leaving their parents and familiar surroundings for a full day of school. The pediatrician may diagnose separation anxiety, which often responds to simple behavioral measures combined with supportive counseling of the parents. Such children may be unusually sensitive to the anxiety that is normal in all children as they begin their grade school experience. In addition, some parents may transmit their anxiety about separating to the child and thereby exacerbate the problem. Such families need to be reminded that school attendance in the first grade is compulsory and that separation from family at this time is a healthy and predictable stage of maturation.

The child's clinician must be sympathetic to the physical complaints and initiate a reasonable medical evaluation. Excessive medical attention to the physical complaints, which may occur when a large number of laboratory tests or specialty referrals are ordered, should be avoided when nonorganic disease is suspected. The clinician must make it clear to the family that the child is to attend school on a daily basis unless the symptoms are severe enough to require a visit to the physician's office. Returning to school will be either diagnostic or therapeutic. The parents may be reassured that the child will usually settle down in school if he comes to understand that his parents expect and will demand school attendance. Often the school can collaborate with the parent in keeping the child in school. Children with separation anxiety disorder become rapidly asymptomatic as their school attendance becomes more regular. When school refusal does not respond to these measures or when pediatric evaluation of the child or family suggests a serious emotional disorder, a specific mental health referral may be indicated.

School refusal in early adolescence often leads to a more extensive differential diagnostic evaluation. If the junior high school student spends school time in community areas, such as malls, and engages in varying degrees of antisocial behavior, one must suspect a conduct disturbance. Those adolescents who remain at home may have physical complaints similar to the 6-year-olds and may be suffering from an anxiety disorder, depression, substance abuse, or teenage pregnancy (see Chapter 21). Some of these youngsters stay home because they are fearful and have been threatened or mistreated by peers. A small number are experiencing the onset of a serious, but usually treatable, psychiatric disturbance, such as depression or schizophrenia. School refusal in adolescence that is not clearly truancy should be carefully examined, and every effort made to prevent a tragic early withdrawal from school.

DATA GATHERING

Children at the age of 6 may not be as candid in providing information to the physician as they once were. Just as the clinician may observe increasing modesty during physical examination at this age, he may also find the child withholding or distorting her answers to questions about personal, school, and family life. Obtaining information with the child and parent present is the most productive technique for 6-year-olds. As with the preschool child, it is important to communicate to the child that you value information provided by the child about her health and feelings. Asking the child first to describe her physical complaints and beliefs about the reasons for the medical examination may provide an opportunity to deal directly with the 6-year-old's lingering misconceptions about the reasons for the medical encounter. In the course of evaluating the child's physical health, the clinician may gather data about the child's development in the areas shown in Table 18-2.

TABLE 18-2 ■ Gathering Data

Cognitive Development	
Questions for Children	**Objective**
Where do you go to school? What grade are you in? What are you learning in school? Are there some things you do at school that you really like? Are there things about school that you don't like?	To assess whether the 6-year-old can provide acceptable answers to nearly all of these questions. Answers may suggest that the child is having difficulty in particular areas. When the child is reluctant to talk about school or provides very little information, the physician should then invite the parent to enter the discussion.
What town do you live in? On what street? Do you know your address? Do you know your telephone number?	To assess the child's attention to basic information important to his well-being as he spends increasing amounts of time away from his family; to assess visual or auditory memory skills.
Ask the child to copy a cross (4-year-old), a square (5-year-old), a triangle (6-year-old), and a diamond (7-year-old).	To observe the child's handedness, his ability to grasp and control a writing instrument, and his competence in increasingly difficult fine-motor and visual-perceptual tasks.
Ask the child to draw a person while you are interviewing the parent.	An estimated mental age may be obtained by using Goodenough's scoring criteria (see chapter 26). In addition, information may be obtained about the child's attentiveness, tendency to cooperate, compulsivity, and even emotional health if the drawing is atypical (see Chapter 26).
What makes the sun come up in the morning? What makes the clouds move in the sky? How can you tell if something is alive?	To assess the child's beliefs regarding causality and to help parents understand that the child remains in a transitional period relative to his cognitive abilities. Most 6-year-olds, regardless of intelligence, will respond to these questions with magical thinking characterized by animism and egocentricity. For example, "The sun comes up in the morning so that I can play."
How do you get to your house from school?	Children at this age continue to be highly egocentric in their ability to give directions and will often leave out important details. This should be interpreted to parents as a normal developmental stage and will help parents understand why it is difficult for children to reverse directions or see the world from another person's perspective.

TABLE 18-2 ■ Gathering Data—cont'd

Cognitive Development	
Questions for Children	**Objective**
Have you seen a recent movie or video? Tell me about the story.	To assess child's capacity for sequencing events, memory, and content of story.
Do you ever have dreams? Do the dreams ever really happen? Where do the dreams take place? What really happens to the people on television who fly or get hurt?	To assess the child's capacity for distinguishing between reality and fantasy, which should be well developed at this age.

Cognitive Development	
Questions for Parents	**Objective**
Does (name) have a problem concentrating or paying attention? Do you think that (name) is more active, less attentive than other children his age?	To assess the parent's perception of the child's ability to attend to a classroom learning environment.
Do you frequently find yourself repeating directions or instructions?	To assess auditory processing maturation.
How is school going? Have you had a conference with teacher? How does (name) fit in with the classroom? What are the teacher's expectations for (name)?	To assess the parent's understanding and involvement with the school; to model the expected close interaction between parent and school personnel.

Social and Emotional Development	
Questions for Children	**Objective**
Do you know the name of the team that plays baseball or football for your city? What is your favorite movie? What is your favorite television show? Where did you go on your vacation?	To assess the child's general fund of information and the child's interest in and retention of information about events that occur outside the home.
Who are your good friends?	To assess the child's relationships outside the home. By this time a child should have formed several close relationships outside the home. The child should name one and preferably more friends close to his age. A child who does not name anybody or who names an adult, a family member, or a much younger child requires further evaluation. The parent may be asked to comment on the child's response.

Continued

TABLE 18-2 ■ **Gathering Data—cont'd**

Social and Emotional Development	
Questions for Children	**Objective**
What games do you like to play?	To assess the child's preferences for solitary versus peer activities. Is he comfortable with the give and take of peer group activities? Does he understand the necessity for and the nature of rules? Is he involved in organized communitywide activities, such as team sports or a religion-based peer group?
Who lives at your house? What do you think about your brother/sister/the new baby?	To assess the child's capacity to express both positive and negative affects relating to family members and the degree of sibling rivalry that may be present.

Social and Emotional Development	
Questions for Parents	**Objective**
How long is (name) in school? What does (name) do after school? What jobs does (name) do around the house? How much television does (name) watch each day? What programs?	To assess the demands on the child's and family's circumstances and arrangements. To assess family responsibilities that the child shares.

ACKNOWLEDGMENT

Nicholas Putnam, M.D., contributed to this chapter in previous editions.

REFERENCES

1. Piaget J: *The origins of intelligence in children,* New York, 1952, International Press.
2. Elkind D: *Children and adolescents: interpretive essays on Jean Piaget,* New York, 1974, Oxford University Press.
3. Hobson RP: Piaget: on the ways of knowing in childhood. In Rutter M, Hersov L, editors: *Child and adolescent psychiatry: modern approaches,* Boston, 1985, Blackwell Scientific Publications.
4. Levine MD, Oberklaid F: Hyperactivity: symptom complex or complex symptom? *Am J Dis Child* 134:409, 1980.
5. Kinsbourne M, Caplan P: *Children's learning and attention problems,* Boston, 1979, Little, Brown & Co.
6. Levine MD: Neurodevelopmental variation and dysfunction among school-aged children. In Levine MD, Carey WB, Crocker AC, editors: *Developmental-behavioral pediatrics,* ed 3, Philadelphia, 1998, WB Saunders.
7. Feldman HM: Attention deficits. In *Gellis and Kagan's current pediatric therapy,* ed 16, Philadelphia, 1996, WB Saunders
8. Conners CK: A teacher rating scale for use in drug studies with children, *Am J Psychiatr* 126:152, 1969.

9. Sleator EK, Ullman RK: Can the physician diagnose hyperactivity in the office? *Pediatrics* 67:13, 1981.

10. American Academy of Pediatrics: The classification of child and adolescent mental conditions in primary care. In American Academy of Pediatrics: *Diagnostic and statistical manual for primary care (DSM-PC), child and adolescent version,* Elk Grove, Ill, 1996, American Academy of Pediatrics.

11. Mannuzza S et al: Hyperactive boys almost grown up, *Arch Gen Psychiatry* 48:77, 1991.

12. Cantwell D: *The hyperactive child: diagnosis, management and current research,* New York, 1975, Spectrum Publications.

13. Levine MD, Brooks R, Shonkoff J: *A pediatric approach to learning disorders,* New York, 1980, John Wiley & Sons.

14. Wender E: Hyperactivity. In Parker S, Zuckerman B: *Behavioral and developmental pediatrics: a handbook for primary care,* Boston, 1995, Little, Brown & Co.

15. Dworkin PH: School failure. In Parker S, Zuckerman B: *Behavioral and developmental pediatrics: a handbook for primary care.* Boston, 1995, Little, Brown & Co.

16. Nader P, Bullock D, Caldwell B: School phobia, *Pediatr Clin North Am* 22:605, 1975.

17. Eisenberg L: School phobia: a study in the communication of anxiety, *Am J Psychiatry* 114:712, 1958.

18. Schmitt BD: School refusal, *Pediatr Rev* 8:99, 1986.

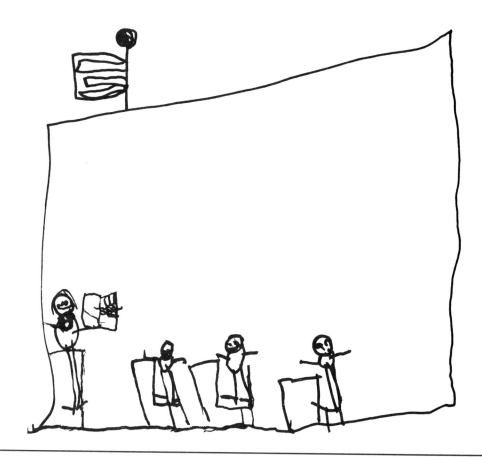

A 6½-year-old boy draws his classroom. The teacher holding the book illustrates the central focus on reading in the first years of school. By Ryan Hennessy.

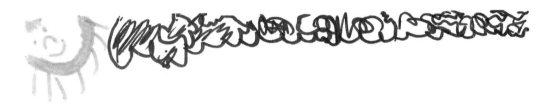

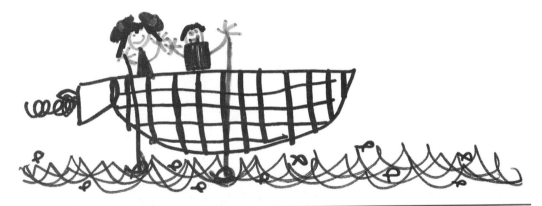

"Fishing with my daddy on Father's Day." A 5-year-old's drawing shows that exploration is always more exciting when the adventure is shared with family.

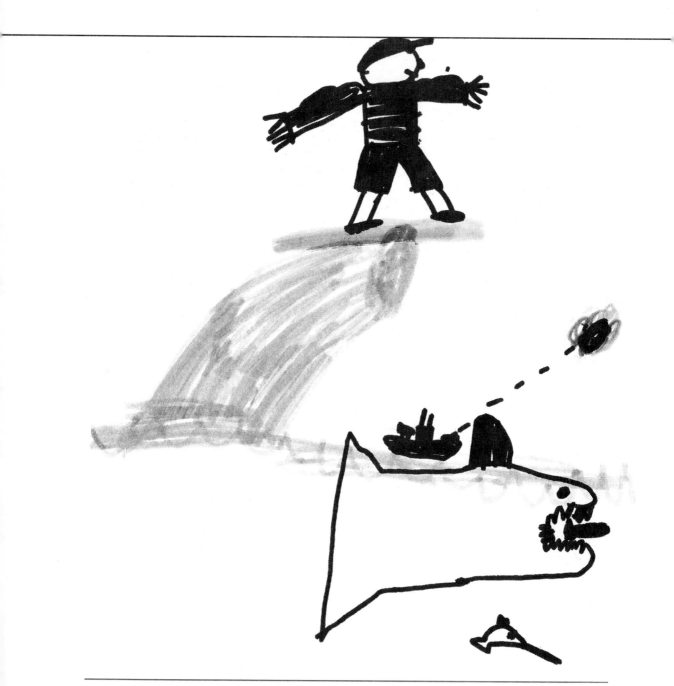

Neil, age 9, shows himself on top of the world, riding a wave above the monster whale, missile-launching ships, and swordfish. A good sense of confidence is conveyed.

CHAPTER 19

SEVEN TO TEN YEARS: WORLD OF MIDDLE CHILDHOOD

■ Robert D. Wells
■ Martin T. Stein

KEY WORDS

Mastery
Moral Development
Conscience
Explorations into Separation
Coping Skills
Activities
Friendships
Stress
School Performance

Aaron, age 9 years, was brought to you after a 1-week history of headaches. He is a fourth grader in a school for gifted children and has been earning excellent grades. You know the family well because he has two younger siblings (ages 3 and 6 years) and because his mother often calls and visits the office with acute concerns. Aaron was born after 5 years of infertility in his parents. His father is an attorney who is even-tempered and serious. His mother is a part-time teacher in computer sciences and has always been intense. She is concerned that Aaron's headaches are the result of a brain tumor because he has also had a major change in his behavior. His paternal grandfather died of an astrocytoma when Aaron was 2 years old. Although Aaron always was an intense but sociable child, he is now withdrawn, irritable, and demanding. He has been out of school for 1 week. His mother is unaware of any specific changes or stressful events but did note that Aaron recently has had problems with friends in the neighborhood. You decide to speak with Aaron alone to assess his developmental and behavioral functioning and determine its potential significance in creating or maintaining his symptoms.

On physical examination, Aaron is a depressed-appearing child with dramatic complaints of headache that are not well localized. A complete examination, including neurological assessment and visual acuity, is normal. The child is afebrile and appears well.

> *When Aaron is interviewed alone, he initially denies with irritation any specific concerns. He easily discusses his baseball card collection. When asked about his strengths, Aaron is unable to tell you what he does well.*
>
> *He says his headache keeps him from doing his schoolwork and admits hating school despite his great success. He admits feeling lonely at times and wishes he had more friends. This is his first year out of the neighborhood school. To attend the gifted program, he must travel to the other side of town and thus far has not met any of his fellow students out of school.*

The middle school-age years are, for most children, a time of robust physical health filled with surges of competencies and vulnerabilities in behavioral and developmental areas. This places the primary care physician in a challenging position because visits become less frequent during a time when many behavior and learning problems may start becoming evident. Self-awareness, control over new feelings and desires, interpersonal engagement, and other psychological processes deepen and evolve. This is not really a "latent" period at all, but one of consolidating and building skills.

A significant number of school-age children face additional obstacles to developing these competencies. Approximately 30% of all children must cope with a chronic illness, of which asthma is the most common. About 5.5% (3.5 million) U.S. children have a chronic condition that limits usual activities,[1,2] and they thus require additional care during a period of heightened independence and self-responsibility. Learning problems, traumatic events, and social and family dysfunctions all pose significant risks for the development of a wide range of behavioral, academic, and psychosomatic disorders. Of school-age children, 15% have a behavior problem severe enough to benefit from a pediatric evaluation and treatment.

DEVELOPMENTAL TASKS
New Cognitive Skills

Mastery, though always a focus of child development, takes on special meaning during the school-age years as a result of the child's increased capacity for making many kinds of determinations. New cognitive skills form the basis of these. At this age, a school-age child is able to consider two or more aspects of a situation simultaneously. In making comparisons, he takes into account more than one variable. He appreciates that a tall, narrow lump of clay can be made short and wide without any net gain or loss of clay (see Chapter 18). Such reasoning extends to the child's capacity for making a variety of judgments. He may appreciate for the first time another child who is clumsy but bright, a teacher who is strict but fair, or medicine that is difficult to swallow but brings down a fever. For the first time the child has the mental capacity to appreciate that a surgical procedure will cause discomfort yet produce a desired result. Children begin to understand that rules in games and in life are the product of mutual consent and respect and that rules may be changed under certain circumstances. Piaget[3,4] demonstrated how children of elementary school age increasingly take context and motivation into account in making moral judgments. Kohlberg[5] (see Chapter 2) found that school-age children have varying levels of **moral development.** Whereas many behave well to earn some tangible reward or to avoid punishment, some are beginning to conform in order to gain approval from peers and adults. Many children at this age focus on clearly defined rules and have difficulty understanding why some people do not behave appropriately. This moral rigidity is developmentally normal.

Identification and Socialization

During this time the child continues to consolidate her identification with important adults in her life. In this process the same-sex parent is an important role model. Other adults inside and outside of the child's family also serve as examples for the child, augmenting the primary organizing force of the immediate family. Freud[6] pointed out the continuing growth during these years of that part of the child's mental life that represents internalized parental values—the superego or internalized **conscience.** Emotional and cognitive growth interact and result in the early development of a more personal conscience with less emphasis placed by the child on adult authority or conventional rules. This growth in conscience is found universally and crosses cultural and religious boundaries. The specific belief systems and norms of behavior are developed within the context of the family and, increasingly, that of society as a whole.

According to Erikson,[7] children this age are negotiating a stage of *contrasting industry and inferiority,* linking achievement with self-concept. The ability to compete productively in academic, extracurricular, social, and family realms in large part determines the child's sense of self-efficacy. Highly self-efficacious individuals believe in the relative ability to master and control the situation to achieve goals and rewards. In the face of failure and disappointment, children with moderate to high self-efficacy will reapply themselves in an industrious fashion and develop a range of skills for overcoming obstacles. In contrast, low self-efficacy may be both the result and the cause of personal failure in developing social and academic skills. Children of this age are always measuring themselves and their achievements against others. This is part of the normal process but may be exaggerated in families or schools that push competition and competitiveness.

Although earlier **explorations into separation** have been experienced, the school-age years are filled with a need to separate from parents for more prolonged periods. The ability to master these outings (e.g., sleepovers, camp) and to use independent **coping skills** when away from home appears critical for healthy development. While the separation process progresses, the child must still manage to function in the home in a manner that allows for recognition of new responsibilities. Chores and homework become frequent testing grounds for conflict resolution skills. These conflicts are really about psychological separation and control. With the child's increased cognitive and verbal sophistication, arguments between parent and child can take on the appearance of a courtroom as each side argues with righteousness over the obvious logic and illogic of the case.

Fantasy and Identification

The psychological work of school-age children involves the *active use of fantasy and identification* with real and imagined characters who do what the child can only wish to do.[8] This

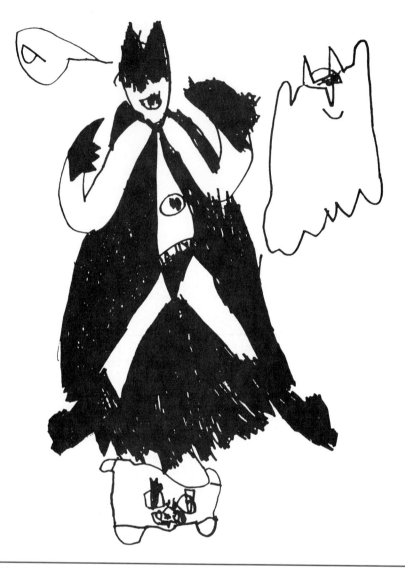

An 8-year-old boy drew this picture, about which he proudly described, "It's me . . . I'm strong and brave and can fly anywhere!" By Ilan Levin.

allows the emotionally healthy school-age child to express feelings without losing self-control. The boy who identifies with a professional athletic team may find expression for aggressive feelings by loudly denouncing a rival team (e.g., "I hate the Raiders!"). Although the child may have only recently outgrown a variety of fears, he may boast of his prowess in the face of the unknown by wearing a superheroes T-shirt. He may communicate to others and to

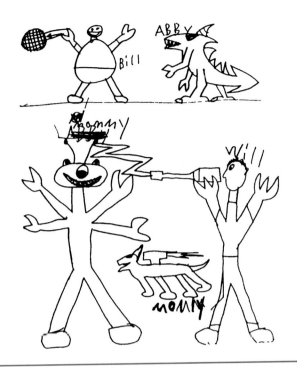

This drawing was done by a 9-year old boy who had been admitted to the hospital on three occasions for severe abdominal pain and vomiting without a detectable organic cause. His parents had separated. In this drawing, the child demonstrates aggression toward his mother and separates his idolized father ("Bill") and a symbolized monster-sister ("Abby").

himself his capacity for aggression by wearing military clothing and engaging in mock but fierce battles with real or imaginary opponents. A school-age girl may identify strongly with the sensuality of a popular actress or singer or with the controlled aggression of a woman tennis champion or ballerina.

The physical, aesthetic, and aggressive actions of these heroes provide an outlet for normal, age-appropriate sexual feelings and drives. Their presence in a child's life can be demonstrated in the clinician's office by asking specific questions ("Who would you most like to be?"), by observing and commenting on the child's clothing and favorite possessions, and by reviewing a child's artwork (see Chapter 26).

It is essential that a child this age be able to spend some of her energy in such fantasy and yet also express herself through active participation in the *real* world. Emotional problems may occur when a child becomes lost in fantasy and fails to gain a sense of competence in dealing with the actual world. The boundary between fantasy and reality should be clear at this age. Behavior problems may occur if a child fails to learn to use fantasy as a means of expressing feelings and instead acts out many of her impulses in real situations, or isn't clear about the effect of fantasy.

Academic Skills

Achievement at school becomes more demanding and complex at this time. Tests, grades, and special classes exert a significant effect on school-age children. Repeating a grade level is one of the most stressful events for an elementary school child, outranking the death of a close friend and just below having a visible congenital deformity.[9] The expectations placed on students by their parents, teachers, and ultimately themselves have a significant impact on learning rate, academic ranking, and the child's sense of self-worth.[10,11] Children with exaggeratedly optimistic or pessimistic expectations will demonstrate significant problems in work motivation and frustration tolerance.[12]

Distinct learning disabilities and learning styles may become most obvious during this time as the cognitive operations required in class become increasingly complex, sequential, and reading based. For mastery to occur, it is important for the child to recognize her capacity to meet the expectations of teachers and parents by assuming responsibility and developing the skills to complete assigned tasks.

By age 7 most children have become proficient in *decoding* basic symbols. Academic demands change qualitatively midway through grade school. A child without any learning disability may develop a "working disability" manifested by low productivity and difficulty in encoding information.[13]

During the *encoding* process, the child may be asked to access previously gained knowledge, organize it, and express it verbally or in writing. Writing an essay and solving a numerical word problem are examples of encoding tasks. Levine et al.[14] have termed disability in such tasks "developmental output failure," which can appear for the first time in some children as late as middle school or junior high. Such children form an extremely heterogenous group with respect to the underlying disorders responsible for their generally poor productivity. Expressive language deficits, attentional deficits, fine motor problems, and even emotional problems may interact to produce the same clinical picture. These children may be seen as "lazy." Although a few students put little energy into their work because of individual temperamental style, many students are handicapped by real neurologically based learning disabilities that can and should be addressed. For example, some children with fine motor difficulties benefit from being given the opportunity to present their work orally, use a computer, or present less work of better quality. The clinician serves such children by helping families, teachers, and the children themselves see the problem in terms of underlying neurodevelopmental disabilities rather than to look at it simply as "work refusal." Through effective advocacy, the clinician can identify these children for further evaluation and educational remediation.

As demand for output increases, so does the complexity of the academic tasks that face the child in grades 2 through 4. Mussen et al.[15] have pointed to five additional aspects of the learning process that are a result of a higher level of central nervous system maturation:

- Perception—the detection, organization, and interpretation of information from both the outside world and the internal environment
- Memory—the storage and later retrieval of information
- Reasoning—the use of information to make inferences and draw conclusions
- Reflection—the evaluation of the quality of ideas and solutions
- Insight—the recognition of new relationships between two or more bits of information

Successful learning requires an ability to attend school and use these cognitive and perceptual attributes. The clinician can examine the child's capacity for such thinking by asking him to tell a story about something that happened to him or about a movie he saw. Alternatively, he can be asked a series of questions that assess increasingly sophisticated educational skills, such as the following:

- Memory—"Where did you go on your vacation?"
- Reasoning—"Why did your family decide to go there?"
- Reflection and analysis—"What did you like best and least about the trip? Why?"
- Insight and creativity—"Where would you like to go if you could go anywhere? Why?"

The nature of the child's answers may reveal the capacity to make use of and communicate the knowledge he has, a task that is increasingly important as the child progresses through school.

Expansion of Activities with Peers

School-age children immerse themselves in sports, clubs, crafts, organizations, music, baseball cards, current fads, and a variety of other activities. These pursuits reflect a drive to master specific motor, social, and artistic skills that are fashioned out of individual experiences and cultural expectations. Some children spend hours drawing, whereas others shoot basketball, write poetry, or build remote-control cars. Doing the "in thing" becomes extremely important at this age, and most school-age children pursue sex-stereotyped activities with same-gender friendship groupings. Every child should have at least one such area of activity to which she, not her parents only, is committed.

Participation in organized athletic and artistic **activities** becomes an important part of the life of most school-age children.[16] By age 6 years, children become aware of their abilities in various areas and in comparison with other children. At this age they may participate in team sports competitively while they rely on adults to structure the activity; at times they may have difficulty in maintaining interest throughout the game. They may even be unclear about the outcome of a game in which they were involved. Nevertheless, by age 10 years, many children have participated in sports and other performance activities that include intense training, commitment, physical risk, and physical contact. The child involved in such activities learns basic skills, rules, and the meaning of teamwork and discipline. She also has fun and develops **friendships,** and this may be reason enough to participate. For the child who is resistant to participation in a team sport, an individual sport (e.g., tennis or swimming) may be encouraged.

Perhaps most central to the school-age years is the *quest for social involvement and social acceptance.* Most children seek to find a place for themselves among a cohesive group of same-sex friends. Their success in maintaining a positive sense of self during the vicissitudes of making and breaking friendships is in part dependent on the resilience of their coping and social skills.[17] Children with positive peer relations tend to give and receive positive attention, conform to classroom rules, and perform well academically. They are also able to initiate social contact in a positive manner and tend to develop pleasant social interchanges with others.[18]

Social skills may encompass a good sense of humor, an ability to make others feel wanted, a willingness to share, a positive mood, creativity, leadership, and negotiation skills.

These abilities are developed typically through observation of others (e.g., peers, parents, siblings, teachers, and even television). For most children, friendships develop naturally as social involvement is pursued. The child's temperament (see Chapter 2) appears to be an important contributor in the school-age child's ability to develop competency at play and in making and losing friendships.[19] Social interactions with peers and teachers in school settings depend not only on the characteristics of the school and the child's abilities and background, but also on the child's temperament.[20] A slow-to-warm-up child may resist social assimilation into the school community. He may appear at first as "anxious" or "insecure." Temperamentally difficult children may appear "immature" as a result of impulsive, disruptive behaviors in class and on the playground.[21] The child with low persistence, a short attention span, high distractibility, and a high activity level is at risk for early unfavorable judgments by peers.[22] Highly impulsive children with attention deficit hyperactivity disorder (ADHD) may experience significant problems with initiating and sustaining desirable social interactions because of their underlying temperament.

On the other hand, scapegoating, teasing, bullying, and self-isolation become social dynamics that can seriously hinder the child with poor social skills.[23] In addition, an intrinsic social-cognitive dysfunction, such as a learning disability, can impair social awareness and skill.[24] An assessment of the components of social cognition can help the clinician focus on the child's specific problems (Table 19-1). A clearer definition of the social deficits may guide management in a primary care setting (Box 19-1).

Children with difficult, *high-strung temperaments* generally show greater mood intensity and lability and have a greater tendency to develop behavioral and psychosomatic symptoms. Children who tolerate frustration poorly, have difficulties with sharing, and stand out as different because of cultural, psychosocial, or physical conditions are at high risk for an array of behavioral, somatic, and developmental conditions. One study found that being labeled by a teacher as a school-age child who "failed to get along" was a more predictive factor of adolescent and adult criminality than any other single factor.[26]

RISK AND PROTECTIVE FACTORS

Adjustment disorders, a condition that describes changes in behavior, mood, or academic performance after a stressful life event, are common in school-age children. Divorce, domestic violence,[27] child abuse,[28] natural disasters, and a serious accident or illness of a family member can also have significant emotional effects on the developmental work of school-age children.[29-31] The impact of any loss is experienced by school-age children with a growing awareness of its permanence and a feeling of being responsible for events around them.[32]

When **stress** exceeds coping resources, maladaptation results. Some children will respond to stress overload by becoming depressed, anxious, or preoccupied with body functions, whereas others may become provocative, angry, and demanding. The array of psychological dysfunctions has been conceptualized as fitting into two broad groupings of disorders—*internalizing and externalizing*[33] (Table 19-2).

Recurrent symptoms of pain, especially head, abdominal, and limb pain, are frequent during the school-age years[33] and in some cases may lead to difficulties in functioning

TABLE 19-1 ■ Social Cognitive Dysfunction: Troubled Subcomponents

Subcomponent	Trouble
Weak greeting skills	Initiating social contact with a peer skillfully
Poor social predicting	Estimating peer reactions before acting or talking
Deficient self-marketing	Projecting an image acceptable to peers
Problematical conflict resolution	Settling social disputes without aggression
Reduced affective matching	Sensing and fitting in with others' moods
Social self-monitoring failure	Knowing when one is in social trouble
Low reciprocity	Sharing and supporting, reinforcing others
Misguided timing or staging	Knowing how to nurture a relationship over time
Poor verbalization of feelings	Using language to communicate true feelings
Inaccurate inference of feelings	Reading others' feelings through language
Failure of code switching	Matching language style to current audience
Lingo dysfluency	Using the parlance of peers credibly
Poorly regulated humor	Using humor effectively for current context and audience
Inappropriate topic choice and maintenance	Knowing what to talk about and for how long
Weak requesting skill	Knowing how to ask for something inoffensively
Poor social memory	Learning from previous social experience
Assertiveness gaps	Exerting right level of influence over group actions
Social discomfort	Feeling relaxed while relating to peers

Modified from Parker S, Zuckerman B, editors: *Behavioral and developmental pediatrics: a handbook for primary care*, New York, 1995, Little, Brown & Co, p 326.

in several areas (Table 19-3). Although most of these recurrent pains are idiopathic with negative physical examination findings,[34-36] many parents of these children have higher rates of depression and somatic preoccupation,[37,38] suggesting a familial pattern of underlying stress. Habit problems are also prevalent in school-age children. Affected children and their parents become increasingly concerned about nocturnal enuresis, encopresis, thumb sucking, nail biting, hair pulling, and other childhood habits as social ostracism becomes more fervent.[39] Recurrent idiopathic pain in school-age children may be a clue to inappropriate anxiety within the child or family.

BOX 19-1	SOCIAL COGNITIVE DYSFUNCTION—MANAGEMENT STRATEGIES

Explain the social skill problems carefully to the child. These may require multiple sessions; not all affected children can process such information readily.

Have the parent of the child who needs social improvement accompany that child to an activity with other children. Then, during a calm and private interlude, the parent can discuss the social interactions (especially any *faux pas* and transgressions that occurred).

Help the child locate one or two companions with whom to relate and begin to build skills. It can be helpful if such peers share interests and perhaps some traits with the unpopular child.

Inform the classroom teacher or building principal if a child is victimized by peer abuse in school. It is the school's responsibility to make every effort to contain this activity. A strongly worded note from a primary health care provider may be vital in such cases.

Help the rejected child develop skills, hobbies, or areas of expertise that can enhance self-esteem and be impressive to other children. The management of such a child should always include the diligent quest for and development of such specialties. Ideally, such pursuits should have the potential for generating collaborative activities with other children.

Never force these children into potentially embarrassing situations before their peers. For example, an unpopular child with poor gross motor skills needs some protection from humiliation in physical education classes.

Manage any family problems or medical conditions through counseling, specific therapies (e.g., language intervention or help with motor skills), and/or medication (e.g., for attention deficits or depression).

Identify social skills training programs within schools and in clinical settings. Clinicians should be aware of local resources that offer social skills training to youngsters with social cognitive deficits. Most commonly this training makes use of specific curricula that are used in small group settings in a school or in the community.

Reassure these children that it is appropriate for them to be themselves, that they need not act and talk like everyone else in school, that there is true heroism in individuality. Clinicians, teachers, and parents must tread the fine line between helping with social skills and coercing a child into blind conformity with peer pressures, expectations, and models.

From Parker S, Zuckerman B, editors: *Behavioral and developmental pediatrics: a handbook for primary care,* New York, 1995, Little, Brown & Co, p 327.

TABLE 19-2 ■ Internalizing and Externalizing Disorders

Internalizing disorders	Externalizing disorders
Psychosomatic complaints	Disruptive behaviors
Depression	Negativism
Withdrawal	Hyperactivity
Anxiety	Conduct disorders

TABLE 19-3 ■ Behavioral-Somatic Symptoms Common During School-Age Years*

Symptom	Psychosomatic Conversion Reaction	Maturational Behavior
Headache	+++	
Recurrent abdominal pain	+++	
Limb pain	++	
Chest pain	I	
Enuresis	+	+++
Encopresis	+	
Thumb sucking	+	+
Hair pulling	+	
Nail biting	+	
Ritual behaviors		+++
Sleep disturbance	+	+

* **Psychosomatic conversion reactions** = symptoms that typically result from situational stress or depression in either the child or parent; **maturational behavior** = residual behaviors seen in some typical children from an earlier stage in development, but not associated with stress or depression; **+++** = common symptom (10%-15% of school-age children); **+** = less common symptom (less than 5% of children).

Matthew is a 7-year-old white boy who has experienced crampy, periumbilical, abdominal pain almost daily for the past 2 months. The symptom had not changed his activity level, appetite, or general behavior, so his mother did not make an earlier appointment for an evaluation. A bright, articulate, and charming child, Matthew has been successful in school and sports and has several close friends; the bellyaches have not altered any of these activities. He denies constipation, diarrhea, nausea, vomiting, dysuria, urinary frequency, trauma, or headaches.

Matthew's birth history and developmental course are uneventful. Described by his mother as a calm baby, he is her first child, and she seems to enjoy nurturing him. An emergency room visit at 2 years of age for a simple chin laceration, a few episodes of reactive airway disease associated with viral illnesses, and an occasional bout with otitis media are the extent of his medical history. A comment in the chart at his 5-year health supervision visit was noted: "Bright and verbal child, inquisitive, enjoys drawing and playing with friends, new sibling past year/appears to have adjusted well."

Family history is negative for gastrointestinal disorders, such as peptic ulcer, inflammatory bowel disease, food intolerance, or irritable bowel syndrome. The parents both work and are successful in their jobs, and no financial stress or marital discord is evident. Matthew, his younger brother, and his parents spend weekends together as a family.

When asked to describe the pain, he points to the periumbilical region and says it is "like the cramps—achy." It lasts from 5 to 30 minutes, occasionally several hours. The pain never radiates, never awakens him at night, and is not accompanied by other symptoms. Lying down or sitting quietly usually resolves the pain.

Physical examination is normal, including a blood pressure determination, growth measurements, and a digital rectal examination. A mental status and neurodevelopmental screening test are normal. Matthew's family drawing (completed while waiting in the office) reveals visual-motor skills and an active imagination, appropriate for his age and gender. Signs of anxiety or depression are not observed. The following laboratory studies are performed, all with normal results: complete blood count, erythrocyte sedimentation rate, urinalysis, and a stool examination for ova and parasites and occult blood.

At the initial visit and before the laboratory studies, the pediatrician emphasizes the normal physical examination findings and the absence of associated symptoms that might suggest a specific cause for his pain. A brief discussion about the connection between "feelings and tummy aches" is initiated. A drawing of a transverse section of the intestinal tract is used to show Matthew how the smooth muscle lining constricts and dilates in response to signals from the brain. Strong feelings, such as anger or sadness, can "change the tightness" of these muscles, causing pain. It is suggested that sometimes kids with bellyaches may feel pain when they are really feeling a strong emotion. Matthew listens attentively and asks a few questions about the illustration of the intestinal tract. Empirical dietary recommendations are written down: limit dairy products and increase fiber and fresh fruits. A follow-up appointment is made for 2 weeks.

> *At the next visit, the abdominal pain pattern and frequency has not changed; it is neither worse nor improved. The pediatrician then interviews the mother alone to explore the family constellation further. This 10-minute interview does not reveal any new information; the mother is given an opportunity to share her concern about her son. The family is emotionally healthy, and Matthew's school performance and social development are on track. Periodic sibling rivalries with his 5-year-old brother are at times troublesome but are manageable and not out of the ordinary.*
>
> *Matthew is then interviewed alone. When asked why he thinks he experiences the pain, he says, "I guess some kids just get it. I don't know why." An assessment of Matthew's affect and interpersonal interactions does not suggest either anxiety or depression.*

Poor **school performance** may be the result of stress overload, sensory-perceptual limitations, learning disabilities, behavioral disorders, retardation, or a host of other potential factors.[40,41] Three percent of elementary-age children have a hearing impairment, almost 25% have visual defects, and 1% have a major speech articulation disorder. In addition, 10% to 20% have a definable learning disability in reading, arithmetic, attention, visual-spatial skills, or other areas of neuropsychological functioning. Children with disabilities that limit their capacity for learning are at twice the risk for developing school avoidance, disruptive behavior problems, depression, and psychosomatic reactions. Concern about poor academic performance may bring a child to the clinician; at other times it is the child's emotional or psychosomatic response to the disability that raises parental concern. Behavioral symptoms and somatic functioning that appear during school days but either lessen or resolve during holidays and weekends may be an important clue to discovering related developmental disorders.

Children with chronic medical diseases carry an additional burden for behavioral and developmental adjustment disorders. Children with central nervous system dysfunction are at three to four times greater risk for behavioral, emotional, and learning problems than is the general population of children.[42] Differences in adjustment capacities do not correlate with the type of illness; they are most affected by family functioning.[43] The quality of the parent-child relationship, emotional disorder in the parents, and marital discord are the strongest predictors of maladjustment for chronically ill and healthy children.[44] In addition, the extent of functional limitation imposed by the illness and its treatment contribute to the risk for maladaptation.[45]

School-age children with greater intelligence, those with easier temperaments, and those from more organized families are at reduced risk for significant behavioral and developmental problems.[46] Flexible coping skills, an internal sense that one can have a positive effect on events and people, and good physical health are also important moderators of stress.[47,48]

Family functioning appears to be both the strongest risk and the strongest protective factor. Genetic predisposition to depression, alcoholism, obesity, learning disabilities, conduct problems, and psychosomatic preoccupations often will become apparent only through a focused family history interview. Of equal importance is the extent to which a family is successful in helping the child develop the necessary skills for social and academic success. Studies of resilience emphasize parental modeling of coping skills and the need to maintain predictable rules and expectations at home. Social support from friends, family, and others exerts significant influence in moderating the range of acute and chronic stress. Although peer friendships are important in helping children become socialized, studies of resilient children suggest that having one healthy, interested, caring, and predictable adult can do a great deal for children facing numerous barriers to their development.[49]

The target for assessment, strengthening, and intervening remains the child's environment, which includes the family unit as always, but also school and outside activities for the school-age child.

ASSESSMENT

Interviewing the school-age child can be a challenge, but certain skills and attitudes will help. In recognition of the child's concerns about competency, the first rule is to focus on abilities and strengths. This will allow the child to present herself in a controlled fashion, which will help in the development of trust. Early questions about stressful events or feelings should be avoided until the child settles down and appears more comfortable. Consequently, questions about the three arenas (family, school, and social functioning) can be ordered such that the least stressful area is discussed first and the most worrisome is left for last. Predictions about this can be made from the information gained from parents, your own observations, and the presenting problem.

Developmental and behavioral assessment of the school-age child should broadly assess the child's functioning at home, in school, with friends, and in the community. The child and parents can be interviewed together, but some time with the child alone will be important to establish your sense of her as an independent and competent individual.

OBSERVATIONS

While the clinician is engaged in developing rapport and expanding her data base, her observations of the child and family will be helpful.
- What are the child's and parent's general mood and level of interaction?
- Is the child's behavior appropriate for age, pseudomature, or delayed?
- How well does the parent allow the child to speak for himself?
- Are there indications of underlying anger, distrust, or worry?
- How age appropriate are the child's basic skills of speech, concentration, attention, and compliance?
- How close do the parents seem with each other, and how close are they with this child?
- How do the parents respond when their child seems anxious, angry, or embarrassed?
- How much do the parents control the child's behavior during the visit?
- How easy or difficult is it to relate to this child and family?

Questions regarding the child's functioning should focus on strengths and successes, as well as concerns and weaknesses. Such terms as *problems* and *failures* should be avoided. Helping the family keep a balanced perspective while discussing the child is extremely important to avoid belittling the child in a disrespectful and potentially harmful fashion. To spend some time with the child alone, explain that this is part of your standard practice with children who are on their way to being teenagers. Showing an interest in getting to know the child and wanting to give him a chance to discuss things in a more private way are also important goals to convey. Clarifying that you will treat him like any competent patient by keeping his communications confidential is also helpful.

DATA GATHERING

The clinician should gather information from the child about all aspects of his life—family, school, and social.

Family Functioning

- Tell me about what the family enjoys doing together.
- What are you allowed to do now that you couldn't do when you were younger?
- What chores do you have at home? How easy is it to do them? What happens if you forget?
- If you have a problem at school or with a friend, who do you talk to about it?
- How much fighting goes on between you and your brother or sister?
- What are the most important rules at home?
- What type of punishment do your parents use?
- How important is it to your parents that you succeed in school, sports, or chores?
- What new freedoms do you expect to get over the next few years?
- What parts of your parents do you wish to be like when you have children?
- Tell me about a usual Sunday. What happens? Who does what with whom?
- What do your parents worry about with you?
- What do you worry about at home?

School Functioning

- What do you like about school the most?
- What do you dislike about school?
- What subjects are easy? Which ones are hard?
- What kind of grades are you getting this year? How about last year? Are you happy with them?
- What is your teacher like this year?
- Do you ever worry that it is extra hard for you to do something the teacher asks?
- Have you ever gotten into trouble for the way you behave at school? What happened?
- How much school have you missed recently?
- Do you ever visit the nurse's office or feel sick in school?
- How do you get along with the other children at school? Do you have friends? Do you have enemies or people who pick on you?
- If you were the principal or teacher, what rules would you change?

- What jobs or careers do you think you would enjoy?
- Do you like to read? Do you read for fun?

Social Functioning

- What kinds of things do you like to do after school and on weekends?
- What are you good at? What types of things do you enjoy and do well?
- Who is your best friend? How long have you known him or her? How often do you get together? What do you like about him or her?
- Can you talk about worries and problems with your friends?
- Have you ever lost a friend? What happened? How did you cope?
- Do you and your friends ever fight or have problems sharing? How do you settle it?
- Do your friends have special problems at their home? Do they worry about their parents?
- Have you slept over at friends' homes? Have they stayed with you?
- What types of things do you wish you could do or learn?
- Have your friends gotten interested in boys or girls? What kind of grades do they get? Are they experimenting with cigarettes, alcohol, or drugs? What are they good at?
- Do you belong to any teams, groups, or clubs?
- How well do you behave when you are out in the neighborhood? Do you get in any fights?
- Has anyone ever hurt you or made you do something you didn't want to do?
- If you could have anything or change anything, what three things might you wish for?
- What is the hardest thing you have ever had to deal with?
- If you could be any age, what age would you pick?
- Is this year going better, worse, or about the same as last year? How come?

ANTICIPATORY GUIDANCE

The child's clinician can offer specific guidance to the child and family directed toward the development of responsible, competent behaviors.

- Counseling about *accident prevention* recognizes the school-age child's cognitive ability to connect an event with an outcome and focuses on the innate interest in controlling one's environment. Thus the need for seat belts, responsible bike riding, skating, rollerblading, and snowboarding should be mentioned because these continue to be the leading causes of death and injury in children.[50]
- When family risk factors for *obesity* are determined, a balanced diet (low in saturated fats, refined carbohydrates, and salt) and regular exercise for all family members should be encouraged.
- Counseling children about *smoking and drinking alcohol* should begin at this age. By encouraging the child's active involvement in these discussions, responsibility and self-control are promoted at an early age.[51] Parents who smoke are more likely to stop when the impact of their smoking on the health of their children is emphasized (e.g., ear infections, allergies, asthma, other respiratory infections, and behavior problems).[52] Questions directed to parents about alcohol and other substance abuse in family members can be re-

vealing (see Chapter 22). Introducing these risks in the context of the parents' habits may encourage a discussion about smoking, drugs, and alcohol with children in the home.

■ Parents can enhance the child's feeling of *responsibility* by having clear expectations of the child for initiating and completing chores and homework.

■ Gradual increases in *independent activities* can be an encouragement for child behaviors that demonstrate trustworthiness and competence.

Extracurricular activities should be supported, but care should be taken to avoid the "hurried child syndrome,"[12] in which the pressures to excel far outweigh the pleasures to explore and experience. This may be particularly true with the school-age child's participation in competitive sports, whether as an individual or on a team. Parents should be encouraged to carefully balance the amount of attention placed on performance and the degree to which the activity is enjoyable and helpful for social maturation. Clearly, some children are very comfortable and ready to participate in competitive sports, whereas others may lack interest, skill, or confidence. Box 19-2 lists the developmental skills required for sports participation.

Parents may be encouraged to maintain reasonable, predictable, and observable boundaries and rules so that the child can accurately predict the parents' positive and negative responses to behavior. Children need to learn a variety of skills, including delay of gratification and frustration tolerance, which can be developed only when negative events are experienced and tolerated. Parents may consult with the child about their concerns, but they

---

BOX 19-2   READINESS FACTORS INFLUENCING SPORTS PARTICIPATION

Cognitive development (Piaget)—Stages of Understanding Game Rules
Egocentric, play using personal rules
Cooperative play
Perception of rules as human productions that can be changed when participants agree

Moral Development (Kohlberg)—Stages of Moral Reasoning
Self-gratification and avoiding punishment
Desire to win approval
Internal sense of ethics (i.e., internalization of a sense of fair play and sportsmanship)

Motor Readiness
Basic prerequisites: running, throwing, hand-eye coordination
Minor prerequisites: height, weight, skeletal age
Specific skills for different sports: e.g., soccer vs. swimming vs. gymnastics vs. baseball

Psychological Readiness—Achievement Motivation and Desire to Perform Successfully
Capacity to evaluate own competence
Capacity to compare own performance with others
Integration of self and comparison evaluations

Modified from Livingood AB, Goldwater C, Kurz RB: Psychological aspects of sports participation in young children. In Camp BW, editor: *Advances in behavioral pediatrics*, vol 2, Greenwich, Conn, 1981, Jai Press, pp 141-169.

are wise to avoid premature suggestions or advice in favor of supporting the child's own problem-solving efforts. The clinician can identify areas of stress for the child and invite family-initiated solutions. Changes in the school and social environments that will support positive growth should be encouraged. Parents must get involved in those environments and understand their impact on the child to effect such positive change.

Clinicians may also anticipate with parents the conflicts that arise in children as they are increasingly exposed to the world outside the family. Children today are aware of violence on a global scale through the media and will almost certainly need help from their parents to deal with the news of events that produce anxiety even in adults and adolescents. Many of today's children are exposed to sexual material that may be perverse or bizarre through television, movies (including videos), and the Internet. Society supports parental guidance in such matters in a number of ways, from the existence of community groups such as the Parent-Teacher Association and the Violence Intervention Project for Children and Families[53] to the movie and television rating system that has been refined to include a "PG-13" rating and the recently introduced "V-chip" that can regulate access to channels. As a children's advocate who is aware of the potential toxicity of exposure to excessive amounts of television (as well as other forms of passive entertainment), the pediatrician has a responsibility to raise the issue of television viewing with parents.[54,55] Parents must understand the confusion and anxiety such material can engender in the child 7 to 10 years old. Parents can be encouraged to limit the child's exposure and provide an atmosphere in which the child feels free to share concerns and clear up misconceptions.

Finally, for those children who experience a major life stress such as a divorce, death, or school failure, the clinician should be an advocate for the child by keeping the child's developmental needs in focus and coping strategies intact. At least one domain should remain a positive area of success for the child as struggles continue in other domains. At the close of each visit, the child and parent should be complimented on their particular strengths. Families will come to anticipate these office visits as an opportunity to share their child's achievements, as well as a place to explore current behavioral and developmental concerns.

The case of Aaron, who had experienced a recent onset of headaches, may be evaluated in the context of developmental issues of a school-age child. Aaron's headaches may stem from stress overload after the loss of a friendship. His social skills appear somewhat limited by his intense preoccupations. His coping style has always been to withdraw and distract by occupying himself with more pleasant stimuli. His parents' responses have often heightened concern and further reinforced his symptomatic behaviors. His social skills in developing and maintaining friendships appear lacking.

After ruling out serious physical illness, his parents were reassured. They were encouraged to decrease the secondary gains (i.e., increased attention, new baseball cards, no chores, no homework) and to return him to school. He was allowed to use acetaminophen for pain analgesia but was also forced to be out of his room and out of his house for approximately 1 hour per day. His father was encouraged to involve Aaron in league baseball and to practice regularly with his son to build up his stamina and sense of resilience. The family was also encouraged to have Aaron arrange to bring friends over to the house. Within 2 weeks Aaron's headaches were gone and his social and academic functioning returned to normal. He continues to be a child of somewhat increased risk as a result of a family history of emotional problems and his own difficult temperament and problematical social skills. On the other hand, his intelligence, his organized and concerned family, and his general competence may serve as important moderators in helping him maintain a positive adjustment.

ACKNOWLEDGMENT

Nicholas Putnam, M.D., contributed to portions of this chapter in previous editions.

REFERENCES

1. Newacheck P, Taylor W: Prevalence and impact of childhood conditions, *Am J Public Health* 82:364, 1992.
2. Perrin EC et al: Issues involved in definition and classification of chronic health conditions, *Pediatrics* 91:787, 1993.
3. Piaget J: *The origins of intelligence in children,* New York, 1952, International University Press.
4. Piaget J, Inhelder B: *The psychology of the child,* New York, 1968, Basic Books.
5. Kohlberg L: *Essays on moral development,* vol 1, *The philosophy of moral development,* New York, 1981, Harper & Row.
6. Freud S: *Introductory lectures in psychoanalysis,* New York, 1965, WW Norton.
7. Erikson EH: *Childhood and society,* ed 2, New York, 1963, WW Norton.
8. Sarnoff C: *Latency,* New York, 1976, Aronson.
9. Heisel JS et al: The significance of life events as contributing factors in the diseases of children, *J Pediatr* 83:119, 1973.
10. Rosenthal R, Jacobson L: *Pygmalion in the classroom,* New York, 1968, Holt, Rinehart & Winston.
11. Samuels S: *Enhancing self-concept in early childhood: theory and practice,* New York, 1977, Human Sciences Press.
12. Elkind D: *The hurried child: growing up too fast, too soon,* Reading, Mass, 1988, Addison-Wesley.
13. Levine MD: *Developmental variation and learning disorders,* Cambridge, Mass, 1993, Educators Publishing Service.
14. Levine MD, Oberklaid F, Meltzer L: Developmental output failure: a study of low productivity in school age children, *Pediatrics* 67:18, 1981.
15. Mussen P, Conger J, Kagan J: *Child development and personality,* New York, 1969, Harper & Row.
16. American Academy of Pediatrics: *Sports medicine: health care for young athletes,* ed 2, Elk Grove Village, Ill, 1991, American Academy of Pediatrics.
17. Asher S, Renshaw P, Hymel S: Peer relations and the development of social skills. In Moore S, Cooper C, editors: *The young child: reviews of research,* vol 3, Washington, DC, 1982, National Association for the Education of Young Children.
18. Ollendick T, Oswald D, Francis G: Validity of teacher nominations in identifying aggressive, withdrawn and popular children, *J Clin Child Psychol* 18:221, 1989.
19. Murphy L, Moriarty A: *Vulnerability, coping and growth,* New Haven, Conn, 1976, Yale University Press.
20. Chess S, Thomas A: *Temperament in clinical practice,* New York, 1986, Guilford.
21. Carey WB, McDevitt SC: *Coping with children's temperament,* New York, 1995, Basic Books.
22. Martin RP: Activity level, distractibility, and persistence: critical characteristics in early schooling. In Kohnstamm GA, Bates JE, Rothbart MK, editors: *Temperament in childhood,* New York, 1989, Wiley, pp 451-461.
23. Asher SR, Coie JD: *Peer rejection in children,* Cambridge, Mass, 1990, Cambridge Press.

24. LeVine MD: *Developmental variation in learning disorders,* Cambridge, Mass, 1993, Cambridge Educators Publishing Service, pp 240-273.

25. Putnam N: Revenge or tragedy: do nerds suffer from a mild pervasive developmental disorder? In Feinstein S, editor: *Adolescent psychiatry: developmental and clinical studies,* Chicago, 1990, University of Chicago Press.

26. Janes CL, Hesselbrock VM: Problem children's adult adjustment predicted from teacher ratings, *Am J Orthopsychiatry* 48:300, 1978.

27. Alpert E, Freund K: *Partner violence: how to recognize and treat victims of abuse—a guide for physicians,* Waltham, Mass, 1992, Massachusetts Medical Society.

28. Ludwig S, Kornberg AE, editors: *Child abuse: a medical reference,* New York, 1992, Churchill Livingstone.

29. Frederick C: Children traumatized in small groups. In Eth S, Pynoos R, editors: *Post-traumatic stress disorders in children,* Washington, DC, 1985, American Psychiatric Press.

30. Pynoos R, Eth S: Children traumatized by witnessing acts of personal violence: homicide, rape or suicide behavior. In Eth S, Pynoos R, editors: *Post-traumatic stress disorders in children,* Washington, DC, 1985, American Psychiatric Press.

31. Williams S, Steiner H: Childhood trauma. In Klykylo W, Kay J, Rube D, editors: *Clinical child psychiatry,* Philadelphia, 1998, WB Saunders.

32. Achenbach TM, Edelbrock C: *Manual for the child behavior checklist and revised behavior profile,* Burlington, Vt, 1983, University of Vermont.

33. Schechter N, Berde C, Yaster M: *Pain in infants, children and adolescents,* Baltimore, Md, 1993, Williams & Wilkins.

34. Appley J: *The child with abdominal pains,* Boston, 1975, Blackwell Scientific Publications.

35. Stein MT et al: Challenging case: recurrent abdominal pain, *J Dev Behav Pediatr* 16:277, 1995.

36. Boyle JT: Recurrent abdominal pain: an update, *Pediatr Rev* 18(9):310, 1997.

37. Hughes M, Zimin R: Children with psychogenic abdominal pain and their families: management during hospitalization, *Clin Pediatr* 17:569, 1978.

38. Routh D, Ernst A: Somatization disorder in relatives of children and adolescents with functional abdominal pain, *J Pediatr Psychol* 9:427, 1984.

39. Schaefer C: *Childhood encopresis and enuresis: causes and therapy,* New York, 1979, Van Nostrand Reinhold.

40. Dworkin P: *Learning and behavior problems of school children,* Philadelphia, 1985, WB Saunders.

41. Wolraich, ML: *Disorders of development and learning: a practical guide to assessment and management,* St. Louis, 1996, Mosby.

42. Rutter M, Tizard J, Whitmore K: *Education, health and behavior,* London, 1970, Longman Group.

43. Breslau N: Does brain dysfunction increase children's vulnerability to environmental stress? *Arch Gen Psychiatry* 47:15, 1990.

44. Lewis BL, Khaw K: Family functioning as a mediating variable affecting psychosocial adjustment of children with cystic fibrosis, *J Pediatr* 101:636, 1982.

45. Stein R et al: Severity of illness: concepts and measurement, *Lancet* 2:1506, 1987.

46. Garmezy N: Stressors of childhood. In Garmezy N, Rutter M, editors: *Stress, coping and development in children,* New York, 1998, McGraw-Hill.

47. Block J, Block J: The role of ego-control and ego-resiliency in the organization of behavior. In Collin WA, editor: *Minnesota symposium on child psychology,* vol 13, Hillsdale, NJ, 1979, Erlbaum.

48. Werner E, Smith R: An epidemiologic perspective on some antecedents and consequences of childhood mental health problems and learning disabilities, *J Am Acad Child Psychiatry* 18:292, 1979.

49. Anthony E, Cohler B: *The invulnerable child,* New York, 1987, Guilford Press.

50. American Academy of Pediatrics: *Manual on injury prevention,* Elk Grove Village, Ill, 1997, American Academy of Pediatrics.

51. Epps RP, Manley MW: A physician's guide to preventing tobacco use during childhood and adolescence, *Pediatrics* 88:140, 1991.

52. Kemper, KJ: Parental drug, alcohol, and cigarette addiction. In Parker S, Zuckerman B, editors: *Behavioral and developmental pediatrics: a handbook for primary care,* Boston, 1995, Little, Brown & Co, pp 378-383.

53. Osofsky JD: Community-based approaches to violence prevention, *J Dev Behav Pediatr* 18(6):405, 1997.

54. Singer DC, Singer JL, Zuckerman DM: *Using TV to your child's advantage,* Reston, Va, 1990, Acropolis Books.

55. Strasburger VC: Children, adolescence and television, *Pediatr Rev* 13:144, 1992.

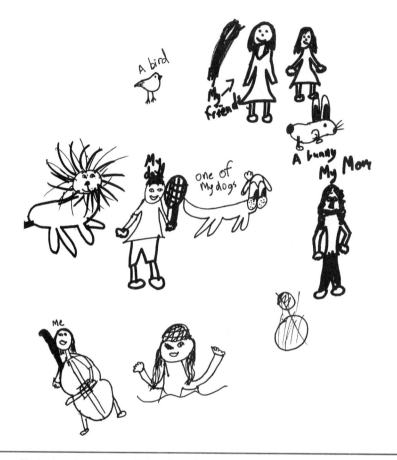

A girl drew herself playing the cello and also drew her mom, dad, two friends (upper right), and several family pets. She fuses her two older sisters into one. By Christina Wright, age 8.

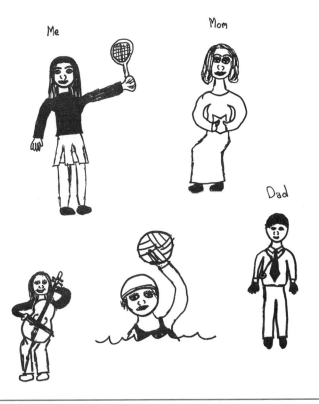

Christina's 12-year-old sister, Alexandra, drew this picture of her family at the same time that Christina drew the picture on page 424.

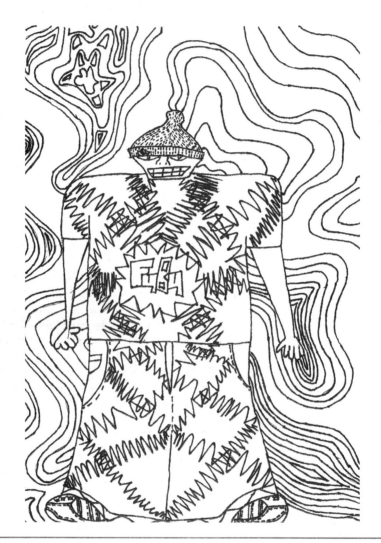

A 15-year-old boy draws an electrified self with baggy pants and cap pulled low. His shoes and labeled T-shirt complete the uniform of many young teens. His turbulent feelings and perceived complexity of the environment are conveyed by the patterned background. The teeth may signal some anger or a need to look fierce. By Brett Blaney.

426

CHAPTER 20

Eleven to Thirteen Years: Early Adolescence—Age of Rapid Changes

■ Marianne E. Felice
■ Jennifer Maehr

> **KEY WORDS**
> Adolescence
> Puberty
> Menarche
> Sexual Maturation
> Nocturnal Emissions
> Masturbation
> Vaginal Leukorrhea
> Peer Group
> Junior High or Middle School Transition
> Substance Abuse
> Gangs
> Concrete Thinking
> Tobacco

OVERVIEW OF ADOLESCENCE

Adolescence is the developmental phase between childhood and adulthood marked by rapid changes in physical, psychosocial, moral, and cognitive growth.[1] This developmental phase consists of three substages: early, mid, and late adolescence. Early adolescence generally refers to age 11 to 13, mid adolescence to age 14 to 16, and late adolescence, as a rule, denotes teenagers 17 years or older and may even extend to youths in their twenties. These age ranges are simply guidelines; many other factors contribute to the adolescent's placement in early, mid or late adolescence, including gender, cultural background, socioeconomic class, and health status. In order to address the pertinent needs of a particular adolescent, it is helpful to first determine in which developmental substage the youngster belongs. This model allows the clinician to tailor the approach to each teen patient.

Certain psychosocial growth tasks are specific to adolescence in general and to each substage of adolescence, as summarized in Box 20-1 and Table 20-1. The key issues are separation and independence, sexual identity, cognitive expansion, moral maturation, and preparation for an adult role in society. In other words, during adolescence, the individual must ask himself, "Who am I, where am I going, and how am I getting there?" For healthy adult-

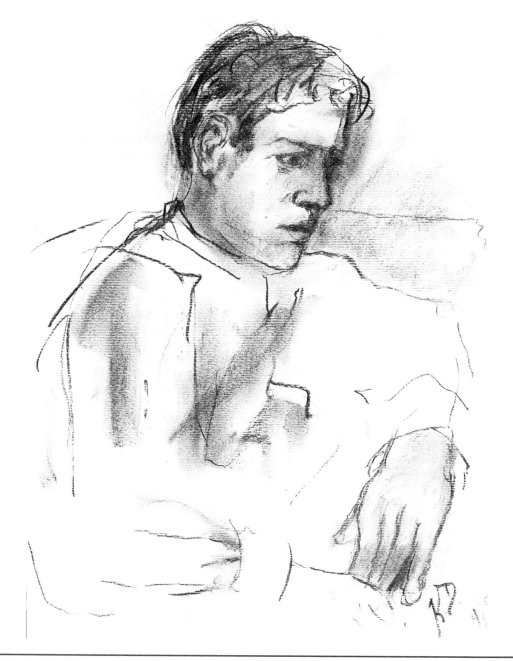

This sketch of a 14-year-old captures some of the anxiety, introspection, and slightly angry or rebellious look of adolescence. Love and consistent support are needed in spite of a cool demeanor. (Original is in charcoal with more definition.)

BOX 20-1	DEVELOPMENTAL GROWTH TASKS OF ADOLESCENCE

Gradual development as an independent individual
Mental evolution of a satisfying realistic body image
Harnessing appropriate control and expression of sexual drives
Expansion of relationships outside the home
Implementation of a realistic plan to achieve social and economic stability
Transition from concrete to abstract conceptualization
Integration of a value system applicable to life events

From Felice M: Adolescence. In Levine MD, Carey WB, Crocker AC, editors: *Developmental-behavioral pediatrics*, Philadelphia, 1983, WB Saunders.

TABLE 20-1 ■ Growth Tasks by Developmental Phase

Task	Early: 10-13 yr	Mid: 14-16 yr	Late: 17 yr +
Independence	Emotional break from parents; prefers friends to family	Ambivalence about separation	Integration of independence issues
Body image	Adjustment to pubescent changes	"Trying on" different images to find real self	Integration of satisfying body image with personality
Sexual drives	Sexual curiosity; occasional masturbation	Sexual experimentation; opposite sex viewed as sex object	Beginning of intimacy/caring
Relationships	Unisex peer group; adult crushes	Begin heterosexual peer group; multiple adult-role models	Individual relationships more important than peer group
Career plans	Vague and unrealistic plans	Vague and unrealistic plans	Specific goals/specific steps to implement them
Conceptualization	Concrete thinking	Concrete thinking fascinated by new capacity for thinking	Ability to abstract
Value system	Drop in superego; testing of moral system of parents	Self-centered	Self-centered idealism; rigid concepts of right and wrong; other-orientated, asceticism

From Felice ME: Adolescence. In Levine MD, Carey WB, Crocker AC, editors: *Developmental-behavioral pediatrics*, ed 2, Philadelphia, 1992, WB Saunders.

hood and personal maturity, mastery of all of these growth tasks is necessary. Like all psychological growth, however, progression through the substages does not occur in a straight line, but is marked by peaks, valleys, and plateaus. Progress in one area may influence progress in another area. For example, "late bloomers" in pubertal development may also be late bloomers in psychosocial development.

Despite the persistent myth that adolescence is tumultuous, most youth will complete adolescence without delinquency, school failure, parenthood, or drug addiction.[2] Rather, it is a developmental period that may baffle parents, frustrate health care providers, and even cause confusion for adolescents themselves. The industrious school-age child who was hard working, compliant, and quiet is suddenly seen as rebellious or unpredictable. The wide-eyed, shy child who was previously in adoration of his parents, teachers, and pediatrician is now viewed as insolent and outspoken. Without trying, adolescents may evoke uncomfortable feelings in the adults around them, often because of memories of the adult's own uncomfortable adolescence. Interaction with teens, however, can be an uplifting experience and a fresh reminder of the idealism of youth. The outspoken young person is actually in the midst of an age of wonderment and is someone who is searching to find herself while learning to make a contribution to society. A practitioner would miss a marvelous experience by not following a cohort of teens, particularly those followed from early childhood, onward as they make the journey toward adulthood.

EARLY ADOLESCENCE AND PHYSICAL DEVELOPMENT

Early adolescence, sometimes called preadolescence, is characterized by the onset of both **puberty** and gradual emergence of independence from the family. As physical changes occur in the body, early adolescents develop sexual curiosity and a heightened body consciousness. It is an important transition time that calls for developmental work by both parents and their growing youngsters. With anticipatory guidance, the health care provider can prepare and support the parent and adolescent in these changes.

To understand the behavior of early adolescents, one must become familiar with the normal pattern of puberty and appreciate the dramatic physical changes that are a part of it.[3] In the United States, pubescence usually begins for girls between the ages of 9 and 11 years with the development of breast buds, and for most boys between the ages of 10 to 12 years with testicular enlargement followed by lengthening of the penis.[4] Further signs of puberty occur over the next 2 to 6 years following a well-described pattern that is summarized in Fig. 20-1 and Table 20-2. In the United States, **menarche** normally occurs between the ages of 10 and 15 years with an average age of onset of 12.5 years.[5] Several factors seem to affect the timing of pubertal events and menarche, such as health, nutrition, ethnicity, and environmental conditions.[6,7] For example, black American girls tend to develop earlier than white American girls.[6] Fig. 20-2 and Table 20-3 demonstrate these differences in **sexual maturation** for more than 17,000 girls seen in pediatric practices across the United States. In this sample population, black girls entered puberty approximately 12 to 18 months earlier than white girls and began menses approximately 8.5 months earlier. The black girls also tended to have pubic hair development *before* breast development and earlier than expected by previous studies on other populations.[6] Given these ethnic differences, a strong argument exists for

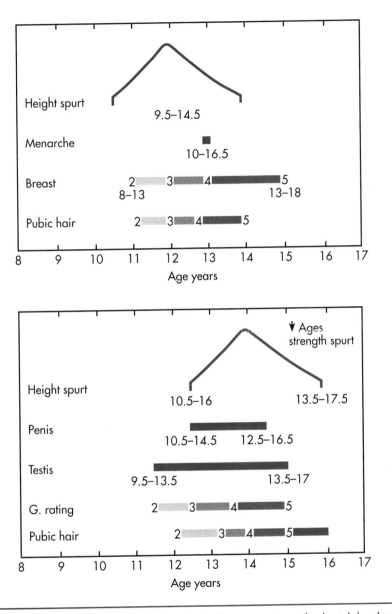

Fig. 20-1   Top, pattern of pubertal development of girls. Bottom, pattern of pubertal development of boys. (From Marshall WA, Tanner JM: *Arch Dis Child* 45:13, 1970.)

TABLE 20-2 ■ **Maturational Staging Criteria for Secondary Sexual Characteristics**

Breast Stage	Female
B1	No visible breast mound
B2	Breast buds: a small amount of subareolar breast tissue
B3	Amount of breast tissue increases
B4	Nipple is distinct from areola; areola forms a mound above breast tissue
B5	Areola recedes to the contour of breast

Genitalia	Male
G1	Infantile genitalia
G2	Scrotal skin reddens and thins; testes increase in size; minimal or no enlargement of phallus
G3	Continued enlargement of testes; phallus lengthens
G4	Continued enlargement of testes; increased length and circumference of phallus and glans penis
G5	Adult-sized testes (>20 cc) and adult-sized phallus; deeply pigmented scrotum

Pubic Hair	Female	Male
PH1	No pubic hair	No pubic hair
PH2	Long, downy hair on labia majora	Long, downy hair at base of phallus
	Coarse, curly hair in small amount on labia majora and mons pubis	Coarse, curly hair in small amount at base of phallus
PH3	Increased amount but not on median aspect of thighs	Increased amount, but not on median aspect of thighs
PH4	Triangular-shaped escutcheon; hair extends to median aspect of thighs	Triangular-shaped escutcheon; hair extends to median aspect of thighs

From Long TJ et al: *Curr Probl Pediatr* 14:1, 1984.

separate standards on normal sexual maturation, precocious puberty, and delayed puberty for white and black girls. Further research is needed to look at differences in pubertal development for girls from other ethnic groups, as well as for boys from various ethnic groups. In general, however, there has been a "secular" trend over the past century toward earlier puberty and larger growth. This change has been attributed largely to better health and nutrition. In North America and Europe, this trend may have leveled off but seems to be continuing in some developing countries where public health conditions are improving.[7]

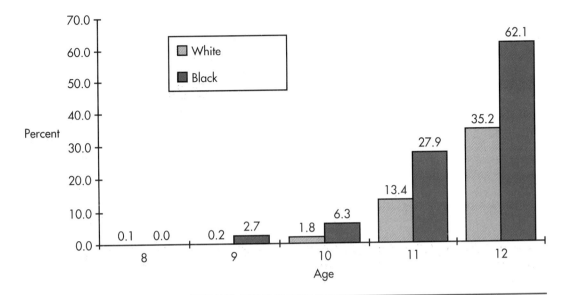

Fig. 20-2 Prevalence of menses by age and race. (Cochran-Mantel-Haenszel X^2 = 55.4, df = 1, P < .001; Breslow-Day X^2 = 4.9, df = 4. P = .295). (From Herman Giddens ME et al: *Pediatrics* 99:505, 1997.)

TABLE 20-3 ■ Mean Ages of Sexual Maturation for Black and White American Girls		
	Black American mean ± SD (years)	White American mean ± SD (years)
Breast: Tanner Stage 2	8.87 ± 1.93	9.96 ± 1.82
Breast: Tanner Stage 3	10.19 ± 1.42	11.30 ± 1.42
Pubic Hair: Tanner Stage 2	8.78 ± 2.00	10.51 ± 1.67
Pubic Hair: Tanner Stage 3	10.35 ± 1.63	11.53 ± 1.21
Any Development† Tanner Stage 2	8.11 ± 2.02	9.71 ± 1.87
Any Development† Tanner Stage 3	9.85 ± 1.59	11.14 ± 1.42
Menarche	12.16 ± 1.21	12.88 ± 1.20

Abbreviations: SD, standard deviation.
*$p < 0.001$ for the comparisons between black and white girls for each stage of development of breast, pubic hair, and menses.
†Denotes the appearance of either breast buds or pubic hair or both.
From Herman-Giddens ME et al: *Pediatrics* 99:505, 1997.

Until puberty, the only bodily changes most youngsters experience are quantitative, steady, and predictable increases in height and weight each year. With puberty, however, physical changes are much more dramatic and rapid, and are qualitatively different from previous ones.[8] Height increases suddenly; hair becomes coarse and appears to grow where it never grew before; major changes occur in the distribution of body fat and musculature; skin becomes oily; apocrine glands begin to secrete; genitals enlarge; and breasts develop.[9]

WORRIES ABOUT PHYSICAL DEVELOPMENT

With adolescence, appearance becomes more critical and may be imagined as much worse than it really is. This is a time for agonizing self-consciousness and painful sensitivity to body changes. Acne may develop, and braces often become necessary. Young adolescents may be unaware or acutely aware of the development of body odor and the need for deodorants and more frequent bathing. Furthermore, the physical changes that occur may be asynchronous, that is, body organs and subsystems may appear to grow at different rates, so that the arms, legs, nose, or chin may seem to enlarge with no apparent respect for overall body harmony.[10] The youngster may not know what to anticipate and may become very anxious about the seemingly out-of-control maturation that he is experiencing. It is not unusual for adolescents to spend hours before a mirror or in the bathroom becoming acquainted with the physical changes that appear to take place on a daily basis. They imagine that the world is as focused on these changes as they are, which is a healthy self-absorption.

Sometimes the physical changes that are observed are worrisome to young teens, who may harbor their own "explanatory models" for these events. For example, the pubertal boy who has gynecomastia (a normal occurrence in many boys during puberty)[5] may be alarmed that he is developing breasts like a girl or may fear that he has breast cancer; the girl who has been inadequately prepared for menstruation may believe that her first period is a result of internal injury or serious illness. All young adolescents are concerned about their bodily changes, whether they easily reveal their worries or not. It is important for the clinician to uncover and allay these concerns.

The young adolescent is well aware that not only is she changing, but also her friends are changing. Not all youngsters grow at the same time or at the same rate. A seventh grade class picture may show 12-year-olds in all sizes and shapes. Youngsters are acutely aware of how their physical changes compare with those of their friends, and they harbor some anxiety about the comparison. Many youngsters feel that they are growing too quickly or too slowly, too soon or too late.[11] These apprehensions are most often revealed by nonverbal or obtuse patterns of communication. Hence, the girl whose breasts are developing more quickly than those of her peers may adopt a hunched posture. The boy whose genitals are not quite as big as those of his friends may suddenly find excuses not to take gym or use the locker room.

The timing of puberty can affect the overall well-being of the adolescent, especially one who develops early or late. For example, boys who develop later tend to have poorer self-image and lower educational goals and tend to do more poorly in school than boys who progress through puberty earlier.[12] It is not difficult to imagine that the former little league star whose body fails to keep pace with the development of his peers may feel incredibly left behind or inferior to his old friends, especially if he is unable to make the varsity or junior varsity teams. Conversely, some girls who develop early, but still within the range of normal, tend to have a poorer self-image than girls who develop later.[11] Even the youngster whose maturation keeps pace with peers may feel out of step.

ADOLESCENT IN THE OFFICE

Jeremy, 12, his mother, and two younger siblings arrive at the doctor's office for his annual examination. When the nurse calls Jeremy, his mother and siblings remain behind in the waiting area. Jeremy follows the nurse, has his vitals measured and is told to undress and change into a gown. Jeremy then waits alone in the examination room; this visit is the first time that Jeremy has seen the doctor alone.

Before entering the room, the physician reviews Jeremy's chart and notices that he has grown 5 inches since the last visit. Jeremy has always been tall, but now he is far larger than most boys his age. The physician enters the examination room and greets Jeremy with a friendly hello. Jeremy meekly replies, "Hi," and looks down at the floor while fumbling with the ties on his gown. When the doctor asks, "What brings you to the clinic today?" Jeremy shrugs and says, "I don't know." Further questioning about school and home brings similar answers—shrugs, nods of head, or a short "yes" or "no" answer. The clinician, who is now feeling a bit uncomfortable, calls Jeremy's mother back to the examination room. Jeremy appears relieved at the sight of his mother and siblings.

Despite Jeremy's mature appearance, he was feeling awkward alone in the examination room with the physician. Jeremy wasn't sure how to answer the physician's questions and was feeling especially self-conscious because he was wearing nothing but an examination gown. It became clear to the physician that Jeremy was feeling uncomfortable. Many young teens like Jeremy have difficulty with the interview process because of their limitations with conceptualization and abstraction; clinicians quickly discover this during the examination process and have to adjust their interview questions to accommodate the developmental stage of the youngster. As with most younger adolescents, it may have been more helpful to have both Jeremy and his mother together initially in order to obtain a more complete history. Waiting to have Jeremy change into the gown until after the history may also have reduced Jeremy's discomfort.

While the physician talks with Jeremy and his mother, it becomes apparent that as Jeremy has grown, more expectations have been placed on him by his family, coaches, and teachers. Most people who meet Jeremy think that he is 14 or 15 years old. Even though he feels more comfortable with his boyhood friends, he often finds himself hanging out with older teenagers who are closer in size to him. Jeremy expresses that he feels under pressure to be the best when he plays sports. Some teachers look to him to be a leader, and when a disruption occurs, Jeremy feels singled out. At home, Jeremy finds himself doing more chores, such as putting away groceries, doing lawn work, and watching his younger siblings. His mother confesses that sometimes she forgets that he is only 12. She has given Jeremy more autonomy to set his own schedule and social and school activities.

People's expectations of adolescents are usually based on their size and appearance rather than on their age. Pointing this out to Jeremy can help validate some of his feelings. His mother may need to talk with teachers and coaches to discuss Jeremy's concerns and to see if any other issues are at play. It appears that Jeremy may appreciate more limit setting and guidance from his mother at this particular point in his life and that his mother may need assistance from the physician and Jeremy in deciding how to make these changes. Jeremy needs to know, however, that as youngsters get older, parents usually do expect more household help from them than in the past. Before Jeremy leaves, the physician takes additional time to discuss with him in private the further pubertal changes, both physical and emotional, that he can expect. The clinician also takes time alone with the mother to provide her with a developmental perspective of early adolescence, specifically for Jeremy, on issues relating to body image adjustment, separation from parents, limitations in the ability to project cognitively, and the importance of supportive friends.

SOCIAL AND SEXUAL DEVELOPMENT

As the young adolescent ponders the various changes taking place in his body, he begins to have an acute interest in sexual matters,[13] but is not usually sexually active and does not usually have a dating partner. The 8-year-old child may scorn romantic movies as "mush" and be embarrassed or even disgusted to see a couple kissing or embracing. The same child as a 12-year-old may now be fascinated by such matters and may even spy on older adolescent couples in order to learn from them. This is the age when parents may find "adult entertainment" magazines hidden under an adolescent's bed. Parents usually are caught off guard by this "early" interest in sexual matters and may believe that the child is already sexually active. As a result, parents may act more restrictively or punitively than in the past. It may be more helpful, however, for parents to turn this discovery into a teachable moment about issues of sexuality. Adolescents often use what they view on television and films, see in magazines, or hear on the radio to help develop their concepts regarding sexuality. For the most part, sexual relationships are portrayed in a nonrealistic fashion in these venues. Women may be sexually exploited; information on issues of safe sex and sexually transmitted diseases may be lacking; and extramarital affairs, multiple partners, and premarital sex may be seen as the norm. In addition, children and adolescents are exposed to numerous and various forms of violence by both audio and visual entertainment, including video and arcade games. Parents ideally need to take the time to watch the television programs or listen to the music that their teenagers are enjoying. In this way, parents can help interpret for the teens and put into context what they are seeing and hearing. This same vigilance also applies to the Internet because teens, who often are more experienced in "surfing the net" than adults, may find themselves with access to sexually explicit material or in potentially vulnerable situations in which they themselves may be exploited.

Early adolescence is the time when teens may begin to masturbate or have **nocturnal emissions** ("wet dreams"). Many myths concerning **masturbation** (e.g., masturbation causes blindness, acne, or hairy hands) exist, and young adolescents need reassurance that those myths are untrue. Occasionally a male adolescent may be frightened by the occurrence of wet dreams because the event happens beyond his control or because he believes the emission to be the result of an infectious disease. Similarly, the female adolescent may note a clear, mucoid discharge in her underpants for about six months before menarche. This discharge is normal and is called **vaginal leukorrhea,** but both she and her parents may be alarmed, erroneously thinking that she has a sexually transmitted disease.

DECLARATIONS OF INDEPENDENCE

Anxiety concerning sexuality may prevent parents from supporting developmental tasks of early adolescence, such as the emergence of independence from the family. During latency, youngsters generally identify strongly with their own families and model their actions after their own parents. In adolescence, youngsters have an appropriate psychological need to separate from their parents and establish their own identities as individuals.[14] It is important to be known as Bobby Jones, rather than "Mr. Jones' son." In most young adolescents, this is generally accomplished quietly, without open rebellion, through the media of clothes, hair, jewelry, music, and the increased importance of close friends. In some families, especially those that are close-knit, this process may still pose difficulties.

> *Erin, 13, prefers being with her friends to joining in family activities. In the past Erin and her mother enjoyed shopping outings together. Weekend picnics and field trips with her parents and little brothers were the norm. Instead of going out with her family, Erin now tries to stay home where she can talk on the phone with friends, watch television, or listen to music. Erin also refuses to shop with her mother; she prefers going to the mall with her girlfriends. When she comes home, however, she and her mother argue over the few clothes and jewelry that Erin has purchased. Now Erin is talking about getting a tattoo or nose ring. Her parents are hurt, and they often find themselves entrapped in futile and potentially harmful arguments with Erin about clothes, cosmetics, and other superficial matters. They know that Erin is doing well in school and is responsible for her age, but cannot risk letting go for fear of loss of influence and control.*

This struggle recalls that of an earlier era, the second year of life. Then the bids for independence heralded the transition from infancy to childhood; now these bids are renewed as the child begins the journey from childhood to adulthood. Most parents need that perspective clearly laid out. In this case, Erin's choice in clothing is a concrete way for her to express her individuality and **peer group** identification. She is appropriately identifying more with peers than family members. Symbols of that identification take on new importance. The more dramatic those symbols, the greater the tensions between parent and child. Limit setting is still necessary, and often compromises can be found. If the parents are opposed to a tattoo or body piercing, for example, they may find a middle ground and allow Erin to wear a temporary rub-on tattoo or clip-on jewelry.

As adolescents separate from parents, they must have the support of a peer group for the safe psychological shelter in which to grow outside the family. The peer group provides a sounding board against which the young teen can test ideas, and it serves as a barometer of her own physical and psychological growth. In other words, the peer group pro-

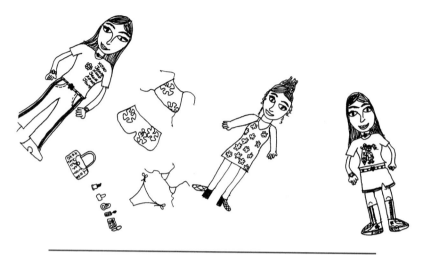

"Dressing for school, party and beach." By Sarah Stein, age 11.

vides an important supportive structure to the adolescent's psychosocial development. The adolescent often must juggle the differences between what friends say or do and what the family's position is on any given issue. Even though the teen must psychologically distance himself from his family, most adolescents do not hate their parents or view their home as an unpleasant place. In fact, adolescents still need reassurance, support, and physical affection from their parents. This comforting may be in the form of frequent hugs, compliments, help with homework, attendance at school or other important events, or simply taking the time to play a game of cards or to talk.

> *Joey, 11, has difficulty settling into his homework. He does well at school, but often becomes anxious with certain assignments or tests. Seeing the frustration in his son one afternoon, Joey's father sits down to play a game of chess with him. After narrowly beating his dad at the game, Joey runs to get his homework and sits down at the kitchen table, where his dad is preparing dinner. Joey pauses from his studies to say, "Dad, when I can do my homework around you, I'm not nervous anymore."*

ROLE OF PEERS

In early adolescence the peer group generally consists of same-gender members who share similar interests and spend a considerable amount of time together.[2] An adolescent may belong to several different groups of friends whose members may or may not overlap; for example, one group of friends at school, another from the home neighborhood or extended family, and potentially others from various social activities (e.g., church, sports, and clubs). Membership in particular peer groups or crowds can be very important to the teen and a means by which to define or label himself and others. An adolescent may not always be able to "get into" the group that he desires and may be forced to accept a peer group of lower social rank.[15] A few teens may not be accepted by any peer group, a condition that can eventually contribute to poor self-esteem, loneliness, and depression.[15] Social isolation or alienation, however, is *not* the norm in adolescence and may be a sign of coexisting psychosocial problems.

> *Robin is a straight-A student, shy and self-conscious. She wears glasses and has braces. She often feels like a nerd and has very few social interactions while at school. Robin is active in a local choir and takes violin lessons. She has a best friend and enjoys going to the movies with friends from choir. Her parents are proud of her. Her primary care provider is impressed with Robin's accomplishments and takes additional time with Robin to talk about issues relating to her self-esteem and self-image.*

Comment: This girl's individuality, her temperament, is being played out during adolescence. She has a friend, acquaintances, and positive family interactions.

> *Ann is a straight-A student, shy and self conscious. She feels anxious around other kids her age, especially at school. She sometimes gets bouts of shortness of breath accompanied by palpitations and sweating. On weekends and evenings, she stays home to study or just sleeps. She cannot identify a best friend. Her primary care provider is concerned about Ann and performs a thorough psychosocial history, including questions about suicidal ideation. She is referred to a specialist for counseling and evaluation for a panic disorder and depression.*

Once in a particular peer group or crowd, the individual members must conform to the norms of the group.[15] Members of the peer group often dress alike. Girls may spend a considerable amount of time together or on the telephone planning outfits and hairstyles. Boys often wear similar clothing, jackets of the same make and color, or T-shirts with the same inscription or insignia. Haircuts are alike. To verify these statements, visit a shopping mall for the afternoon and observe a group of youngsters walking by. The tendency to dress alike continues through all of adolescence, but is most exaggerated in early adolescence. It signals the important work of separation from parents and peer-group identification and in that sense is an indicator of developmental progress.

Depending on the particular peer group, conformity pressures can be either beneficial or counterproductive to family values, school performance, and overall well-being of the adolescent. Many peer groups encourage individual achievement, for example, in sports and academics, but some may encourage delinquent behavior, such as **substance abuse** or criminal acts. Teens with the lowest self-esteem are the most vulnerable to peer group pressure and may knowingly do things against their better judgment and their parents' wishes. These conformity pressures are felt most strongly during the junior high or middle school years.[15] **Gangs** are an extreme example of this type of peer pressure. In general, gangs become appealing when other, healthier peer group options are not available. The setting for gangs is most commonly a poor inner city area, where gangs offer perceived protection from outside threats or a means to social and economic advancement. Once in a gang where violence is part of the culture, the individual members have no alternative but to acquiesce and perform as expected, whether it be burglary, weapon carrying, fighting, or homicide.

SCHOOL MILIEU

Early adolescents are usually in middle or junior high school (grades six, seven, and eight). For most teens, this is a new social experience with a completely different milieu from elementary school. The youngster must adapt to changing classes, multiple teachers and teaching styles, and variable homework loads and testing schedules.[16] This may be the first time that a young person is exposed to youngsters outside his neighborhood. He may meet others of different races, religions, and socioeconomic status. These new experiences may make him uncomfortable. Most young people make this transition with minimal anxiety, tempered by the comfort of knowing that grade-school companions are in the same predicament. Those youngsters who must attend a new school with all new classmates may be more anxious and frightened. This anxiety may manifest as psychosomatic complaints, school avoidance, or school difficulties. Hence, all adolescents with school dysfunction must have a social, as well as physical, neurological, and academic evaluation.[17] **Junior high or middle school transition** should last weeks, not months. Continuing school difficulty must be taken seriously and evaluated broadly.

COGNITIVE DEVELOPMENT: IMPLICATIONS FOR CLINICAL INTERVIEW

Because of a young adolescent's assumption of pseudoadult mannerisms or the emulation of older models, it is easy for both parents and clinicians to overestimate their cognitive abilities.[18,19] When evaluating a child in early adolescence, one must realize that 11-year-olds usually still engage in **concrete thinking;** that is, they do not yet have the cognitive ability to think abstractly, to develop contingency plans, or to conceptualize. They may still be in Piaget's *concrete operational stage* of cognitive development and may still have difficulty in organizing large bodies of data or inferential tasks (see Chapter 2).[20] As a result, they may not relate present actions with future consequences. This inability has important implications for health counseling and the management and treatment of illnesses. Explicit linkages and short-term consequences must be spelled out clearly for the young adolescent.

Physicians who care for young adolescents frequently proclaim that they are difficult to interview. Teens may answer questions with only monosyllabic answers. In these instances, the physician is probably not being specific enough for a concrete-thinking youngster. For example, instead of saying, "Tell me about yourself," the clinician may be more successful in saying, "Tell me what you do on the soccer team." Because of limitations in conceptualization, young adolescents may be unable to sustain lengthy verbal interviews. Other youngsters may view a physician's questions as a test and interpret the medical interview as an examination at school, with right or wrong answers. In those instances, the physician may glean more information by interacting with the young teen through playing checkers or drawing pictures. This may be much more efficient in terms of getting to the core issues than more "standardized" interviews. Some children of age 11 or 12 may talk more freely in such a play environment. In addition, the young adolescent may be more able to describe specific behaviors, beliefs, and attitudes in her peer group than in herself. The clinician will do well to respect these distancing maneuvers and may even use these approaches in data gathering.

DATA GATHERING

Adolescents should be seen annually by a health care provider.[21,22] At these health maintenance visits, the clinician may perform a history, including a thorough psychosocial history and physical exam, as well as any needed immunizations, health education, and anticipatory guidance. Table 20-4 presents components to be included in the examination of the child in early adolescence.

GENERAL GUIDELINES
Separate but Equal

At the very first visit with the young teen, ground rules should be established for both the patient and the parents. Let them know that teenagers are interviewed separately from parents but that parents will also have an opportunity to discuss their concerns privately with the physician. Separate interviews not only enable the clinician to obtain sensitive information from the adolescent and parents in private, but also emphasize the emerging independence of the youngster and help to establish rapport.

Sex and Drug Issues

Parents and teens should be notified that the information shared between the clinician and teen is confidential, including issues about sex and drugs. Exceptions to this rule exist and will vary depending on the practice, but normally confidentiality is broken only if the teenager discloses a history of abuse or is at risk of harming herself or someone else (e.g., suicidal or homicidal ideation).

> Sam, I wanted to explain to you and your parents that my role here is as your physician. Therefore the things that you and I talk about, even if it's about sex or drugs, are just between you and me. Of course, I would encourage you to discuss these matters with your parents or at least allow me to tell your parents for you. Nonetheless, I will not break this rule of confidentiality without your permission except in two situations: 1) if you are at risk of seriously hurting yourself; for example wanting to kill yourself; or 2) if you are at risk of hurting someone else; for example wanting to shoot someone. Knowing that our conversations are confidential may make you feel more at ease about talking to me and also may make your parents rest easy knowing that you have someone to turn to if you can't talk to them.

Setting the Stage

It is important to try to make the teenager feel comfortable. If the setting is in a general pediatric practice, it is helpful to have a separate room that is age appropriate in which to in-

TABLE 20-4 ■ Components of Examination of Early Adolescent

What To Observe	Objective
Interactions between adolescent and parent	To assess whether they communicate well or if the mother/father answers all the questions for the adolescent or allows the youngster to answer for himself; these interactions may reveal the status of the separation process
The adolescent's willingness to be interviewed and/or examined alone without parental presence	To determine the adolescent's willingness to begin to act independently from his parents

What To Ask	Objective
Inquire about the young adolescent's school activities (e.g., "Tell me what happens to you on an average day at school. What is your favorite class? Why is that class so special? Who is your favorite teacher? What's so special about that teacher? Is yours a friendly or a not so friendly school? If you were having difficulty in school to whom would you go to talk? How far away from your home is your school?")	To determine whether the youngster is in the right grade for his age and to begin the interview on generally neutral grounds To assess the youngster's attitude toward school
Inquire about the adolescent's function with a peer group (e.g., "Do you have a best friend? What is his name and age? What kind of things do you do together? What's so special about Tommy? How long have you known him? Do you ever spend time at each other's homes? Do you and Tommy belong to a group of friends? How long have you known these friends? What do you do together? Is there another group you wish you belonged to, but do not?")	To determine whether the patient is beginning to develop independence from the family; to assess patterns of interaction outside the family from the youngster's perspective
Inquire about the adolescent's function in his family (e.g., "Are you the oldest or youngest? What's it like being the oldest, youngest, or only child in your family? Do you have your own room? What kind of duties do you have around the house? Who are you closest to in your family—your mother or father, brother or sister? What do you do if you become angry? What happens in your family if someone is angry with you? How are you punished?)	To assess this child's role in the family; to assess patterns of interaction within the family from the youngster's perspective

TABLE 20-4 ■ Components of Examination of Early Adolescent—cont'd

What To Ask	Objective
Inquire about the adolescent's feelings about himself and his body (e.g., "In your class, are you the tallest, shortest, or in between? What is it like being the tallest or shortest in your class? As most young people grow up, their bodies change. . . . Is there anything about your body's changes that has you worried? Is there anything about yourself that you wish were different?")	To determine the youngster's concerns about his body; to determine the youngster's information about the physical changes that are taking place or will soon occur

Physical Assessment	Objective
Height, weight	To have a baseline to mark the adolescent's percentile on a growth chart
Blood pressure	As a baseline to rule out hypertension if symptoms develop later
Tanner maturational staging (see Table 20-3 and Fig. 20-1)	To determine baseline and progress for physical maturation
Check carefully for scoliosis	Scoliosis is most apparent during the adolescent growth spurt and should be carefully assessed as early as possible in this phase of development
Note the presence of gynecomastia in boys	Gynecomastia is common in pubertal boys and is generally a source of concern
Careful palpation of thyroid gland	Adolescent goiter is common and may be pronounced in this age group

Psychosocial Assessments	Objective
The adolescent's comfort during the physical examination	To assess the adolescent's feelings concerning his body
Affect regarding this visit (anger, fear, anxiety, sulking)	May help explain responses or actions in this patient
The report of the importance of peer group; the style of hair or dress	To assess the important identification with a peer group

terview and examine the patient. Reading materials, such as pamphlets, magazines, and posters that are geared toward adolescent issues, should be provided. In this way, the teen may be more inclined to bring up sensitive issues or may even find answers to questions that were not addressed during the visit.

Questionnaires

The clinician may also want to make use of health survey questionnaires as an adjunct to the patient-physician interview. The use of questionnaires can be reassuring to the teen because it implies that other adolescents have similar problems and concerns.

Choice of Clinician

It is not unusual at this age for the teenage patient to develop a preference for a same gender health care provider, and if possible, this desire should be respected.

Sensitivity in Examination

The examination must be done with sensitivity and awareness of the young adolescent's shyness and perhaps exaggerated embarrassment.[1] For example, the clinician should give clear directions concerning disrobing and gowning in preparation for a physical examination. If the underwear should be removed, the clinician must say so. The examination should be undertaken behind closed drapes or in a secure room to protect the adolescent's privacy. If the teen wishes, a parent or support person may be present during the examination, or the teen may prefer to be examined alone.

Narrating the Examination

During the examination itself, it is important to affirm normal physical findings especially of sensitive areas like the genitals. The clinician's narration during the physical examination demystifies the clinical encounter and involves the patient while providing valuable information.

Throughout the health visit, the health care provider must use active listening skills to pick up on the patient's underlying concerns. Showing interest and giving nonjudgmental counseling also lets the teenage patient know that she is taken seriously.

SPECIAL REFERRALS
Endocrine Issues

Boys and girls who do not follow the normal pattern of pubertal development (e.g., advanced pubic hair development with little or no breast development) warrant an endocrine evaluation.[23] In addition, adolescent boys who have not begun pubertal development by the age of 14 and adolescent girls who have not begun breast development by the age of 13 or had menarche by the age of 16 should be evaluated for pubertal delay.[24]

Chronic Illness

The teenager who has a chronic illness, such as asthma, cystic fibrosis, diabetes, or sickle cell disease, may have delayed or atypical psychosocial development because of dependence on parental support, medical personnel, and therapeutic regimens. Physical development, including puberty, may also be delayed secondary to the disease process.[25] With the limitations imposed by the illness, either physically or mentally, adolescence can be an excruciatingly difficult time for the child with a chronic disease. Independence, a positive body image, and a supportive peer group may be difficult to obtain.[25] As a result, some adolescents with a chronic illness may become depressed, angry with parents and medical staff, and noncompliant with medical therapy. Teens with a mental health condition may experience similar problems with obtaining independence and a healthy self-esteem. Adolescents with a chronic physical or mental health condition usually require counseling for support through this difficult transition time and may need a referral for further assistance with adjustment.

Poor School Adjustment

Children who are adjusting poorly to middle or junior high school after 6 weeks may need special psychological or educational assessments, tutoring in special areas, or counseling to assist in social interactions. Declining school performance should never be attributed to benign causes.

Friendless Youth

Youngsters who do not have a peer group of friends need careful psychological or psychiatric evaluation. This signals significant social isolation and is a serious matter.

Family Conflict

Families that have persistent conflict during this time may need additional sessions to identify areas of disagreement and to put patterns of mutual respect in negotiation. Family counseling may be indicated. Some turbulence is expected in all families, but a decline in functioning or prolonged conflict is not to be expected.

ANTICIPATORY GUIDANCE FOR EARLY ADOLESCENT
Physical Development

Young teenagers need reassurance and education about their bodies. Explain the pattern of physical and sexual maturation to each youngster. For example, if a girl has not begun to menstruate but has breast development, the clinician can outline for her the expected pattern of growth, including approximate time of menarche. The physician may say,

"Mary, I notice that you have begun to develop as a young woman. Have you been wondering what happens next? or Jack, when I did your physical examination, I noticed that you are starting to have pubic hair. Have you wondered what would happen next?"

Menstruation

All girls should receive an explanation of menstruation whether they have started menses or not. It is usually helpful to ask the teenager what she already knows about menstrual periods and the menstrual cycle and then to build on her knowledge. Teens often appreciate being told that it is normal for their periods to be irregular for some time after menses start. They also need to know that once menarche occurs, it is possible to become pregnant, a natural lead-in to a first discussion about contraception. It is important that young women be exposed to a positive rather than negative attitude toward menstruation. Pamphlets do not substitute for personal counseling by the health provider.

Masturbation and Nocturnal Emissions

Adolescents may need reassurance concerning masturbation, and adolescent boys may also need education about nocturnal emissions. It is often very embarrassing for a teen to be asked about these issues directly. It is usually more helpful to say,

"Many boys your age start to notice more sexual urges now than they did when they were younger. Sometimes these urges occur at night, resulting in a sticky, white discharge in their pajamas. Boys may also have an ejaculation from feeling their own penis; this is called masturbation. I don't know if this has happened to you yet, but I want you to know that this is normal."

Pubertal Development of Opposite Sex

Adolescents may be ignorant of the development of the opposite sex. Some teens may be too embarrassed to ask questions concerning this topic. It is usually helpful to say,

"What have you learned at school about the changes that boys (or girls) experience at your age? Is this something you'd like to learn more about?"

A brief explanation accompanied by pamphlets is usually sufficient.

Tobacco, Alcohol, and Drugs

It is never too early to begin counseling about the health risks of using **tobacco,** alcohol, or illicit drugs. Alcohol and cigarettes are the drugs most frequently used by adolescents, followed by marijuana, smokeless tobacco, and inhalants.[26] Initiation to cigarette use usually occurs between grades 6 and 9. In fact, close to 20% of eighth graders say that they are now smoking.[27] Likewise, peak ages for initiation to alcohol use are in grades 7 to 9, with almost one third of students reporting that they first drank alcohol before they were 13.[27] For marijuana, more than 7% of students have tried it before the age of 13, and one third of "marijuana users" started using the drug by the time they were 14 years old.[27]

Although these rates may seem high, many teens who try drugs, including tobacco and alcohol, will not continue to use them on a regular basis.[26] It is the health care provider's job to provide information on these drugs so that the teen will understand the risks involved. Young teens may not care about health risks that will occur decades from now, such as cancer, heart disease, and emphysema, and they often don't appreciate the addiction potential. Discussing short-term effects on health and appearance may be more beneficial. For example, smoking affects physical endurance and may lower sports performance; it also yellows teeth and fingernails, causes bad breath, and increases the risk of getting upper respiratory infections. With the support of the clinician, teacher, parent, or all three, the teen may be better equipped to resist peer pressure to engage in drug use and therefore be less likely to become a regular user.

ANTICIPATORY GUIDANCE FOR PARENTS
Pubertal Development

Parents should be informed when a youngster has begun the process of puberty, a fact that may not be obvious to the parent. A simple explanation concerning the expected progression of pubertal development is usually appreciated by most parents, with specific emphasis on those matters that will be most noticeable to parents rather than to someone outside the family. For example, let parents know that when doing the laundry, they may notice leukorrhea in a girl's underpants for 4 to 6 months before the onset of menarche. This knowledge will prevent misconceptions about the discharge and will enable the parent to be prepared for menarche to occur, so that sanitary pads or tampons will be available. Also, point out that sexual interest is appropriate at this age and does not necessarily indicate sexual activity. Assumptions of inappropriate behavior may become a self-fulfilling prophecy.

Need for Privacy

Parents should be informed that with the onset of puberty, young adolescents must have privacy. This is best accomplished by allowing the teen to have his own room; if this is not possible, he should have his own section of a room where he can go and be by himself and not be bothered by siblings or by parents.

Sensitivity to Teasing

Parents should be advised that it is not appropriate to tease youngsters about their pubertal development. Most teenagers are exquisitely self-conscious about their development and may be acutely embarrassed by this teasing. This advice is best given in two ways: 1) by asking the parent if anyone is teasing the youngster about pubertal changes; and 2) by asking the parent about his or her own early adolescence. In that context, most parents will recall their own self-consciousness and will be more likely to show increased sensitivity to their child's needs. Parents may also need to restrain siblings from making comments.

Quest for Independence

Parents must be reassured that the teenager's quest for independence is normal and should not be interpreted as rejection of the parent. Give examples of this situation. For instance, young teenagers may not want to join the family on all family outings or may not want the parents at school or social functions in a chaperone capacity. If possible, another authority figure may do better. Young teens may begin to confide in an adult outside the family rather than in their parents, possibly a change from previous years. Parents should avoid arguments about trivial things. It is best to concentrate on basic hygiene, physical safety, and school attendance when deciding which behaviors to address.

REFERENCES

1. Felice ME: Adolescence. In Levine MD, Carey WB, Crocker AC, editors: *Developmental-behavioral pediatrics,* Philadelphia, 1992, WB Saunders.
2. Weiner IB: Distinguishing healthy from disturbed adolescent development, *J Dev Behav Pediatr* 11:151, 1990.
3. Tanner JM: *Growth at adolescence,* ed 2, Boston, 1962, Blackwell Scientific Publications.
4. Marshall WA, Tanner JM: Variations in the pattern of pubertal changes in boys, *Arch Dis Child* 45:13, 1970.
5. Kulin HE, Muller J: The biological aspects of puberty, *Pediatr Rev* 17(3):75, 1996.
6. Herman-Giddens ME et al: Secondary sexual characteristics and menses in young girls seen in office practice: a study from the pediatric research in office settings network, *Pediatrics* 99:505, 1997.
7. Kreipe RE: Normal somatic adolescent growth and development. In McAnarney ER et al, editors: *Textbook of adolescent medicine,* Philadelphia, 1992, WB Saunders.
8. Fujii CM, Felice ME: Physical growth and development: current concepts, *Prim Care* 14:1, 1987.
9. Garn SM: Physical growth and development. In Friedman SB, Fisher M, Schonberg SK, editors: *Comprehensive adolescent health care,* St. Louis, 1992, Quality Medical.
10. Stone LJ, Church J: Pubescence, puberty, and physical development. In Esman AH, editor: *Psychology of adolescence,* New York, 1975, International Universities Press.
11. Hamburg BA: Psychosocial development. In Friedman SB, Fisher M, Schonberg SK, editors: *Comprehensive adolescent health care,* St. Louis, 1992, Quality Medical.
12. Litt IF: Pubertal and psychosocial development: implications for pediatricians, *Pediatr Rev* 16(7):243, 1995.
13. Freud S: The transformation of puberty. In Esman AH, editor: *Psychology of adolescence,* New York, 1975, International Universities Press, pp 86-99.
14. Erikson EH: *Identity, youth and crisis,* New York, 1968, WW Norton.
15. Ladd GW: Peer relationships. In Friedman SB, Fisher M, Schonberg SK, editors: *Comprehensive adolescent health care,* St. Louis, 1992 Quality Medical.
16. Black JL, Nader PR: Academic achievement. In Friedman SB, Fisher M, Schonberg SK, editors: *Comprehensive adolescent health care,* St. Louis, 1992, Quality Medical.
17. Sandler AD, Levine MD: Learning and attention deficit disorders. In Friedman SB, Fisher M, Schonberg SK, editors: *Comprehensive adolescent health care,* St. Louis, 1992, Quality Medical.
18. Elkind D: Understanding the young adolescent, *Adolescence* 13:127, 1978.
19. Elkind D: Cognitive structure and adolescent experience, *Adolescence* 2:427, 1967.
20. Piaget J: The intellectual development of the adolescent. In Caplan G, Levovici S, editors: *Adolescence: psychosocial perspective,* New York, 1969, Basic Books.
21. American Academy of Pediatrics, Committee on Practice and Ambulatory Medicine: Recommendations for preventive health care, *Pediatrics* 96:373, 1995.
22. American Medical Association: Guidelines for adolescent preventive services (GAPS), *Recommendations monograph,* ed 3, 1996.
23. Copeland KC: Variations in normal sexual development, *Pediatr Rev* 8(2): 18, 1986.

24. Neinstein LS, Kaufman FR: Abnormal growth and development in adolescence. In Neinstein LS, editor: *Adolescent health care: a practical guide,* ed 3, Baltimore, 1996, Williams & Wilkins.

25. Britto MT et al: Risky behavior in teens with cystic fibrosis or sickle cell disease: a multicenter study, *Pediatrics* 101(2):250, 1998.

26. National Adolescent Health Information Center, UCSF: Fact sheet on adolescent substance abuse, *Adolescent Fact File,* November 1995.

27. Ozer EM et al: America's adolescents: are they healthy? San Francisco, 1997, National Adolescent Health Information Center.

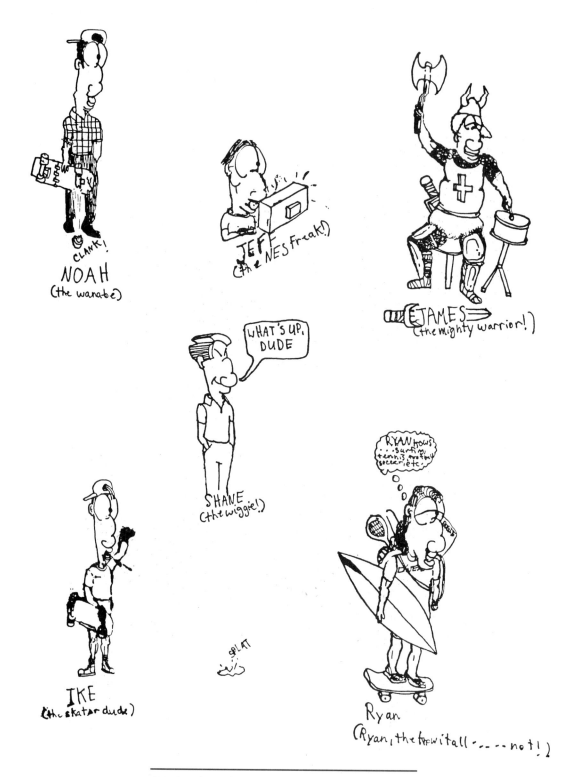

"My brother's friends." By Colin Hennessy, age 11.

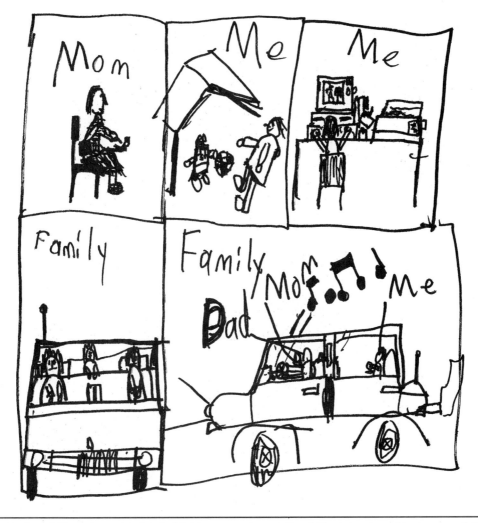

This 11-year-old boy shows his family highly compartmentalized. The intrusion of technology into his life is clear.

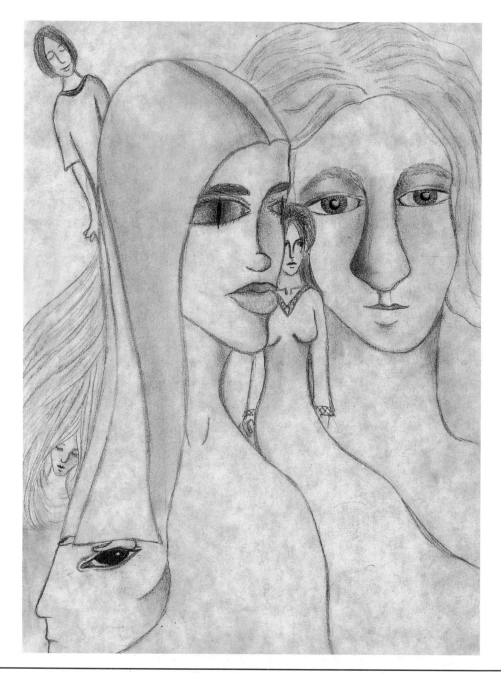

A 16-year-old girl draws her world, a blend of identities, sophistication, and physical maturation. This gives us a sense of the complexities of relationships and personae at this age. By Carmen Goodheart. (Original in charcoal.)

FOURTEEN TO SIXTEEN YEARS: MID-ADOLESCENCE — DATING GAME

- Marianne E. Feli
- Jennifer Maehr

The major developmental task of mid-adolescence, approximately 14 to 16 years of age, is the achievement of sexual sense of self. This means becoming comfortable with one's sexuality, as well as learning to express sexual feelings in an appropriate manner and to receive sexual advances from another in a comfortable way. It means the assumption of culturally defined sexual roles, including behaviors and activities.

REFINEMENT OF THE SELF-IMAGE

For the adolescent to become comfortable with her sexuality, she must be comfortable with her body. Most mid-adolescents have already experienced puberty, but they may not yet be

453

comfortable with the results. Hence, mid-adolescent girls and boys spend much time, money, and energy on their appearance. Teens may experiment with clothing, hair, jewelry, makeup, tattoos, and body piercing in an effort to "try on" different images and find the real self (see Chapter 16 for the preschooler's similar developmental work). It would not be surprising to observe a 15-year-old girl in pigtails at one medical visit and see her with a sophisticated hairstyle or dramatically changed hair color 2 weeks later at another visit. This experimentation is evidence of developmental work.

The emphasis on bodily development is one part of the pervasive self-centeredness of many mid-adolescent teenagers. Because they are spending so much time thinking and looking at themselves, they presume that others are thinking about them and looking at them as well. This preoccupation with self may seem to border on paranoia, hysteria, or frank narcissism, but it is completely normal. An example of this self-absorption can be easily observed by watching a group of same-sex adolescents in a public place being approached by a group of adolescents of the opposite sex. Each teenager will act and feel as if all attention is focused on him or her, that everybody is looking directly and completely at him or her. No wonder then that so much effort is spent on the development of an image. This self-centeredness and heightened self-awareness may account for the continual hair grooming, clothes straightening, and makeup activities that take place in any gathering of mid-adolescents.

SOCIAL DEVELOPMENT: THE ENLARGING WORLD OUTSIDE HOME

The supportive approval and combined efforts of the peer group fuel self-confidence under the imagined scrutiny of the opposite sex. Even when not **dating,** adolescents benefit from interactions with members of the opposite sex as they learn to expand the peer group from a unisexual group to a heterosexual one, from a local neighborhood clique to selected groups with individuals of similar interests or talents. Frequently these interactions are initiated through school-based activities, such as team **sports,** clubs, theater, academic societies, or elected positions. In these organizations the mid-adolescent has the opportunity to socialize even when not actually dating. For many teens this is a safer, more comfortable environment than a formal dating situation.

Not only are relationships with members of the opposite sex expanded, but all relationships outside the family are expanded. Mid-adolescents, typically high school freshmen, sophomores, and juniors, usually make some new friends of the same sex, frequently develop a strong attachment to one or two adults, and begin to care about and for younger children. These are important interactions and expose mid-adolescents in depth to life-styles and philosophies different from those of their own families. During mid-adolescence, teens may begin to try on different life-styles in dress, manner of speech, and political viewpoints to the chagrin of parents. But these excursions are normal developmental explorations, and by young adulthood, adolescents usually have political and philosophical opinions similar to those of their parents. In fact, for most adolescents, constant conflict and recurrent turmoil are the exception rather than the rule,[1] and most adolescents love and respect their parents in spite of disagreements about everyday issues.[2]

SEXUAL DEVELOPMENT

Some say that sexual and aggressive drives are stronger during adolescence than at any other time of life. Learning to express and control these drives is a major and formidable task of the teenage years, and the need to master these drives is felt most acutely during mid-adolescence, a time when the individual may seem least equipped to control them. Responding to strong sexual drives, most mid-adolescents begin to date members of the opposite sex. However, one characteristic of mid-adolescent sexuality is that the opposite sex is often viewed as a sex object, and both boys and girls may see the relationship as an opportunity for social gain. The degree of attractiveness of one's sexual partner provides an important measure of one's own self-worth.

Most mid-adolescents engage in some aspect of sexual experimentation, the extent of which varies from adolescent to adolescent and from one socioeconomic group or subcultural group to another. Overall, more than half of teenagers will have had sexual intercourse by the age of 17.[3] Some teens are having sex at earlier ages and some with multiple partners.[4,5] In spite of these figures, one cannot presume that all mid-adolescents are sexually active, but one can assume that all mid-adolescents are interested in sexual issues.

SEXUAL ABUSE

Not all sexual activity in adolescence is consensual. This is especially true for the younger, more vulnerable teenager. In fact, about half of girls who have had intercourse before the age of 15 report having had nonvoluntary sex at the first or subsequent sexual encounters.[6] Although statistics vary, as many as one in four high school girls and one in ten high school boys report having been physically or sexually abused; these abused teens are at higher risk than others for substance abuse, alcohol use, smoking, depression, and **eating disorders**.[7] Girls with a history of **sexual abuse** are also more likely to become pregnant, engage in earlier sexual activity, have more sexual partners, and not use **contraception**.[8,9] It is important to inquire about a history of abuse in order to help ensure the future safety of abuse victims. Teens who have been abused often benefit from ongoing counseling with a trained professional experienced in working with adolescent abuse victims. Any history of abuse of a minor should be reported to Child Protective Services regardless of the teenager's wishes.

ADOLESCENT PREGNANCY

Of those female adolescents who are sexually active, each year approximately 20% of them become pregnant, accounting for about 1 million teen pregnancies annually in the United States.[4,5] Of these pregnancies, 85% are reported as unintended.[4] Almost half of all pregnant teens will opt to keep the infant, whereas 13% will miscarry, and 40% will have an induced abortion.[4] Many factors contribute to unintended teen pregnancies, including lack of contraceptive use, improper contraceptive use or contraception failure, lack of health education, and barriers to family planning services. Many teens cannot afford care or contraception because of a lack of insurance. Others may be too embarrassed to buy contraceptive supplies or too shy to discuss issues of sexuality with their health care provider. The issues underlying teen pregnancy and parenthood are complex.[10] Certain characteristics have been identified that put a teen at an increased risk for teen parenthood—early school failure, early behavior problems, family dysfunction, and poverty.[6] The more risk factors in a teen's life, the more time a health care provider needs to spend with the teen in order to discuss family planning and life options other than early parenthood.

Unfortunately, up to 40% of teens do not use any form of birth control at their first sexual encounter, and the percentage of sexually active teenagers who do report current use of any contraception ranges from 32% to 75%.[4] Adolescents often have misconceptions about birth control, especially hormonal contraception. Some teenagers believe that they cannot become pregnant, for instance, because of a past genital infection or a failure to conceive in the past. Even if an adolescent chooses a contraceptive method with the help of a health care provider, she may use it incorrectly or not at all, especially if she is worried about a perceived health consequence, such as weight gain, infertility, or irregular menstrual bleeding. These concerns often stem from comments made by friends or family members. The sexual partner is also very influential in whether the chosen contraception will be used. In some subcultures, condom use or hormonal contraception is not looked on favorably. Fortunately, condom use seems to be increasing, most notably among younger adolescents.[11,12]

After several discussions with her clinician, Erica decides to start taking birth control pills as her contraceptive method. She is dispensed four packs with verbal and written instructions. Erica, however, is also given advice by her girlfriend on how to take the pills. Whenever Erica begins her period, she stops taking the pill and does not start a new pack until the Sunday after her bleeding stops. In 6 months, Erica is pregnant.

Judy refuses any form of hormonal contraception. She is afraid of needles and therefore does not want Depo. She does not want to gain weight or "be changed" by the pill. The thought of something in her arm is "freaky," so Norplant is out. She is consistently given condoms and vaginal contraceptive film by the clinic. Several months later, Judy is pregnant. She hadn't been using the condoms. She just shrugs, "I didn't think that I would really get pregnant. I had chlamydia; doesn't that make you infertile?"

Another result of teen sexuality is **sexually transmitted diseases** (STDs), such as gonorrhea, chlamydia, syphilis, herpes, trichomonas, human papilloma virus (HPV), hepatitis B, and human immunodeficiency virus (HIV). Adolescents run a greater risk of obtaining STDs than people of other ages because of various biological and behavioral reasons.[13] In fact, each year approximately 25% of sexually active teenagers will become infected with an STD.[4] As in the adult population, acquired immune deficiency syndrome (AIDS) is becoming more prevalent in the heterosexual adolescent population. Of the new adolescent AIDS cases, 46% involve females, the majority of whom acquired HIV from heterosexual sex, often with a partner who used drugs intravenously.[11]

HOMOSEXUALITY

Similar to adults, some adolescents are **homosexual**.[14,15] It is difficult to determine the actual number of adolescents who are homosexual or who have homosexual tendencies. Many mid-adolescents may not yet realize or are not able to admit that they are homosexual; this realization may not be faced until late adolescence or early adulthood.[16] Information from adult homosexual men and women shows that most perceived themselves as being different from their same-sex peers as early as childhood but did not develop feelings of being *sexually* different until sometime during adolescence (see Chapter 16).[16]

In the process of establishing a sexual sense of themselves, many adolescents may wonder if they are homosexual. Adolescent girls commonly develop crushes on girlfriends or female teachers, and it is certainly not unusual for adolescent boys to experience an erection in the company of other males. Same-sex arousal or experimentation with same-sex sexual activity does not necessarily indicate that an adolescent is homosexual nor does it predict future sexual orientation.[17] With time, a teenager's sexual preference will become clear.

Teens who are homosexual, however, are at increased risk for psychosocial problems, such as deteriorating school performance, mental illness, substance abuse, homelessness, **delinquency,** suicide attempts, and prostitution.[15,18,19] Homosexual adolescents may feel isolated and hate themselves.[19] They often face peer ridicule and physical violence.[18] Without the support of family and peers and without information from knowledgeable adults, such as health care providers, teachers, or adult homosexual role models, adolescence for the homosexual teen can be an incredibly lonely and terrifying time.

With the knowledge that mid-adolescents are heavily invested in sexual issues, the clinician must be capable and willing to discuss sexual issues with the adolescent patient. This means that the clinician must be comfortable with his own sexuality, as well as comfortable with and knowledgeable about the subject of sex. Clinicians must be aware of their own limitations and biases in this area and must try not to impose their biases on the adolescent patient.

COGNITIVE AND MORAL DEVELOPMENT

Mid-adolescence is usually characterized by a shift in cognitive abilities. Most mid-adolescents have developed the capacity for **abstraction** and are usually capable of introspection. In other words, they can think about thinking and can now reflect on their own thought processes in an "objective" manner. This stage of cognitive development is known as **formal operational thinking** and is a giant step in mental development.[20] The mid-adolescent may become fascinated with his newfound intellectual tool, and this aspect of growth may be another factor contributing to the self-centeredness of mid-adolescence: they can now think about themselves thinking.[21] A marvelous sense of self-cleverness may contribute to a positive self-image or a slight disdain for the archaic thought processes of adults.

With the development of abstract thinking, adolescents have new capacities for moral decision making.[22] In younger years, children are in a stage of moral growth in which good behavior results in reward and misbehavior results in punishment. Hence, good or bad is determined solely by the consequences. A second level of morality is marked by the need to meet the expectations or follow the rules of one's family, peer group, or nation. In fact, maintaining the rules of the group becomes a value in itself for the youngster in mid-childhood. The third stage of moral development consists of a major thrust toward autonomous moral principles that have validity apart from the authority of the group and are based on the individual's own beliefs and conclusions concerning what is right or wrong. This is called **adult morality.** This last stage of morality usually begins in mid-adolescence, although not all individuals make this shift.

The mid-adolescent may be capable of making moral judgments based on the principles of a moral code, but, unfortunately, the self-centered behavior of mid-adolescents also results in a narcissistic value system, "what is right is what makes me feel good," and "what is right is what I want." This self-centered attitude partially explains the sexual exploitation described previously. Indeed, many activities during the mid-adolescent years may be impulsive, with little thought about consequences. Hence, other psychosocial processes may supersede cognitive capacities. For example, **risk-taking behavior** is typical of mid-adolescence. It is therefore not surprising that injuries that include motor vehicle accidents, homicides, suicides, and drownings are the leading cause of death for adolescents.[4] Many factors contribute to these deaths, including drugs and alcohol, fighting, weapon use, and poor judgment on the part of automobile drivers and passengers, such as not wearing seat belts or driving while intoxicated.[4,23,24] Even though not all teens engage in risky behaviors, violence, alcohol, and other drugs affect the lives of almost all teens sometime during their adolescence.

COUNSELING PARENTS

During the child's mid-adolescent years, the physician may begin to see the adolescent patient regularly without a parent present, but this does not mean that the role of the parent is unimportant. Indeed, the mid-adolescent years are considered the "heart" of adolescence and may be the most difficult time period for parents to face. Children in the mid-adolescent years are characteristically ambivalent about their relationship with their parents as they struggle with self-identity. Having already progressed through *early* adolescence, they have declared their need for independence in one way or another. But being wiser than their younger selves, they realize that complete independence from parents may be frightening. So, typically, the mid-adolescent "flirts" with a close relationship with his parents, sometimes asking for help and at other times rejecting all offers of assistance for fear that the parents' assistance will engulf him and suffocate his independence. This back-and-forth is normal. Parents must realize that to be of most benefit to a teenager, they must remain a constant and consistent figure, willing to be a sounding board for the youngster's ideas without overtaking and dominating the teen. Mid-adolescents must learn to think through problems to evolve solutions, and parents are a valuable resource to assist in that task.

> *Karen, 16 years old, comes alone and on time for her appointment at the doctor's office. She tells the nurse that she is here for birth control. With family planning forms in hand, Dr. Smith walks into the examining room to see Karen. Although Dr. Smith has been her physician for several years, Karen suddenly seems more mature and independent. Sitting at the small table in the exam room, Karen works diligently on her school assignments. Her nails are long and painted with intricate designs. Dressed in a purple suit with matching shoes, Karen very much looks like the young adult. After Dr. Smith compliments her for working on her homework, Karen replies that she has auditions for the choir after this and is worried that she won't finish all her work by tomorrow.*
>
> *At past visits, Karen had not yet been engaging in sex. Because she came for birth control, Dr. Smith assumes that she has become sexually active. During the interview Dr. Smith asks Karen, "Are you sexually active now?" Karen hesitates in thought for a few moments and then answers, "No." Surprised by this response, Dr. Smith adds, "Do you have a boyfriend now?" to which Karen answers, "Yes." With further questioning it becomes clear that Karen has indeed been sexually active for several months now and wants birth control pills because she doesn't want to get pregnant. When Dr. Smith asked about being "sexually active," Karen thought the doctor was asking her if she is really active, physically, when she has sex.*

A health care provider can easily be fooled by the appearance of a teenager. Karen seemed very mature and was indeed taking responsibility for herself and her body. However, Karen did not understand what Dr. Smith meant by "sexually active." Many teens don't. To some, being sexually active means having multiple sexual partners; having sex recently, for example in the past month; or frequently, for example multiple times per week or per day. Being "sexually active" may imply to the teen a heightened sexuality, such as being more physically active during sex or engaging in more risqué sexual acts.

One can never assume that the teenager understands what is being said or implied when it comes to sex. A health care provider needs to use easy-to-understand language in a nonthreatening manner and may need to give examples of what is meant:

- Many teens your age are starting to have boyfriends or girlfriends. Are you involved with anyone?
- Have you done any kind of sexual activity with this person, like kissing, touching, or having sexual intercourse?
- Do you know what I mean when I say sexual intercourse?
- Are you using anything to protect yourself from pregnancy or sexual infections, like condoms?
- Some teens are homosexual, that is, some boys (or girls) are attracted to other boys (or girls). Are you interested in being involved in a sexual way with boys, girls, or both? Are you wondering if you are homosexual?

Questions should be open ended so that teens don't feel impelled to answer questions in a certain way. Broaching and discussing the subject of sex with the teenage patient can be challenging for the practitioner. If done well, however, the teenager will feel supported by the health care provider, who has now become a valuable and trusted source of information on confidential and sensitive matters.

DATA GATHERING
Some Guiding Principles

The mid-adolescent needs to be seen on an annual basis for health maintenance and may need additional visits for follow-up of other issues and conditions.[25,26] Table 21-1 outlines components to be included in the history and physical examination. Following are additional principles to keep in mind:

■ As part of the adolescent health visit, it is essential to take a sexual history from every teen patient. Before asking questions about sexual activity, it may be helpful to inquire about sexual development, such as menstruation or testicular changes. These questions can lead into more sensitive areas, such as sexual activity, contraception, and symptoms of STDs.

■ Adolescents should be asked questions about sexuality only in private, not in the presence of parents. All adolescents should be assured of confidentiality concerning sexual matters, and the clinician should be aware of the laws governing informed consent and treatment of minors without parental consent in the local community.

Many states now permit clinicians to provide health care to teenagers without parental knowledge or consent for contraception, diagnosis and treatment of sexually transmitted diseases, diagnosis of pregnancy, abortions, and, in some states, treatment for drug use and abuse. Because these laws vary from one community to another, it is important that the physician know what the regulations regarding the treatment of minors are in a particular locale.

SPECIAL REFERRALS
Teenager with Multiple Sexual Partners

Although many teenagers are sexually active, their activity is usually confined to one partner at a time and is an expression of affection. Adolescents who have multiple partners at the same time are outside normal behavior. Promiscuity may be a sign of difficulties in the adolescent's life and may be the means by which an adolescent tells the adults around her that she is having difficulties. For example, an adolescent girl with very poor self-esteem and self-image may seek many sexual partners to affirm that she is worthwhile, or a young woman who is not getting along well at home may deliberately flaunt her newfound sexual prowess in an effort to antagonize her parents.

Homeless youth or teens in desperate situations may depend on sex for their own survival, so-called survival sex, or may have sex in exchange for drugs. In other words, sexual intercourse may be used for nonsexual reasons, such as hostility, rebellion, self-destruction, survival, or in a search for comfort and love.[27] Any teen, male or female, who has multiple sexual partners deserves a thorough psychosocial history to explore the family dynamics, the teen's financial situation, and risk factors for depression, suicide, or drug abuse. In addition, promiscuous teens should be asked about past history of sexual or **physical abuse.**

TABLE 21-1 ■ Components of the Examination (Mid-Adolescence)

What To Observe	Objective
Relationship between teen and parent if parent accompanies teen to the physician	To determine the nature of the relationship and interactions of the mid-adolescent and the parent
Who made the appointment?	Knowing this may explain some of the adolescent's behavior and attitude during interview and examination
Dress and clothing style of the patient	Observing clothing styles of the adolescent may give insight into how he sees himself at the present time

What To Ask	Objective
Ask how the adolescent is doing in school (e.g., in what activities is he engaged? Does the patient belong to any clubs or play any sports? What is the most fun about being in school? Who is the favorite teacher and why? What are the social activities that take place at school? Are there any areas at school that give the patient difficulties?)	To determine the adolescent's perception and function in the school setting, as well as involvement with a social group
Ask about the adolescent's function in the family ("Are you involved in many activities with your family? Do you accompany the family on many outings? What are your responsibilities around the house? Most adolescents have curfews, do you? Do you feel that your parents are fair in their treatment of you concerning dating and outside events? Most adolescents and their parents disagree on certain issues. What issues do you and your parents disagree on? What do you do if you disagree with your father or mother on a certain issue? Who are you the closest to in your family?")	To determine relationships in the family

Continued

TABLE 21-1 ■ **Components of the Examination (Mid-Adolescence)—cont'd**

What To Ask	Objective
Ask questions about the peer group and dating ("Do you have a best friend? How long have you been friends? What kind of activities do you do together? Do most of your friends have a steady girlfriend or boyfriend? How are your friends different from you? Do you have a steady boyfriend or many boyfriends? Some teenagers your age have begun to be sexually active—what are most of your friends doing about sexual activity? Have you ever felt forced to have sex when you didn't want to? Many adolescents today find that at school they are exposed to drug usage—is this true at your school? What are most of your friends doing about drugs? Have you ever felt that you were forced to take drugs when you didn't want to?")	To determine the adolescent's function in his peer group and his comfort with dating and sexual issues
Ask about the adolescent's feelings about himself ("Most young people your age have experienced a lot of changes in their bodies. Are you satisfied with the way your body has turned out? Is there anything about yourself you wish you could change?")	To determine the adolescent's comfort with himself

Physical Assessment	Objective
Height and weight	To follow the progress on a growth curve
Blood pressure	Hypertension often begins in adolescence
Sexual maturation by Tanner staging (most mid-adolescents are Tanner III-V)	To mark progress on the maturational curve

Psychological Assessment	Objective
Comfort during the physical examination	To determine the adolescent's comfort with his adultlike body
Maturity in answers to questions (e.g., monosyllabic responses to questions vs. complete sentences, or even paragraphs; formal thinking; moral dilemma)	To determine cognitive development

Adolescent Who Is a Loner

Adolescents should have several close friends and engage in multiple social activities. Those who do not belong to a peer group are defined as loners and are worrisome. Adolescents who are loners may be depressed and at risk for suicide[28]; they may be involved in truancy and drugs[29]; or they may be in the early stages of psychosis, such as schizophrenia, which may begin to manifest in mid to late adolescence.[2]

Decline in School Performance

Deterioration of an adolescent's grades should not be viewed lightly; it may be the result of one of the following[29,30]:

- Learning disability
- Drug use or abuse
- Clinical psychosis
- Family dysfunction
- Sexual or physical abuse
- Family crises
- Excessive stress or pressure

     Poor grades in high school may be the first clue to emotional disturbance because neurobehavioral disorders characterized by disturbances of thoughts or emotions may be first identified by a marked change in school performance.[2] These maladaptive thought processes may interfere with cognitive function to such an extent that a young person is unable to sustain his usual grades.

Serious Delinquent Behavior

Adolescents who are in trouble with the law need careful evaluation.[2] Although many adolescents are arrested each year, most offenses are minor and are not repeated. Minor offenses (e.g., shoplifting) by young adolescents may not signify a major psychosocial problem and may reflect the young adolescent's struggle with independence and peer group approval. Nonetheless, this behavior should not be ignored. Young people who commit major crimes against people or property, or minor crimes repeatedly, may be having severe difficulties, including sociopathic tendencies.[28]

Out-Of-Home Youth

Out-of-home youth refers to adolescents who are in foster care, run away, are homeless, or are incarcerated. They are at higher risk for health and psychosocial problems than the general adolescent population. Many of these problems existed before they were out of the home. Although their problems will vary, these teens are more likely to have chronic medical problems, such as mental illnesses; a history of being abused or neglected; school problems, including learning disabilities, truancy, and higher drop out rates; and higher rates of emergency room use, substance abuse, unsafe sex, and pregnancy.[31-34] When an out-of-home teen seeks medical care, the health care provider will probably have to set aside additional time to deal with all the issues presented. The clinician may not have the luxury of follow-up visits for these teens, and referrals to specialists may not be kept. The clinician must therefore attempt to cover all the most pertinent problems and treat any suspected illness before the teen leaves the clinic. This can be quite a challenge!

Amira has recently run away from home and is now living with various friends and relatives. She is seeking medical attention today because of painful lumps in her genital area. The clinician seeing Amira has never met her before but can tell from her unkempt and tired appearance that issues besides medical concerns should be addressed. During the history, Amira reveals that she has had many sexual partners and wonders if she has an infection; the clinician wonders if she has been prostituting. In the course of the examination, it is clear that Amira has enlarged, tender inguinal lymph nodes and a purulent vaginal discharge. Cervical testing for gonorrhea and chlamydia is performed, and blood is drawn for syphilis and HIV testing. A urine pregnancy test is negative. The clinician is concerned that Amira has cervicitis and syphilis. Rather than wait for test results, the physician gives Amira medication to complete treatment for gonorrhea, chlamydia, and syphilis before she leaves the office. Also, she receives the first vaccination for hepatitis B. Amira is urged to return to the clinic in 1 week for results and contraceptive counseling. She refuses all offers for psychosocial counseling today. The clinician calls Child Protective Services to see if a case has been opened on Amira. No name matches her name, and the address and phone number that Amira has given are false. Amira does not show for her follow-up appointment. She is positive for gonorrhea and syphilis; the health department is notified. Her HIV is negative.

ANTICIPATORY GUIDANCE FOR ADOLESCENT
Issues Relating to Sexual Activity

Sexual Intercourse

It is not unusual for adolescents to have questions about sexual intercourse, although they may be embarrassed about asking or about what terminology to use. Young people who are unskilled in lovemaking may not know whether their experiences are normal. They may simply need information about anatomy or physiology or they may actually require counseling concerning sexual dysfunction. To discuss sexual intercourse with adolescents, the clinician must be comfortable with the topic itself and with her own sexuality, as well as knowledgeable about sexual issues. If this isn't the case, she should be aware of other resources in the community.

> *Jan's chief complaint at her clinic appointment is pain with sex. A full pelvic examination is normal. On further questioning, it becomes apparent that she and her partner are not adequately lubricated when they have sex. They use condoms every time, but often with no foreplay. The nurse practitioner recommends a lubricating liquid. Jan is embarrassed, but relieved that nothing is wrong with her.*

Sexually Transmitted Disease

Adolescents should be informed about the different infectious causes of STDs and the disease processes associated with them, such as cervicitis, urethritis, epididymitis, pelvic inflammatory disease, urogenital ulcers and warts, genital cancers, AIDS, tubal infertility, and ectopic pregnancy. The teen should be instructed on how to recognize the signs and symptoms of STDs, but also should be told that many men and women with cervicitis or urethritis are asymptomatic. In this way, teens will understand the need for consistent condom use and annual screening for STDs. Although condom use is to be encouraged to prevent disease spread, it is only fair to tell the teenager that condoms will not protect them from all risk of STDs. Only abstinence can ensure that a teen will not acquire STDs. Many clinicians find it helpful to have pamphlets in the waiting room for adolescents to take home and read. However, these do not substitute for the clinician's direct invitation for questions in this area or an open attitude on these issues.

Birth Control, Contraception

The words *birth control* have different connotations for different adolescents. To some it simply means the birth control pill. When an adolescent girl requests birth control pills, it may signify that she has already been sexually active for many months. Any inquiry should be met with a positive response. The adolescent should be commended for taking responsibility for her actions. It is usually helpful to have a contraceptive kit available to use in discussions with teenage girls and boys. The kit should include various forms of contraception—barrier methods, such as condoms and the diaphragm; spermicides, such as vaginal contraceptive film, spermicidal jellies, and foam; the intrauterine device (IUD); and hormonal contraception, including birth control pills, Depo-Provera, and Norplant. It is often helpful to show adolescent boys and girls how to properly use a condom; they can practice putting a condom on by using a plastic model or their own fingers. The discussion of birth control should include information on emergency hormonal contraception so that the teen knows that this option exists as a backup for contraceptive failure. The physician or nurse should clearly present the pros and cons of each method and provide informational pamphlets.

Sometimes teenagers know immediately what they want to use, but others are more timid and need to talk the decision over with a boyfriend or girlfriend. It is inappropriate to push a teenager into accepting one form of contraception over another or to demand that a teenager use contraception. Although remaining abstinent should be highly recommended as an option to the teenager, abstinence-*only* education has not been shown to be effective in reducing the rates of teen pregnancy or STDs.[35,36] It is important to teach teens about contraceptive options.

After the initial discussion on contraception, it is often helpful to arrange for a follow-up visit in a week or two so that the adolescent may express her wishes concerning birth control. It is often enlightening to invite teenagers to bring the partner to the follow-up appointment. The discussion of birth control should be seen in the broader context of individual decision making, taking responsibility for one's actions, and planning for the future. These developmental skills have obvious applicability in many areas.

Teenage Pregnancy

A mid-adolescent girl may be seen by the clinician for the first time when she is actually pregnant. The physician should be prepared to make the diagnosis of pregnancy and to discuss the adolescent's options with her. Once a teen is told that she is pregnant, she may be incapable of rationally thinking about what she would like to do. It is therefore helpful to sit down with the adolescent before obtaining the test result in order to think through a possible pregnancy scenario with her:

- Does she want to be pregnant?
- Would she keep the baby?
- How does she feel about abortion?
- How does she feel about adoption?
- What does her partner want?
- What would her parent(s) say?
- If she wants to keep the baby, who would help her take care of the baby, and who would financially support her? Would she be able to go back to school?

All options should be presented to the pregnant adolescent, who should be encouraged to make her own decision with the help of information provided by the clinician. How to handle the pregnancy is always the *adolescent's* decision, not the physician's. She should be encouraged to discuss the pregnancy with her parents, and this can often be done in the office of the physician, who may play an important mediator role in this setting. The teenager should also be encouraged to involve the father of the baby in the decision process, to explore his wishes and capacity for emotional or financial support.

Issues Relating to Good Health Habits

Several preventive health topics are important to discuss with adolescents during health care visits:

- Pap smear
- Breast examination
- Testicular examination
- Nutrition
- Exercise or athletics
- Drugs, smoking, alcohol
- Driving

Routine Papanicolaou Smear

When teenagers become sexually active is a good time to instill good health habits concerning their own bodies. For those girls who are sexually active, a Papanicolaou (Pap) smear and screening for genital gonorrhea and chlamydia should be performed yearly. Annual screening for syphilis and HIV is also recommended for those at risk. For women who are not sexually active, routine Pap smears are recommended after the age of 18 years. The first **pelvic examination** can be a frightening experience, even for the sexually active teen. Every woman should be educated about the pelvic exam and female genital anatomy before the examination. The purpose of the Pap should be explained in simple language, not to scare a teenager but to educate her about her body and to encourage her to take responsibility for it.

Breast Examination

Most mid-adolescent girls have reached Tanner stage IV breast development and are ready to be taught to do a breast self-examination (Cromer et al, 1989).[37] Although breast cancer is uncommon in teenage girls, this practice instills good health habits at an early age and supports the process of being comfortable with one's own body. Show the girl what her breast feels like by having her palpate her breast after you. To explain what an abnormal lump feels like, have her place her tongue in her cheek and feel her face over that area; it will feel like a firm rubbery lump or very much like an abnormal breast mass. Models are available from medical supply houses.

Testicular Examination

Testicular cancer is rare, but when it does occur, it often occurs in the adolescent male. Hence, boys should be taught how to perform a testicular self-examination and instructed that if they find lumps or bumps on the testis or in the scrotal sac, they should have an immediate checkup by a physician.[38] This discussion itself acknowledges and verifies a new attitude toward the genitalia. Sexually active adolescent males should also be screened yearly for genital gonorrhea and chlamydia, and if indicated, HIV and syphilis.

Nutrition and Exercise

During adolescence, it is important to develop healthy habits, such as eating right and staying fit. Many teens have concerns about their body, proper nutrition, and exercise; the health care provider can offer guidance in these areas. The media, and hence society, portray the ideal body as thin, attractive, and muscular, but also promote fast food, caloric sweets, and alcoholic beverage or soda consumption. The following statistics should not be suprising:

- 12% of teens are overweight[39]
- 62% of female and 20% of male adolescents in grades 7 through 12 have dieted in the past year[40]
- up to 10% of postpubertal females have some form of an eating disorder that presents a threat to their growth and development[41]

In addition, many teens skip breakfast and avoid lunch while at school, preferring to eat snack foods and perhaps one large meal at the end of the day. During mid-adolescence, some teens will opt to become vegetarians, often without the knowledge of how to meet their nutritional needs. Mid-adolescents may choose their diet as a mechanism to gain control and independence from their parents. If, however, the adolescent meets the criteria for an eating disorder, such as anorexia nervosa or bulimia nervosa, that youngster should be referred to an interdisciplinary team experienced and skilled in working with this special group of adolescents.[41]

> *Tiffany is 16 years old. Her parents have recently become concerned because they have noticed that Tiffany's clothes are fitting loosely. In addition, Tiffany avoids eating with the family and has eliminated sweets, dairy products, and meats from her diet. She wakes up at six in the morning to take a run every day. Although Tiffany continues to do well in school and in her extracurricular activities, her parents have decided to bring her to the family doctor. Tiffany weighs 15 pounds less than she did a year ago at her last visit. Her heart rate is 50 at rest, and her body temperature is sub-normal. She has not had a period in the past 3 months and is not sexually active. Tiffany denies using any laxatives or diet pills and states that she does not make herself throw up because it hurts too much. Tiffany likes to weigh herself before each meal in order to know how much food she can eat. Although Tiffany is concerned about some recent hair loss, she does not think that she has an eating disorder and would actually like to lose 10 more pounds. Tiffany's doctor appropriately diagnoses anorexia nervosa and discusses the referral and treatment options with Tiffany and her parents.*

During the history and exam, the clinician can ascertain whether the teen has body image, diet, or weight concerns. It may be helpful to ask the following:
■ Does the teen like the way her body looks?
■ Is there anything the teen doesn't like or would like to change about herself?
■ Would the teen like to weight a particular amount?
It is important to identify those teens who are actively dieting, skipping meals, restricting certain foods, or exercising excessively. It is also important to identify those teens who are eating excess amounts of fast foods or fried foods, who are not engaging in any form of exercise or physical activity, and who have a family history of hypertension, hyperlipidemia, or heart disease. Triglyceride and cholesterol screening may be warranted for some teen patients. A teen should be told if she has a weight, diet, or exercise problem, and the clinician should help make a plan about how to correct the problem. It is usually helpful to involve a parent in this discussion so that assistance can be given in menu preparation, shopping, or planning an exercise program. Parents often share similar problems and may benefit from the discussion.

Adolescent patients need reassurance about their bodies, especially adolescent females who are not overweight but think that they are fat. Even those teens who are doing well may have questions about their dietary intake and may appreciate information on how to meet their nutritional needs, especially for protein, calcium, and iron. The clinician can help every teen create an individual wellness plan for healthy living and can be supportive in the development of a positive body image.

Athletics

Many teens participate in organized sports at school or on teams outside of school. Most adolescent athletes can successfully combine sports, schoolwork, and a social life into a healthy balance and reap benefits in health and morale from the experience. Some, however, become obsessed or driven by coaches and parents to perform beyond their capabilities and to the exclusion of other activities. These teens may not realize to what extent their sport involvement has consumed their life. They may need someone to provide this perspective. Serious adolescent athletes who are aiming for athletic scholarships need to know that a minimum grade point average is required. They may not have considered the possibility of an unintended injury that would jeopardize their athletic career; they should be encouraged to develop themselves in other ways in case they become unable to compete in sports. Frequent injuries, stress factors, and chronic pain may be signs of overuse injury and a signal to the clinician that the teen is overexerting. Prolonged amenorrhea or extreme dietary measures to gain or lose weight may be a sign that the teen is overinvested in the sport at the cost of his own health.

Another extreme scenario is the use of performance-enhancing substances, such as caffeine, amphetamines, anabolic steroids, and creatine. Teens more frequently use more benign products to boost performance and physique, such as protein and energy mixes, bars, and drinks available in most health and nutrition stores. Teens, parents, and coaches, however, should understand the dangers associated with the use of amphetamines and anabolic steroids. Although creatine is used by many professional athletes, its potential effects on kidney function are still debated. When addressing the use of drugs in sports, the media focus on college, Olympic, and professional athletes. The use of performing-enhancing substances by adolescents, however, is a real problem. In fact, the 1995 Youth Risk and Behavior Surveillance System shows that 4.9% of males and 2.4% of females in grades 9 through 12 across the United States have used anabolic steroids at least once in their lives.[42] This is not to say that adolescent athletes need to be screened for anabolic steroids or other drugs, but the clinicians, coaches, and parents should be aware of the potential for abuse.

Illicit Drugs, Cigarettes, and Alcohol

Although children are exposed to drugs even in grade school, the pressure to use them is not usually as threatening as it is in mid-adolescence. When adolescents begin dating, they may also begin substance use and misuse. Many adolescents experiment with drugs (especially alcohol), but they may be reluctant to admit using these substances if an authority figure asks them directly. Sometimes it is productive to ask about peer group usage of substances rather than about the individual teen's use and to provide factual information on the possible effects of these substances on health.

"Tommy, I know that many teens your age are using drugs. What about in your school or in your neighborhood? Are your friends using drugs or smoking on a regular basis? Do you ever feel pressured into trying drugs, smoking cigarettes, or drinking alcohol?"

Although it is common for adolescents to experiment with alcohol and marijuana, it is not normal for adolescents to be habitually drunk or "stoned," and it is not normal for adolescents to use "hard drugs," such as cocaine, phencyclidine (PCP), or amphetamines.

Half of the students in high school have used illicit drugs, most commonly marijuana and inhalants.[43] Many teens don't understand that infrequent use can be toxic if large quantities are ingested. When adolescents do admit using alcohol or other drugs, it is appropriate to ask about the frequency and amount. The experienced clinician will usually double or quadruple the figure given by the adolescent.

Some signs of drug abuse are a drop in school performance, accidents, family stress, legal problems, and noticeable changes in behavior, dress, or peer group.[43] These substance-using teens need special help.[29] Adolescents who abuse drugs should be referred for drug counseling with mental health workers experienced in drug counseling of youth. Frequently this requires residential treatment, and pediatricians should become familiar with drug rehabilitation agencies in their area of practice. Drug usage that alters a youngster's functioning cannot be dealt with in an ordinary pediatric office setting.

For those teens who remain abstinent, positive reinforcement is a must. Compliment the teen on his decision to stay away from cigarettes, alcohol, or other drugs. "Good for you! You are really doing the best thing for your body." Encourage the teen to remain abstinent. "I know it may be difficult to not smoke, drink, or use drugs with some friends, but I feel that you are a very strong person and don't need to do those things to feel good about yourself." Leave the door open for future discussions if the need arises. "I hope that you can come to me if you have any concerns about drugs, tobacco, or alcohol or if you are worried about someone you know who is using these substances."

Teenage Driver

The mid-adolescent is usually a newly licensed or about to be licensed driver and, as such, is inexperienced in the skill of driving. The motor vehicle fatality rate is higher for adolescents than for any other age group. In fact, drivers who are 16 years old are more than 20 times as likely to have a crash as the general population, when compared on a per-mile-driven basis.[23] Teenagers tend to drive more at night and have a much higher nighttime crash fatality rate. In addition, adolescents use seat belts only 35% of the time. The combination of high risk-taking behavior and lack of driving experience accounts for the increased risk of a **teenage driver** crashing.[23]

It is unclear whether a discussion on automobile safety between the adolescent patient and health care provider is helpful in preventing motor vehicle accidents. Most sensitive adolescents, however, will give at least transient thought to the clinician's observation that more teenagers die from accidents than from any other cause. The clinician should encourage the adolescent to avoid driving while under the influence of alcohol or other drugs and to avoid riding in a car driven by someone who is intoxicated. Parents and teens may want to discuss the availability of a nonjudgmental, noninquisitional, safe adult from whom the teen may request a ride home if she finds herself in an unsafe situation.[23] Teens should be urged to always wear a seat belt and to be especially careful while driving at night.

Helmet Usage

Many teenagers ride motorcycles and bicycles and yet do not use helmets. A clinician may ask if the teenager uses a helmet and then explain that the most common result of not wearing a helmet when riding a bike or motorcycle is serious head injury, with paralysis and permanent disabilities. Again, it is not helpful to preach to the adolescent, but merely to give facts with which he can make his own decisions.

ANTICIPATORY GUIDANCE FOR PARENTS
Limit Setting Versus Power Struggle

It is not unusual for mid-teens to "test" all authority figures, including parents, but this does not mean that they do not need or want rules or regulations. Indeed, most mid-adolescents appreciate reasonable parental limit setting as evidence of parental concern and as a safe, bounded area in which to function. But there is a difference between limit setting and power struggle. Limit setting refers to rules and regulations concerning behavior; power struggle occurs when authority itself is at stake regardless of the issue being discussed. Limit setting is necessary; power struggles should be avoided because someone (usually the teenager) always loses face and is inevitably resentful and bitter. One example of limit setting is the curfew. Teens and their parents should decide together on a reasonable curfew; also, in advance, the parent and teen should discuss the consequences that will follow the curfew's being missed. In contrast, a power struggle may involve an argument over one person being "right" and the other person "wrong." Usually the subject matter is unimportant; being "right" is all that counts. Because limit setting consists of rules, these may need to be modified as the adolescent matures or the situation changes. Adolescents and parents should be encouraged to communicate as these changing needs arise.

Cross-Sex Parent Attachments

As adolescents cope with sexual issues, it is common for them to experience renewed attraction for the opposite-sex parent. This is the reemergence of the "Oedipal complex" (see Chapter 16). In healthy families, this attraction may be used to bolster the adolescent's self-esteem and provide reassurance to the young person that he is developing into an attractive normal adult. In most families, this phenomenon is expressed in normal parental-filial affection and pride. In other families, the cross-sex parent attachment is a threatening experience or a source of conflict or pain. In such instances, the conflict is almost always the result of a parental problem. Some parents become frightened by their child's attentions, particularly because it occurs at a time when the youngster is sexually blossoming. A parent may become aloof and distant from a youngster who, in turn, finds such action confusing. For example, a father may tell his daughter that she's "too big to be hugged anymore," even though he continues to hug the younger children. Another father may inappropriately respond to his daughter's attentions by taking sexual liberties in the form of incest. It is normal for parents to find their adolescent children attractive. In fact, the son or daughter usually resembles the parents at a younger age or looks like the spouse looked when the parents married. Given this similarity, it is not unusual that the teenage youngster is also seen as attractive. It is *not* normal to act on that attractiveness or to take advantage of the teen's stage of development for personal sexual gratification. All cases of suspected incest should be referred to the appropriate authorities for investigation.

Vicarious Satisfaction in Adolescent's Activities

Sometimes the parents of adolescents unconsciously encourage adolescents to misbehave so that the teenager will act out the parent's own fantasies. For example, a mother may warn a daughter to remain a virgin until marriage, yet buy her revealing or provocative clothing. If so, this area should be explored and brought to the parent's attention.

Effect of Parenting an Adolescent

It is not easy to be a parent, and the mid-adolescent years may be the most difficult for some parents. They should be prepared for the commonly experienced conflicts involved in raising adolescents. For example, for the first time, parents may face unresolved issues from the adolescent's childhood and unresolved issues from their own adolescence, and they may find their authority as parents repeatedly challenged. Parents should be reassured that the best approach to their teenagers (and to themselves) is to keep lines of communication open. Parental connectedness—that is the adolescent's perception of warmth, love, and caring from parents—and parental availability to the adolescent are key to the successful development and health of every adolescent.[5] In most families, parents find themselves growing in wisdom as they struggle with the issues that teenage children force them to face.

REFERENCES

1. Offer D, Ostrow E, Howard K: Adolescence: What is normal?, *Am J Dis Child* 143:731, 1989.
2. Weiner IB: Distinguishing healthy from disturbed adolescent development, *J Dev Behav Pediatr* 11:151, 1990.
3. Alan Guttmacher Institute: *Sex and America's teenagers,* New York, 1994, Alan Guttmacher Institute.
4. Ozer EM et al: *America's adolescents: Are they healthy?,* San Francisco, 1997, National Adolescent Health Information Center.
5. Resnick MD, et al.: Protecting adolescents from harm—findings from the National Longitudinal Study of Adolescent Health, *JAMA* 278(10):823, 1997.
6. Moore KA et al: *Facts at a glance,* Washington, DC, October 1997, Child Trends.
7. Schoen C et al: *The Commonwealth Fund survey of the health of adolescent girls,* New York, 1997, The Commonwealth Fund.
8. Luster T, Small SA: Sexual abuse history and number of sexual partners among female adolescents, *Fam Plann Perspect* 29(5):204, 1997.
9. Stock JK, et al.: Adolescent pregnancy and sexual risk-taking among sexually abused girls, *Fam Plann Perspect* 29(5):200, 1997.
10. East PL, Felice ME: *Adolescent pregnancy and parenting—findings from a racially diverse sample,* Mahway, NJ, 1996, Lawrence Erlbaum Associates.
11. Collins C: Dangerous inhibitions: how America is letting AIDS become an epidemic of the young, *Monograph Series #3,* San Francisco, February 1997, Center for AIDS Prevention Studies.
12. National Adolescent Health Information Center, UCSF: Fact sheet on adolescent sexuality, *Adolescent Fact File,* San Francisco, March, 1996, National Adolescent Health Information Center.
13. Irwin CE, Shafer MA: Adolescent sexuality: Negative outcomes of a normative behavior. In Rogers DE, Ginzbert E, editors: *Adolescents at risk: medical and social perspectives,* Boulder, Colo, 1992, Westview Press.
14. Remafedi G et al.: Demography of sexual orientation in adolescents, *Pediatrics* 89:714, 1992.

15. Remafedi G: Homosexual youth: a challenge to contemporary society, *JAMA* 258:222, 1987.
16. Troiden R: Homosexual identify development, *J Adolesc Health Care* 9:105, 1988.
17. Ehrhardt AA, Remien RH: Sexual orientation. In McAnarney ER et al, editors: *Textbook of adolescent medicine,* Philadelphia, 1992, WB Saunders.
18. Nelson JA: Gay, lesbian, and bisexual adolescents: providing esteem-enhancing care to a battered population, *Nurse Pract* 22(2):94, 1997.
19. Radkowsky M, Siegel LJ: The gay adolescent: stressors, adaptations, and psychosocial interventions, *Clin Psychol Rev* 17(2):191, 1997.
20. Piaget J: The intellectual development of the adolescent. In Caplan G, Lebovici S, editors: *Adolescence: psychological perspectives,* New York, 1969, Basic Books.
21. Elkind D: Egocentrism in adolescence, *Child Dev* 38:1025, 1967.
22. Kohlberg L, Gilligan C: The adolescent as a philosopher: the discovery of the self in a post-conventional world. In Kagan J, Coles R, editors: *12 to 16: Early adolescence,* New York, 1972, WW Norton.
23. American Academy of Pediatrics, Committee on Injury and Poison Prevention and Committee on Adolescence: The teenage driver, *Pediatrics* 98(5):987, 1996.
24. Schwartz DF: Violence, *Pediatr Rev* 17(6):197, 1996.
25. American Academy of Pediatrics, Committee on Practice and Ambulatory Medicine: Recommendations for preventive pediatric health care, *Pediatrics* 96(2 Pt 1):373, 1995.
26. American Medical Association, Department of Adolescent Health: Guidelines for adolescent preventive services (GAPS), *Recommendations Monograph,* ed 3, Chicago, 1996, American Medical Association.
27. Cohen M, Friedman SB: Nonsexual motivation of adolescent sexual behavior, *Med Aspects Hum Sex* 9:31, 1975.
28. Wolraich ML, Felice ME, Drotar D, editors: *The classification of child and adolescent mental diagnoses in primary care,* Elk Grove Village, Ill, 1996, American Academy of Pediatrics.
29. American Academy of Pediatrics: *Substance abuse: A guide for health professionals,* Elk Grove Village, IL, 1988, American Academy of Pediatrics.
30. Black JL: Adolescents with learning problems, *Prim Care* 14:203, 1987.
31. Ensign J, Santelli J: Health status and services use: comparison of adolescents at a school-based clinic with homeless adolescents, *Arch Pediatr Adolesc Med* 152:20, 1998.
32. Ensign J, Santelli J: Shelter-based homeless youth, *Arch Pediatr Adolesc Med* 151:817, 1997.
33. National Adolescent Health Information Center, UCSF: Fact sheet: Out-of-home youth—foster care, incarcerated, homeless/runaways adolescents, *Adolescent Fact File,* San Francisco, August, 1996, National Adolescent Health Information Center.
34. Szilagyi M: The pediatrician and the child in foster care, *Pediatr Rev* 19(2):39, 1988.
35. Cagampang HH et al.: Education Now and Babies Later (ENABL): Life history of a campaign to postpone sexual involvement, *Fam Plann Perspect* 29(3):109, 1997.
36. Kirby D et al: The impact of the postponing sexual involvement curriculum among youths in California, *Fam Plann Perspect* 29(3):100, 1997.
37. Cromer BA, Frankel ME, Keder LM: Compliance with breast self-examination instruction in healthy adolescents, *J Adolesc Health Care* 10:105, 1989.
38. Klein JF, Berry CC, Felice ME: The development of a testicular self-examination instructional booklet for adolescents, *J Adolesc Health Care* 11:235, 1990.
39. Berg FM: Three major U.S. studies describe trends, *Healthy Weight Journal* 11(4):67, 1997.
40. Johnston PK, Haddad EH: Vegetarian and other dietary practices. In Rickert VI, editor: *Adolescent nutrition—assessment and management,* New York, 1996, Chapman & Hall.

41. Kreipe RE: Eating disorders among children and adolescents, *Pediatr Rev* 16(10):370, 1995.
42. Yesalis CE et al: Trends in anabolic-androgenic steroid use among adolescents, *Arch Pediatr Adolesc Med* 151:1197, 1997.
43. Knight JR: Adolescent substance use: screening, assessment, and intervention, *Contemp Pediatr* 14(4):45, 1997.

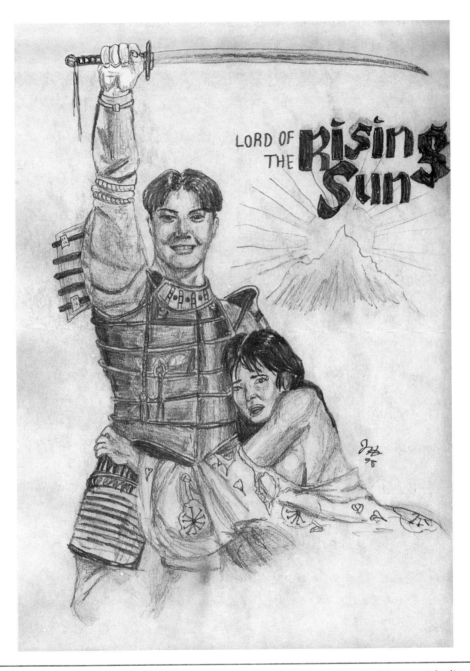

A 15-year-old boy draws himself as a superhero warrior, like a comic book character. Idealized stereotypes such as this testify to the struggle to define a gender identity and develop cross-gender relationships. These stylized pictures often are used as a safe presentation of self. By John Henry.

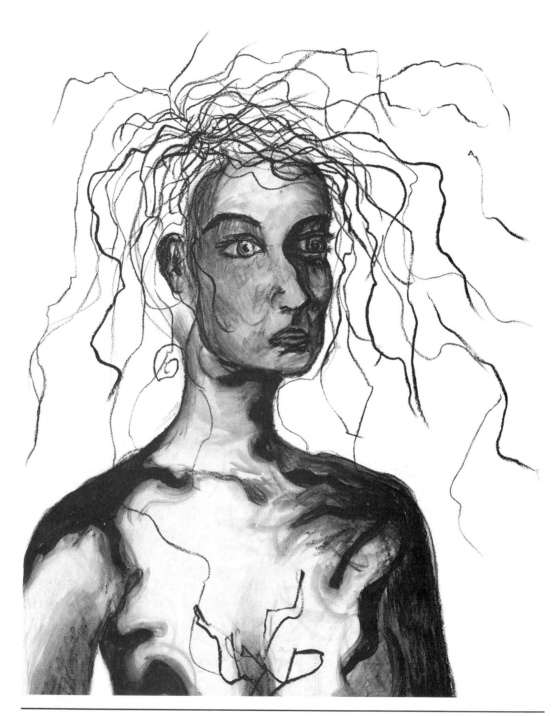

A 17-year-old's self portrait conveys outward calm and sophistication, hiding the anxiety, tension, and confusion that mark this important transition time. By Jessie Boilek. (Original 16″ × 20″ charcoal significantly better than reproduction.)

CHAPTER 22

LATE ADOLESCENCE

■ Lawrence S. Friedman

KEY WORDS
Vocation Planning
Critical Life Transitions
Intimate Relationships
Homosexuality
Substance Abuse
HIV/AIDS

Betsy, an 18-year-old high school senior, with below average grades, but above average performance on college entry examinations, has decided to forego application to college and apply for a job in the retail fashion industry. In spite of pressure from her mother to attend a local community college, Betsy wants to be financially independent and live with her boyfriend.

Three years earlier, Betsy's parents divorced. She currently lives with her mother and her mother's boyfriend. Gradually, since her parents' divorce, Betsy has become moody, has withdrawn from family activities, and has developed a new set of friends who are older and no longer in school. Several months ago her mother discovered a small amount of marijuana and an empty bottle of vodka in Betsy's bedroom. Betsy's father, who now lives in a neighboring town, thinks that his daughter may have a drinking problem, but her mother thinks that she is just behaving like a lot of other teenagers.

Late adolescence is the final stage in transition from childhood to adulthood. The defining issue of this developmental period is realistic awareness of "who I am." The integration of family, peer, educational, social, cultural, and community experiences comes into clearer focus and is grounded in enhanced behavioral, emotional, and cognitive maturity. Many adolescents are now less dependent upon peers and are able to develop realistic vocational goals, pursue monogamous interpersonal relationships, and embrace individual ethical and moral standards. Although the independent "self," defined by vocation, relationships, and values, takes form during late adolescence, realistically these are lifelong evolving processes. Similarly, by late adolescence almost all teenagers have accommodated themselves to adult physical stature but will continue adjusting to evolving physical appearance throughout adulthood.

As with earlier stages of adolescence, not all teenagers progress at similar physical or emotional rates. For example, although an 18-year-old boy is physically capable of fathering a child, he may not be emotionally capable of responsible fatherhood. In addition, many factors interfere with normal development. For instance, teenagers who heavily abuse alcohol or other mind-altering substances frequently have delayed emotional, behavioral, and cognitive development. Likewise, the psychopathology of anorexia nervosa, which commonly afflicts girls during mid-adolescence, at least in part involves fear of sexual and emotional maturity and delays transition to adulthood. In general, teenagers given progressive independence and responsibility by supportive family, peers, school, and community are the teens most likely to achieve timely developmental hallmarks. Conversely, individuals who do not appropriately address the issues of early, middle, and late adolescence will likely grapple with these issues into adulthood.

VOCATION PLANNING

As teenagers prepare to enter the adult world, **vocation planning** becomes a preoccupation. Vocational options usually depend on a combination of cognitive ability, educational achievement, financial resources, and career goals. Superimposed on these factors may be other responsibilities, such as marriage or parenthood. As they enter late adolescence, most teenagers will be in the final stages of completing secondary education. However, some will be attending alternative schools, be school dropouts, or be incarcerated.

Under the best of circumstances, vocational decisions are made after consideration of competing options and when individual abilities and aspirations are satisfied. However, it is common for teenagers to make choices under considerable influence of friends, family, and counselors. Although vocational choices made under such circumstances may work out, they may lead to regret later in life. Delaying a decision for a year or two may in the long run be the best choice.

> *Betsy, who has the intellectual capacity to attend college, has for now decided on other plans. With questions about a drinking problem and perhaps depression, the decision to put off higher education may be correct. With those issues unresolved, the likelihood of Betsy's failing in college is greater. A timely medical and psychosocial evaluation, possibly followed by intervention and treatment for substance abuse and mental health issues will give Betsy the best opportunity to make the proper decision about what is best for her.*

For clinicians, discussion with a patient about future vocational plans may be useful as a catalyst to assess health risk behaviors and provide health education and anticipatory guidance. Almost all teenagers will be eager to have such a discussion if it occurs in a nonthreatening, nonjudgmental, and confidential manner. Common transition options are discussed in the following sections along with vocation-oriented suggestions for health-related discussions.

CRITICAL LIFE TRANSITIONS
Transition to College

Approximately 12 million American teenagers or young adults are currently enrolled in post-secondary school education. Of Americans between the ages of 18 and 24, approximately one half are enrolled in some sort of educational program or have already attended college. Although some believe that college may delay confronting issues of adulthood, significant variability of postsecondary educational experiences makes generalization difficult. Social and psychological adjustment may be more difficult for those attending college because of parental or social pressure and may predispose to greater degrees of substance abuse and depression. For some teenagers, college may represent the first extended time away from home. In some instances, heavy drinking and drug use, as well as suicidal thought, are related to stress associated with the difficulty of reproducing high school performance in a more competitive college environment.

Transition to Work or Unemployment

Teenagers enter the workforce under a variety of circumstances. Those who have dropped out of school before completing high school will generally have greater difficulty entering the workforce and have lower-paying unskilled jobs. A chronic illness or parenthood interrupts the education of a significant number of American teenagers. For some intelligent and capable teenagers, work may be an appropriate choice because on-the-job training may offer sufficient career preparation. Many successful individuals in business, professional sports, entertainment, and the arts never went beyond high school.

Transition to the Military

The military offers structure, discipline, excitement, education, and travel. Traditionally it has been a route of upward mobility for lower socioeconomic populations. The military may be a stepping stone, offering vocational training before entering the workforce, or may be a long-term career choice. Because comprehensive health care is provided, concern about health insurance and accessing health services is unwarranted.

Transition from Incarceration

A growing number of teenagers spend their adolescence (and often childhood) under social service or juvenile justice authority. At least 510,000 juveniles are incarcerated in the United States every year with a daily census of at least 65,000.[1] Nearly 90% are male, 60% are black or Hispanic, and between the ages of 14 and 17.[1] Juvenile delinquency is a complicated subject but is receiving increased study and community awareness. Teenagers who have been in the juvenile system for prolonged periods usually face daunting social, psychological, family, and career obstacles. These obstacles become magnified as teenagers transition from the juvenile to adult justice system. Because the criminal justice system generally treats minors more leniently than adults, incarcerated adolescents should be made aware that their changing legal status will change their legal consequences. Theoretically the juvenile justice system places greater emphasis on counseling, rehabilitation, and "second chances," whereas the adult system tends to be more punitive. Although health services provided to incarcerated youth are often superior to ones they might receive elsewhere, their health risk behaviors are generally greater than those of their peers. Compounding the problem is that many of these teenagers are neglected, disenfranchised, and have no health insurance. Most, but not all, are from lower socioeconomic strata. Health problems of this population often include substance abuse, family and interpersonal violence, sexually transmitted disease, poor dentition, and a variety of mental health problems.[2] Transition from incarceration back to society should be guided by the probation system. However, this system is often seriously overburdened, and health issues frequently receive low priority. It should not be assumed that probation officers have the knowledge to anticipate health issues or are aware of health care options. Minors should be informed about the adult legal and incarceration systems.

Transition from Homelessness

The problems of homeless and runaway youth are often similar to those who are incarcerated. A subgroup of homeless youth, but not all, will have been incarcerated or involved with legal authorities. Some teenagers are homeless along with their families; some are homeless for short periods of time and may live with friends or relatives; and others are homeless because they have run away from home and do not plan to return. In the last group, almost all have been victims of physical, severe psychological, or sexual abuse. Two thirds to three quarters of all runaways have experienced sexual or physical abuse, with such abuse reported more commonly among girls.[3] The needs of these teenagers may seem daunting but can be managed effectively when they are prioritized. A stable housing situation is most important because it is difficult to address issues of substance abuse or even a medical problem as simple as a respiratory infection if the teenager is constantly uncertain about shelter, food, and a place to keep medications.[4]

DEVELOPING INTIMATE INTERPERSONAL RELATIONSHIPS

Well-balanced transition from adolescence to adulthood includes the ability to develop **intimate relationships** with members of both genders. Some of these relationships will be emotional and others will be emotional and sexual. The ability to develop both emotional and sexual interpersonal relationships is inextricably intertwined with the definition of "who I am." By late adolescence, the security found in activities that are group centered gives way to activities that are individual centered. Like other developmental tasks, past collective experiences with family, peers, teachers, and community often define the degree to which intimate relationships develop. Individuals with poor self-esteem, inadequate or inappropriate role models, poor peer group acceptance, depression, or thought disorders may have difficulty developing mature intimate relationships.

> *Betsy has developed an "intimate" relationship with her boyfriend, but her seemingly unresolved issues about her parents' divorce, substance use, and depression put her at risk for unstable interpersonal relationships.*

Historical trends redefine interpersonal relationships within a constantly changing cultural context. Over the past half century the nature of marriage and family has changed dramatically in American culture (see Chapter 23). Early in the twentieth century, for instance, it was common for American teenagers to marry and begin raising families, often before finishing high school. Those living in rural farming communities were encouraged to have large families to help with household and farm chores. At the same time, out-of-wedlock pregnancy was a personal and family embarrassment and usually resulted in adoption or marriage. Today, marriage is often delayed because cohabitation is culturally acceptable and because both individuals want to continue their education so that each can obtain full-time employment. Concurrently, improvements in family planning and economic necessity have prevented many unwanted pregnancies and have decreased the size of the average American family. Also, unmarried teenagers who are pregnant or are parents are no longer ostracized. Although new strategies are constantly being developed to decrease unwanted teenage pregnancy, the status of these adolescents is discussed openly and they are accommodated with special schools and parenting programs.[5]

The nature of marriage, as well as the permanency and definition of interpersonal relationships, continues to change. Over half of marriages in the United States currently end in divorce. Many teenagers today are raised in households of divorced parents, and research indicates that they are at risk for repeating this pattern of marital behavior (see Chapter 23). The long-term effects of these changes in social patterns are not clear. However, the next 50 years may see continued remodeling of the American family and new roles for religion and other social institutions. Evidence of social change is probably no better demonstrated than in the current dialogue about the characteristics and legitimacy of homosexual relationships, marriage, and families in American society.

GAY AND LESBIAN YOUTH

Only two decades ago, **homosexuality** was defined within the context of psychopathology by national mental health and medical organizations. It was rarely a subject of public discussion. Since the 1980s, when the American Psychological Association and psychiatric and other medical societies redefined homosexuality as a normal psychological variant, a greater national dialogue and gradual acceptance of this alternative life-style have taken place.[6-8] The last few years have found major corporations offering health insurance and other benefits to homosexual partners, national figures disclosing their sexual orientation, and a variety of governmental and religious organizations actively debating the legitimacy of homosexual adoption, partner rights, and marriage.

The etiology of homosexuality is the subject of ongoing research, but it likely involves some blend of environmental and genetic factors.[9] It is estimated that between 5% and 10% of adults identify themselves as exclusively homosexual, and a greater percentage have had periodic homosexual thoughts or experiences.[10,11] Some studies indicate that up to 20% to 30% of the male population has had at least one same-sex sexual experience, usually sometime during adolescence.[10] These experiences may lead to anxiety, shame, and guilt and do not alone indicate a homosexual orientation. Although homosexual teenagers' acknowledging their sexuality is still fraught with the risk of social isolation and physical violence, greater social tolerance in recent years has made many feel more safe about doing so. Like other teenagers, however, homosexual teens become aware of their sexual feelings during early or middle adolescence and often have a variety of sexual experiences before making a definitive life-style choice.[12,13]

Gay and lesbian teenagers can benefit from informed, supportive, and nonjudgmental health care providers. Although many positive role models and institutions now exist that can help homosexual youth build self-esteem, in many cases, tremendously negative pressure still comes from family, peer community, and society. The social isolation and poor self-esteem many of these teenagers experience may lead to depression, suicide, or increased rates of alcohol and drug use.[14] Health care providers should assess the level of self-acceptance in homosexual teens and also assess potential external stressors, such as parents, church, school, and peers. It is important to become aware of peer support groups for teenagers and their families so that referral can be made when appropriate. Most regions have support groups for gay and lesbian youth, and they are usually listed in telephone books or affiliated with colleges or universities. Parents frequently find support in the local Parents and Friends of Lesbian and Gay Youth (PFLAG), which has a chapter in most urban areas. For social and emotional support, teenagers and young adults who so desire should be referred to a gay and lesbian youth group in their area. If no such group exists, a local college or university may have or know of an appropriate group.

CHRONIC DISEASE

Approximately 2 million teenagers in the United States have a chronic illness or disability. This is a diverse group, entering adulthood with a variety of medical expectations, needs, and concerns. Like other teenagers, their concerns usually center around physical, social, and sexual development. Ideally, during earlier adolescence, these concerns have been honestly addressed while, at the same time, parents and care providers have allowed the teenager a progressively greater role in making medical decisions. Additionally, realistic identification of academic, vocational, and social capabilities is important to enhance self-esteem and peer relationships. As this vulnerable population enters adulthood, it is especially important for health care providers to assess the capability to navigate a complicated health care system. Probably the most important task is assessing whether health insurance benefits will continue after leaving adolescence. Most teenagers who have relied on parents or the government for health insurance will need guidance about these issues and possible referral to knowledgeable experts.[15] Teenagers who discontinue their education, move out of their parents' house, and work at low-wage jobs are most at risk for losing all health insurance coverage.

Unless health insurance is an employment benefit, Betsy's decision to enter the work force may jeopardize her health benefits if she has been getting them under either parent's policy. Staying in school frequently allows continuation under a parent's policy.

One of the greatest challenges may be the transition to a new set of health care providers for adults. In many cases, patients and parents will have grown up with and become dependent upon the same team of pediatric nurses, social workers, and physicians. Separation may be difficult for patients, parents, and providers, and the process can be managed most successfully over a period of time that allows for several office visits. Ease of transition will depend on parental trust and the patient's ability to assume and demonstrate responsibility for self-care and sensible decision making.

ALCOHOL AND OTHER SUBSTANCE ABUSE PROBLEMS

Natural history studies indicate that most adolescents who use alcohol and other drugs will, as they assume adult roles and responsibilities, spontaneously quit using drugs and develop controlled patterns of alcohol consumption.[16] However, a small proportion will be seriously affected by use during adolescence. Motor vehicle and pedestrian accidents, interpersonal violence, date rape, suicide, and decreased use of condoms are all associated with alcohol or substance use.[17,18] In addition, approximately 20% of adults become dependent upon substances and with few exceptions, harmful patterns of use begin to appear during adolescence. The section in this chapter on interviewing should assist in identifying those who need special attention and intervention (Box 22-1).

Working with substance-abusing patients frequently frustrates health care providers. Frustration comes because treatment often seems futile; treatment resources are limited; patients and their families are in denial; and patients often do not ask for help. These issues can be addressed partially by learning about appropriate community referral sources, treatment programs, and counselors, including Alcoholics and Narcotics Anonymous groups specifically for teenagers and young adults.[19] The local telephone directory is usually the best source for local self-help groups such as Alcoholics Anonymous, Cocaine Anonymous, Narcotics Anonymous, and Alanon (for individuals and families living with someone with a drinking problem). Inquiry should be made about local groups specifically for teenagers and young adults. If age-appropriate groups don't seem to exist, local college or university health centers can frequently provide referral assistance. Denial frequently interferes with patients' and families' abilities to recognize the connection between alcohol or substance use and adverse consequences. Denial is a recognized adaptive mechanism often used by patients and their families to avoid the discomfort associated with admitting a substance abuse problem. It is predictable and can be addressed through multiple visits. In time, denial can be overcome by a respectful, empathic, and supportive clinician. Patients will not change their behavior until they are ready. Although a drinking or drug problem may be obvious, advice to change will be

BOX 22-1	RISK FACTORS FOR SUBSTANCE USE AND ABUSE AMONG ADOLESCENTS

Characteristics
Family History
Low Self-Esteem
   Learning disabilities
   Poor body image
   Gay/lesbian identity
   Chronic disease
   Physical, psychological, or sexual abuse
Depression/Thought Disorder
Antisocial Personality
Peer and Cultural Pressure
Repeated Thrill and Risk-Taking Behavior
Young Age of Initiation

Diagnostic Clues
Change in Peer Group
Increased School or Work Absences
Decline in Grades or Work Performance
Increased Interpersonal Turmoil and Arguments

futile if the patient is not ready. Assessing the stage of change (Table 22-1) and working with patients at their current "level" make the process easier and more assessable for the provider and patient.

     Chemical dependency is a chronic medical condition with lifelong implications. Like other chronic medical conditions, it has periods in which symptoms are well controlled and periods of relapse. Because of this, successfully intervening with an adolescent does not preclude periods of relapse in adulthood.

Drug Testing

Bioethical principles about patients' rights apply to drug testing.[20] Testing should be performed only for the benefit of the patient and only with the patient's consent. This is often a point of contention between parents of minors and providers. For patients who are no longer minors, it is less of an issue. To begin with, it is important to know what is included in the drug test done at an individual laboratory or facility. Urine drug testing never includes the most commonly abused substance, alcohol. Many laboratories do not include tetrahydrocannabis (THC—the active ingredient in marijuana) in their screening drug panel. Moreover, the ability to detect drugs depends upon the dose and frequency of drug use in question.

TABLE 22-1 ■ Stages of Change: Preparing Adolescents to Change Addictive Behavior

Stage	Description	Motivational Task
I. Precontemplation	No acknowledgment of a problem or a need for change. Physician should present "evidence" of a problem and raise patient's awareness. Do not expect patient to agree with diagnosis or plan.	Create doubt, increase awareness of risks and problems with current patterns of substance use.
II. Contemplation	Patients are ambivalent about having a problem or needing to change. Physicians should help patients become aware of their ambivalence. Help patients reflect on their comments such as: "You said at times you feel like you should stop drinking. Tell me why you feel that way."	Help weigh relative risks and benefits of changing substance use, evoke reasons to change and risks of not changing, strengthen self-efficacy for changing current substance use.
III. Determination	Accepts problem and willing to attempt treatment. Treatment options (day program, evening program, Alcoholics Anonymous or other 12-step programs) should be provided, and patient must participate in choosing the most appropriate.	Help determine best course of action to change substance use from available alternatives.
IV. Action	Attends treatment program and attempts to change behavior.	Help establish clear plan of action toward changing substance use.
V. Maintenance	Requires skills to maintain sobriety and is usually dependent on positive experience and treatment and its effects. Positive reinforcement by health provider, family, and social and work environment is important.	Help identify and use strategies to prevent relapse.
VI. Relapse	Recurrence of substance abuse. Some may slip back into contemplative stages. Possibility of relapse should be discussed with patients and, as with other chronic disorders, should not be unexpected.	Help renew process of change starting at contemplation.

Modfied from: Samet JH, Rollnick S, Barnes H: A brief clinical approach after detection of substance abuse. *Arch Int Med* 156:2287, 1996.

Many parents request drug testing as a substitute for teenager-parent communication. Because of this, it is important to explore reasons for the test request. Before a test is performed, parents should be asked the following questions:

- "Why and what do you suspect your teenager is using?" If the answer is something obvious, such as drugs or empty bottles discovered in the teen's bedroom, testing is rarely helpful.
- "What do you plan to do if the test is positive?" It is important that a plan is in place beforehand and that both parents agree on the plan. If the drug in question is used infrequently or in relatively low doses, it is quite possible that the test will be negative.
- "What will you do if the test is negative?" This is not a trivial issue because it becomes more difficult to change the behavior of a substance-using teenager who receives a negative test result.

Testing is always justified if the teenager consents. It can also be helpful to satisfy parental concern before the teen is allowed to get a driver's license or to continue use of the family car. It can also be a way for those in recovery to prove and maintain abstinence.

 Betsy should be evaluated to assess her "stage" of substance use or abuse and to determine what type of intervention, if any, is appropriate. At the same time, she should be assessed for depression. Because substances themselves or the effects of withdrawal can mimic mental health problems, coexisting mental health problems are best evaluated when the patient is known to be substance free for several weeks.

TAKING A MEDICAL HISTORY

As with all teenagers, the clinician must ensure confidentiality before beginning the interview. Because the questions may seem embarrassing, intrusive, or trivial from the patient's perspective, it is important to reassure patients that all questions are asked to provide advice about maintaining health and avoiding disease. Patients 18 years or older are legally adults.

Betsy is 18. Legal statutes require that all decisions about health care be her own. This is the case even though her parents may be "paying the bills."

For those who recently became adults, it is important to reaffirm legal provisions of consent and disclosure. This is especially true if the patient is accompanied to appointments by a parent. Most teenagers want to discuss and receive information about health-related behaviors, such as sex, drugs, protection against human immunodeficiency virus (HIV) and sexually transmitted disease (STD), and pregnancy prevention.[21] Most teenagers or young adults, however, will not initiate such discussions. They depend on the care provider to begin a dialogue.

HIV/AIDS

HIV risk assessment, counseling, and testing have become routine among those providing health services to teenagers and young adults. Although teenagers constitute a relatively small proportion (approximately 1%) of AIDS cases nationally, the long incubation time (approximately 10 years) and large proportion of AIDS cases affecting individuals in their third decade of life indicate that adolescents are at substantial risk of HIV infection.[22] Adolescent rates of unprotected sexual intercourse, as measured by unwanted pregnancy and STDs, substantiate this concern.[23] Clinicians should be knowledgeable about which groups are at highest risk and know local HIV seroprevalence among teenagers. National data indicate that minority females, gay males, and those practicing survival sex (having sex for money, food, drugs, or shelter) are at greatest risk.[24] Having sex with older partners, who themselves may have had multiple partners or used intravenous drugs, is the thread that connects the highest risk teenagers (Figs. 22-1 and 22-2).[25] Many teenagers are concerned about their risk for HIV and are often encouraged to be tested without thought to the potential consequences. Reasons for requesting an HIV test frequently include health concern, guilt or anxiety about sexual experiences, media messages, school curriculum, and peer group pressure. Everyone should be counseled that HIV does not preferentially infect stereotypical groups but is spread only by specific behavioral practices, all of which involve exchange of body fluid. Intravenous drug users should be advised to use sterile needles exclusively, and condom use should be advised for all who are sexually active. Special attention should be paid to the most vulnerable patients because they are usually the least able to handle the implications of HIV infection. It is always hoped that those who are HIV infected will alter behavior to stay healthy and prevent others from becoming infected. This may not apply to those who are substance dependent, homeless, or runaways. These teenagers are often disenfranchised, angry, and have difficulty trusting adults. In this population, consideration about substance abuse treatment, housing, case management, social services, and availability of medical services should be given before HIV testing.

DATA GATHERING
Life Transitions

College. Ask about reasons for attending college, vocational goals, and whether attendance is self-motivated. Discuss separation fears and potential benefits about moving away from home.

Employment/unemployment. Ask about reasons for entering the work force and about preparedness to accept financial independence and responsibility. Ask pregnant or parenting teenagers about plans to reenter school or the workplace.

Military. Ask about reasons for enlisting and whether this is a career path or a means to developing a skill set. Discussion about exposure to alcohol, drugs, and sex should be similar to that for those attending college.

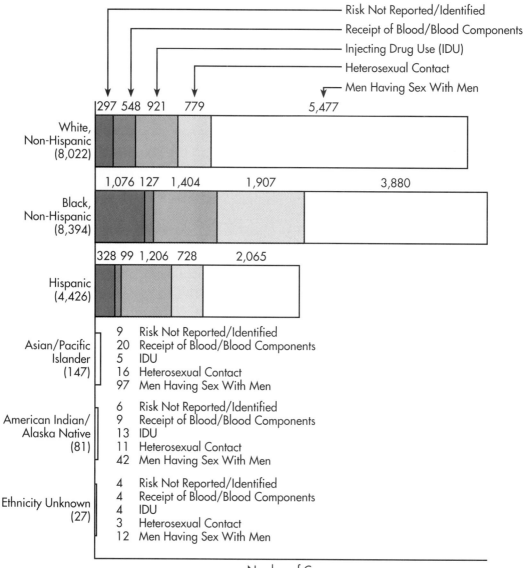

Fig. 22-1 Young adult AIDS cases by race or ethnicity and exposure category for ages 20 to 24 from 1981 to 1996. (From Centers for Disease Control and Prevention, National Center for HIF, STD, TB Prevention: HIV/AIDS surveillance report, year-end edition, Atlanta, 1996, Public Health Service.)

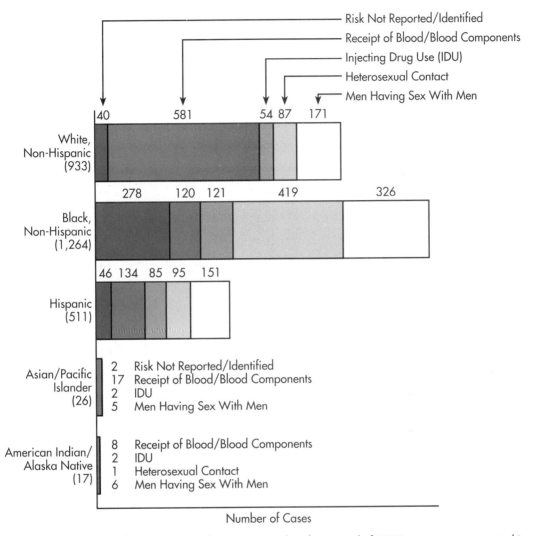

Fig. 22-2 Adolescent AIDS cases by race or ethnicity and exposure category for ages 13 to 19 from 1981 to 1996. (From Centers for Disease Control and Prevention, National Center for HIF, STD, TB Prevention: HIV/AIDS surveillance report, year-end edition, Atlanta, 1996, Public Health Service.)

Incarceration. Inquiry should be made about whether and where routine health care is obtained in the community.

Homelessness. Ask about the circumstance that led to homelessness.

Organizing History

For organizational ease and consistency, to address current and potential health risk behaviors and to provide health education, many recommend that the history be organized to follow the *HEADS format—H(ome) E(ducation) A(ctivity) D(rugs) S(ex).*[26] Although most practitioners still depend on gathering data by using a verbal history, recent investigation suggests that a history obtained via interactive computer software may be even more accurate.[27]

Home

Goal: Determine whether patient lives independently, with family, with friends, in cohabitation with significant partner, or at home with parents temporarily.

For college students, determine living situation while at school and during vacations. If the patient is living with roommates, inquire about the household use of cigarettes, alcohol, and other drugs. It is generally difficult to live in a house with peers who use alcohol or other drugs heavily and have no personal use. Also, determine degree of financial independence, conflict resolution skills, and existence of household violence. If violence is present, determine whether the patient is victim or perpetrator.

Questions: "Where are you living now?" and "Who else lives where you live?" Ask whether the living situation is satisfactory and whether the patient is exposed to potential health-compromising behavior. For instance, cigarette smoking by roommates may explain recurrent asthma exacerbations, or financial hardship may prevent proper diet and nutrition. Questions about household violence should include "What happens when people in your household argue?" and "Does anyone ever get hurt during arguments?" This should be followed by "Do arguments ever happen when someone has been drinking or under the influence of drugs?" Ask about meals served at home (quality and availability of food). Is health care available when you need it?

 In Betsy's case, the reasons for her parents' divorce should be explored to determine whether alcohol, drugs, or physical abuse was involved. Additionally, Betsy's relationship with her mother's boyfriend needs exploration.

Education and Vocation

Goal: Evaluate current achievements, strengths, and weaknesses and their realistic connection to future plans. Assess for unrecognized learning disabilities and stress or anxiety related to college admission or separation from family, school, and community.

Questions: Discussion about educational or vocational status can initially be directed according to patient's age. For those still in school (high school or college) ask "What classes are you taking? How are your grades? How do your grades compare to last year?" Without specific questioning about classes or grades, most will typically respond that everything is "OK." Falling grades may indicate a mental health condition, a substance abuse problem, or a conflict with the development of a personal identity (see Chapter 2). Generally speaking, teenagers who are performing well in school are less likely to participate in multiple health risk behaviors.

For those not in school, ask "Have you graduated from high school?" If not, ask "What is the last grade you completed? Why did you drop out of school? Do you have any plans to complete high school?" The spectrum of reasons why youngsters drop out of school includes some that relate to physical and mental health conditions. Answers to these questions may help uncover learning disabilities, severe family disruption, or abuse by family or peers. For instance, an unrecognized learning disability may result in school termination because of recurrent poor performance, low self-esteem, and ridicule. Teenagers may leave home before completing high school because they have been sexually victimized or because they reveal gay or lesbian sexual orientation and become ostracized by family, school, and peers.

Activity

Goal: Evaluate social interactions, interests, and self-esteem.

Questions: "What do you do for fun?"or "Are you involved in any clubs, organizations, religious groups, sports, or hobbies?" Because activity participation is often linked to self-esteem, this may be a nonthreatening way to assess social skills, peer group, and community connections. Adolescents who participate only in solitary activities may have difficulty with social skills, feel alienated, or be depressed. Evidence is strong that teenagers who feel closely connected to family, school, and community are less likely to participate in health-compromising or delinquent behaviors than peers who are not well connected.[28] Depending on circumstances, also ask "Do you belong to a fraternity or sorority or to a gang?" These activities, to varying degrees, provide a sense of community and belonging. They also may be sources of extreme peer pressure and result in inappropriate drug and alcohol use, sexual behavior, or interpersonal violence. Gangs are a powerful source of identity for those who feel disempowered, disenfranchised, and alienated.

Drugs

Goal: Determine personal, environmental, and genetic risks for substance use and abuse and current habits. Identify those whose substance use is likely to interfere with social, mental, and physical performance. Injection drug use, uncommon in early and middle adolescence, usually begins in late adolescence or early adulthood, and identification is crucial. Reinforce the behavior of those who have chosen not to use drugs or alcohol (Table 22-2).

Questions: By late adolescence, most American teenagers have had some personal experience with cigarettes, alcohol, or other drugs. Among many teenagers, the use of substances is not considered abnormal or dangerous. In spite of this, questions about substance use may seem threatening and intrusive. For that reason, initiating the discussion by asking first about use by peers is often preferable. Begin by acknowledging that it is common for teenagers to have some drug or alcohol experiences. Then ask "Do any of your friends ever smoke cigarettes, drink alcohol, or use other drugs?" This should be followed by "Have you

TABLE 22-2 ■ Advice to Adolescents about Substance Abuse

Drug Use Status	Clinician's Action
Nonuser	Praise decision
Potential user	Praise decision and offer alternatives
Experimental user	Encourage quitting and set date
Committed user	Encourage quitting, set date, and ask again at next encounter

ever tried any of these substances?" Those whose friends use are more likely to use themselves. Even if the answer is negative, permission has been given to ask questions in the future. Inquiry should address specific substances, such as cigarettes, alcohol, marijuana, stimulants (cocaine, crystal methamphetamine), hallucinogens (LSD, mescaline, ecstasy), prescription pills, anabolic steroids, and opiates, as well as routes of ingestion such as intravenous, nasal, or inhalation. If the patient reports use, ask for each substance, "How often do you use (daily, weekly, occasionally, rarely)? When was the last time you used? How much do you use at a time? Is your use increasing (to determine whether tolerance is developing)? What are the circumstances of your use (parties, friends, alone)?" Determining level of use and whether a substantial problem exists can challenge the most experienced clinician. Recognition of a problem depends on patient's willingness to share and clinician's willingness to receive information about the use of drugs. Box 22-1 lists common risk factors and diagnostic clues associated with substance abuse.

Prejudicial statements and negative body language or facial expression by a provider will hinder the diagnostic process. Evaluation should initially focus on adverse consequences associated with use. Ask "Have you ever had any physical consequences such as vomiting, blacking out, or losing consciousness from use? Have you gotten into family, school, or legal trouble because of use? Have you found it difficult to drive when using a drug?"

Most chemically dependent teenagers are polysubstance users. Untreated, polysubstance use will generally continue into adulthood with the development of preference for a particular substance.

It is most important to differentiate teenagers at highest risk for developing adult problems from those whose use will moderate with time. Differentiation can often be achieved by searching for patterns of use common in adult users. Some classes of drugs, such as the stimulants (cocaine, crack, crystal methamphetamine) and the opiates (heroin), have had the bases of their addiction defined at the level of molecular receptors in the central nervous system.[29] On this basis, physical addiction, defined by tolerance and withdrawal, develops in anyone who uses opiates or sympathomimetics at high enough doses for long enough periods of time. Anyone who becomes a regular user is likely to become dependent. Predicting who may try using these drugs can be difficult. The same is not necessarily true of alcohol. For instance, many people consume wine daily and do not develop any signs or symptoms of alcohol abuse or dependency. Males who have a family history of alcoholism and those who begin use in early adolescence are at especially high risk for alcohol problems.[30,31] These individuals should be identified by asking "How old were you when you first began using, and how old were you when you started using regularly?" Obtaining an accurate family history isn't always easy. Rather than asking whether a parent or grandparent has a drinking problem it may be more efficient to ask, "Do your mother or father ever drink alcohol?" If so, "Have you ever seen either one intoxicated? Has either parent ever received treatment for a drug or alcohol problem or ever attended Alcoholics Anonymous?"

Convincing evidence exists that many alcoholics have high alcohol tolerance, are relatively insensitive to the effects of alcohol, and can consume extraordinary amounts without perception of adverse consequences.[30] This should be evaluated by asking, "What is the most that you have drunk at one time? When you drink, can you stop after one or two drinks, or is your goal always to get drunk? Can you feel the effect of one or two drinks?" Although no data support counseling's efficacy or prevention benefit, those at high risk because of family history should receive it and be told of their risk. They should be advised that if they don't drink, they will not develop an alcohol problem. A variety of diagnostic tools are available to identify substance abusers. Although all have advantages and disadvantages, perhaps the most widely tool used in the office setting is the *CAGE* questions (*Cut down, Annoyed, Guilty, Eye-opener* [Box 22-2]).

Affirmative answers to two or more CAGE questions strongly suggest an alcohol or drug problem. Although their predictive value in teenagers is still uncertain, the sensitivity and specificity of CAGE questions in adults are high enough to suggest that they might be integrated into every medical interview of young adults.[32]

Table 22-2 provides focused and timely counseling advice, developed for cigarette smoking, that can be used for other substances.

> *Betsy's change to an older peer group, withdrawal from family activities, moodiness, and the discovery of an empty alcohol bottle in her room—indicating nonsocial drinking—collectively suggest strongly a substance abuse problem. Whether a concurrent depression is present is important to know so that it can be treated. However, treatment of depression will be hampered by continued substance use.*

Sex

Goal: Evaluate and counsel about sexual behavior, family planning, sexually transmitted diseases, HIV, and sexual abuse. Reinforce the decision of those who have decided to remain sexually abstinent.

Questions: Open-ended questions that do not assume sexual orientation, such as "Have you ever been involved sexually with anyone?," are a nonthreatening way to begin a discussion. For those who report sexual involvement, to determine use of condoms and birth control, ask "How do you protect yourself from sexually transmitted diseases and pregnancy?" Ask females "Have you ever been pregnant?" and ask males "Have you ever fathered a child?" For those answering affirmatively ask "What was the pregnancy outcome?" Ask about the age of the sexual partner. Those with older partners may be at greater risk for sexually transmitted diseases, including HIV. If condom use is reported, ask "Do you use condoms some of the time or all of the time?" Because it is surprising how often a history of pregnancy or STD exists even in older teenagers who report always using a condom, it is

BOX 22-2	"CAGE" QUESTIONS FOR IDENTIFICATION OF ALCOHOL AND DRUG ABUSE

Pattern of Use

Have you ever felt the need to **CUT DOWN** on drinking (or drug use)?

Probe

What was it like? Were you successful? Why did you decide to cut down? Have you ever limited substance use in order to please someone?

Consequences

Have you ever felt **ANNOYED** by criticism about your drinking? (Drug use)?

Probe

Can you give me an example? What led to the criticism?

Consequences

Have you ever felt **GUILTY** about your drinking (drug use)? Or Have you ever felt **GUILTY** about something you said or did while you were drinking (using drugs)?

Probe

Tell me more about that. What happened? Can you give me an example of a specific event?

Pattern/Tolerance

Have you ever taken a morning **EYE-OPENER?**

Probe

Have you felt shaky or edgy after a night of heavy drinking (drug use)? What did you do to relieve the feeling? Have you ever had trouble getting back to sleep early in the morning after a night of heavy drinking (drug use)?

From Cyr MG, Sherman SE: Screening, assessment, making the diagnosis. In Bigby J, editor: *Substance abuse education in general internal medicine,* SGIM, HRSA and ADAMHA contract 240-91-0053, 1993.

worth reviewing safer sex, condom use, and effective methods of pregnancy prevention with all teenagers. Also ask, "Do you ever have sex while under the influence of drugs or alcohol?" It is important to inform patients that condom use diminishes significantly, even among those with excellent HIV prevention knowledge, when they are intoxicated. In addition, patients should be informed that almost all date rape occurs while one or both dating partners are under the influence.

Although it is important to reinforce the decision of those who have chosen sexual abstinence, they should be allowed to ask questions and be reassured that if their sexual behavior changes, they have a source of information, advice, and prevention resources.

PHYSICAL EXAMINATION

The *Guidelines for Adolescent Preventive Services*[33] recommend that adolescents who have no disease or symptom-specific complaints receive a health maintenance visit to discuss disease-related and prevention behaviors once during each period of adolescence—early, middle, and late. In the adolescent with symptoms or signs of drug use, depression, and other mental illnesses, more frequent office visits for an interval history, physical examination, or counseling are usually necessary. The American Academy of Pediatrics' *Guidelines for Health Supervision III*[34] recommend annual visits for health supervision and emphasize that social, psychological, educational, and vocational screening and counseling is a major part of the visit. In addition, these guidlines recommend that (1) all menstruating adolescents be screened once with laboratory evaluations of a hematocrit or hemoglobin, (2) a urine dipstick for leukocyte esterase and nitrate be performed once as a screening test for sexually transmitted diseases, and (3) a pelvic exam and Papanicolaou (Pap) smear be done as part of preventive health maintenance for patients between 18 and 21 years of age. During an examination of a late adolescent, attention should be directed to general condition, height, weight, blood pressure, and pulse rate. General appearance and cleanliness often provide clues about self-esteem, and type of clothing may indicate with which group or clique the teenager identifies. Look for tattoos and body piercing. Although tattoos are currently popular among many teenagers, pay attention to large tattoos of numbers or neighborhood names because they may indicate gang membership. Body piercing sites should be inspected for signs of infection, and inquiry should be made about whether piercing was self-inflicted or performed professionally. If self-inflicted, assess risk of hepatitis B or HIV transmission. Tanner staging should be performed, and any signs or symptoms of delayed puberty identified and evaluated. If not done in earlier adolescence, girls should be taught breast self-examination, and boys be taught testicular self-examination. Sexually active girls should receive a pelvic examination with Pap smear yearly. Those with multiple partners should have a Pap smear every 6 months.

Laboratory Examination

Routine laboratory evaluation in an asymptomatic late adolescence is usually unnecessary. Sexually active teenagers should routinely be screened for sexually transmitted diseases. Recent advent of urine screening using PCR and LCR for chlamydia and gonorrhea means that this evaluation can be performed accurately (high specificity and sensitivity) without requiring urethral swab or pelvic examination.[35,36]

Cholesterol screening is controversial. Those with a family history of hypercholesterolemia or early adult heart disease should be screened at least once during adolescence. However, screening should always be accompanied by counseling about diet and exercise. Vision testing should be performed periodically, once every 3 years for youth without symptoms. Audiometry is recommended when a hearing loss is suspected.

ANTICIPATORY GUIDANCE
Vocation Planning

For clinicians, discussion with a patient about future vocational plans may be useful as a catalyst to assess health risk behaviors and to provide health education and anticipatory guidance. Almost all teenagers will be eager to have such a discussion if it occurs in a nonthreatening, nonjudgmental, and confidential manner.

Betsy undoubtedly would benefit from a discussion about many issues, including family, parents, future plans, goals, and educational possibilities.

Transition Events

College. Pressure to use alcohol and other substances, along with pressure for sexual relationships, should be discussed and integrated into conversation about disease prevention and health maintenance. All youth, especially those who excel scholastically, should be cautioned about school-related stress and anxiety.

Parenthood or Teen Pregnancy. Rapid return to school or work should be encouraged because this strongly decreases the likelihood of repeat pregnancy and increases the ability to achieve financial and social independence.[37]

Incarceration. If a regular source of medical care does not exist, suggestions should be offered for where care can be obtained. This is especially important for minors requiring chronic medication, such as those with mental health problems. Compounding these problems, in most communities, the medical and mental health systems are often difficult to navigate, making follow-up and prescription refills problematic.

Homelessness. Solving problems of homeless youth always requires help from social service and counseling organizations. Providers should be aware of local agencies with which they can work before providing care to homeless or runaway youth.

REFERENCES

1. US Department of Justice: *Conditions of confinement: juvenile detention and corrections facilities,* Washington, DC, 1994, Office of Juvenile Justice and Delinquency Prevention.
2. US Department of Justice: Public juvenile facilities, *Juvenile Justice Bulletin,* 1991.
3. Anderson B, Farrow J: Incarcerated adolescents in Washington state: health services and utilization, *J Adolesc Health* 22:363, 1998.
4. Pennbridge J, MacKenzie R, Swofford A: Risk profile of homeless pregnant adolescents and youth, *J Adolesc Health* 12:534, 1991.
5. Morey MA, Friedman LS: Health care needs of homeless adolescents, *Curr Opin Pediatr* 5:395, 1993.
6. Alan Guttmacher Institute: *Sex and America's teenagers,* New York, 1994, Alan Guttmacher Institute.
7. American Psychiatric Association: *Diagnostic and statistical manual of mental disorders, 4th edition (DSM IV),* Washington, DC, 1994, American Psychiatric Association.
8. Ernol FKE, Innala SM, Whitan FL: Biological explanation, psychological explanation and tolerance of homosexuals: a cross-national analysis of beliefs and attitudes, *Psychol Rep* 65:1003, 1989.
9. American Academy of Pediatrics: Homosexuality and adolescence, *Pediatrics* 92:631, 1993.
10. Friedman RC, Downey JI: Homosexuality, *N Engl J Med* 331(14):933, 1996.
11. Kinsey AC, Pomeroy WB, Martin CE: *Sexual behavior in the human male,* New York, 1948, WB Saunders.
12. Kinsey AC, Pomeroy WB, Martin CE: *Sexual behavior in the human female,* New York, 1953, WB Saunders.

13. Remafedi G: Adolescent homosexuality: psychological and medical implications, *Pediatrics* 79:331, 1987.
14. Ryan RC, Futterman D: Lesbian and gay youth: care and counseling, *Adolescent Medicine: State of the Art Review* 8(2):211, 1997
15. Remafedi G, Farrow JA, Deiswas RW: Risk factors for attempted suicide in gay and lesbian youth, *Pediatrics* 87:879, 1991.
16. Robertson LM, Middleman AB: Knowledge of health insurance coverage by adolescents and young adults attending a hospital-based clinic, *J Adolesc Health Care* 22:439, 1998.
17. Johnston L, O'Malley P, Bachman J: National survey results on drug use from the Monitoring the Future study, 1975-1995, Rockville, Md, 1995, National Institutes on Drug Abuse.
18. American Academy of Pediatrics Committee on Substance Abuse: Role of the pediatrician in the prevention and management of substance abuse, *Pediatrics* 91:1010, 1993.
19. Friedman LS, Stronin L, Hingson R: A survey of attitudes, beliefs, behaviors and knowledge about AIDS and HIV testing by adolescents and young adults enrolled in alcohol and drug treatment, *J Adolesc Health Care* 14:442, 1993.
20. Wheeler K, Malmquist J: Treatment approaches in adolescent chemical dependency, *Pediatr Clin North Am*, 34(2):437, 1987.
21. Rawitscher LA, Saitz R, Friedman LS: Adolescents' preferences regarding human immunodeficiency virus (HIV)-related physician counseling and HIV testing, *Pediatrics* 96(1):52, 1995.
22. Garl MH, Brookmeyer R: Methods for projecting course of the acquired immunodeficiency syndrome epidemic, *J Natl Cancer Inst* 80:900, 1988.
23. Centers for Disease Control: Summary of notifiable diseases, United States, 1993, *MMWR* 42(53), 1994.
24. Rosenberg PS, Biggar RJ: Trends in HIV incidence among young adults in the United States, *JAMA* 279(23):1894, 1998.
25. Futterman D et al: Human immunodeficiency virus–infected adolescents: the first 50 patients in a New York City program, *Pediatrics* 91:730, 1993.
26. Goldenring JM, Cohen E: Getting into adolescents' heads, *Contemp Pediatr* 5:75, 1988.
27. Turner CF et al: Adolescent sexual behavior, drug use and violence: increased reporting with computer survey technology, *Science* 280(5365):867, 1998.
28. Blum WR, Geber G: Chronically ill youth. In McAnarney ER et al, editors: *Textbook of adolescent medicine*, New York, 1992, WB Saunders, p 222.
29. Koob GF, Bloom FE: Cellular and molecular mechanisms of drug dependence, *Science* 242:715, 1988.
30. Schuckit MA: Genetics and the risk for alcoholism, *JAMA* 254:2614, 1985.
31. Rogers PD, Adger H Jr.: Alcohol and adolescents, *Adolescent Medicine: State of the Arts Review* 4:295, 1993.
32. O'Connor PG, Schottenfeld RS: Patients with alcohol problems, *N Engl J Med* 338(9):592, 1998.
33. Elster AB, Kuznets NJ, editors: *AMA guidelines for adolescent preventive services*, Baltimore, 1994, Williams & Wilkins.
34. American Academy of Pediatrics: *Guidelines for health supervision, III*, Elk Grove Village, Ill, 1997, American Academy of Pediatrics.
35. Marrazzo JM et al: Community based urine screening for chlamydia trachomatis with a ligase chain reaction assay, *Ann Int Med* 127:796, 1997.
36. Bass CA et al: Clinical evaluation of a new polymerase chain reaction assay for detection of chlamydia trachomatis in endocervical specimens, *J Clin Microbiol* 31:2648, 1993.
37. Stevens-Simon C, Parson J, Montgomery C: What is the relationship between postpartum withdrawal from school and repeat pregnancy and adolescent mothers? *J Adolesc Health Care* 7:191, 1986.

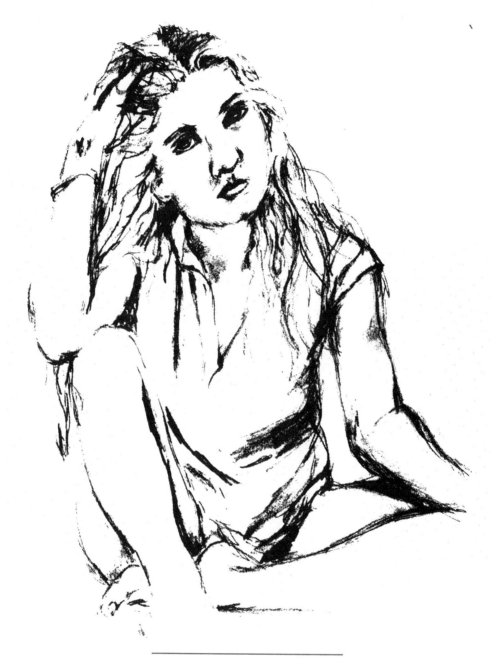

"Self portrait." By Eileen Fitz, age 18.

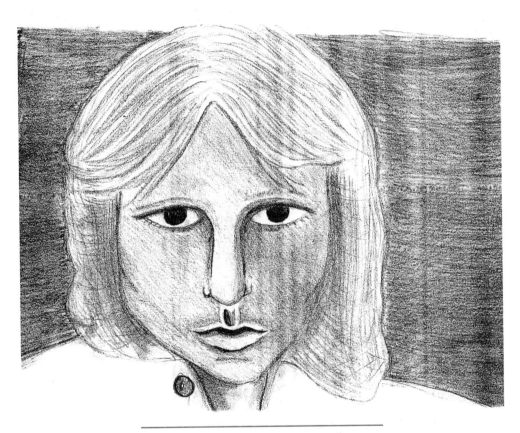

"Self-portrait." By Carmen Goodheart, age 16.

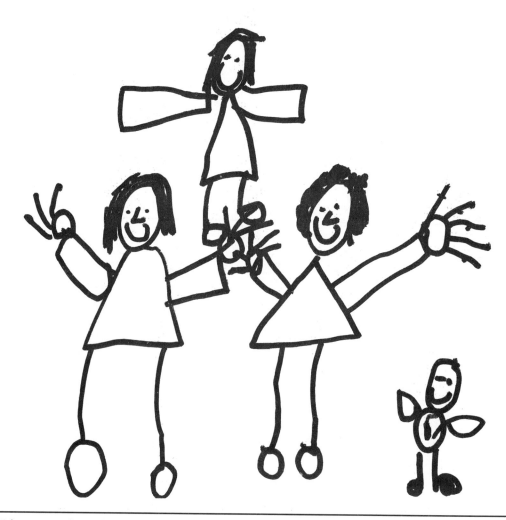

Girl, age 5½, draws her two-mother family, with herself depicted on top of the world, safe in the middle. Her little brother is shown below, happy. (Original in green marker.)

CHAPTER 23

SPECIAL FAMILIES

- Robert D. Wells
- Martin T. Stein

KEY WORDS

Divorce Process
Stepfamilies
Serious Illness of Parent
Single Parents
Adoption
Foster Care
Gay or Lesbian Parent
Homeless Children

 Shelly, an 11-year-old girl, was seen by her pediatrician for recurrent abdominal pain. She lived with her mother, a 52-year-old nurse administrator, and her father, a 63-year-old retired physician. Shelly had been complaining of abdominal pain almost daily for the past year. At first her parents had dismissed it as "just nerves." When she was sent home from school, her parents became more concerned. Shelly was evaluated by her pediatrician, who did not find an apparent cause for her pain after an initial history, review of symptoms, and complete physical examination. Results of screening laboratory tests, including a complete blood cell count, erythrocyte sedimentation rate, urinalysis, chemistry panel, and a stool examination for occult blood and ova and parasites, were normal. While performing the medical assessment, her pediatrician was impressed by Shelly's depressed and anxious demeanor. She was fidgety and often rolled her hair around a constantly moving finger. When a question was directed to Shelly, eye contact diminished, she looked down, and a sad appearance came over her.

When Shelly's mother was questioned alone, she quickly became tearful and disclosed that her husband was severely disabled by multiple sclerosis and was abusing opiates to control his pain and depression. Marital conflict was extremely high, and she admitted to being involved in an extramarital affair, which Shelly had known about for 1 year. She also wondered how Shelly was coping with taking care of her dad after school.

Interviewed alone, Shelly indeed appeared quite depressed and worried. She described a recurrent fear that she would return home from school to find her father dead or severely injured. She hated having to take care of him and longed for her moth-

er's return from work. She did not volunteer any information about her mother's affair but did admit to worrying about her mother's adjustment. She saw her as a "workaholic who was always stressed out" and quick to anger. It was clear that Shelly experienced a tremendous amount of stress and anxiety related to her special family circumstances.

The pediatrician referred Shelly and her mother to a pediatric psychologist. The mother was eventually referred to an adult psychiatrist for psychopharmacological treatment of a significant depression. Through counseling, she made a decision to place her disabled husband in a chronic care facility. She recognized that she and Shelly were unable to sustain him at home.

Shelly was responsive to individual counseling. In the context of a warm, supportive relationship, she enjoyed the mutual detective work of understanding and modifying her stress and pain. After the third visit and without direct interpretation, Shelly verbalized the belief that her anxious state and frequent stress were associated with her abdominal pain. As she was helped to see the special nature of the stressors in her family, her feelings of anger, worry, and sadness were now viewed as a natural outcome of stress overload. Her love for both parents was constantly reaffirmed in the counseling sessions, but she was also helped to get in touch with her anger and frustration at their excessive demands on her. Her abdominal pain declined steadily and resolved completely shortly after the nursing home placement of her father. She continued to visit him in the nursing home, where he was able to resolve his substance dependency.

Rapid changes in family constellation in the United States over the past 50 years have created great diversification in the makeup of families. The divorce rate has doubled since 1965, as have the number of mothers who are working full time. If our definition of the typical family is restricted to homes with two parents, the majority of children come from special families. The most recent census indicates that 25% of children are raised by single parents and greater than 50% experience a divorce; demographers predict that 33% of children will live with a stepparent before turning 18 years old. It may well be that over the next decade, the child with both birth parents present will be seen as unique.

No evidence proves a particular family constellation is either "good" or "bad" for children. However, the way in which a family functions to support the growth and development of its children is important. Several family characteristics are important for children, regardless of the specific constellation:

- Regular provision of life necessities, including food, housing, clothing, and medical care
- Demonstrated warmth, unconditional love, and constructive limit setting for the child
- Continuity and stability in caregiving for the child
- Appropriate models of the development of healthy sexuality
- Cooperation among involved caretaking adults
- Lack of violence toward, and respect for, all members in the family
- Lack of excessive stress, such as significant physical or mental illness of the caretaking adults, including depression, alcoholism, and drug abuse

- Adequate support for caretaking adults from relatives, friends, neighbors, and community
- Stimulation of cognitive development
- Capacity for meaningful interpersonal relationships, good communication, problem-solving capacity, and motivation to achieve
- Fostering of socialization by helping children function as cooperative members of society

These basic aspects of family functioning are necessary if children are to acquire a sense of security and self-esteem, learn to socialize, respond to rules, and limit and control their anger and aggression.

All families provide varying levels of concrete resources, discipline, expectations, modeling, and emotional support to their children. After significant acute or chronic loss, most families appear somewhat less able to meet the needs of their children. When the functional capacity of these special families is assessed, it is important to avoid value-laden expectations in favor of a more objective appraisal of relative strengths and weaknesses. Specifically, it is not important how different from the norm the family is, but how well it goes about meeting the needs of the various family members while remaining effective in the wider community.

The term *special families* is used in this chapter to delineate a variety of family constellations that may affect child health, behavior, and development. Such a definition includes foster, adoptive, stepparent, and single-parent families, in addition to families facing severe strain because of poor parental health or adjustment. Although differing from each other in important ways, the families' commonality lies in the effects of loss on the children. In this manner, intact, nuclear families can be seen as "special" if they indeed subject the child to certain risks as a result of loss or threatened loss. Farm families who are facing bankruptcy, inner-city homeless families, and immigrant families who have had to flee their homelands should be considered special because of the uniqueness of loss that their members experience. For clinicians, recognition of these special circumstances focuses our behavioral and developmental assessment on each family and promotes individually tailored anticipatory guidance for greater effectiveness.

The assessment of children in special families must take into account the extent of loss experienced, the amount of time that has elapsed, the child's age, the degree to which stressors are acute, chronic, or recurrent, and the adaptive capacity of the child and parenting figures. Although the clinician should be restrained from letting personal values and beliefs enter into the equation, the values of the family's community should be considered. Unique family constellations are more or less acceptable in certain contexts. Teenage pregnancy in some middle-class neighborhoods is associated with greater ostracism than in a neighborhood where it is more common and acceptable. Similarly, having homosexual, adoptive, or disabled parents will be less of a strain on those children living in communities where it is not considered unusual.

Even when large numbers of families experience similar losses (e.g., after natural catastrophes), the actual experience in terms of severity of the loss is highly subjective. Some parents find that the **divorce process** is a considerable strain, whereas others find it energizing and liberating. Death of a family member is typically stress producing, but a study of

Amish families has documented those families' relative ease of adjustment.[1] Loss and stress clearly are subjectively determined experiences.[2] The implication for clinicians is that the family and child must be asked about their sense of the severity of loss or upheaval rather than the clinician's relying on her own impression.

The amount of time that has elapsed since the change or loss is also important in determining the nature of an individual child and family's adjustment. Studies of bereavement and divorce indicate significant upheaval during the first year after the loss, with the majority of children returning to baseline functioning during the second year.[3] Consequently, disruptions in a child's behavior or academic functioning during the first year after divorce are not unusual and may not signify serious maladaptation, whereas such behavior after the second year is far more serious.

Age and developmental skills also play an important role in determining the child's state of adjustment to special family circumstances. Infants require responsive and predictable caregiving behavior, and the biological relatedness of the caregiver is relatively unimportant. Separations or changes in caregivers are particularly stressful between about 8 and 18 months, when the developmental theme of attachment is prominent. Similarly, losses because of divorce or death during infancy and the preschool years are less obviously sensitizing than those that occur during the school-age and adolescent period.[3] Divorce itself may not be so stressful for the preschool child, but the necessity to live in two homes may require significant adjustment and provoke behavioral stress. In general, children will be more vulnerable to special family circumstances from elementary school age to middle adolescence.

The effects of multiple, chronic, and severe stressors on children appear most dramatic and disabling. Ongoing domestic violence, parental substance abuse, and dire poverty are particularly devastating and appear to have longstanding effects on child development and adjustment.[4] Acute stressors, such as natural catastrophes, divorce, sudden loss of income, and death of a parent can also pose a profound challenge to the child and family. Longitudinal studies suggest that a period of adaptation follows the initial shock. For children and parents alike, this may lead to decreases in academic and occupational functioning, moodiness, depression, anger, behavioral problems, and sleep disturbances.

After the initial trauma, the quality of a child's adaptation is determined primarily by the parent's ability to model effective coping strategies while maintaining family rules and expectations.[3,5-8] When the child's clinician focuses family energy toward the augmentation of parental recovery, she encourages the child's adaptation and recovery as well. Self-help groups, religious organizations, and more formal mental health services may be helpful, especially when the parent and the child have few friends or available family.

Prediction of the developmental outcome of a particular child reared in one class of special families is usually not possible. However, some generalizations about the ways in which families influence children can be made from the available literature. Clear evidence exists that children can be successfully reared in special families despite some evidence that an intact family with both biological parents present and reasonably compatible provides children with the best opportunity for healthy growth and development. One study concluded that poor, single-parent families have the highest risk of social maladaptation and psychological problems in their children.[9] The presence of second adults in these families did have important ameliorative functions. Families headed by mother and grandmother were nearly as effective in producing socially and emotionally healthy first graders as were mother-father families. The powerful ameliorative effects of social support have clearly been documented.

Developmental and behavioral problems in children may not be related directly to the loss of the nuclear family. Rather, it is family discord and harsh parental discipline, associated with isolation, financial stress, and parental mental states, that seem to lead to delinquent behavior in children.[10] Family discord may occur, of course, in either an intact family or a special family.

These general principles of understanding and determining the specific needs of the individual family and child should assist the child's clinician. The following sections provide more specific information about different types of special families.

DIVORCING FAMILIES

The effects of the divorce process on the development of children has been studied extensively.[3,11,12] Approximately 50% of children experience a divorce of their parents by the middle of adolescence. Most children respond to the initiation of separation and divorce with significant feelings of depression, anxiety, and anger.[13] Infants and preschool-age children appear less affected than their older counterparts. Notable declines in academic performance may occur in both boys and girls during the first year after the separation. Boys tend to respond to this loss with increased emotional outbursts, noncompliance, and other external behavior problems (Fig. 23-1). Withdrawal, sadness, and anxiety, characterized as internalizing behaviors, are more commonly observed in girls, and their difficulties may be overlooked for longer periods of time. Some data also suggest that some young women suffer from a "sleeper" effect, whereby an initial adjustment is realized, but when the women enter young adulthood, a reawakening of anxieties regarding male-female relationships may occur.[14]

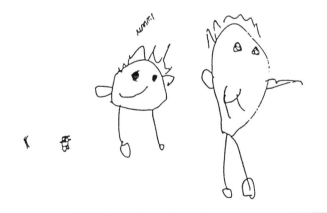

Fig. 23-1   Joey, age 7, has drawn himself as a very small person next to his mother and her new boyfriend. When his mother saw the drawing, she became convinced that Joey should receive counseling to help him adjust to his parents' separation and probable divorce (see page 507. From Stein MT: *J Dev Behav Pediatr* 18:334, 1997.)

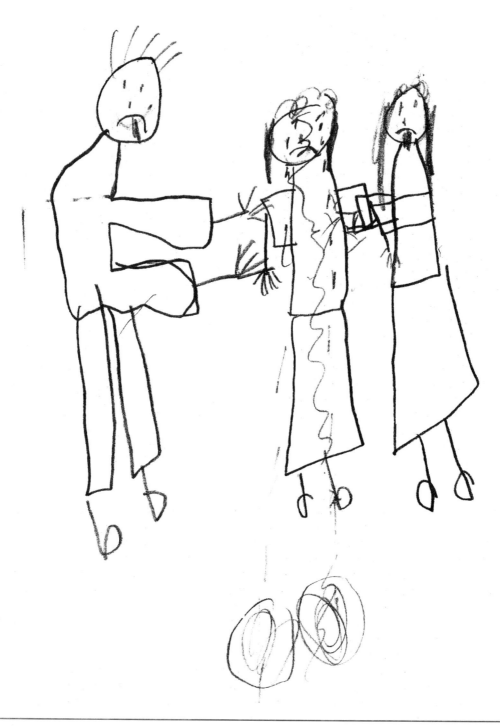

A girl shows us what it feels like to be in the middle of a contentious divorce, literally being torn down the middle, both parents pulling her apart. No one looks happy. By Heather Davis, age 9.

When Joey's mother made an appointment for his health supervision visit just before his seventh birthday, she talked about his recent behavior change. During the past 6 months, his teacher phoned on several occasions with concerns about Joey's disruptive classroom behavior. He hit other children on two occasions, offered comments when not called on, and frequently wandered aimlessly around the class, talking to other students and upsetting their work. He often did not complete his assigned work in school or at home. This behavior pattern was in contrast to his cooperative, interactive, and productive style of learning and social interactions before this time.

The pediatrician discovered that Joey's parents had separated 6 months earlier. The marriage had been conflictual during the past 3 years. Verbal battles between the parents were common, and Joey witnessed physical spousal abuse on two occasions. Joey saw his father on weekends, but the parents' lingering distrust and anger surrounded the visits with ambivalence and stress. Joey would not talk to the pediatrician about the visits with his father. He was subdued and answered questions with a single word and limited eye contact. His physical examination was normal. When the pediatrician recommended a brief period of counseling to help Joey explore his feelings about the separation and his new living situation, his mother adamantly refused. She declared that "therapy would harm him more."

While Joey was waiting for the doctor, he was asked to draw a picture of his family. When the pediatrician showed the drawing to his mother, she cried immediately, followed by "Of course, you're right. Joey needs counseling to help him."

Joey drew himself as a very small person next to his mother and her new boyfriend (see Fig. 23-1). The visual image of a diminutive person with poor self-esteem helped his mother to overcome her resistance to counseling by associating his behavior with a poor self-image. The drawing acted as a nonverbal trigger to seek help. After five sessions with a therapist, Joey's classroom behavior improved, and he was once again responsive to learning.[14]

From Stein MT: Challenging case: the use of family drawings by children in pediatric practice, *J Dev Behav Pediatr* 18:334, 1997.

Recent evidence refutes the general belief that by the second year the majority of children adjust to their altered family circumstances. In a longitudinal study, 37% of children were doing poorly (i.e., academic underachievement and behavior problems at school, home, or both) at 5 years after divorce. At the 10-year follow-up, 41% were still maladjusted, which suggests that the years following a divorce continue to be stressful for many children.[15]

Investigators studying the 10-year period after a divorce reported that only one of seven children saw their parents happily remarried, 50% experienced a new divorce, 60% felt rejected by at least one parent, and 50% grew up in families in which the parents remained intensely angry at each other. The economic consequence of a divorce is also quite significant, with 25% of children who experienced a divorce living with a parent with significantly reduced financial resources. How the divorcing parents as individuals and as partners in parenting make social, psychological, and economic adjustments after the divorce determines the long-term effects on children.

The degree to which families are unable to develop their own parenting plan and custody decisions is an important predictor of child adjustment. When parents continue to litigate with emotional viciousness after divorce and children have frequent access to both parents, the children appear more depressed, withdrawn, aggressive, and prone to psychosomatic complaints.[16] Child transfers in a neutral setting (e.g., school or church), where parents need not be in direct contact with each other, may help reduce the extreme stress associated with this activity.

> *Quinn was 3 years old when his parents arranged an appointment with the pediatrician to discuss different approaches to Quinn's child rearing. An abrupt separation had occurred 2 months before the visit. The parents expressed anger and hostility toward each other. Before the separation they worked with a marriage and family therapist for 3 months without resolution of differences. Quinn's mother did not want Quinn spending time with his dad, who was now living with another woman and her two children. Quinn's dad expressed a desire to continue his role as a father and wanted Quinn to stay with him at least 2 days each week.*

A number of factors may predict the relative risk of maladaptation after divorce. Children exposed to continuing family discord either before or after a divorce are at much greater risk for developing conduct disturbances.[17] If open family conflict decreases after divorce, better outcomes are predicted. In contrast, children who have been sheltered from parental conflicts and awaken to open conflict during and after the divorce are often the most grievously injured. Children whose parents demonstrate aggressive styles of resolving conflict with each other tend to have continued difficulties with behavioral problems and poor coping skills.[18] Those children who are able to experience a trend toward family stabilization after a divorce are more likely to return to their baseline functioning.[19]

The emotional availability of one or both parents is often diminished during the separation and divorce process. If this continues unabated, children face tremendous obstacles in meeting their own, their siblings', and their parents' needs. Although age (younger) and sex of the child (female) are predictors of a better outcome in general, appropriate ongoing relationships with both parents are the most important factor in predicting resilience. An easy child temperament, social support, physical health, and intelligence also contribute to better outcomes.

The clinician's role in helping families who experience divorce should precede the actual separation. During regular pediatric health supervision visits, families should be made aware of the clinician's interest and need to know about significant family events that might affect the child. Periodic focused questions that serve to update the clinician about family function will both inform and cement the relationship between the parents and the clinician. If marital separation occurs, specific guidelines can be offered regarding how and what to tell the child. Attention can be focused on ways to support the child's coping skills and to maintain appropriate contact with parents, friends, and concerned others. Parents frequently need help in controlling their own emotional state, and the clinician should directly address this.

> Quinn's pediatrician recognized that both parents would benefit from individual counseling in order to learn strategies to manage their emotions at this difficult time. The pediatrician saw this as an opportunity not only to suggest an appropriate mental health referral, but also to emphasize the parents' mutual desire to help Quinn through the family crisis and to be effective parents.

Parents' distinguishing their own needs and feelings from those of their child is also important. Predicting the types of reactions they and their child may experience is usually helpful. Monitoring subsequent responses of child and parent is then critical for effective clinical assessments, and at times referral to a mental health professional may be appropriate. Anticipatory guidance for a child whose parents have separated or divorced can be guided by recognition of predictable responses at each developmental stage (Table 23-1).

STEPFAMILIES

As the divorce rate remains high and that of remarriage continues to increase, **stepfamilies** have become an important part of our culture. Although these reconstituted families usually function as effectively as nuclear family units, a number of salient differences should be appreciated by responsive clinicians.[20] Each member of the family has experienced significant losses. Children who are depressed and anxious after a parental separation now must cope with sharing their biological parent with a new adult. The biological parent, who may also be functioning with diminished coping resources, must contend with playing a "middle man" role, leaving neither side satisfied. The stepparent will quickly appreciate that parent-child bonds precede his involvement; issues of loyalty and alliance in the biological parent may lead to a sense of isolation and rejection in the stepparent. Most stepchildren continue to visit the other biological parent. Differences in rules between the households and jealousies between the biological noncustodial parent and the stepparent may lead to further disruption.[21]

Despite these challenges, studies suggest that children from stepfamilies do not differ significantly from children in other family structures.[22] They can achieve effective family functioning with developmentally appropriate levels of adjustment and are equally prone to maladaptation in the face of family discord. Family functioning is optimal with positive marital adjustment, strong parent-child attachment, generalized family cohesiveness, and effective problem solving.[23,24] When stepfamilies are dysfunctional, they are characterized by strong parent-child coalitions (rather than parent-parent coalitions) and a lack of mutual decision-making skills. Adolescents appear particularly vulnerable to developing problems when their stepfamilies are characterized by chaotic rules, punitiveness, excessive dependency, and frequent major life changes.[25]

The sensitive and alert clinician may at times become confused about the nature of the alliance between natural parents, stepparents, and children. Attempts should be made to maintain contact with all adults who serve as psychological parents while complying with the legal rights and restrictions to information stipulated in custody agreements. Keeping in

TABLE 23-1 ■ Responses of Child to Parents' Divorce Within the First Year

Developmental Status	Child's Response	Primary Care Clinician's Role
Preschool	Regressive behavior Sleep disturbance Tantrums Aggressive behavior Bowel and bladder difficulties Clinging Fears of abandonment	Encourage stable, predictable meal and bedtime routines Develop consistent patterns of joining and separating from child Continue contact with noncustodial parent Provide reassurance
Younger school age	Sadness Fearfulness Loyalty conflicts Attempts to determine responsibility Hopes for family reconciliation Declining school performance	Empathize with child's feelings Provide regular opportunities for child to talk Support child's continuing relationship with both parents Offer reassurance
Older school age/ prepubertal	Grief, intense anger Declining school performance Disrupted peer relationships Attempts to clarify responsibility for divorce Caretaking of a parent	Express interest in and availability to the child Support child's school and peer involvement Provide clear acknowledgment and support for child's working through feelings about the divorce
Adolescence	Depression Anger Premature emancipation Increase in adolescent acting out Sleeper effects, particularly in females	Provide opportunities for discussion Offer appropriate supports within and outside the family, including peer involvement (such as in school-based family transition groups).

Modified from Wallerstein JS: Separation, divorce and remarriage. Levine MD, Carey WB, Crocker AC, editors: *Developmental-behavioral pediatrics,* ed 2, Philadelphia, 1992, WB Saunders. In Parker S, Zuckerman B: *Behavioral and developmental pediatrics: a handbook for primary care,* Boston, 1995, Little, Brown & Co.

mind the nature of loss experienced by children in reconstituted families, expect some early adjustment difficulties with eventual remission in the majority of cases. Specific attention should be paid to developing well-recognized rules of behavior in the home. Stepparents can be counseled to develop a role as an independent caregiver in addition to supporting the spouse's actions. Parents, children, and the clinician should maintain hope that, over time, rules and roles will become more comfortable and acceptable. The clinician should express clear support for the importance of the noncustodial parent's right to visit, obtain information about the children, and discuss concerns. Finally, the stepparent and biological parent should be encouraged to maintain nonparental, romantic, and supportive roles with each other so that the alliance between the adults remains balanced and strong. When adjustment problems predominate or become chronic, or when fixed maladaptive roles and alliances have developed, referral for family counseling is indicated and often helpful.

Stepparents and adoptive parents may need considerable external validation of their roles as parents, and the child's clinician is often in a unique position to provide such support. In her role of advocate for the child's development, the clinician may assist parents through timely support and guidance in understanding the changes the family is experiencing in terms of the best interest of the child or children, as well as the needs and emotional responses of the parents.

SERIOUS ILLNESS OF PARENTS

The psychosocial effects of growing up with a parent who has a serious, life-threatening physical illness is perhaps one of the least studied stressful childhood events. In contrast, the effects of parental mental illness on children have been more extensively studied.[26,27] Children who have a schizophrenic parent benefit significantly when they have a healthy relationship with a caring and predictable adult. This was also the conclusion for families with mothers who were diagnosed with breast cancer, diabetes, or fibrocystic breast disease.[28] Children in these families showed the most adaptive behavior when fathers maintained frequent interactions with their children. Not surprisingly, marital harmony was also correlated with improved child functioning.

For the clinician treating children who have highly stressed, physically ill parents, special attention should be directed to guilt reactions in children. Psychosomatic conditions, school avoidance, separation anxiety, and depression are common responses to a sudden threat to a parent's health. A temperamentally easy child may show a tendency to develop "pseudomaturity," appearing to be the psychological parent for the family. Extra effort is needed to keep the child out of the family's decision-making process so that she experiences and benefits from a normal period of growth and development. Parents may have to be explicitly informed not to seek counsel from children acting in pseudomaturity, and they should be encouraged to develop more adaptive and supportive relationships with other adults and health care providers. Children should be encouraged to continue their normal scholastic and extracurricular activities. Family communication about the parent's illness and treatment should be encouraged, particularly when the focus is on the feelings and reactions that are naturally evoked.

The clinician may find it useful to maintain contact with the ill parent during the course of illness. The questions on the minds of the well parent and the ill parent are often different regarding what, how, and when to tell children about predictable and frightening events. In the majority of circumstances, open and honest communication with children is the best advice. Concerns about the death of a parent must be addressed to minimize the child's tendency to fantasize catastrophic outcomes or miraculous cures. Most important, the clinician should take the time to empathize with the child regarding her worries about the parent. She should be encouraged to ask questions about her parent's condition and to call for an appointment if she becomes confused, overwhelmingly anxious, or depressed (see Chapter 25).

SINGLE-PARENT FAMILIES

Financial concerns are a serious problem faced by most **single parents.** Earning a living and caring for the needs of children can easily consume the full-time energy of more than one adult. Remarkably, many single parents find ways to spend as much or more time with their children than they would if they were in a marriage, although certain sacrifices must be made. Frequently, single parents have to sacrifice some "adult time" that would ordinarily be spent meeting their own emotional needs to meet their financial and family obligations. When appointments are broken or arrival to the office is late, when anxiety levels are heightened or payment for medical service is delayed, the child's clinician should be sensitive to these added stresses among single parents.

Clinicians can be helpful to single parents by accepting their families as healthy units that are capable of providing for the needs of their children[29] while being sensitive to the special pressures felt by single parents. Isolation from other adults is a particular problem for some single parents, and at times they need to share their experiences with another adult. The child's clinician may be the most respected and available adult. The physician can use this position therapeutically by providing feedback, empathy, and validation of the parental role. More explicit directions, detailed action plans, and direct feedback may be needed (Fig. 23-2).

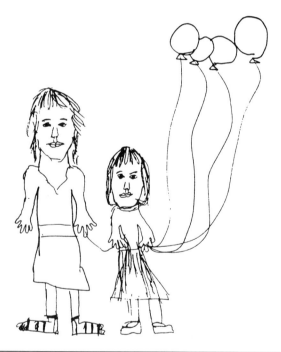

Fig. 23-2   A drawing by Joy, age 11, reveals that her relationship with her mother may be too close. After talking about the drawing, the mother agreed with the pediatrician that she and her daughter should explore ways to separate more psychologically. (From Stein MT: *J Dev Behav Pediatr* 18:334, 1997.)

Joy was 11 years old when she drew this picture (Fig. 23-2) during a visit for a mild acute illness. She had lived with her mother in a single-parent family since birth. She had no siblings. On the surface, her physical health, schoolwork, and social development were satisfactory. However, clues revealed restricted interpersonal and social development. Joy made friends slowly. She was unusually cautious about leaving her mother to go to a friend's house. She preferred to have a friend come to her house and play in her mother's presence.

Joy's pediatrician had been concerned that the close bond between Joy and her mother had limited their emotional separation. Separation and individuation, the gradual process from dependency to autonomy, had not been completed.[30] At several previous office visits, the pediatrician unsuccessfully looked for an opportunity to discuss this observation with Joy and her mother. This drawing was an opening. When her mother was asked, "What do you think about this picture?" she initially responded with pride in her daughter's drawing skills. Then she said, "We are rather close, aren't we?" The pediatrician encouraged the mother to explore that observation further. After 10 minutes alone with the pediatrician, Joy's mother was motivated to help her daughter (and herself) to discover ways to psychologically separate while maintaining their loving and close relationship.

Single parents can be encouraged to share some of their parenting obligations with other responsible adults. Depending on the situation, this might mean encouraging contact with grandparents or noncustodial parents or using the support of various social agencies, such as Big Brothers and Big Sisters organizations and single-parent clubs. The pediatric office can make available a directory of single-parent support groups in the community. Finally, a number of joys and strengths can result from single-parenting experiences (e.g., learning self-sufficiency as a parent), and those positive aspects of single parenting can be emphasized to members of single-parent households.

ADOPTIVE FAMILIES

Adoption provides a caring and responsive home and family for about 2% of U.S. children, who might not otherwise have a home, and provides children for couples who wish to parent. Like other special families, children and adults each bring their own unique strengths and liabilities together to create a warm environment for healing prior losses and developing new capacities. Although most adoptions are formulated when relatives become the adoptive parents, many unrelated families are adopting infants and older children with the help of adoption agencies and private attorneys. The clinician may be asked to help review birth and health information of the soon-to-be adopted child. The parents may have many questions regarding ways to best help their infant or child's transition to a new family be as smooth and enjoyable as possible.

Adoptions outside the family involve at least three participants, referred to as "the adoption triangle."[31] At one corner of the triangle is the biological parent or parents, often a

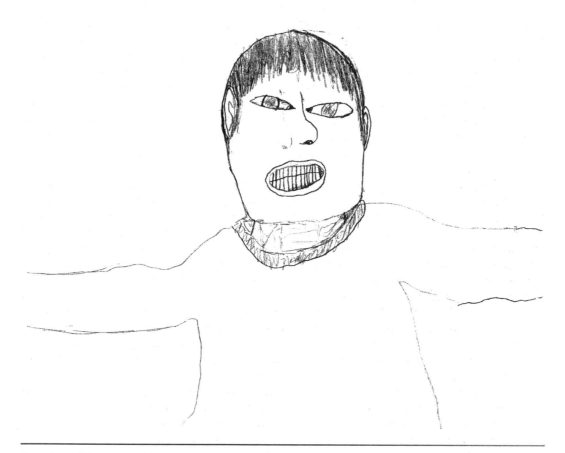

James, adopted at age 9, is settled into his new home two years later and is getting the help he needs in school. The teeth, cut-off arms and hands, and solo appearance suggest some residual anger and a personal sense of ineffectiveness. These characteristics are on all of his drawings of himself as "a person." By James Haviland, age 11.

single woman in her early 20s who has chosen adoption for her fetus or newborn. Frequently she is under considerable emotional stress, supported by neither the biological father of the baby nor her own parents. Although many adoptions are arranged during pregnancy, a significant number of babies are placed after birth as a result of neglect or abuse. To avoid a tendency to blame or stigmatize the biological parent, the clinician should bear in mind the difficult circumstances in which many parents live. In general the decision to relinquish a child demonstrates the parent's capacity to recognize the predominance of the child's needs. The biological parent's adjustment is aided by having the opportunity to know her neonate and "say good-bye." Reassurance of the child's well-being from the clinician also aids adjustment.

At another corner of the triangle are the adoptive parents, who have long dreamed of and contemplated the wonderful experience of raising a child. Although many families have been counseled by the time adoption becomes a reality, private adoptions may be completely free of counseling. Some couples may have unresolved feelings related to their decision to adopt, and most parents worry about their own reactions to the parenting role. Grief over infertility or unresolved anger at a spouse may also be operative. Over the years, adoption has become far less stigmatized, though some parents may still not experience supportiveness in extended family members and friends.[32] Adoptive parents also live with many unanswered questions about the child's biological and genetic background and the possibility of intrauterine substance exposure or other unknown pregnancy complications.

The adopted child forms the final part of the triangle. This child brings a particular genetic endowment that includes intellectual, temperamental, and physical factors. The child may have experienced many prenatal stresses related to the biological mother's age, emotional state, and physical health and habits during pregnancy. Placement for varying periods of time at critical ages in one or more foster homes may have occurred with its accompanying stress and disruptions of attachments. When adoption takes place within the first 6 months of life, the infant is likely to avoid the experience of significant loss that is often apparent in older children. The quality of care that children experienced before placement has significant effects on the level of trust they exhibit. Children with a background of abuse, neglect, and unpredictability will come to the adoption setting with a very different set of expectations, and parents may find the attachment process to be lengthened and more complex. The child's temperament is also an important aspect to consider when determining risk factors and level of adjustment, with easier temperaments leading to more rapid family integration. Ethnic differences, in appearance and cultural identification, may be additional challenges for the racially mixed adoptive family.

When caring for adopted children, clinicians should realize that all three parties in the adoption process have their own emotional needs and civil rights. Open adoptions are now becoming the norm, and all three members of the triangle are encouraged to maintain contact. In open adoption, the biological and adoptive parents agree beforehand on the level of involvement that each will have with the child.[33] This can range from sending a picture during Christmastime to regular weekly visitations. In general, full awareness and select visitation with biological parents appears to be beneficial to all three parties involved; however, research on open adoptions is limited, and long-term effects on children are not documented. In an open adoption, the biological parent may be helped to assuage concerns about the child's circumstances, and the adoptive parents may come to appreciate the character and heritage of their child. Just as with divorce, the child may be powerfully influenced by the ability of the biological and adoptive parents to form an effective alliance and to function without insecurity and jealousy.

Helping parents feel comfortable in talking with a child about his adoption is a matter in which physicians can be quite helpful (Table 23-2). Families should be encouraged to include the child's adoption as an important part of the family's story. When parents tell a child about an adoption by age 3 or 4, the adopted child will grow up with true knowledge about his birth status. Children's books can be used to help portray the adoption process. Even when children grow up with early knowledge of their adoption, it is in the school-age years that many first become aware that adoption meant loss and relinquishment by their biological parent. The child may demonstrate signs of mourning and will be helped by sensitive questions from the adoptive parent after either subtle or overt behaviors or questions.

TABLE 23-2 ■ Issues of Adoption at Different Ages

Age	Issue
Preschool	"Where did I come from?" Life and death issues Generally accepting of being adopted
School age (7-11 years)	"Why was I adopted when most people aren't?" Worried that their value as a person is less because they are adopted Concerns about being different Aware that they have lost someone who played an extremely important role in their life Imagines birth parents as rich, famous, and more attractive than adoptive parents
Adolescence	Task of developing an identity and discovering how they are different and how they are connected to "their people" Concerns about family illness, such as insanity and talents, and physical appearance of birth family Interest in meeting birth parents

From Parker S, Zuckerman B: *Behavioral and developmental pediatrics: a handbook for primary care,* Boston, 1995, Little, Brown & Co.

Physicians will occasionally come in contact with school-age and adolescent patients who were adopted but have not yet been told, and parents will at this point seek consultation on when and how to break the news to their child. In most instances, families should be encouraged to share this information at the earliest opportunity to avoid a sense of rejection and mistrust. These exchanges should be done as a process over time and should be responsive to the types of questions asked by the child. The clinician can be particularly useful in helping adoptive parents find ways to explain the reason for adoption and difficulties experienced by the biological parent. Avoidance of the idea of having "been chosen" by the adoptive parents is important because this concept can introduce the thought that one can be "unchosen." Clinicians should avoid such pejorative terms as "natural" or "real" mother. The adoptive parents are real and natural; the term "birth mother" is preferred when referring to the biological mother.

FOSTER FAMILIES

In the United States, approximately half a million children receive **foster care** services. Foster care provides children with a home and family life when the child's parents are unable to do so, usually in the child's known community. At one time, foster care was used primarily to serve the needs of temporarily displaced children. Currently, children in foster care are likely to have been placed there because of severe psychological, social, or behavioral problems in the child, in the parents, or in both. Unlike adoption, the goal of foster care placement is to preserve and hopefully improve the child's relationship with the biological parents. Like adoption, this creates a triangle consisting of the child, the foster parents, and the biological parents. Like the stepchild, the foster child may feel as though she is a member of two (or more) homes and families concurrently and that this circumstance is beyond her control.

Foster parents volunteer to take children into their homes and are infrequently given specific training in the complexities of foster parenthood. Foster parents must attempt to provide for the present needs of and perhaps even rehabilitate the children entrusted to their care. They must also make room in the family for the new child. The birth children of foster parents may experience feelings akin to sibling rivalry on the arrival of a foster child in their home. Conversely, they may benefit by exposure to children less fortunate or to infants who are the result of irresponsible behavior on the part of others. Foster parents must also maintain a collaborative relationship with the foster care agency and be open to investigation and periodic evaluation of their intimate family life. They must often fight for services and deal with mounds of paperwork. The foster family must establish a relationship with the birth parents of the child, and such relationships are often quite challenging. Finally, foster parents must work through issues of attachment and separation with their foster children and within themselves related to the continuous process of bonding with and separating from foster children.[34]

When foster children present the foster family with challenging problems, a variety of reactions can occur. Some foster parents distance themselves from these problems, citing the child's lack of biological relationship, as well as the previously poor conditions in which the child lived. Other foster families assume that the child's maladaptive behaviors are a response to the foster family and feel frustrated or rejected. In working with these parents, the clinician should help them realize that children bring a significant history into foster family relationships. In fact, perhaps after a brief "honeymoon," the child may test to the limit the structure provided by the foster family. In some cases it may even appear that the child has set out to prove that he is unmanageable in any home and therefore should be returned to his biological parents. With a high rate of physical and mental illness and often unmet needs for care, these children meet these challenges with diminished resources.[35]

In helping a foster child the health care provider must understand the effects of separation from natural parents on children at various developmental levels. Most children react to the loss of their relationship with the biological parent in the same ways that children react to the loss of a parent through divorce or death. Reactions include a period of grief, a sense of failure, angry feelings toward the present caretaker, and perhaps behavioral acting out or depression and withdrawal. Many children will develop somatic complaints, and a loss of previously achieved developmental milestones may occur. Children who are placed in foster care between the ages of 6 and 18 months may show the classic pattern of reaction to separation from parents that is described by Bowlby.[36] This includes reactions of protest, despair, and finally a period of "detachment," in which the child may appear to have adjusted to the new home but has become dangerously superficial in his relationships to important adults. These signs of infantile depression must be recognized, and a permanent placement sought with urgency. The clinician should advocate for no further changes, if possible, and certainly not during this critical period in affective development.

A clinician may have a relationship with a child that continues despite the child's various living arrangements with natural or foster parents. Whenever possible, the clinician should develop a relationship with the child that allows the child to express feelings about foster placement and allows the clinician to help the child and foster parents deal with a variety of problems. The physician may act as the child's advocate in her relationship with the foster parents and the foster care placement agency in helping to determine the individual child's needs and current state of development. The foster child's clinician should encourage continuity of medical records as the child moves from one foster home to the next or into an adopting family. Physicians should be supportive of the children in foster care by seeing them with priority, delineating their physical and mental health needs in detail, and communicating these to the child welfare agency. The tendency to avoid these complex, often recordless cases should be resisted to advocate for the best interests of these at-risk children.[37]

GAY AND LESBIAN FAMILIES

Currently 6 to 14 million children live with a **gay or lesbian parent**[38] with wide variations in the type of openness demonstrated to children and to the wider community. Some homosexual couples may become parents using surrogates and insemination techniques, and these children grow up within the context of having two same-sex parents. Other families may develop through adoption and foster parenting. Additionally, a number of children may have been initially raised in a more conventional family, but after separation, divorce, or death, one parent may acknowledge his or her homosexuality. Some of these families have full-time custody, whereas others may share custody with an ex-partner. As children grow up within these family units, they may face some of the same issues experienced by children in other special families, including concerns about being accepted by others in the wider community.

Health care professionals must be especially conscientious to avoid being insensitive to these new family constellations.[39] Increased awareness and acceptance are needed in order to allow families and children to receive the same quality of care given to more mainstream families. Homophobia (fear and disapproval of homosexuality) and heterosexism (a belief that only heterosexual families are the appropriate setting for raising children) should be avoided to reduce the risk of insulting these individuals or of isolating them from health care services. Parents are more likely to be open about their concerns if they perceive that the health care provider is nonjudgmental and open to nontraditional family structure. Gender-neutral terms such as "parent" or "family member" may be preferred on office forms and questionnaires to avoid the appearance of bias and prejudice.

In the past, common misconceptions were that children raised in gay- or lesbian-headed families would have increased risks of emotional disorders or sexual dysfunction later in life. Recent research has demonstrated that children raised in these families are similar to children in traditional families and are equally likely to be well adjusted and to have positive self-esteem. Patterson,[40] in her review of 12 studies of more than 300 children of gay and lesbian parents, concluded that these children are not more likely to establish a homosexual preference than children raised in heterosexual-led families.

Children who are raised in communities that are tolerant of these differences probably experience less stress and concern about the reaction of others. The scientific literature suggests that they adjust to being raised by two same-sex parents by creating names to help distinguish them (e.g., Mommy Kate and Mommy Jane). When openness is encouraged at home, children may show very little concern about the different characteristics of their family. As adolescence approaches, issues of sexual identity and exploration can be discussed with the same sensitivity and openness that one hopes to find in more traditional families. It is likely that over time, health care professionals and our society at large will become more aware and sensitive to the needs of these children and their parents.

HOMELESS FAMILIES

Families are the fastest growing segment of the homeless population in America.[41] As such, more and more children are living in cars, vans, low-cost hotels, shelters, or simply on the street. They are exposed to severe poverty, violence, and profound deprivation. Approximately one half of these children suffer from severe depression, anxiety, and learning and behavior problems.[42] Their parents are typically aware of these problems but do not have resources for dealing with them.

When treating **homeless children,** the clinician should pay particular attention to their school attendance and functioning. Collaboration with teachers, public health nurses, social workers, and mental health personnel is useful. Concrete recommendations for the parents about community resources and customary guidance about growth and development are important. With the high rates of violence and substance abuse among the homeless, these children should be screened carefully for developmental delays, depression, post-traumatic stress disorder, conduct problems, and substance exposure.

As a result of the tremendous disorganization commonly found among homeless families, clinicians may become frustrated by the lack of follow-up during planned medical visits. It is useful to keep in mind Maslow's hierarchy,[43] whereby motivation for higher goals of achievement, self-esteem, and identity is based on achieving earlier goals of safety, comfort, and love. As with all special families, issues of safety, predictability, and organization can help overcome the effects of prior losses. It is likely that more children will be growing up in these disruptive environments, and clinicians will need to be particularly sensitive to the frustration experienced by parents who are unable to meet their child's needs because of extraordinary social circumstances.

CONCLUSION

The needs of children living in specific forms of special families (stepfamilies, single-parent, adoptive, foster care, homeless, and families with gay or lesbian parents) have been described. Other types of special families in which a child's development may be affected in unique ways are increasing in contemporary America. These include children living with a grandmother as a primary parent and live-in situations. Openness, respect, and a desire to talk about the effect of these special family environments on the development of children should be the goal of the child's clinician. Helping parents to guide the development of children who live in special families is an appropriate goal—and challenge—in a developmentally focused clinical practice. The generic functions of a family unit must be kept clearly in mind when the circumstances in which a child lives, no matter how "special" they seem, are evaluated.

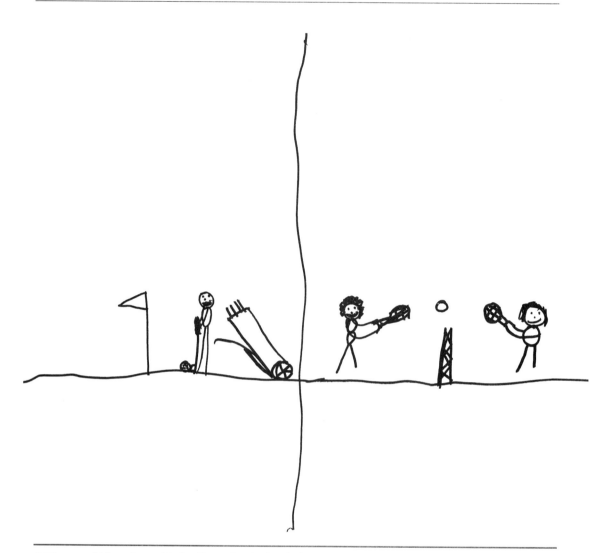

A 10-year-old boy draws his family as clearly divided. His parents are divorced. His father goes on the left while his mother plays tennis with her new husband. The boy is left out of the picture.

REFERENCES

1. Bryner KB: The Amish way of death: a study of family support systems. In Moos RH, editor: *Coping with life crises: an integrated approach,* New York, 1986, Plenum Press.
2. Lazarus RS: *Psychological stress and the coping process,* New York, 1966, McGraw-Hill.
3. Wallerstein J, Kelly J: *Surviving the breakup: how children and parents cope with divorce,* New York, 1980, Basic Books.
4. American Medical Association: Violence: a compendium, *JAMA, American Medical News* and Specialty Journals of the American Medical Association, 1992.

5. Block JH, Block J: The role of ego-control and ego-resiliency in the organization of behavior. In Collins WA, editor: *Development of cognition, affect and social relations: the Minnesota symposia on child psychology,* vol 3, Hillsdale, NJ, 1980, Lawrence Erlbaum Associates.

6. Murphy LB, Moriarty AE: *Vulnerability, coping and growth,* New Haven, Conn, 1976, Yale University Press.

7. Sameroff AJ, Barocas R, Seifer R: The early development of children born to mentally ill women. In Watt NF et al, editors: *Children at risk for schizophrenia: a longitudinal perspective,* New York, 1984, Cambridge University Press.

8. Werner EE, Smith RS: *Vulnerable but invincible: a longitudinal study of resilient children and youth,* New York, 1982, McGraw-Hill.

9. Kellam S, Ensminger M, Turner R: Family structure and the mental health of children, *Arch Gen Psychiatr* 34:1012, 1977.

10. Patterson GR: Stress: a change agent for family process. In Garmezy N, Rutter M, editors: *Stress, coping and development in children,* Baltimore, 1988, Johns Hopkins University Press.

11. Heatherington EM, Cox M, Cox R: Long-term effects of divorce and remarriage on the adjustment of children, *J Am Acad Child Psychiatry* 24:518, 1985.

12. Kappelman MM, Black J: Children of divorce: the pediatrician's responsibility, *Pediatr Ann* 9:48, 1980.

13. Hoyt LA et al: Anxiety and depression in young children of divorce, *J Clin Child Psychol* 19:26, 1990.

14. Stein MT: Challenging case: the use of family drawings by children in pediatric practice, *J Dev Behav Pediatr* 18:334, 1997.

15. Wallerstein JS, Johnston JR: Children of divorce: recent findings regarding long term effects and recent studies of joint and sole custody, *Pediatr Rev* 11:197, 1990.

16. Johnson JR, Kline M, Tschann JM: Ongoing postdivorce conflict: effects on children of joint custody and frequent access, *Am J Orthopsychiatr* 59:576, 1989.

17. Rutter M: Families. In Rutter M, editor: *Helping troubled children,* New York, 1975, Brunner-Mazel.

18. Radovanic H: Parental conflict and children's coping styles in litigating separated families: relationships with children's adjustment, *J Abnorm Child Psychol* 21:697, 1993.

19. Wallerstein JS: Separation, divorce and remarriage. In Levine MD, Carey WB, Crocker AC, editors: *Developmental-behavioral pediatrics,* ed 2, Philadelphia, 1992, WB Saunders.

20. Herndon A, Combs LG: Stepfamilies as patients, *J Fam Pract* 15:917, 1982.

21. Visher EB, Visher JS: Stepfamilies are different, *J Fam Ther* 7:9, 1985.

22. Ganong LH, Coleman M: The effects of remarriage on children: a review of the empirical literature, *J Appl Fam Child Studies* 33:389, 1984.

23. Anderson JZ, White GD: An empirical investigation of interaction and relationship patterns in functional and dysfunctional nuclear families and stepfamilies, *Fam Process* 25:407, 1986.

24. Papernow Q: *Becoming a stepfamily: patterns of development in remarried families,* San Francisco, 1993, Jossey-Bass.

25. Garbarino J, Seves J, Schellenbach C: Families at risk for destructive parent-child relations in adolescence, *Child Dev* 55:174, 1984.

26. Anthony EJ: Children at risk for psychosis growing up successfully. In Anthony EJ, Cohler B, editors: *The invulnerable child,* New York, 1987, Guilford Press.

27. Garmezy N: Children under stress: perspectives on antecedents and correlates of vulnerability and resistance to psychopathology. In Rabin AI et al, editors: *Further explorations in personality,* New York, 1981, John Wiley & Sons.

28. Lewis FM et al: The family's functioning with chronic illness in the mother: the spouse's perspective, *Soc Sci Med* 29:1261, 1989.

29. Wessel MA: The pediatrician and adoption, *N Engl J Med* 262:446, 1960.

30. Mahler MS, Pine F, Bergman A: *The psychological birth of the human infant: symbiosis and individuation,* New York, 1975, Basic Books.

31. Sorosky AD, Baran A, Pannor R: *The adoption triangle,* New York, 1978, Doubleday.

32. American Academy of Pediatrics, Committee on Early Childhood, Adoption, and Dependent Care: Families and Adoption: The pediatrician's role in supporting communication. In American Academy of Pediatrics: *Policy reference guide of the American Academy of Pediatrics,* Elk Grove Village, Ill, 1997.

33. American Academy of Pediatrics: Issues of confidentiality in adoption: the role of the pediatrician, *Pediatrics* 93(2):339, 1994.

34. Schor ED: Foster care, *Pediatr Clin North Am* 35:1241, 1988.

35. Dubowitz H et al: The physical health of children in kinship care, *Am J Dis Child* 146:603, 1992.

36. Bowlby J: Loss: sadness and depression. In *Attachment and loss,* vol 3, New York, 1980, Basic Books.

37. Sokoloff B: Adoption and foster care: the pediatrician's role, *Pediatr Rev* 1:57, 1979.

38. Gold M et al: Children of gay or lesbian parents, *Pediatr Rev* 15:354, 1994.

39. Spock B: *Dr. Spock's baby and child care,* ed 7, New York, 1998, Pocket Books, pp 685-688.

40. Patterson CJ: Children of lesbian and gay parents, *Adv Clin Child Psychol* 19:235, 1997.

41. Edelman MW, Mihaly L: Homeless families and the housing crisis in the United States, *Child Youth Services Rev* 11:91, 1989.

42. Bassuk EL, Rubin L: Homeless children: a neglected population. *Am J Orthopsychiatry* 57:279, 1987.

43. Maslow AH: *Motivation and personality,* ed 2, New York, 1970, Harper & Row.

ACKNOWLEDGMENT

An early draft of this chapter was written with contributions from Nicholas Putnam, M.D.

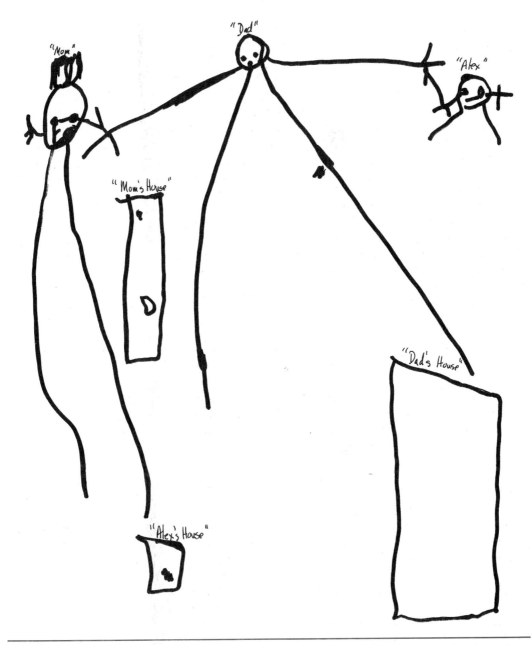

Alex, a 4-year-old boy, draws his family and circumstances as he sees them. He is in joint physical custody with both parents. He's the smallest and is aligned with dad. Mom's shown also attached to Dad (perhaps a wish) and with more detail, including breasts, which is not atypical for an "oedipal" (4- to 6-year-old) child. Alex also imagines his own house, separate from his parents, perhaps a more constant place than the two different ones in which he lives. He was referred for evaluation because of serious aggressive behavior resulting in expulsion from preschool.

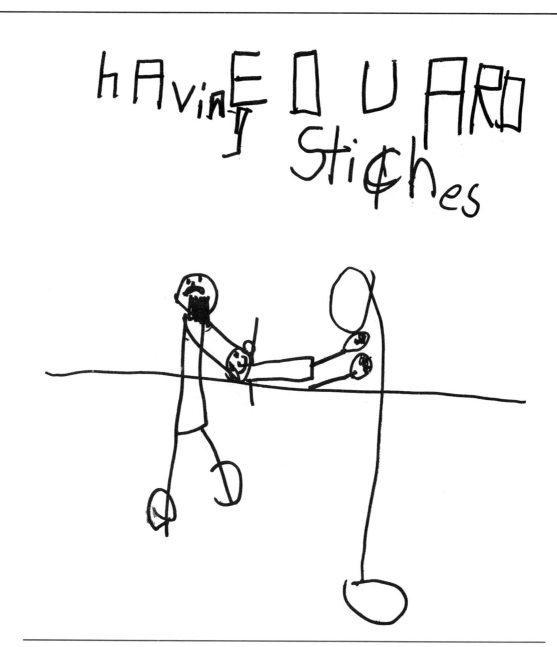

"Having stitches." A boy, age 6, shows his doctor fixing him up. The nurse is less well drawn and is faceless. The lack of hands and disconnected leg might suggest a sense of losing control, of powerlessness in the situation.

CHAPTER 24

ENCOUNTERS WITH ILLNESS: OPPORTUNITY FOR HEALTH PROMOTION

■ Martin T. Stein

KEY WORDS

Acute Illness
Chronic Disease
Social Competence
Developmental Regression
Patient and Parent Agenda
Solution Building–Family Model
Object Constancy
Separation Experience
Protest-Despair-Denial
Explanatory Models of Illness

Accurate diagnosis of an acute physical illness is the hallmark of a pediatric clinician. It is accomplished hundreds of times each year as clinical experience generates greater precision. In addition to disease recognition and appropriate treatment, attention to the way patients (children and parents) perceive a disease and the behaviors and emotional feelings that are a result of their perceptions are important components of comprehensive care. By considering a child's development, behavior, and the psychosocial profile of the family, the clinician not only broadens the data base on which to make decisions, but brings a new dimension to the encounter. An "illness" (in contrast to the physical "disease" state) can be viewed in the context of a particular child's development, as well as the family's experience with symptoms and disease and their expectations and resources. Parmelee has made the insightful observation that in some families ". . . one may have a disease and not feel ill or feel ill and not have a disease."[1] Although an illness may interfere with normal developmental processes, it may also be an opportunity for mastery and the enhancement of self-esteem. Once this concept is appreciated, the emphasis may no longer be limited to the disease process but can include perceptions and reactions to the diagnosis, treatments, stresses that accompany the illness, and coping mechanisms of the child and family.

In primary care pediatric practice, at least 50% of the office visits are for an **acute illness;** about 10% to 15% of children have a **chronic disease;** and at least a few children are hospitalized each month. The impact of a disease on a child's behavior and developmental expectations is not limited to chronic disorders (see Chapter 26). Opportunities for the appli-

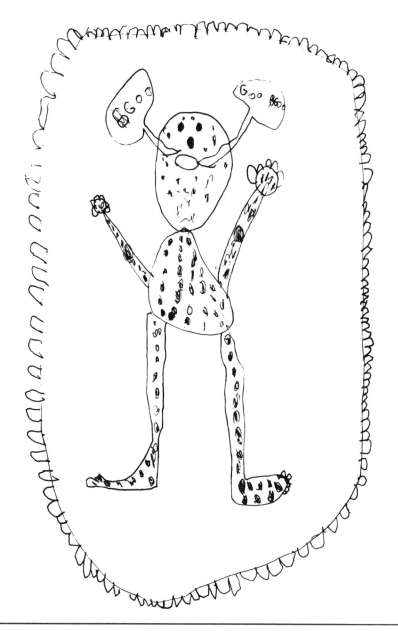

A boy, age 7, draws his baby brother with the chicken pox. The blanket serves as an enclosure, perhaps reflecting the boy's distancing himself from the baby's predicament.

cation of useful pediatric principles about our responses to and counseling about disease and illness are equally important during acute illness visits for common problems. Whether a child has a well-defined, limited illness (e.g., streptococcal pharyngitis) or a complicated, chronic disorder (e.g., asthma in poor control in a child with multiple hospitalizations), office management should make use of fundamental principles of child development and the importance of family interactions. Doing this, as well as recognizing the distinction between disease and illness, is more likely to lead to success in meeting a child's and family's needs.

ACUTE MINOR ILLNESS

Acute illness is a part of childhood. It occurs frequently and is usually self-limited or responsive to medical therapies. During the first 3 years of life, most children experience between six and nine illnesses each year; most illnesses are respiratory or gastrointestinal infections. Between 4 and 10 years old, children average four to six illnesses annually.[2] The high transmission rate throughout a family means that a family with two adults and two children will average 21 illnesses per year.[3] A child's early experiences with these inevitable parts of childhood potentially shape several aspects of her development.

Every pediatrician who enters an examination room has one major objective, to get the diagnosis right and prescribe the appropriate treatment. This goal, coupled with courtesy, empathy, and the recognition that at least two patients are being treated (see Chapter 3), make up the core components of pediatric practice. The next level of understanding is to ask the question: What is the child's understanding of her symptoms and the reason she has been brought to the doctor? The child may think or say: "Why is mommy or daddy being asked all these questions? Why is the doctor putting a tube on my body and a popsicle stick in my mouth? Am I going to get better? Will I get a shot? Do I have to take off my clothes?"

An understanding of a child's perspective on the acute illness visit is crucial for two reasons. First, it generates age-appropriate ways to communicate with children, a core pediatric value. Equally important is the clinician's recognition that *the experience of the office visit itself shapes the way a child learns about the body, physical symptoms and illness, and the healing process.* Although limited research has been done in this area, it seems reasonable to assume that the cumulative experience of the way parents manage illnesses and the experience at the doctor's office may contribute substantially to subsequent adult perceptions of symptoms and response to illness and health care.

Stacy, a 13-year-old, came to the office with a concern about a sore throat of 3 days' duration without fever or other symptoms. This was Stacy's seventh office visit during the past year for the same symptoms. Physical examinations demonstrated mild erythema of the pharynx and tonsils without fever or adenopathy; at other times the oropharynx was normal. Throat cultures were consistently negative for group A beta-hemolytic streptococcus, and Stacy was given a handout about viral respiratory illness.

This situation is familiar to all pediatric clinicians. An early adolescent comes to the doctor with frequent sore throats that are either mild and self-limited viral infections or exaggerated concerns of a mild irritation of the throat. These office visits may reflect a parental perspective of this child as fragile and vulnerable. Or, she may be growing up in a family where somatic complaints for minor problems among other family members are frequently brought to medical attention. She and her family may really be worried about something serious, a concern that isn't stated. Either situation is an opportunity to go beyond taking yet another throat culture and labeling the problem viral pharyngitis. A focused medical history may reveal one or more encounters with illness that were perceived by Stacy's parents to be more serious than implied by the diagnosis. Alternatively, a family history may suggest a pattern of somatization among a parent and other members of the extended family. In this situation, chronic stress or acute situational stressors may trigger the onset of physical or emotional symptoms that are repeatedly brought to the attention of the clinician. A pediatric intervention might start with recognition that there is a problem in addition to a sore throat. The next step, depending on the intensity of the problem and the particular family, might be a few brief follow-up appointments with the pediatrician to explore the associations between minor physical symptoms and the family's responses. A referral to a mental health specialist would be useful when frequent visits for minor symptoms of a sore throat continue even after pediatric education, probing, and counseling. A brief dismissal of each episode never really gets at the core issues and is unlikely to break a pattern of care for such minor complaints.

Clinicians who care for children are generally empathic individuals. They care for children and have a genuine regard and understanding of the experience of their patient and his parents. To strengthen the capacity for empathy, it is useful to analyze the components of a child's experience as he encounters illness in his home and at the doctor's office (Table 24-1).

Periodic analyses of a patient's psychological and social responses to an illness will bring refreshing clinical insights into the process of providing primary care. These insights usually point to both strengths and vulnerabilities in a particular child and family. They also suggest language to use to strengthen a therapeutic alliance and help children adapt to illness. Most children adapt effectively to illness. Through a greater understanding of the emotional and social context that surrounds illness, clinicians will discover those children and families who experience greater stress or a sense of ongoing vulnerability during each episode.

Children perceive the nature of their illness in a manner consistent with their cognitive level of development. The level of understanding of symptoms moves during childhood through a rapid developmental change from the magical responses ("You get sick because you ate too much candy.") of preschool children to early school-age children ("You get sick because you go out in the cold.") to older school-age children, who are able to generalize symptoms and show some understanding of the role of a germ in causing disease, as well as a beginning awareness of their contribution to the nature of the experience (Table 24-2).

As clinicians incorporate a better understanding of a child's internal emotional response to an illness, they are in a better position to offer individualized helpful suggestions. In addition, this knowledge strengthens the therapeutic alliance with children and their parents. Knowledge about frequently used coping strategies during an acute illness will bring some of these insights to the medical encounter. For example, it is important to understand

TABLE 24-1 ■ Components of the Experience of Acute Minor Illness

Child's Experience	Parents' Experience
Physical discomfort of the illness and treatment	Increased child care responsibilities
Emotional responses: guilt, fear, anger, depression, lethargy	Expense of illness
	Interference with employment
Fantasies about illness	Sleep deprivation/fatigue
Loss of social contacts	Decreased recreation
Restrictions (bed rest, diet)	Effects on marital relationship
Decreased or altered sensory input	Fear, anger, guilt
Change in relationship with parents (indulgent or hostile)	Depression
Worry about body integrity	Distortions and misconceptions
Fear of serious illness	

Modified from Carey WB: Acute minor illness. In Levine MD, Carey WB, Crocker AC: *Developmental-behavioral pediatrics,* ed 2, Philadelphia, 1992, WB Saunders, pp 295-296.

that a child under 5 years old often runs away from a clinician and hides behind or under an examination table. She may ask for a bandage or a kiss on a "boo-boo." These are direct coping mechanisms that reflect the child's magical thinking rather than logical consequences of events. For the school-age child who may perceive a set of symptoms in concrete terms and may begin to show some evidence of the development of causality, the astute clinician can make use of the new coping skills. Allowing the child to listen to his heart with a stethoscope and to ask questions about a medicine or an x-ray film and encouraging him to talk about his perceptions about the illness will give him an opportunity to use age-appropriate coping skills, as well as enhance the therapeutic relationship. The *TEACHER* mnemonic is a useful technique to improve the quality of communications with children and their parents at the time of a pediatric illness visit (Table 24-3).

Further probing of the case of Stacy, the 13-year-old girl with the sore throat, revealed several family members with irritable bowel syndrome, tension headaches, and chronic low back pain. Her maternal grandfather had acute rheumatic fever as a child, and her mother grew up in a family that feared the medical consequences of acute pharyngitis. A pattern of somatization, coupled with an exaggerated fear of a mild sore throat, suggested to the clinician that to break the generational transmission of vulnerability to minor illness, a referral to a behavioral-developmental pediatrician or a family therapist was indicated.

TABLE 24-2 ■ Growth in Child's Understanding of Illness

Age	Understanding	Examples
4-6 yr	Circular, magical or global responses	"I got a boo-boo on my head because I didn't eat my soup!" (A child's reaction to a scalp laceration caused by his falling and hitting his head on a table shortly after lunchtime, when his mother unsuccessfully encouraged him to eat tomato soup)
6-8 yr	Concrete, rigid responses with a "parrot-like" quality; little comprehension by the child; enumeration of symptoms, actions, or situations associated with illness	"The cough is a bug that tickles my throat and makes me stay home and in bed. The bug can't play with my friends."
8-11 yr	Increased generalization, with some indication of child's contribution to the response; quality of invariant causation remains	"I get these headaches sometimes because I fight with my sister and won't let her play with my things." When asked about his symptoms during a mild gastroenteritis, Sammy responded, "I got it because I ate some poison, just like last year when we all got sick at the restaurant."
11-13 yr	Beginning use of an underlying principle; greater delineation of causal agents of illnesses	"Kids get sick when germs like a virus get into their body. It's the virus that makes us feel lousy, causes a fever, and makes us want to sleep more."
Over 14 yr	Organized description of mechanism(s) underlying illness and recovery; abstract principles	"Last year I had mono along with three of my friends. I know it's caused by a virus that makes you sleepy and not want to eat and zaps energy. But my friends got better quickly. I stayed out of school for a month. It seems that the mono virus was harder on my body and tougher to get rid of. My mom thinks it's because we've had a lot of stress in the family. She may be right because I know I get better quicker from a cold when things at home are cool."

Modified from Perrin EC, Gerrity PS: *Pediatrics* 67:841, 1981. In Levine MD, Carey WB, Crocker AC: *Developmental-behavioral pediatrics*, Philadelphia, 1992, WB Saunders, p 306.

Pediatric clinicians can practice a form of preventive medicine in order to limit adverse psychosocial responses during the course of acute minor illnesses. Several strategies are available. Overdiagnosis of benign, often transient, physical findings may lead to excessive parental concern or unnecessary restrictions. For example, a benign functional cardiac murmur may be managed in several ways: (1) do not mention it because it is so frequently found and inconsequential; (2) explain to the parents that it is a sound heard when listening to a normal

TABLE 24-3 ■ TEACHER—Method for Enhancing Communication With Pediatric Patients and Their Parents

T	Trust	Build trust and rapport with the child by asking nonthreatening questions not related to illness.
E	Elicit	Elicit information from parent(s) and child regarding parental fears and concerns and the child's understanding of the reason for the visit.
A	Agenda	Set an agenda early in the visit to help ensure that the parents' concerns are addressed.
C	Control	Help the child feel control over the visit (e.g., knowing what will and will not happen) to help decrease fear and increase cooperation.
H	Health plan	Establish a health plan with child and parent to meet the child's needs and limitations.
E	Explain	Explain the health plan to the child in a way he can understand.
R	Rehearse	Have the child rehearse the health plan as a way of assessing understanding; reinforce the child's jobs related to health care; explore any potential problems in the plan with the child and parent.

From Bernzweig J, Pantell R, Lewis CC: Talking with children. In Parker S, Zuckerman B, editors: *Behavioral and developmental pediatrics*, New York, 1995, Little, Brown & Co., p 7.

heart in a healthy child, does not reflect any cardiac problems, and will disappear as the child grows; (3) tell the parents that "he has a murmur coming from the heart that is called a functional murmur . . . it's not really important and we won't worry about it." The latter explanation for some vulnerable families may predispose to "cardiac nondisease," a condition in which the parents leave the office uncertain of their child's cardiac status because of the vague explanation. Some parents may inappropriately restrict the child's activity or develop an inappropriate sense of vulnerability about the health of the child.[4] Other physical findings that require clear explanation in order to prevent a "nondisease" problem include mild (physiological) adenopathy, tibial torsion, hydrocele, strawberry hemangioma, and umbilical hernia. This preventive behavioral work may begin in the newborn period.

Juan was moderately jaundiced during his first office visit for a weight check, following an early discharge from the nursery. At 60 hours of age, his serum total bilirubin was 18 mg/dl. Plans were initiated to begin home phototherapy and to assist his mother with techniques for optimal breast feeding.

This case is an opportunity to educate parents about a problem that may appear serious or even life-threatening to a parent, but is characteristically benign and limited to the early neonatal period. Diagnostic and monitoring interventions (blood tests) and therapy (phototherapy accompanied by daily home nursing visits) are often overmedicalized by clinicians, nurses, and other medical personnel. In part this is because hyperbilirubinemia can be associated with serious consequences in some circumstances. However, a pediatrician should be able to manage the diagnosis and therapy of this condition with information for the parents that leaves little room for exaggerated worry. It is most likely a benign condition that will resolve spontaneously or with a few days of phototherapy, will not recur, and will not have any lasting effect on the baby's growth and development. Without this kind of focused parent education, a simple problem like neonatal hyperbilirubinemia can induce in the new parents a lasting sense of vulnerability about the baby.[5]

Direct, age-appropriate, and honest explanations during acute-illness visits help children and parents understand and adapt to each situation. Dishonesty ("the shot the nurse will give won't hurt you"), belittling a child's feelings ("your belly really doesn't hurt that much"), and preoccupation with the disease (medical diagnosis) demonstrate limited attention to the patient's perceptions and style of coping with disease and are risk factors for adverse behaviors in children. Separation of children from their parents during a procedure should be avoided. A parent's presence usually serves to anchor a frightened child.

Donnie came to the office for a health supervision visit at 3 years of age. His mother remarked that his behavior had changed dramatically in the past month.

After a year of feeding himself and learning to use a cup and spoon, he now wanted her to help feed him. His language became "like a baby," and he used fewer words than before. He wanted to be held more often and cried when left with a sitter or about simple frustrations that he had managed with less emotional upset in the past.

His pediatrician, at first alarmed by the recent history of acute regression in social, motor, and language milestones, asked a critical question, "Did anything out of the ordinary occur to Donnie just prior to the changes in his behavior?" In fact, he had been to the emergency room for treatment of a small scalp laceration from a fall onto a coffee table. Restraints were used during the procedure, and his parents (inappropriately) were asked to leave the treatment room.

Following a normal physical examination, the pediatrician explained to Donnie's mother that Donnie most likely reacted to the stressful emergency room encounter with a developmental regression ("He lost some of his skills as a way to cope with the stressful experience of the E.R. visit."), which is one of the few coping mechanisms available to a toddler. The pediatrician guided Donnie through a play experience with a doll (available in a drawer in the examining room) "who went to the doctor to get a hurt fixed up." His mother was encouraged to use the play technique at home a few times. She phoned the pediatrician 2 weeks later and reported resolution of the regression and reestablishment of his previous developmental skills.

POSITIVE ASPECTS OF ACUTE ILLNESS

Parmelee has suggested that the multiple experiences with acute illness, a characteristic of everyone's childhood, guides the process of **social competence.**[1] The manner and style of each family's response to an illness shapes the child's sense of self and his coping strategies. From an experience with overindulgence in response to a simple cold to the denial of the symptoms when a child is uncomfortable or in pain ("let's move on, get well, and return to school"), children are exposed to a variety of adult responses to symptoms as they experience an illness associated with fatigue and vulnerability (Box 24-1). Discovering the nurturing value of chicken soup must be balanced against the risk of overindulgence.

Children often regress in their development in response to even minor illness. Those milestones that have been achieved most recently are vulnerable to temporary loss. Expressive language and self-regulation skills, such as feeding, sleeping, and toilet training, are most vulnerable. Parents can be guided to anticipate some degree of **developmental regression** in all children during an illness to help them achieve a balance between reasonable indulgence and maintaining a goal of recovery. It is a delicate balance that should encourage the healing process while the child learns about the value of being cared for by another individual. For many families, various healing rituals that are transferred through generations provide positive expectations that teach coping mechanisms through social relationships.

Social competency begins with the family and the thousands of interactions with others experienced during childhood. An illness event that is misinterpreted with regard to severity and duration of adverse effect may have the effect of creating an aura of vulnerability.

CHRONIC ILLNESS

Compared to acute illness, primary care pediatric clinicians have considerably less experience with chronic illness in children. With the exception of asthma and attention deficit-hyperactivity disorder (ADHD), conditions that have a prevalence of 5% and 5% to 8% among children, respectively, clinicians who care for children typically do not see specific chronic disorders frequently. However, most pediatric practices are filled with children with various disorders managed by the pediatrician along with specialists. Care of the psychosocial needs of children with chronic illness and their families can be guided effectively by a set of principles that simultaneously account for developmental considerations and the biol-

BOX 24-1	**WHAT CHILDREN CAN LEARN DURING ACUTE ILLNESS**[1]

An important social lesson learned is that there is an appropriate time to let others take care of us so that we may recover as rapidly as possible and resume our usual activities. Making the decision to let others care for us in a timely fashion is essential to restoring wellness. Learning when and how to do this is one of the aspects of general social competence that is learned in childhood.

ogy of the disease. A biopsychosocial approach to chronic illness does not require specific knowledge of a particular disorder's impact on a child. Substantial clinical benefits are derived from a generic approach to children and families with chronic disorders rather than an approach that views each disorder as distinct.[6] Certain characteristics are common to all chronic health conditions; they transcend the specific nature of the illness. For example, behavioral problems and psychological disorders occur twice as often in children with most chronic illnesses as in children without a chronic illness. Effects on parents' work schedules, job stability, marriage, and family finances are seen to variable degrees regardless of the specific illness. A family's adjustment to a child with a chronic illness does not correlate with the severity of the illness. Individual, family, and community factors have a tremendous impact on adaptation and adjustment.[7]

To establish a therapeutic alliance, in which mutual trust guides the clinical dialogue and decision-making process, following guidelines for working with children and their families facing chronic illness can be useful (Table 24-4). Following the initial assessment it is critical that the child's clinician begin to convey the effect of a chronic disorder on a child's

TABLE 24-4 ■ Biopsychosocial Approach to Chronic Disease

Approach	Action
Recognition of a chronic disorder	Help child and family understand fluctuating symptoms, good days and bad days, amelioration of symptoms (vs. cure)
Treatment that should fit pattern of child's and family's daily activities	Use knowledge about family life, family members, schedules, roles, decision making, who provides care at various times
Assisting child and family in identifying major concerns, priorities in care and outcome	Child, family, and clinician have shared agenda
	Ask "What would you like to see changed?" Initially address only 3 concerns
Valuing and building on small successes	Set small goals, specific measures of progress
Effective use of a clinician's:	
Skill	Help child and family to articulate problems, strengths, and goals
Patience	
Ability to set realistic goals	View the illness as chronic disorder for biological and psychosocial aspects of illness
Persistence	Plan follow-up visits, phone calls, periodic assessment

Adapted from Stein MT, Meltzer EO, Stein REK: Challenging case: recurrent episodes of asthma in a 10 year old, *J Dev Behav Pediatr* 19:44, 1998.

patterns of living (at school, at home, with friends, and with the family). When a cure is not the goal, realistic expectations for the amelioration of symptoms and adaptations to living should be made clear, even if only a short time frame is known. For treatment strategies to be effective, they must fit the patterns of a child's and family's daily activities. The primary care clinician can negotiate and adapt schedules and regimens that are stressful or impossible without unduly compromising the quality of care. To be effective, this kind of planning requires knowledge about family life, family members, and those who provide child care at different times.

Although the identification of parental concerns (the parent's agenda for the visit) is critical to all pediatric clinical encounters, it is especially important when working with a child who has a chronic disorder. Ask the parent and child to identify those things that they most want to see changed. Ask them to establish the care priorities. Encouraging them to identify three concerns often leads to the discovery of one that can be relatively easy to address.

> *Eric, a boy with autism, was becoming increasingly disruptive in school and couldn't participate in his speech program. His family was fearful of working on a medication change with the psychiatrist because Eric's sleep had been disrupted by medication in the past. They felt they couldn't cope at all if Eric didn't sleep at night. The primary care physician helped them start a sleep diary and wrote a note to the psychiatrist about the family's priority and the school's concern.*

Success in working on a problem that the family perceives as important improves the opportunity to then work on more difficult problems and those that are important to the clinician as well.[8] A clinician's sensitivity to treatable symptoms, whether they are physical, psychological, or social, brings further opportunities to achieve these goals. Building a therapeutic relationship with a family through successful negotiations of realistic goals leads to small and large gains. Encouragement and reinforcement of each small success improves adherence to therapies and problem-solving skills.

POOR COMPLIANCE

When working with some parents of children with chronic disorders, it is not uncommon to find either poor adherence to a treatment or suboptimal adaptation to an illness after appropriate medications, advice, and education have been tried. This means it's time to pull back and approach the situation differently. These situations are opportunities to reframe the nature of the problem. Returning to the **patient and parent agenda** model, it is useful to discuss with the child and family their perceptions of the illness and their experiences with trying to solve specific problems. The goal is to reframe the individual problems of the child with a disease as family problems that require a joint effort. Epstein has observed that "just as rapport and empathy facilitate self-disclosure and trust with individual patients, developing rapport by 'joining' the family and demonstrating understanding of each family member's perspective on a problem can facilitate collaborative problem solving. By adopting an

TABLE 24-5 ■ Comparison of Approaches to Patients

Issue	Biomedical	Solution-Building with Family
Patient role	"Sick" patient; passive partner	Equal and active participants
Patient focus	Problems, dilemmas	Solutions
Expert	Clinician	Clinician, patient, and family as problem-solvers and solution-builders
Encounter focus	Deficits, pathology of individual; extended history of the problem	Strengths, competence of family system; brief history of the problem; detailed history of goals and solutions
Therapeutic focus	Clinician's decisions	Clinician, patient, and family develop solutions

Modified from Stein MT, Coleman WL, Epstein RM: We've tried everything, and nothing works: family centered pediatrics and clinical problem solving, *J Dev Behav Pediatr* 18:118, 1997.

attitude of active curiosity in learning each member's point of view, the clinician can convey a genuine interest in the family."[9] This is the foundation for better compliance for any care plan or therapeutic effort. Participation of the family in the problem-solving process is illustrated when the traditional biomedical model is contrasted with a solution-building model that relies on the strength and competencies of the family (Table 24-5). Finally, if clinicians are sensitive to their own emotional reactions to families of children with a chronic illness, their self-awareness helps them to use their own particular strengths as they work within the **solution building–family model** of communication (see Chapter 3).

HOSPITALIZATION AND PROCEDURES

The hospitalization of a child involves the removal of that child from a characteristically safe and nurturing environment within the home to a place populated by strangers, to a crib or bed that is unfamiliar, to a place with walls and floors that are different from home colors, and to sounds that are new and, at times, cacophonous. The child may see people in uniforms for the first time. Procedures, examinations, and treatments may be perceived as frighteningly invasive or affrontive. Any hospitalization, no matter how well managed, is stressful for the child. That stress can be a source of growth in experience and competence[10] or can create additional illness complications and delay healing in its broadest sense.

The behavioral patterns of hospitalized children have received increasing attention in the past 50 years from research, clinical, and child advocacy vantage points.[11] In association with the emergence of hospitals and wards designed specifically for the needs of children, more attention has been given to the emotional needs and developmental capacities of children in hospitals. The American Association for the Care of Children in Hospitals has provided leadership in making these changes. Hospitals in general are better able to respond to the unique needs of children now than ever before. Family visiting and involvement, child life programs, school involvement, and attention to psychosocial needs are now nearly routine. However, the clinician cannot rely on the institution alone to be supportive of the patient during the stress of hospitalization.

Impact of Hospitalization

The impact of hospitalization is significant when viewed from the perspective of a sudden environmental change. A hospital environment brings predictable alterations to a child's relationships with family members, peers, and school activities. Perhaps most significantly, going to the hospital means a loss of independence that is appropriate to the child's developmental level. Because the quest for independent activity and psychological autonomy begins at birth and is the energizing force that fuels development, most children are affected by the loss of independence when hospitalized. In addition, they may be stripped of their usual patterns of coping with stress (e.g., withdrawing to the bedroom, a temper tantrum at dinnertime, asking for and receiving more nurturing time from parents). This leaves them in a vulnerable, psychologically naked position. We expect their behavior to be altered.[12]

Children develop attachments to important people throughout childhood. A child relies on these attachments to carry him through developmental hurdles and times of stress. The hospitalization experience varies among children, depending upon the quality of those attachments and the developmental level of each child. In this context, the experience of separation (from mother, father, or another significant caretaker) is the major psychological event that occurs when a child is hospitalized.[13] She is deprived of the trust and security of having the loving person or persons present and responsive at all times of need. The psychological and physiological effects of separation are mediated to some extent by the child's ability to maintain the image of primary caretaker or caretakers in her mind. This milestone in development is known as **object constancy** (see Chapters 2 and 11). It is a necessary cognitive skill, but it is not sufficient help for the child to weather the separation without stress. With this skill the child may be able to call forth the image of the primary caretaker without experiencing an overwhelming feeling of abandonment. The attachment figure's presence is maintained throughout the separation if the separation is relatively short and if the bond has been a strong one. These concepts can be illustrated by expressing the development of object relationships and separation reactions in terms of the primary developmental theme at each age group from infancy to adolescence (see Table 3-1).

Infant. At less than 6 months of age, most infants seem to tolerate hospital experiences with minimal long-term behavioral or physiological reactions to **separation experiences.** Very young infants do distinguish parents and strangers in social interactions, so some transient change in behavior and responsiveness should be expected. The clinician will appreciate behavioral differences in the child when cared for by the parent rather than a nurse. These differences are data to support or refute the attachment between the parent and child. Although the close bond with the mother is described as "symbiotic,"[14] the infant less than 6 months old has not reached the stage of perceiving herself as an independent being to the point that separation appears threatening. A young infant may show behavioral reactions (fussiness, inconsolability, sleep disturbances) or physiological reactions (vomiting, constipation, poor weight gain, poor feeding) in response to a hospital experience. Young infants will begin to establish new relationships with sensitive, consistent caretakers and will build on these very quickly. Similarly, they will reestablish patterns of interactions with parents quickly after the separation, if it is brief. Alterations in sleep patterns and feeding may show the impact of hospitalization on the child's schedule and state regulation.

Toddler. Behavioral changes in the toddler are more dramatic and require a longer recovery phase. As she develops independence, the child has an accompanying awareness of the stress of separation. This response is particularly acute between age 8 months and 18 months. The toddler's concern is, "Will mommy come back?" She appreciates cognitively and emotionally that a strange environment without the parent's presence is threatening and overwhelming. She also lacks a sense of time, so she cannot appreciate a promise of a prompt return by the parent. Her anxiety remains chronically high. Temper tantrums, listlessness, refusal to eat, and sleep disturbances are characteristic responses of the normal toddler to a hospital setting without the presence of the parent. It is testimony to appropriate psychological growth. Regressive behavior in this situation should be seen as adaptive and appropriate because it allows for conservation of energy and a bid for help during this "crisis" situation. It usually subsides after hospitalization as long as the separation experience has not been too intense or prolonged and the attachment process has evolved normally before the hospitalization.

Normal toddlers who experience abrupt or prolonged separation from parents undergo a progression of behavioral patterns. Originally described by Bowlby, these phases allow the clinician to monitor the child's response to stress.[15] They are the following:

- **Protest** reaction—tantrums, refusal to eat, aggressive behavior
- **Despair**—a quiet, withdrawn, sad appearance
- **Denial**—the previously depressed, despairing toddler now appears outgoing and responsive to everyone indiscriminately and shows no differential response to familiar care providers.

This third stage attests to severe stress for the child, who is now resistant to engaging in deep relationships or unwilling to risk wide excursions into either negative or positive emotions. It is a conservative psychological mechanism and is evidence of the severity of the insult. Red flags should appear when a child becomes the favorite of every nurse on the floor, offers no objection to examinations, or makes extraordinary efforts to elicit interactions with every passerby. A sad, withdrawn toddler or one who is "too good" is a warning that there has been a serious psychological assault.

Language may play an important role in the toddler's reaction to hospitalization. Before age 18 months, the child's expressive language is limited; he may not understand hospital personnel, or they may not understand him. After age 1 year, the toddler becomes acutely aware of this dissonance. After age 18 months to 2 years, the acceleration of expressive and receptive language provides the toddler the equipment to interact with others in a more advanced form and therefore to understand, at least in part, some of the strange people and events around him.

Preschooler. In contrast to the toddler's experience, the preschool child's response to hospitalization may call forth newly developed skills of imagination, verbal questioning, and magical thinking to understand and deal with the acute stresses of a strange environment.[15] The 4- to 5-year-old can tolerate the absence of parents for a longer period of time because she now understands that out of sight is not out of mind. Her memory is better developed, and she can use words to call up images, talk about planned events, and elicit conversations with hospital personnel. At the same time, cognitive thinking may produce distortions about causality,[16] with associated fears, fantasies, and body distortions. Children at this age may feel personally responsible for their illness or that they did something wrong that caused their parents to bring them to the hospital.[17] Causal relationships may depend on the child's perception of the temporal or spatial placement of events. Linkage occurs automatically as the child generates her own hypotheses regarding events around her. These "**explanatory models**"[18] may be resistant to change, no matter how many "facts" the parents or clinician provides.

The preschool child has the emotional and developmental equipment to tolerate separation experiences with increasing competency. He can exercise newly developed capacities for memory and imagination to learn new coping skills and to emotionally grow from hospitalization. This will depend on the strength of primary attachments, past history of separation, and environmental supports. The provision of a supportive environment, appropriate preparation, and outlets for expression of feelings will assist the preschool child in adapting to the hospital experience.

School-Age Child. The hospitalized school-age child is often able to develop peer-group friendships and attachments to nurses, physicians, and other personnel that may buffer the feelings arising from a new environment. Increasing verbal skills and the capacity to understand causality allow the school-age child to gain more control over the situation. He understands the basic causes of illness and the logic of treatment. Multidimensional causal models will be beyond his understanding. In addition, the child may be able to exercise more options in his treatment and participate in his own care if these are concrete, specific, and make some sense to him.

The hospital experience may become stressful for the school-age child because she may experience a lack of control and feelings of guilt and anger. A loss of internal controls, with subsequent behavioral manifestations of either depression or anxiety or behavioral regression, can be expected. The concept of *locus of control* (a feeling of either internal or external control of events or an illness) at times may be useful in understanding and navigating a child through a stressful hospital experience.[19] This approach encourages greater clarity of what's happening and what control and choices she has. The loss of school relationships and fear of getting behind scholastically and socially may add to the distress for a child of this age.

Adolescence. As the child reaches adolescence, the toddler theme of independence versus dependence takes on a more advanced stage of negotiation in the form of a quest for personal identity separate from the family. A hospital experience, as well as the disease process, confronts the adolescent's identity directly. The loss of an idealized self as a result of the disease, coupled with an abrupt separation from peer group and activities, may bring about psychological conflict in the hospitalized teenager. The disease process, coupled with invasive hospital procedures, may distort the adolescent's concept of body image and disrupt future plans, real or imagined. Although the adolescent possesses the cognitive ability to understand multiple and somewhat abstract causality with regard to illness and the need for hospitalization and procedures, the psychological turmoil may be dominant. Fantasies of the future may be encroached on by visions of deformities and disabilities. Age-appropriate in-

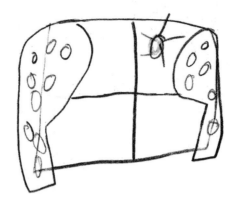

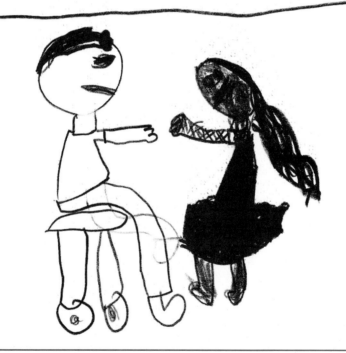

A girl shows a doctor applying an arm cast. The doctor is drawn only in outline whereas the patient has long brown hair, a purple dress, red lips, blue eyes, and a summer tan. Detail and color often signal importance, and the patient is clearly the center here. By Louise Dixon, age 7.

dependence may be distorted by the need for care, increased dependence, and disruptions of social support.

Developmental Regression

Children of all age groups can be expected to demonstrate a loss of some developmental milestones during and after a hospital experience (see Table 24-3). The intensity and duration of developmental regression are controlled by several determinants that have both preventive and therapeutic implications for the clinician:

- The child's developmental level with regard to social and language skills
- Personality and temperament—what kind of child was she before hospitalization? The quality of the reaction to a separation experience will vary not only with developmental level but also with the unique temperament of each child.
- Previous styles of coping with new situations
- Characteristics of the illness—duration, acuteness, severity, invasive procedures, immobilization, isolation
- Family's response to illness—the behavioral reactions of close relatives may influence the child's behavior. Is denial, rejection, or overpermissiveness apparent?[20]
- Fears and fantasies—Ask the child, "What do you think is wrong with you?" or "Why are you in the hospital?" Observation of play or review of the child's drawings may uncover the fears or fantasies that are based on her own explanatory model of the illness.

In an attempt to lessen the adverse reactions of children to the hospital experience, pediatric professionals should not lose sight of the fact that *developmental regression symbolizes both a stress and a protective maneuver* to defend against the loss of parent or parents and settle into the hospital experience. In this sense, behavioral alterations in the hospital may be adaptive and represent a healthy response to the experience. For example, a toddler's mild to moderate protest is an appropriate adaptation to a strange new world, inhabited by a new crib, an intravenous line, and numerous nurses and physicians. Preparing parents for these responses to hospitalization may help them to understand their adaptive significance.[21]

MEASURES TO HELP CHILDREN WITH HOSPITALIZATION

Pediatricians and other providers of health care for children may be advocates for their patients when hospitalization is considered by attending to the following issues (see Table 24-3):

- *Avoid hospitalization when possible.* When diagnostic or therapeutic procedures can be accomplished without hospital admission, do not hospitalize the child. Outpatient procedures usually allow more parent participation, which may lessen the stress on the child. Outpatient surgical units for children provide the child a hospital experience without an overnight stay. Short stays with home nursing follow-up will also lessen the impact.
- *Provide parents and the child with an age-appropriate explanation for the hospitalization.* Ask the verbal child, "Why do you think you must come to the hospital?"
- *For elective procedures (e.g., hernia repair, cardiac catheterization, myringotomy), provide the child with a description of the hospital setting and the procedures that will be encountered before anesthesia.* Children's books, coloring books, and doctor-nurse toys may assist the child in pre-

paring for the new experience. Some hospitals arrange tours through the children's facility to acquaint parents and children with the setting, uniforms, and routines before hospitalization. Tours have been shown to lessen fears, fantasies, and behavioral symptoms during the following year.

▪ *Encourage a rooming-in policy for parents and encourage family members to be present as much as possible.* The parent's presence in the hospital may assist the child in his adaptation to the new setting by helping him master separation anxiety and self-control. Rooming in may give parents the opportunity to assist in the care of the child and may lessen parental feelings of losing control over their child. Parent participation in hospital care is so beneficial to the well-being of children that it outweighs the occasional problems that parents may bring to the nursing or medical staff. When one nurse from each shift cares for the child during the entire hospitalization, the child and the parents may benefit by developing feelings of attachment and trust. It is the practice in some hospitals that serve children to involve parents during the induction of anesthesia. This is carried out in a special room adjacent to the operating room. Although it is difficult to document a beneficial behavioral effect from these child-oriented interventions, they deserve consideration in planning hospital policies along with further careful study.

▪ *Hospitalize children in a pediatric setting that is appropriately designed for children.* Colors and pictures on the walls should be child oriented. Toys in a play room that provide flexibility of movement should be available; play is the "work" of childhood, and in this role it provides children with an opportunity for symbolic expression of concerns and fantasies. The mere act of playing can be therapeutic.

▪ *Encourage the parents to bring a few familiar toys and books or a lovey* as a way to lessen the effects of the separation. Keep as many things as possible the same.

▪ *Be truthful about procedures.* Children are not helped by statements such as, "It won't hurt," if it will. Mistrust builds anxiety. When painful procedures are planned, an explanation just before the procedure that "it will hurt for a moment" prepares the child older than 2 in an honest manner.

▪ *Provide realistic options for the child and age-appropriate opportunities for her to participate in her own care by making as many choices as possible.* Set clear, simple limits and expectations on behavior as much as possible. For anxious parents, clear directions for their participation can ease anxiety.

▪ *When possible, allow the child to participate in medical care.* Child-centered health care allows children to feel that they have some control over their bodies, even at a time of illness. For example, ask the older child, "Which arm would you like the blood test from?" "What color gown do you want today?"

▪ *Sensory information and coping strategies.* A description of each part of a planned procedure and the purpose behind it may focus on particular sensations that the child will experience. Relaxation techniques, self-talk, and distracting imagery can be combined to block out unpleasant sensations.[22,23] In some pediatric centers, pain management has reached sophisticated levels in the form of hypnosis[24] and other distraction-relaxation techniques.[25,26] Many of these techniques can be adapted to pediatric office practice.[27] Children are very amenable to these techniques. These will be particularly helpful if children need recurrent painful or aversive procedures (e.g., cancer treatment, renal dialysis).

The desired outcomes for the hospitalized child are that the child heal as quickly and completely as possible, that he be supported in an appropriate manner through recognition of his developmental needs, and that he be given the opportunity to grow from the experience. The clinician's role is to understand and support the child's developmental work while caring for the child's physical illness. The clinician must monitor the environment to assure that it is providing the appropriate support. The parents must be provided with expectations for their child's physical and psychological recovery. They should emerge from the experience of their child's hospitalization as better parents, better observers of their child's physical and mental health, better participants in the healing process, and with an enhanced sense of competency as guardians of their child's health. The child's physician must support these processes through knowledge and sensitivity.

REFERENCES

1. Parmelee AJ Jr: Illness and the development of social competence, *J Dev Behav Pediatr* 18:120, 1997.
2. Dingle JH, Badger BF, Jordan WS Jr: *Illness in the home: a study of 25,000 illnesses in a group of Cleveland families*, Cleveland, 1964, Western Reserve University.
3. Valadian I, Stuart HC, Reed RB: Studies of illness of children followed from birth to 18 years, *Monogr Soc Res Child Dev* 26:9, 1961.
4. Bergman AB, Stamm SJ: The morbidity of cardiac nondisease in school children, *N Engl J Med* 276:1008, 1967.
5. Kemper KJ, Forsyth BW, McCarthy PL: Persistent perceptions of vulnerability following neonatal jaundice, *Am J Dis Child* 144:238, 1990.
6. Perrin EC et al: Issues involved in the definition of chronic health conditions, *Pediatrics* 91:787, 1993.
7. Perrin JM: Chronic illness. In Levine MD, Carey WB, Crocker AC: *Developmental-behavioral pediatrics*, ed 2, Philadelphia, 1992, WB Saunders, pp 304-308.
8. Coleman WL, Howard BJ: Family-focused behavioral pediatrics: clinical techniques for primary care, *Pediatr Rev* 16:448, 1995.
9. Stein MT, Coleman WL, Epstein RM: "We've tried everything and nothing works": family centered pediatrics and clinical problem solving, *J Dev Behav Pediatr* 18:117, 1997.
10. Parmelee AH: Childhood illness as a source of psychological growth, unpublished presidential address, Society for Research in Child Development, 1985.
11. Vernon DTA et al: *The psychological responses of children to hospitalization and illness: a review of the literature*, Springfield, Ill, 1965, Charles C Thomas.
12. Thompson RH, Vernon DTA: Research on children's behavior after hospitalization: a review and synthesis, *J Dev Behav Pediatr* 14:28, 1993.
13. Rutter M: Separation experiences: a new look at an old topic, *J Pediatr* 95:147, 1979.
14. Mahler M: *The psychological birth of the human infant: symbiosis and individuation*, New York, 1975, Basic Books.
15. Robertson J: *Young children in hospital*, ed 2, London, 1970, Tavistock.
16. Perrin EC, Gerrity PS: There's a demon in your belly: children's understanding of concepts regarding illness, *Pediatrics* 67:841, 1981.
17. Bibale R, Walsh M: Development of children's concept of illness, *Pediatrics* 66:912, 1980.
18. Klineman A, Eisenberg L, Good B: Culture, illness and care, *Ann Intern Med* 88:251, 1978.
19. Lefcourt HM: *Locus of control: current trends in theory and research*, Hillsdale, NJ, 1976, Lawrence Erlbaum Associates.
20. Azarnoff P: Parents and siblings of pediatric patients, *Curr Probl Pediatr* 14:1, 1984.

21. Visintainer MA, Wolfer JA: Psychological preparation for surgical pediatric patients: the effects on children's and parents' stress responses and adjustment, *Pediatrics* 56:187, 1975.
22. Peterson L, Shigetomi C: The use of coping techniques to minimize anxiety in hospitalized children, *Behav Ther* 12:1, 1981.
23. Siegel LJ, Peterson L: Stress reduction in young dental patients through coping skills and sensory information, *J Consult Clin Psychol* 48:785, 1980.
24. Olness KN, Kohen DP: *Hypnosis and hypnotherapy with children*, ed 3, New York, 1996, Guilford Press.
25. Zeltzer LK et al: A randomized, controlled study of behavioral intervention for chemotherapy distress in children with cancer, *Pediatrics* 88:34, 1991.
26. Zeltzer LK, Jay SM, Fisher DM: The management of pain associated with pediatric procedures, *Pediatr Clin North Am* 36:1, 1989.
27. Sugarman LI: Hypnosis: teaching children self-regulation, *Pediatr Rev* 17:5, 1996.

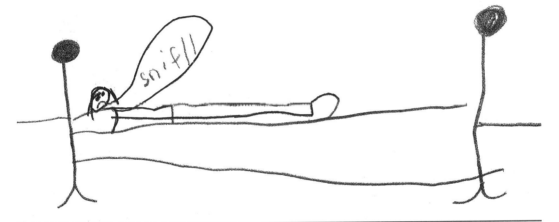

A girl draws a picture of what it is like to be sick with a cold. The bed seems stark and confining and the expression very sad. These "cinema noir" pictures are typical of children with acute illness. A brighter picture and a more sophisticated figure would be expected when she recovers. By Louise Dixon, age 7.

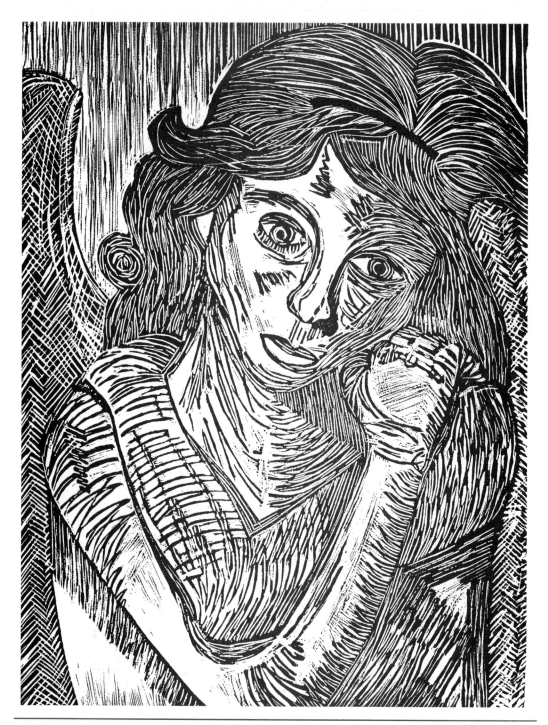

An 18-year-old girl depicts herself, with her evident sense of loss after the death of her father. She used her substantial artistic talent to explore and express this monumental loss in her life. A woodcut by Loni Blankenship, age 18.

546

STRESSFUL EVENTS: SEPARATION, LOSS, VIOLENCE, AND DEATH

■ Maria Trozzi
■ Suzanne Dixon

KEY WORDS

Children's Understanding of Death
Grief Reactions
Suicide
Sibling Loss
Parental Loss
Violence and Trauma

Losses are an inevitable part of the landscape of childhood. Examples are the first time an infant is aware of her mother's momentary absence, the toddler's struggle with separation and autonomy at bedtime, and the preschooler's brave leap from a safe, known environment to the bigger world of a classroom. But with each loss comes an opportunity for growth. In each successful resolution and adaptation to loss come increased coping skills and a greater sense of self.

In contrast to the normal losses we expect as part of development, a death—even though an inevitable part of the life cycle—represents a true crisis to a child. The Chinese express the concept of crisis well when they write the word as a combination of two pictographs—one representing danger and the other, opportunity. A child will need help to realize the opportunity in a loss situation. The following are some forms of such help:

■ Realistic perception of the loss: having adequate and age-appropriate information about what happened
■ Help in expressing immediate feelings
■ Adequate situational supports: having a network of people currently or potentially in the child's life to assist with the variety of the practical needs that arise
■ Adequate coping mechanisms: having in place well-functioning ways of dealing with the anxiety generated by the loss[1]

It is the role of the clinician to see that a child has these in place when faced with an ordinary or an extraordinary loss. This chapter focuses on the conceptual assumptions, interventions, and insights that will help clinicians provide monitoring and assistance to bereaved children and their families.

<table>
<tr><td>BOX 25-1</td><td>INDIVIDUAL FACTORS THAT INFLUENCE ABILITY TO COPE WITH LOSS</td></tr>
</table>

The child's ability to make sense of the death from the perspective of his own development
The child's history of loss and death
The child's normal ability to cope with change, temperament, and situational stress

CHILDREN'S UNDERSTANDING OF DEATH: DEVELOPMENTAL PERSPECTIVE

> A simple child
> That lightly draws its breath
> And feels its life in every limb
> What should it know of death?
> —Wordsworth

For adults, death is a disruption in their usual "steady state" and results in a sense of disequilibrium. **Children's understanding of death** is different, however. For children, death can represent a developmental interference that results in a suspension of their ongoing (cognitive and emotional) growth. The goal of clinical intervention with children is to get them "unstuck," to help them get through, over, under, or around a temporary barrier to their normal and healthy forward movement.[2] The health provider should view the child's ability to cope with a significant loss or death in relation to specific factors (Box 25-1).

DEVELOPMENTAL FRAMEWORK

Although Piaget (see Chapter 2) did not specifically address children's ability to understand death, much of the current thinking about how children perceive death comes from his theories about children's cognitive development. This framework is helpful in assessing a child's reaction to the death of a loved one. Remember, however, that children regress under a stress such as a major loss, and the age and stage boundaries are meant as broad guidelines only. Table 25-1 presents these stages.

Infants (0-2 Years)

Before age 3, infants and toddlers have no cognitive understanding of death. However, Bowlby, who made a significant contribution to current thinking about attachment and loss, argued that even infants and toddlers who experience (maternal) separation grieve:

> If a child is taken from his mother's care at this age (18 to 24 months), when he is so possessively and passionately attached to her, it is indeed as if his world has been shattered. His intense need of her is unsatisfied, and the frustration and longing may send him frantic with grief. It takes an exercise of imagination to sense the intensity of this distress. He is as overwhelmed as any adult who has lost a beloved person by death. To the child of 2 with his lack of understanding and complete inability to tolerate frustration, it is really as if his mother had died. He does not know death, but only absence; and if the only person who can satisfy his imperative need is absent, she might as well be dead.[3]

It seems indisputable that infants and toddlers react strongly to the loss of a meaningful person and show their **grief reactions** in conformity with Bowlby's three stages: protest, despair, and detachment. However, what is more controversial is whether the very youngest child is capable of mourning without the mature understanding and meaning of the loss. Behavioral change indicative of stress is expected. The following suggestions can be useful:

■ If the deceased was the infant's primary caregiver, identify a permanent surrogate caregiver as soon as possible.
■ Learn the deceased caregiver's routines; keep the same as much as possible.
■ Provide a consistent, nurturing, dependable environment.
■ Be prepared for regression in behavior and developmental competency.

TABLE 25-1 ■ Children's Understanding of Death at Different Ages

Age	Understanding
Infants	Have no cognitive understanding of death
0-2 years	Respond to changes in routine, caregivers, emotional chaos of family situation
	Experience separation anxiety
Preschoolers (3-5 years)	Death is temporary, reversible, living under different circumstances
	Concrete and literal thinking
	Use magical thinking to explain death
School-aged (6-8 years)	Death is final, irreversible, but not universal
	See death as a person or spirit that catches you
	Death "catches" the elderly, disabled, klutzes
	May be contagious
	Concerned with safety, predictability
	Need for details
Preadolescents (9-12 years)	Adult understanding: Death is final, irreversible, universal
	Understand the biological aspects of death
	Interested in rituals
	Understand causality: may feel guilty
	Intellectualize death: thoughts more available than feelings
Adolescents (13-18 years)	Adult understanding: Death is final, irreversible, universal
	Engage in high-risk activities (challenge own mortality)
	Understand existential implications of death
	Reject adult rituals and support

Preschooler (3 to 5 Years)

Preschoolers view death as temporary or reversible,[4] as going someplace else.

 Four-year-old Alexandra, whose grandfather died the previous Christmas, proudly showed her aunt a picture she had drawn on Christmas Eve and said, "Last year Papa was very sick and he died. But this year he's coming back on Christmas." With that said, she placed her little drawing under the Christmas tree, awaiting his return.

Children this age want and expect to continue a relationship with their deceased loved one via prayers, writing, or engaging in one-sided conversations. They think the person is coming back. Children this age often place the deceased loved one in heaven. They want to visit, call, or write to him. Their thinking tends to be egocentric, making their own unique sense of each situation. They often attribute magical thinking to the death, making spurious associations.

 When a 3-year-old child died in day care after choking on a grape, her little classmates concluded that, "Sally died because she ate her dessert before her sandwich."

Preschoolers need simple, straightforward explanations of death. "Grandpa died. His body totally stopped working." At this time, many preschoolers will help you operationally define death. "Can he eat? Can he sleep? Does he still dream? Does he go to the bathroom? Will he breathe under the ground? Can he hear me in heaven? Does he need his wheelchair still?" Be particularly careful to respond with concrete, simple explanations. Avoid euphemisms like "lost," "sleeping," "gone to heaven," "with the angels." At best they confuse young children. At worst, they terrify them.

Adults, in explaining death to their very young children, often jump to their own spiritual

A bereaved parent told her 5-year-old child that "the angels came down and took your baby sister," after the baby had died of Sudden Infant Death Syndrome (SIDS) during the Christmas season. Six weeks later, 5-year-old Jeffrey was taken to a counselor because of an inability to sleep at night. When asked to tell the counselor about his baby sister, he said, "I don't want to talk about her. I want to talk about angels. There's two things to know about angels. There are lots of them, and they're on the loose at Christmas. And, they don't have headlights. So you can't see them coming and you have to stay awake at night so they won't get you."

beliefs. Although this can be comforting, it is also confusing. For instance, preschool children are confused by how the body and spirit can simultaneously be in the grave and in heaven.[5] One preschooler found for himself an adequate explanation: "The insides go up, and the outsides go down!" However, adults should resist elaborate stories about heaven that suggest a composite of Disneyworld and Nintendo, or stories about Uncle Henry dancing with angels.

School Age (6 to 8 Years)

Children this age understand death to be final and irreversible but *not universal.* They know that people who die stay dead, but they don't think that they themselves will die. Death is often personalized, perceived as a male Darth Vader-like character who can grab you at any unsuspected time. Those who are vulnerable can't run (e.g., elderly, physically disabled). All the others who get caught must be klutzes.[2] This explanation works at this age to allow the child to distance and defend himself, from death. But, unlike younger children, a death presents him with the challenge of questioning his and other's safety. "Is life still safe?" becomes an overriding question. An ongoing sense of impending disaster or unpredictable happenings exists unless the safety issue is addressed.

> *Six-year-old Beth was vacationing with her parents when, while crossing a Vermont country road at dusk, her mother was struck by a car and died. Beth reasoned thereafter that crossing the street led to disaster. Understandably, she refused to cross any streets following her mother's death. At the September start of school, her teachers were perplexed as to how to handle this issue, especially because the temporary playground was across a busy street. Their solution was to allow her to stay in at recess with the school nurse. After a consultation with a mental health professional, they understood that being motherless is isolating enough; any further separation would not only exacerbate the isolation, but would ultimately lead to the challenge of weaning her from this temporary solution. They decided instead to "normalize" her fear of crossing the street and allow her and her classmates to strategize ways to stay safe while crossing. This plan was not only successful the first day of school, but within the first week, Beth had taken on the role of "crossing guard" for her class! What an opportunity for healing!*

Predictability, that is, what will be the same versus what will be different because of this death, is an inescapable concern confronting the school-age child. The child needs direct, simple answers to what changes will happen that will affect her life. She may ask after a sibling's death, "Will I have my own room now? Can I have Jimmy's Nintendo?" Although adults may initially view these questions as egocentric and completely unfeeling, the child is really asking how his world will change fundamentally because of this death. Both the specifics and the general concern should be answered directly with support and assurance.

Typical of this age are underlying concerns such as, "If Beth's mom died, are you (i.e., the parent) going to die also? Who will take care of me? Am I safe? Will I be safe?" Parents, particularly those in single-parent households, should face these important questions directly and seriously. It would *not* be useful to respond, "Don't worry about that" or "I'm too healthy to die." Remind the child that *everyone* dies someday, but that, unlike Beth's mom, most people live to be very, very, very old. "If I were to die, your Aunt Susie is prepared to care for you until you are grown up." Children are generally satisfied with that response, and it teaches them that you can talk about even "the unmentionable death of self." Although discussing details of a death, particularly the gross and grubby ones (e.g., what happens to the body? was there blood? what did she look like?), is difficult for adults, most school-age children have a need for some details about these events to help them feel more in control of the overwhelming event. What seems to be morbid curiosity to the adult is really the way for the child to get a handle on an incomprehensible situation. The emotional response will come later. Adults in the child's life have an opportunity to face these questions with her and by doing this, they are telling their child that they can face stressful life events together. In contrast, to refuse to discuss issues or to give flip answers sends the wrong message. "If it's unmentionable, it's unmanageable." Children are left with uncertainty, fear, and no place to go to get their questions answered and their needs met.

Preadolescents (9 to 12 Years)

Preadolescents have an adult understanding of death: It is final, irreversible, and universal. Most youngsters this age understand that everyone dies someday, even them, and it's forever. They may view death as a punishment for bad behavior as they begin to explore moral development at this age. They are able to understand the biological aspects of death, such as what happens if the heart has a blockage or what the effect of a brain tumor is on life function. Furthermore, they can understand the concept of specific and possible multiple causes and effects. That leads them to wonder about what part, if any, they may have played that contributed to a death. They may feel guilty in ways that they may not even understand; adults need to help them process such complicated emotions.

Preadolescents are fascinated with the religious and cultural rituals that surround death and display a curiosity about topics such as cremation, burial, embalming, and the afterlife. Adults in their life may find these questions disarming. However, if approached in a straightforward way, youngsters are reminded that they can trust adults to give them useful information about "difficult to talk about" topics.

Many preadolescents respond without a display of emotion or may even be sarcastic when faced with a loved one's death. They intellectualize death because *their thoughts are often more available to them than their feelings.* This bewilders and concerns most adults, who think that their typically sensitive and caring 11-year-old has been replaced with an insensitive creep. Feelings are typically buried under a very unattractive demeanor at this age. It takes a long time to identify and let out feelings.

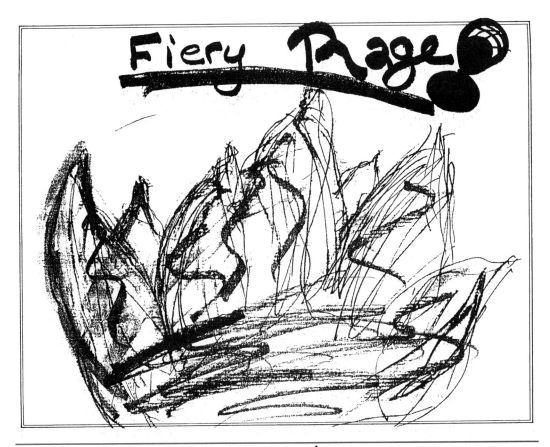

A 12-year-old girl expresses her feelings after her sister had been killed by a drunk driver. Drawing gives children a safe way to express feelings. (Original is in vivid red, purple, and black.) By Sara, age 12.

The Smiths were vacationing in Florida when they learned from their adult baby-sitter that their 4-year-old child had died after running into the street and being hit by a car. Bewildered and overcome with grief, they returned home on the next plane. When 12-year-old Christine faced her parents at the door, she smiled and asked, " What did you bring me from Florida?" This response, although infuriating to her parents, protected her from a display of overwhelming grief. Christine knew how to handle her parent's anger because she had probably seen it before; she was less prepared to respond to their presumable expression of overwhelming grief. "After all, if they fall apart, then who will take care of me?" was her unconscious motivation for turning around the emotional climate of the family.

The 12-year-old's comments brought more predictable attention and energy from her parents. The preadolescent is dependent on the adults in her life to make life feel safe for her, especially in times of crisis, such as a death. It is critical when helping loved ones to know how to help their children through a loss. Parents and other support people should remember to do the following:

- Be authentic. Kids pick up platitudes, gloss-overs, and ambivalence like radar.
- Verbalize that, in spite of your grief, you are still able to care for them. Help them feel that they are safe and that their lives will go on.
- Give them repeated opportunities to discuss the death, but don't push too hard. It will take weeks to months to get at feelings. Provide openings and then wait.
- Talk about your own grief and how your feelings influence your own behavior.

> *One winter morning, shortly after her father had died, Terry was removing a gallon of milk from the refrigerator door when it slipped out of her grasp and crashed to the floor. The children, seated at the kitchen table, were shocked to hear their mother scream and then sob. They quickly started to help with the cleanup. When Terry stopped crying, she faced her children and explained, "I'm having a bad morning. I am missing your Grampa terribly." She proceeded to help the children with the cleanup, and together they sat down to breakfast.*

Children can face intensely difficult emotional times if the adults in their life continue to make them feel safe throughout. If this mom had run out of the room, leaving them without breakfast and without an explanation, the children may have felt abandoned by her. Explaining her display of emotion and continuing to care for them (in spite of her feelings) teaches them that grief and its intense emotions can be faced with the adults in their life.

Adolescents (13 to 18 Years)

This period brings in several new cognitive abilities, emotional processes, and developmental processes that touch on the experience of death.

- Adolescents are actively engaged in the normal developmental task of separation from the significant adults in their lives. A significant death, such as the death of a parent or a sibling, can derail this individual separation-individuation process, making the maturational process scary and overwhelming.
- Adolescents typically engage in high-risk behavior, almost as though they need to "flirt with death." They are fascinated with death, but may be overwhelmed when it intrudes more closely on their lives.
- Paradoxically, adolescents intellectually have an adult's understanding of death, but behave as though they themselves were immortal. Many adolescents will, during this period, face the death of a peer, and it shatters all their fantasies of immortality. The intellectualization that is typically seen may make it harder to get at the devastating developmental and emotional experience.

- Adolescents are capable of understanding the existential implications of death as they gain the ability to think abstractly. They may not have formed their understanding at this level before it is forced upon them.
- Adolescents are interested in exploring society's attitudes about life and death. They will monitor how their immediate circle of family and friends, as well as the broader society, respond to, explain, and grieve a death. They look to others to help make sense of these overwhelming events while seeming to ignore the usual conventions or to challenge beliefs.

Although they often reject traditional adult rituals surrounding death and create their own with the help of their peers, they do need adults in their life to help them sort out the often colliding feelings of sadness, anger, disbelief, and isolation. Adults often feel rejected when attempting to provide emotional support at this age. However, just their continued presence and availability during the crisis are therapeutic. Adults must interpret this distancing as developmentally appropriate and respect it, while remaining available for reassurance and support.

> *Brendan, 16, became furious when his parents said they would attend the funeral of his beloved teacher, who had died suddenly. The parents would have liked to attend the ceremony because they too knew the teacher. Brendan insisted that he was going with his friends and preferred that his parents not go. That evening he asked to play cards with his mom and just "hang out" at home. He said the service was "fine."*

SPECIAL CASE OF SUICIDE

Adolescent **suicide** is an increasing phenomenon. In fact, statistics reveal that every day in this country, many youth between the ages of 13 and 25 will attempt suicide, and many will succeed. Why do so many adolescents attempt to kill themselves? Why, if they have an adult understanding of death, can they see "ending their lives" as an option? Unfortunately, adolescents deny the *physical* consequences of suicide. They often are unable to look beyond the act itself and fail to understand that the consequences of death are final and irreversible.

> *Seventeen-year-old Amy was a senior at a prestigious prep school. She was bright and popular and had recently been accepted at her first-choice Ivy League college. One afternoon, three of her girlfriends betrayed her in a powerful secret. She was humiliated. That evening, she slashed her wrists in an attempted suicide. When the therapist asked her what she was thinking when she was hurting herself, she replied, "All I could think was 'won't my friends be upset when they walk by the casket and see me lying there.'"*

Adults who care for, teach, and live with adolescents must help them face the stark reality of the act of suicide through clear discussion with them whenever a suicide is in the news or happens in their school or neighborhood. Conversation should emphasize facts such as the following:

- It is killing yourself.
- People who commit suicide don't know how to get help to solve problems.
- You don't come back.
- It will not glorify your memory.
- It is a permanent solution to a temporary problem.
- Adolescents need to look for help with problem solving.
- No problem is solved by suicide.

CHILDHOOD BELIEFS ABOUT DEATH

Another predictable influence on a child's understanding of death that transcends developmental processes is magical thinking. Although the psychological literature suggests that magical thinking occurs only during the early childhood years, ample empirical evidence suggests that magical thinking about death and loss occurs even as late as adolescence.

> *Bob, 15, and his older brother, Ted, 17, were playing basketball against the side of their grandmother's brick apartment building. Several times she opened the window of her third floor apartment and asked them to stop. Finally, she angrily yelled to them, "For the last time, stop. You boys will be the death of me!" Sadly, the next day, grandma suffered an aneurysm and died. In therapy, one of the boys revealed that he thought that they had killed their grandmother.*

At any age, magical thinking should be uncovered and challenged. Simply ask the question, "What made your (mother, father, friend, pet) die? Why do you think he died?" Offer a simple statement of your own belief around the issue. And then wait or leave it. The child or an adolescent has been given fuel to reconstruct his thinking and a supportive place to discuss it.

CHILDREN'S GRIEF REACTIONS—SPECIAL CHARACTERISTICS

Children's *grief responses* are different than adults'. Their behaviors must be understood as indicating grief so that appropriate support can be provided.

- First, *children grieve in spurts*, fluctuating between expressions of anger, sadness, anxiety, and confusion, and then, in a moment, resumption of their normal behavior. They do not continuously show overt signs of grieving such as seen with adults. This leads some to believe that children do not recognize the loss or understand its implications and therefore do not grieve. The behavior is adaptive, however, because children have a limited capacity to tolerate emotional pain and will pull away from it when it all becomes too much for them. Adults may mistrust the child's intermittent display of intense feelings and see them as disingenuous. However, children, even very young children, experience intensely painful responses that adults must understand, legitimize, and help them through.[6]

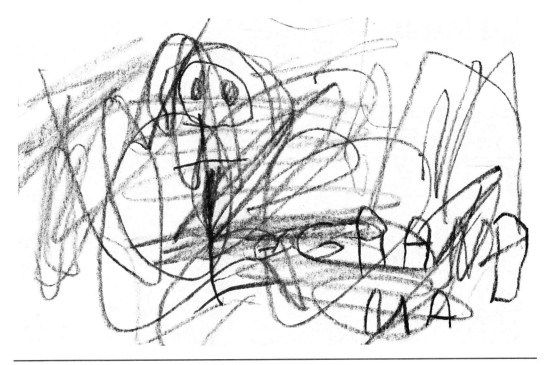

A 4-year-old-girl draws her grandmother in the year after her death. The figure is primitive compared to the writing beside it. It is orange, but scribbled all over with grey. Drawing level often goes down when stressful emotions are being expressed. Scribbled over scenes often mean depression or sadness. By Louise Dixon, age 4.

The availability of *one* significant adult and a safe physical and emotional environment in which to mourn are the two most significant predictive factors of the child's successful outcome after suffering a loss. Children will work through their grief over time if they have this emotional space and support to do so. This is a cyclical task that needs sustained support.

■ *Children grieve longer than adults, contrary to popular thinking.* They *regrieve* the loss over and over again at each new stage in development as they change their perspective on themselves and the world around them, making more mature meanings of the significance of the past loss.

Kate was barely 5 when her mother died of lung cancer. Her only memories of her mother were of the illness. Now, 6 years later, she and her brother have adjusted to life with dad as the primary caregiver. However, when 11-year-old Kate brought home the school notice for the mother-daughter "Learning About Our Bodies" evening, she angrily threw it on the kitchen counter and said, "I'm not going!" When her father offered to go with her, Kate began to cry inconsolably. She ran upstairs to her room, slammed her door, and refused to talk to her father for the rest of the evening.

As Kate grows through each developmental stage, being a "motherless daughter" takes on a new meaning. Each event that marks her growing up, such as the first signs of puberty, the prom, graduation from high school, marriage, pregnancy, and giving birth also restimulates her grief of mother-loss.

■ Childhood grief is manifested in *qualitatively different ways.* Adults often think the child is not grieving following a loss, but they notice marked changes in the child's behavior. Difficulty concentrating, heightened sibling squabbles, inappropriate and aggressive behavior, moodiness, withdrawal, disorganization, and temper tantrums are normal symptoms of grieving in childhood. Because of differences in cognitive ability and personality structures, children are apt to use more primitive defense mechanisms than adults, particularly denial and regression. Common psychosomatic symptoms include headaches, stomachaches, bowel and bladder difficulties, and sleep disturbances. The clinician can interpret these behaviors as manifestations of grief for baffled families and school personnel.

MONITORING GRIEF PROCESS

Prolonged duration or intensity of these normal behaviors and symptoms may indicate the need for a clinical intervention, whereas brief periods of turmoil are usually evidence of expected grief work. Chronic depression or hostility, longing to join the deceased, persistent fear or panic, chronic loss of appetite or ability to sleep indicate the need for a professional referral. For the school-age child, regular communication with the teacher regarding the child's classroom behavior is recommended because this should show gradual normalization after a brief period of disruption. Especially during the first several months following a loss, caring adults can help the grieving child significantly by providing a stable environment and well-defined behavioral boundaries, but doing so with empathy. Well-intentioned teachers who become more permissive do not serve the grieving child, particularly because the school environment is often the only place that feels the same for the child. Similarly at home, the same level of expectation, routine, and pattern is more supportive than a more permissive or lenient approach.

INHIBITORS OF SUCCESSFUL GRIEVING

For a child to grieve a loss, he must perceive his world to be safe and "back to normal." Sometimes one loss leads to secondary losses that may, in effect, have a more profound immediate influence on a child's sense of loss. For example, when a parent dies and the surviving parent goes to work full-time or when the family must move. A deceased parent may be fantasized as away on a trip, but the immediacy of moving, leaving friends, changing schools, etc., goes beyond the child's ability to use denial in coping. It is the stress of these immediate changes that fuels the crisis because they are unavoidable in spite of any defense mechanism. Especially during the first few months following a loss within the family unit, family dynamics are apt to change because of explosive emotions, significant depression, financial stress, and new schedules. This is all part of the predictable "grief" landscape and will normalize with time. However, certain factors can significantly derail the child's mourning process and require a clinical intervention:

■ The inability of the significant adult in the child's life to mourn. Stony silence is devastating to a child's sense of safety.

 When Brian's father committed suicide, Brian's world and that of his three brothers changed forever. The day after the funeral, all family photos that included dad were put away; mom never talked about dad again. Shortly after dad died, mom went to work for the first time, took a computer course at night, and moved the family from the only home that Brian had ever known.

■ The significant adult's inability to tolerate the child's expression of grief. "Stiff upper lip" is not to be encouraged.

 Julie's eighth birthday would be especially bleak this year because her twin sister had died 6 months earlier. When she cried while discussing party plans with her parents, dad immediately started in with his routine response, "Let's not be sad; we must be grateful to be alive!"

■ Forced hypermaturity of the child; requirement to exemplify adult behavior, such as to take care of the siblings and prepare meals.

 Fourteen-year-old Charlie refused free tickets to the Red Sox game that evening; he knew his mom would be alone if he went.

■ Overwhelming secondary losses or a history of unresolved losses.

 Seven-year-old David no longer cried when he left his foster family. After all, this family was the third one he had had in 2 years.

■ Ambivalence towards the deceased person or confusion about the details of the death.

Dad's drinking had finally hurt everyone for the last time. He killed himself and an innocent couple in an oncoming car when he veered over the yellow line. Sixteen-year-old Paul was flooded intermittently with rage, relief, and shame.

■ Inability to make meaning of the loss, lack of ability to accept the finality of the loss. Fantasy ideas beyond a few weeks.

Each time 9-year-old Rebecca looked at the video of her family's vacation, it assured her that her baby brother would be at the cottage when the family returned next summer.

CONTEXT OF GRIEVING: RELIGIOUS AND CULTURAL IMPLICATIONS

Clinicians must view a child's conception of death and grief reaction in religious and cultural contexts that are determined by the child's family and tradition. McGoldrick et al warn that "clinicians should be careful about definitions of 'normalcy' in assessing families' responses to death, [since] the manner of, as well as the length of time assumed normal for mourning differs greatly from culture to culture."[7] It is important for the clinician to learn from the family what the child has been taught to believe about illness, death, and mourning and especially the rituals surrounding death. It is equally important for the clinician to learn what the child has "caught" with regard to his own idiosyncratic logic about death and the afterlife.

The child in the movie My Girl felt comforted after her best friend died from an allergic reaction to a series of bee stings when she reasoned that now her deceased mother, who "resided" in heaven, would take care of him.

Most bereavement specialists agree that it is of assistance to children to attend funerals and other rituals associated with the death of a loved one[9]. However, an adult, not necessarily a member of the immediate family but a familiar and supportive person, should prepare the child for the experience directly and without euphemisms, accompany the child, and be available to answer questions. A child should be told what her role will be and that she can leave if she needs to do so (this rarely happens). For a child to benefit from this experience, she must be old enough to make sense of the event and be assured of an adult for direct support. Keeping a child separate from the family and community during this time may be threatening to the child. Abandonment at a time of family upheaval can be stressful for a young child. Her fantasies may be more scary than anything that will happen in reality. Participation in all or part of the grieving ritual is to be supported in the vast majority of cases.

SPECIAL SITUATIONS

Pet Loss

Few if any children will grow up without facing the painful experience of "losing" their pet. Some parents, in an effort to shield their children from the pain, mistakenly disallow the child the opportunity to face the grief that is a necessary by-product of affection and connection to their beloved pet. How many adults can remember being told as children that Rover was sent to a "farm in Iowa where he can run and breathe fresh air." Why did parents think that information would not be equally devastating? No better are all-too-familiar stories of children returning home from school to learn that while they were gone, Rover was brought to the veterinarian's and "put to sleep." The unexpected and hidden aspect of the event makes it difficult for a child to profit from this learning opportunity (or to sleep securely themselves!).

In fact, the death of a pet provides a rich opportunity for a youngster to strengthen coping skills and learn how to face losses. Furthermore, the family can grieve together, naming the feelings and recognizing and respecting each family member's individual way of dealing with feelings. Lastly, the family can engage in the rituals involved in saying good-bye. Parents and other caring adults serve their children by not trivializing or denying their feelings of grief, but at the same time not being overwhelmed by them or exaggerating them. Simple, clear, and short rituals and discussions are best.

Sibling Loss

The death of a sibling presents an enormous challenge to the surviving child. She has weathered the loss of her brother or sister, a contemporary whose loss will continue to be felt throughout the life cycle. She also has lost her parents as she knew them because the complicated mourning process that parents face is more intense and prolonged than any other.[6] Marital conflict, depression, guilt, social isolation, and possible resentment toward the perceived more brief adjustment for the surviving children exacerbate parents' grief and may inhibit their ability to be emotionally available to their surviving children. To gain affection and ease their parents' pain, the surviving child may attempt to "replace" a deceased sibling, thereby compromising the youngster's own identity development. Too often the tendency to idealize the dead also makes it difficult for surviving siblings to deal with their ambivalent feelings (e.g., unresolved sibling rivalry) or with anger at the deceased or at their parents (e.g., for not preventing the death or for seeming to care more about the deceased child). Finally, a survivor's guilt is commonly felt by the surviving sibling and must be challenged. Many times brief counseling is needed to explore these issues, separate from any group family therapy. Sibling survivor groups may be an additional help.

Parental Loss

It is not clear exactly how many children experience the death of a parent; Kilman[10] estimates that 5% of children in the United States—1.5 million—lose one or both parents by age 15; that proportion may be substantially higher in lower socioeconomic groups. The death of a parent affects the child's development of a sense of trust and self-esteem. When a young child experiences the loss of that significant relationship, the core of his existence is shaken. Trust in the consistency and constant source of support and comfort is disrupted.[6]

In addition to the child's developmental age at the time of death, the next most important consideration is the emotional availability of the surviving parent, who has the seemingly impossible task of managing her own grief while providing a consistent, stable, and "normal" environment for her children. Children can only do their necessary grief work if and when life feels safe again, and sometimes that is delayed if a lot of family disruption takes place. The acute grieving period, usually 2 to 3 years, is a period of adjustment because each family member feels a real need to be understood and has the least capacity to give understanding.

> *A month after 9-year-old Molly's mother died of amyotrophic lateral sclerosis (ALS), Molly and her dad were at a drive-through at McDonald's. When he grabbed for his wallet, he realized that he had left it at home and had no money to pay for dinner that night. Molly became hysterical, thinking that they were poor now that mommy had died.*

Children may idealize and overidentify with the deceased parent while distorting their view of the remaining parent. They are particularly concerned about any perceived vulnerability of the remaining parent. Depending on the cause of death, safety or health issues may become exaggerated. A common concern for the surviving parent is whether the very youngest children will remember their deceased parent. Looking at family photos and videos and storytelling is not always welcomed by the children, who may fear the surviving parent's strong display of emotion. Although family members are all grieving the same person, he or she had a unique relationship with each of them.

The Dying Child

When a child is diagnosed with a serious or life-threatening illness, parents turn to their child's primary care clinician, with whom they already have a trusting relationship. Special care should be taken by the primary care clinician to share updated information regarding the diagnosis and prognosis. Furthermore, continuing communication with the child and his family throughout the course of the illness and eventual death is recommended. In particular, siblings may benefit from increased communication or appropriate referrals during particularly stressful periods of the illness. Before the 1970s, most professionals employed a protective approach regarding the disclosing of information to the dying child. However, today most researchers and clinicians agree that an open approach promotes coping skills and adaptive behavior. Children should be given information that allows them to understand, as much as they can, the experience they are undergoing. The child may vacillate between denial and acceptance of the disease. With some people the child may practice mutual pretense, and with others he may be open about the seriousness of his illness and his fears and fantasies of impending death. Listening to the child and taking cues from him mitigate his sense

BOX 25-2	FACTORS TO CONSIDER BEFORE DISCUSSING DEATH WITH A DYING CHILD

1. Parents' **philosophical stance** on death. What are their religious and cultural views about life, death and the afterlife?
2. Parents' **emotional stance** on death. Is either parent in denial about death as an eventuality? Is either parent likely to be stoic or hyper-emotional?
3. Child's **age, experience, and level of development**
4. Family's **coping strategies.** What history of crisis or illness can predict its ability to cope with this illness?
5. Child's **perception of process over content.** Does the child require detailed information about procedures or treatment? Can she look at "the big picture"?

of isolation.[11] Spinetta et al[12] suggest five factors that should be considered by caregivers before discussing the illness or death with the dying child (Box 25-2).

Today the child is often actively involved with the treatment team. Because many children will die at home, the parents play a much more active role in treatment as well. When curative therapy has been replaced by palliative therapy, the treatment team should take special care not to abandon the child or family. The primary care clinician's ongoing communication with the family at such a stressful time is suggested.

GETTING HELP

When a child faces a family death or the death of a friend, parents often turn to their primary health care provider for guidance. She should be aware of the resources available within the community to assist the bereaved child. Developmentally appropriate grief groups are outstanding supports for children and the parent(s) who bring them. Children can be helped to express their grief through individual and group play, artwork (see the artwork in this chapter), journaling, and sharing time. Selected books and videos can be particularly helpful to the bereaved child. The Good Grief Program at Boston Medical Center offers an annotated bibliography that catalogs books by the type of loss, the reading level, and a summary.[13]

CHILDREN AND TRAUMA

Children in the United States are exposed to **violence** in epidemic proportions. Each day in the United States, 9 children are murdered, 30 children are wounded by guns, and 307 children are arrested for violent crimes.[14] If children are not victims of violent behaviors directly, they are often witnesses to domestic or community violence. The media have brought school violence home to every household in America. Domestic violence occurs in rural and urban areas without regard to class or ethnicity. Interviews with parents of children ages 6 years and younger, showed that 1 in 10 children had witnessed a stabbing or shooting.[15] Young children are deeply affected by witnessing violence, particularly when the perpetrator or victim is a family member.[16]

What is the effect on children who live with violence in their world? Lenore Terr[17] defined childhood **trauma** as "the mental result of one blow or a series of blows, rendering the young person temporarily helpless and breaking past ordinary coping and defensive operations." The child's reaction to violence will depend on a number of factors, including her age, prior exposure to violence, whether the perpetrator and victim are known, and whether the violence is a single incident or chronic. Children are usually more affected than adults suspect. Most children will communicate their fear and uncertainty about their lives through behavior rather than language.

The following are cues that a child may have witnessed violence that has been overwhelming:
- Hypervigilance
- Hyperactivity
- Nightmares
- Separation anxiety
- Risk-taking behavior
- Withdrawal
- Emotional numbing

A small percentage of children who experience severe violence will develop posttraumatic stress disorder (Box 25-3). Studies of precursors to PTSD in children have shown that witnessing domestic violence is as traumatic as being the victim of sexual abuse.[10] Clinical experience suggests that PTSD can be a chronic problem and a source of problems in school, relationships, and emotional development.[16] One of the unmistakable symptoms of chronic exposure to violence is the child's foreshortened view of the future.

> *Although Jeremy was legally old enough to take driver's education classes, he couldn't see the point. His best friend, Joshua, had not lived long enough to get his license; his older brother, Reme, was also killed before he was able to buy a car that he was saving to buy. What were the chances he would live long enough to have a car the way things were going in his neighborhood?*

Because the scars carried by children who are chronically exposed to violence are invisible and because their immediate caregivers may also be victims, it is often incumbent on the clinician to recognize symptoms and ask questions that can lead to first-line intervention. Asking about violence takes little time, doesn't require special expertise, and demonstrates concern. The following are indications that a referral to a mental health specialist should be made:
- The child's safety is at immediate risk.
- Symptoms have persisted for more than 6 months.
- The trauma was particularly violent or involved the death or departure from the home of a parent or caretaker.
- The child's caretakers are unable to empathize with the child.

BOX 25-3 DIAGNOSTIC CRITERIA FOR POSTTRAUMATIC STRESS DISORDER

A. The person has been exposed to a traumatic event in which both of the following were present:
  1. The person experienced, witnessed, or was confronted with an event or events that involved actual or threatened death or serious injury, or a threat to the physical integrity of self or others.
  2. The person's response involved intense fear, helplessness, or horror. Note: In children, this may be expressed instead by disorganized or agitated behavior.
B. The traumatic event is persistently reexperienced in one (or more) of the following ways:
  1. Recurrent and intrusive distressing recollections of the event, including images, thoughts, or perceptions. Note: In young children, repetitive play may occur, in which themes or aspects of the trauma are expressed.
  2. Recurrent distressing dreams of the event. Note: Children may have frightening dreams without recognizable content.
  3. Acting or feeling as if the traumatic event were recurring (includes a sense of reliving the experience, illusions, hallucinations, and dissociative flashback episodes, including those that occur on awakening or when intoxicated). Note: In young children, trauma-specific reenactment may occur.
  4. Intense psychological distress at exposure to internal or external cues that symbolize or resemble an aspect of the traumatic event.
  5. Physiological reactivity on exposure to internal or external cues that symbolize or resemble an aspect of the traumatic event.
C. Persistent avoidance of stimuli associated with the trauma and numbing of general responsiveness (not present before the trauma), as indicated by three (or more) of the following:
  1. Efforts to avoid thoughts, feelings, or conversations associated with the trauma
  2. Efforts to avoid activities, places, or people that arouse recollections of the trauma
  3. Inability to recall an important aspect of the trauma
  4. Markedly diminished interest or participation in certain activities
  5. Feeling of detachment or estrangement from others
  6. Restricted range of affect (e.g., unable to have loving feelings)
  7. Sense of a foreshortened future (e.g., does not expect to have a career, marriage, children, or a normal life span)
D. Persistent symptoms of increased arousal (not present before trauma), as indicated by two (or more) of the following:
  1. Difficulty falling or staying asleep
  2. Irritability or outbursts of anger
  3. Difficulty concentrating
  4. Hypervigilance
  5. Exaggerated startle response
E. Duration of the disturbance (symptoms in criteria B, C, and D) is more than 1 month
F. The disturbance causes clinically significant distress or impairment in social, occupational, or other important areas of functioning.
Specify if:
  Acute: duration of symptoms is less than 3 months
  Chronic: duration of symptoms is 3 months or more
Specify if delayed onset: onset of symptoms is at least 6 months after the stressor.

Ideal intervention is multifaceted and usually involves mental health clinicians, health providers, schools, law enforcement, and the court system. It is unclear why some children who are exposed to chronic violence do not develop PTSD. However, resiliency factors such as the presence of a strong role model and activities that promote competence and self-esteem[23] remind us that an understanding, nurturing parent, a dedicated coach, or a youth minister can positively change the child's view of the world.

SUMMARY

Because losses are an inevitable occurrence in the lives of children and their families, and because the pediatric clinician cares for the child in the context of these losses, she has a unique ability to assist the family through the losses over time. The pediatric clinician who can offer anticipatory guidance to parents, accompanied by an empathetic ear at the time of an acute loss and at *significant times thereafter* is esteemed.

Equally treasured is the clinician who wisely "checks in" with the young patient who has experienced a serious loss at pivotal times in his development. Connecting with both parents and young patients around these challenging life events can be daunting for the clinician, but the rewards are plentiful. A parent reflects on her special relationship with her pediatrician nearly 19 years after the birth of her second son.

> *When Dr. J. came into my room and told me that Michael had Down's syndrome, for just a minute I couldn't remember what that meant. I guess I was in shock. But then I looked into his eyes and saw that they had "filled up," and I knew that Michael and I were not alone, that we would face this together with Dr. J. He has been with us every step of the way, acknowledging the grief, the challenges, and the joys of having a child like Michael.*

REFERENCES

1. Aguilara DC: *Crisis intervention: theory and methodology,* St. Louis, 1974, Mosby.
2. Fox S: *Good grief: helping groups of children when a friend dies,* Boston, 1988, New England Association for the Education of Young Children.
3. Bowlby, J: Grief and mourning in infancy and early childhood, *Psychoanal Study Child* 15:9, 1960.
4. Nagy M: The child's theories concerning death, *J Genet Psychol* 73:3, 1948.
5. Saravay B: Short-term play therapy with two preschool brothers following sudden paternal death. In Webb NB, editor: *Play therapy with children in crisis: a casebook for practitioners,* New York, 1991, Guilford.
6. Rando T: *Grief, dying and death,* Champaign, Ill, 1984, Research Press, p 155.
7. McGoldrick M et al: Mourning in different cultures. In Walsh F, McGoldrick M, editors: *Living beyond loss: death in the family,* New York, 1991, Norton.
8. Webb NB, editor: *Helping bereaved children: a handbook for practitioners,* New York, 1993, Guilford.
9. Kastenbaum RJ: *Death, society, and human experience,* ed 4, New York, 1977, MacMillan.

10. Kliman G: Death: some implications in child development and child analysis, *Adv Thanatol* 4:43, 1980.

11. Blubond-Langer M: Meanings of death to children. In Feifel H, editor: *New meanings of death*, New York, 1977, McGraw-Hill.

12. Spinetta JJ: The dying child's awareness of death: a review, *Psychol Bull*, 81:256, 1974.

13. Books and Videos on Loss for Children and Adolescents: An Annotated Bibliography, Boston, 1996, The Good Grief Program, One Boston Medical Center Place, Boston, MA 02118.

14. Children's Defense Fund: *Annual report: the state of America's children*, Washington, DC, 1993, Children's Defense Fund.

15. Taylor L et al: Witnessing violence by young children and their mothers, *J Dev Behav Ped*, 15:120, 1994.

16. Groves, BM et al: Silent victims: children who witness violence, *JAMA* 269:262, 1993.

17. Terr LC: *Too scared to cry: psychic trauma in childhood,* New York, 1990, Harper & Row.

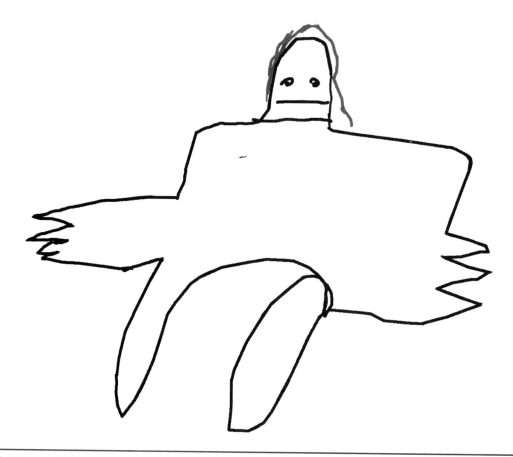

A 5½-year-old boy draws his sister, who recently died from leukemia. He depicts her morphing into an angel in line with his family's beliefs. He draws her hair carefully in bright pink, almost like a halo. He says, "She has beautiful hair now; she's in heaven." He had a healthy resolution to his grief.

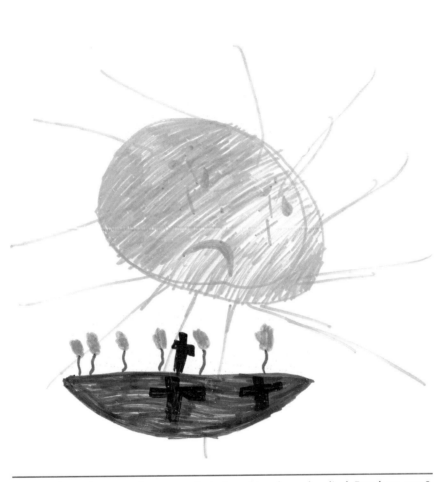

A sun is frowning over the grave of a beloved teacher who died. By a boy, age 8.

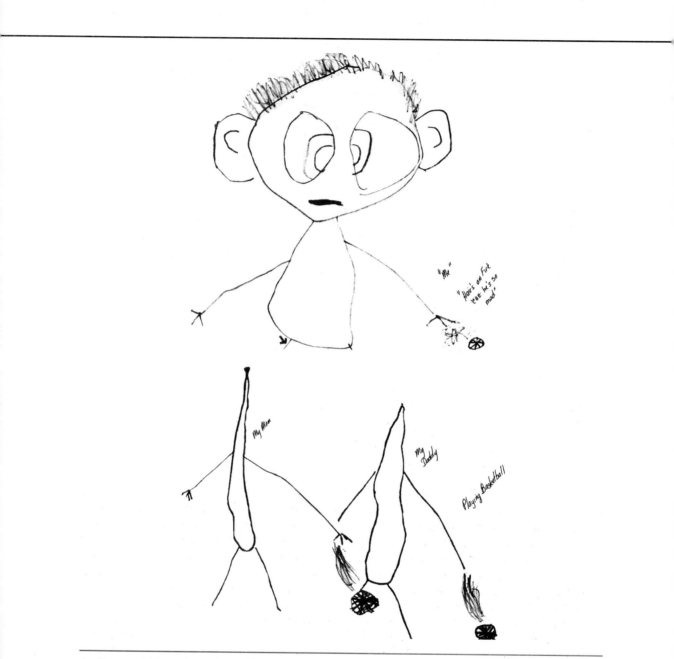

An 8-year-old boy shows himself wearing glasses, playing dynamic basketball. His cropped hair is more than it seems as he says, "He's on fire 'cuz he's so mad," shifting to the third person to convey this strong emotion. He shows us where his anger is directed when he draws his parents nearly headless. "We each have our own ball," he explains.

CHAPTER 26

USE OF DRAWINGS BY CHILDREN IN THE PEDIATRIC OFFICE

■ John B. Welsh
■ Susan L. Instone

The regular use of drawings can make a number of contributions to a child's visit to the pediatric office. These productions create a nonthreatening, relaxed ambience in the office setting and allow clinicians to make meaningful observations of the child at the same time. The manner in which the pencil is held and manipulated by the child to copy geometric shapes or draw pictures can be observed to assess fine-motor skills, visual perception, and visual-motor integration beginning at 18 months and continuing through adolescence. A child's drawing is often an opportunity to engage parents and children in a discussion of an important event or concern that does not surface during the medical interview. Sequential drawings should be part of the medical record to mark the child's development, to monitor both ordinary and extraordinary adaptive stress, and to serve as a developmental screen.[1]

DEVELOPMENTAL ASPECTS

A definite sequence, beginning with basic linear scribbles that progress to more complex diagrams and designs, such as suns and mandalas, is seen early in the drawings of toddlers and young preschool children.[2] The human figure emerges by the time the child is 3½ to 4 years of age. These drawings seem to be universal and cross-cultural in their progression toward meaningful, symbolic representation of the human figure.[3]

The emergence of visual-motor integration skills can be monitored by pediatric clinicians in formats suitable for office practice. Well-established norms have been documented for the sequence of copying simple geometric forms (Fig. 26-1). The Draw-A-Person (DAP) Test extends the information gained from geometric figures and correlates with mental age. It is used for children above 3 years of age and has proved to be reliable for nearly 60 years as a general screening test for well children.[4,5]

The evolution from subjective to objective realism marks cognitive maturation as the figures drawn progress from depicting the world as it seems to the child to the objective reality of the world as it really exists.[6] These changes correlate with the child's evolving cognitive structures from *intuitive* or *egocentric* to those of a logical *concrete* thinker (see Chapter 2). The "distortions" seen in early drawings reveal the child's view of the world, often

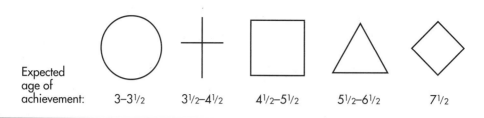

Fig. 26-1   A screening test for visual-motor integration and fine-motor coordination and the expected developmental sequence for copying geometric forms.

enlightening parents. More accurate, realistic drawings come from grade schoolers. Abstractions, conscious distortions used to convey concepts, coincide with the emergence of abstract thought in the adolescent.

The development of a third dimension, depth perception, and visual occlusion (not seeing the parts of a figure through another object, so-called x-ray visibility), are marks of an intellectual maturity that gradually develops between the ages of 7 and 8 years through 10 and 12 years. Developmental psychologists acquire insight from observation of the changes as seen in this progression toward photographic reality. Although the emergence of these elements is quite standard, their utilization by any given child remains the unique product of that individual. Temperament, family, culture, and sociopolitical influences shape how these emerging skills are employed.

PROJECTIVE ELEMENTS

Drawings used as a projective technique, in which the child reveals inner feelings about himself and his world, significantly strengthens their utility. This necessitates a wide range of symbolic interpretations of the drawings, and its effectiveness varies with the skill and experience of the viewer. Certain literature supports this approach to children's drawings.[7,8] Of particular importance are family drawings, especially kinetic family drawings.[9] The child is directed to draw a picture "with everyone in your family, all doing something." Considerable sophistication and objective verification of the family drawings have established this technique in child development. Several components of these drawings call for attention because they reveal a great deal about family dynamics:

■ Where individual members are placed in the picture
■ Relative size and position on the paper
■ Distortion of members or parts of members
■ Omitted members
■ Force lines between members
■ Relative sophistication of specific members

Studies employing grid analyses and computer evaluation add considerable sophistication to the analysis of these components.[10] But that isn't usually needed. Clinically, the child lays out his internal perception of his family through these drawings. Such information can be enormously helpful to the child's clinician in the process of assessing the child's self-image, patterns of communication, and relationships with others in the family.

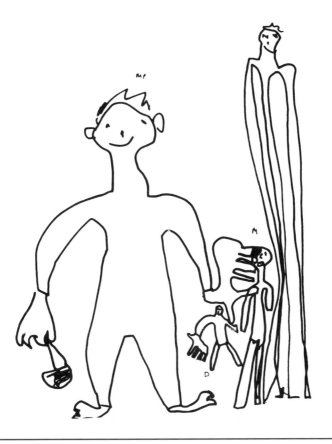

Fig. 26-2   A kinetic family drawing (KFD) by a 6-year-old boy who had a particularly close relationship with his mother. The mother is attached to a magnified left hand of the child, whereas the father (described as emotionally distant) is placed below the powerful hand and drawn as a smaller figure. An older brother is at the right side of the picture.

Psychological insights may be especially helpful for the drawings of children who are younger than than 7 or 8. These extend the child's language ability and allow access to his subjective reality. The threatening parent of the opposite sex; exaggeration of size; siblings missing; the magnified, nurturing mother; or the threatening, menacing father occur with such regularity as children go through important social and emotional stages that these are seen readily in drawings (Fig. 26-2). Occasionally parents can gain insight from these drawings into these special stages of development in ways that may not be apparent from the child's behavior. The drawing tells more about deep-seated emotional issues than the child can tell in words or the parent can see in behavior or speech (Figs. 26-3 and 26-4). When the child is able to describe his drawings, his verbal reflections can assist in the interpretation and should be encouraged.[10]

Parents are often interested in interpretation of these drawings. Caution must be used to not overextend their meanings. At times, however, they can shed illumination on

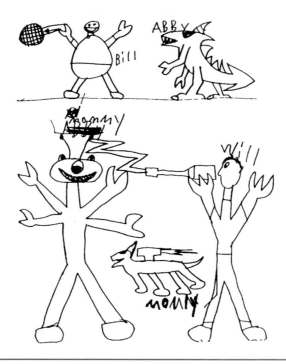

Fig. 26-3 This drawing was done by a 9-year-old boy who had been admitted to the hospital on three occasions for severe abdominal pain and vomiting without a detectable organic cause. His parents had separated. In this KFD the child demonstrates aggression toward his mother and separates his idealized father ("Bill") and a symbolized monster-sister ("Abby"). The child appeared depressed in the office, and his mother was concerned that "he wants to sleep all the time."

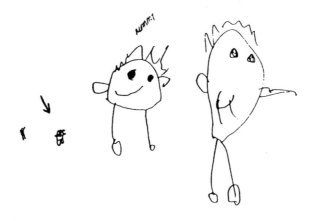

Fig. 26-4 A 7-year-old boy, depicted by the arrow, drew this picture during an office visit initiated as a result of disruptive behaviors and diminished school performance following his parents' emotionally conflictual divorce. He had witnessed several moments of spousal abuse; his symptoms developed when his father left the home 6 months before the office visit. A brief period of counseling was recommended for behavior management and to help the boy to gain a better understanding of his parents' separation, but his mother adamantly refused. The mother in the drawing is on the boy's right side, and her new boyfriend is next to her. The boyfriend's young son is at the far left. As the mother looked at the drawing, she cried for several minutes and said she could now see the need for counseling. The diminutive figure of her son was sufficient for her to recognize his poor self-esteem. The drawing was a nonverbal trigger to seek help.

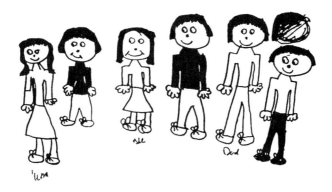

Fig. 26-5   A 9-year-old girl with several months of nonorganic, recurrent abdominal pain drew herself, her parents, and three siblings with a uniformity that lacked individuality. These "cookie-cutter" drawings are seen among school-age children with limited ability to express their feelings associated with perfectionistic, achieving patterns.

situations that would be otherwise obscure. The drawing, like a urinalysis or electrocardiogram, is only one piece of data at one point in time and must not be overinterpreted. However, the appearance of recurring themes in drawings collected over time can contribute to the validity of their meaning.

Making the child's drawing a regular part of the medical record gives it an individual identification, which extends over a period of time. Children naturally like to draw; their creations are given recognition and encouragement in an office setting. Drawing and symbolic representation lead naturally to writing and reading and may be useful precursors to the latter. Children are interested in their previous drawings; adolescents, in particular, are impressed with what they have done in the past, and this thread of continuity helps in their seeking a personal identity. A sense of control and ownership in the medical visits builds a foundation for involvement in and responsibility for health and health care.

DRAWINGS AND MEDICAL CONCERNS

Of specific importance to pediatric practice are certain drawing configurations of children with psychosomatic complaints, such as recurrent abdominal pain and headache syndromes. The regularity with which these children produce characteristic pictures can be of considerable diagnostic aid in these clinical situations. Following are such characteristics:
■ Rigid, stiff body images
■ Fixed, uniform smiles
■ Perfect symmetry
■ Short stubby fingers
■ "Cookie-cutter" figures
These features often correlate with perfectionist, achieving children with significant need for approval and limited ability to ventilate feelings (Fig. 26-5). These styles represent a

predisposition to the internalization of stress and pressures, which may result in recurrent somatic complaints. Reviewing these drawings with the child or family often serves to open up discussion of the background and dynamics of the symptoms without an organic etiology.

Assessing school readiness and appraisal of neurodevelopmental status is an important part of pediatric practice. A child's drawing adds a dimension to this evaluation (Fig. 26-6). Studies of drawings of preschool children have identified particular characteristics that correlate with subsequent school dysfunction. Examples at this age are poor integration of torso, absence of eyes or ears, unusual placements or size distortions, wobbly lines with over- or under-connections, reversals, and difficulty sustaining effort with the early part of the drawing coming out significantly better than the last part. Age-appropriate visual-motor integration in association with distortion of body image or other atypical features may point to psychosocial or emotional problems rather than visual-motor integration difficulty. Figure copying may be aberrant at this age in high-risk populations who may otherwise appear developmentally normal in gross motor, expressive, language, and social skills. Difficulties seen at this time call for early and specific assessment before school entry.[12]

Many studies have been made of the drawings of seriously ill and abused children in hospital and community settings; interpretation of these drawings may be therapeutic for the children and give useful clues to the developmental stage of the illness. Ill children or those undergoing procedures often show cognitive regression, emotional disintegration, and signs of stress. The drawings of children with a serious chronic condition can illuminate the child's understanding of the illness, perceptions of being sick or injured, and feelings of isolation.[13] Specific indicators in the drawings can help the clinician evaluate the child's degree of psychosocial adjustment. For example, the unusual treatment of certain parts of the body in drawings may suggest feelings of anxiety or worry (Fig. 26-7). Themes of threatening weather may suggest feelings of distress about the illness that the child may be unable or unwilling to verbalize (Fig. 26-8). Drawings of seriously ill children may demonstrate a sense of social isolation (Fig. 26-9) or feelings of being overwhelmed by the illness (Fig. 26-10). Recovery, in a psychological sense, can be seen in subsequent drawings (Fig. 26-11). Jungian analysts emphasize the importance of colors used in the drawings and of subtle changes occurring in the course of succeeding pictures as evidence of internal state changes within the child that may precede clinical changes in the course of the illness. The drawings used in this book serve to emphasize the communicative power of these creations in identifying developmental issues, hurdles, and progress.[14]

In summary, children's drawings regularly lessen the stress of the visit to the pediatric office and may provide useful information about the child's developmental status and family relationships. The drawings often open up a discussion among parents, child, and clinician. Children can be asked routinely to "draw a picture of your family" at all well-child visits beginning at 4 or 5 years of age.

DRAW-A-PERSON TEST

The purpose of the DAP Test is to give the clinician an approximation of the mental age of a particular child. The test assesses three areas of visual-motor development: (1) visualiza-

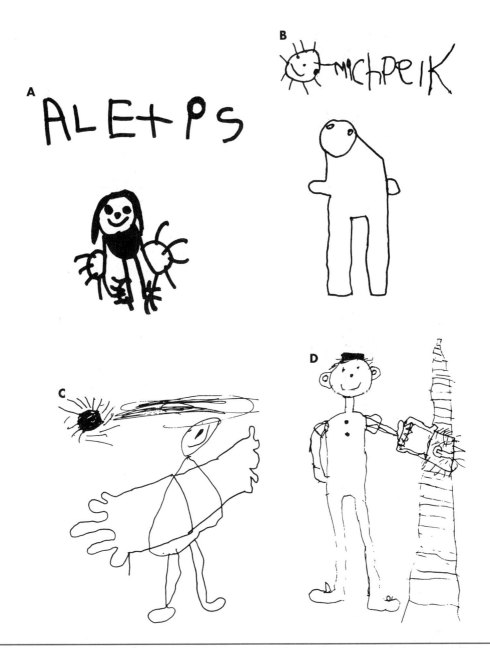

Fig. 26-6 **A.** Drawing by a girl, 3 years, 10 months old, with advanced school readiness skills in language, social, and motor areas. This drawing indicates a mental age of 5 years, 6 months. **B.** Drawing by a 6-year-old boy who was small for gestational age and whose perinatal period was associated with distress and tremulousness in the nursery. Discipline problems characterized his early development. His drawing is atypical at school entry; it demonstrates a constricted sense of self with limited body parts, especially a paucity of facial features. Mental age assigned to drawing is 4 years, 9 months. **C.** Drawing by a 6-year-old boy with attention-deficit disorder associated with aggressive behavior and hyperactivity. At 4 years old, he had viral encephalitis with a residual abnormal electroencephalogram. Mental age assigned to drawing is 6 years. **D.** Drawing by a boy, 6 years, 4 months old, which he described as "an engineer that signals to the train." He demonstrates advanced school readiness skills in areas of fine motor, spatial, and conceptual skills. Mental age assigned to drawing is 7 years, 6 months. (A follow-up visit 20 years later revealed that he had completed a degree in architecture and was studying to become a stage designer.)

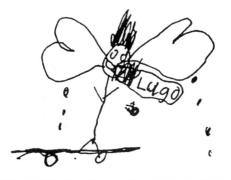

Fig. 26-7   In some cases, a parent's wish to protect a child from the prognosis of a terminal diagnosis can have unintended results. This picture by a bright 9-year-old hemophiliac boy with asymptomatic HIV infection was drawn during a routine visit to the HIV clinic. His mother had not told him about his HIV diagnosis and prohibited everyone else from discussing it with him. The figure on a skateboard is spitting and has exaggerated ears that appear to be crying, suggesting feelings of distress and a need for reassurance about his diagnosis.

tion of the human figure, (2) organization and interpretation (i.e., abstract conceptualization of form, etc.), and (3) reproduction through motor skills of the visualized image as it is seen and interpreted.

The child is given a large blank piece of paper and a pencil and is instructed to draw the picture of a person. She is told to take her time and to draw as complete a picture as possible. The child is left alone to make the drawing, because it is not unusual for a concerned parent to offer help or criticism. The tendency for adults to hover over the child can also produce a degree of anxiety that might cause the child to make a less complete drawing. The test is most suitable for children between 3 and 10 years of age.

Scoring

The child receives 1 point for each of the items that is present in his drawing. One point is equivalent to 3 months of developmental age. For each 4 points, 1 year is added to the basal age, which is 3 years. Thus, if the child scores 9 points, his mental age is $5\frac{3}{12}$ ($2\frac{3}{12}$ + 3) years. The criteria are shown in Box 26-1. Other scoring schemes have been developed but do not really add or change this basic and easily remembered scheme.

In addition to measuring mental age, the test can serve as a diagnostic aid, as previously mentioned. Very poor drawings, rather than representing low intelligence, may indicate neurological or psychological difficulties, and the child should be examined carefully for physical or neuromuscular defects and emotional symptoms. Beyond the cognitive elements of the drawings, projective psychological elements, as described by Burns and Kaufman[9] and as shown in Table 26-1, may become apparent (Fig. 26-12). Primary care clinicians should be cautious about overinterpreting psychological aspects in the drawings. They are

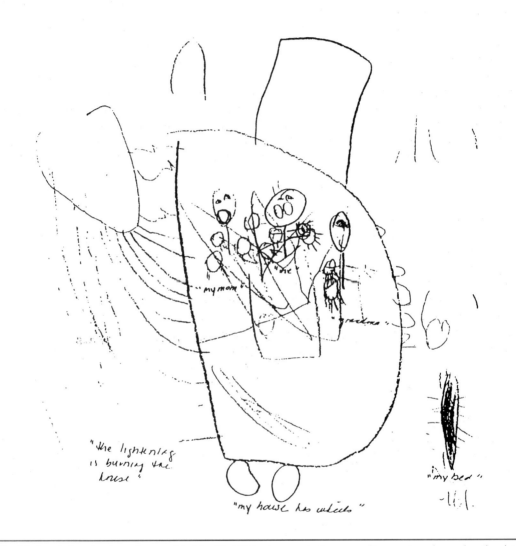

Fig. 26-8 A drawing by a 6-year-old girl with AIDS who was in the care of her maternal grandmother because her mother was ill. She drew herself in her house with her mother and grandmother during a lightning storm, depicted by the curved lines on the left. She described the lightning as "burning the house . . . it hit the door . . . it's trying to get in . . . and it shot me," suggesting significant emotional distress.

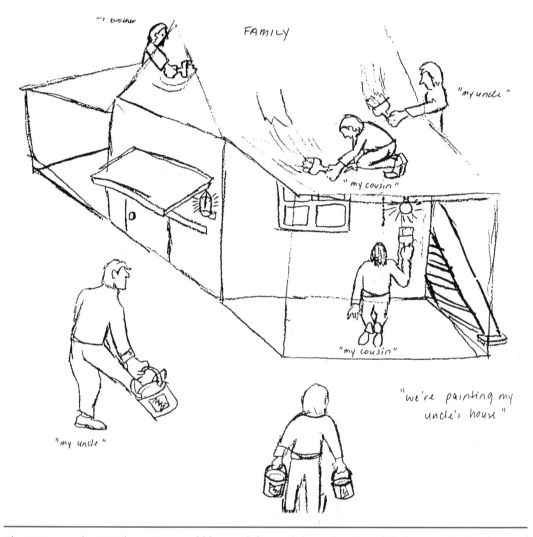

Fig. 26-9 In this KFD by a 12-year-old boy with hemophilia and AIDS, subtle barriers (the buckets and walls of the house) lie between the child and other family members, suggesting feelings of separation and isolation. In addition, the absence of facial features on most of the family members, the absence of his maternal aunt (his primary guardian), and the child's depiction of himself with his back to the viewer reinforce this interpretation.

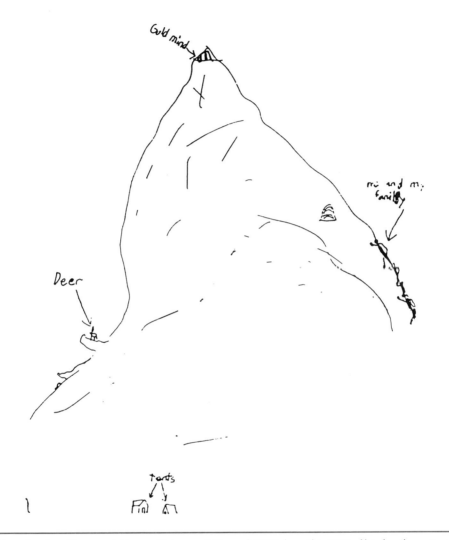

Fig. 26-10   Another 11-year-old boy with hemophilia and AIDS drew this KFD of his family on a camping trip. The minuscule size of individual family members (his father, mother, younger brother, and himself) drawn climbing the side of a mountain toward a "gold mine" suggests a struggle against enormous odds. He rarely spoke about his illnesses during office visits and usually said that everything was "fine."

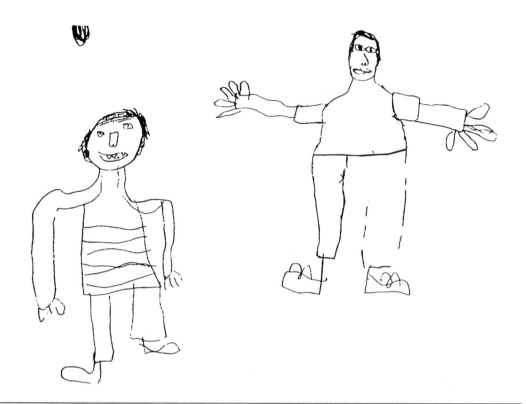

Fig. 26-11   An 8-year-old boy drew the self-portrait on the left that illustrates his perception of his spastic left hemiparetic cerebral palsy. After 1 year of intensive physical therapy and some improvement in function, he drew a picture of himself that reflects a different perception of his neurological impairment.

not diagnostic in themselves. They open opportunities for discussion and further evaluation. Often, a parent will recognize a theme or event in the child's drawing that may trigger further discussion and assessment.

KINETIC FAMILY DRAWINGS: SYMBOLIC INTERPRETATIONS

The older preschooler and grade-school child can be asked to do a family drawing as previously described. Colors can be used. The danger of overinterpretation and misinterpretation of symbols can be prevented by considering the totality of the individual who made the drawing. Viewing the drawings with a pediatric medical and developmental perspective that is comprehensive should prevent these mistakes.[9] Some possible interpretations have been found to recur in kinetic family drawings. Repeated drawings, each with the context clearly laid out, are useful when employed with regularity in a pediatric setting. They provide suggestions and support for diagnostic formulations. They are not diagnostic in them-

BOX 26-1	SCORING CRITERIA FOR DRAW-A-PERSON TEST

1. Head present
2. Neck present
3. Neck, two dimensions
4. Eyes present
5. Eye detail: brow or lashes
6. Eye detail: pupil
7. Nose present
8. Nose, two dimensions (not round ball)
9. Mouth present
10. Lips, two dimensions
11. Both nose and lips in two dimensions
12. Both chin and forehead shown
13. Bridge of nose (straight to eyes; narrower than base)
14. Hair I (any scribble)
15. Hair II (more detail)
16. Ears present
17. Fingers present
18. Correct number of fingers
19. Opposition of thumb shown (must include fingers)
20. Hands present
21. Arms present
22. Arms at side, or engaged in activity
23. Feet: any indication
24. Attachment of arms and legs I (to trunk anywhere)
25. Attachment of arms and legs II (to trunk anywhere)
26. Trunk present
27. Trunk in proportion, two dimensions (length greater than breadth)
28. Clothing I (anything)
29. Clothing II (two articles of clothing)

selves. Some drawings may have no symbolic meanings.[15] Interpretive elements are laid out in Table 26-2. For the clinician interested in further exploration of this topic, the references here will expand the presentation of this area of research.

SUMMARY

Children's drawings are a delightful, cost-effective, low-technology way of highlighting a child's developmental progress, emotional and social concerns, and need for further evaluation. This low-cost diagnostic aid adds vitality, veracity, reflection, and insight into every pediatric encounter. Facility with this tool should be in every black bag.

TABLE 26-1 ■ Draw-a-Person: Clinical-Projective Interpretation

Element	Interpretation
Arms	Controllers of the physical environment; *arm extensions* as aids in controlling the environment may include cleaning implements (mops, brooms, vacuum cleaners), paint brushes (paddles?) and weapons; *long and powerful arms* reach out to control the environment; *lack of arms* represents feelings of helplessness; *folded arms* are usually produced by suspicious and hostile persons.
Belt, heavily emphasized	Suggests conflict between expression and control of sex or impulses
Bilateral symmetry	If overemphasized, suggests an obsessive system of emotional control
Broad shoulders	Need for physical power
Buttons	Usually reflect dependency
Cartoons, clowns	Self-deprecation, defensive attitudes
Cross-hatching	"Controlled shading" attempts to control anxiety through obsessive methods
Disproportionately small body parts	Feelings of inadequacy in specific areas, denial, or repression
Elevated figures	Numerous techniques will be used to elevate various figures, occasionally a dominant sibling will be elevated or it may represent children striving for dominance.
Erasures	Ambivalence, conflict, or denial
Exaggeration of body parts	Enlargement or exaggeration of parts suggests preoccupation with the function of those parts.
Eyes	Facial features that refer primarily to social communication; large eyes scan the world for information, whereas small eyes exclude it and may be paranoid in their wariness or crossed out in guilt.
Facial expressions	Faces depicting various emotions were believed by Machover to be one of the more reliable signs of inner feelings.

TABLE 26-1 ■ Draw-a-Person: Clinical-Projective Interpretation—cont'd

Element	Interpretation
Feet, long	Need for security
Feet, tiny	Dependency, constriction, instability
Figures on back of page	Many children will have difficulty with certain figures and may finally ask whether they can put the person on the back.
Figures hanging, leaning, or falling	Figures seen in precarious positions are usually associated with tension.
Mouth	Emphasis may be associated with feeding difficulties or speech disturbances; in children, overemphasis is frequently associated with dependency.
Neck, long	Usually reflects dependency in children; because the neck connects the impulse-laden body with the controlling mind, the neck is a frequent area of conflict expression.
Omission of body parts	Suggests denial of function; conflict
Omission of figures	Conflict; the figure cannot be drawn on either the front or the back of the paper; often seen with a new baby
Precision, orderliness, neatness	Often reflects a need for a structured environment; overconcern with structure may be viewed as an attempt to control a threatening environment.
Pressure	The pressure used in drawing suggests outward or inward direction of impulse, i.e., the depressed person presses lightly, whereas the acting-out individual uses excessive pressure
Rotated figures	Feelings of being different; demanding attention
Shading or scribbling	Shading in a drawing suggests preoccupation, fixation, or anxiety.
Size	Size suggests diminished or exaggerated view of the self; persons who feel inadequate usually draw a tiny person.
Teeth, prominent	Anger

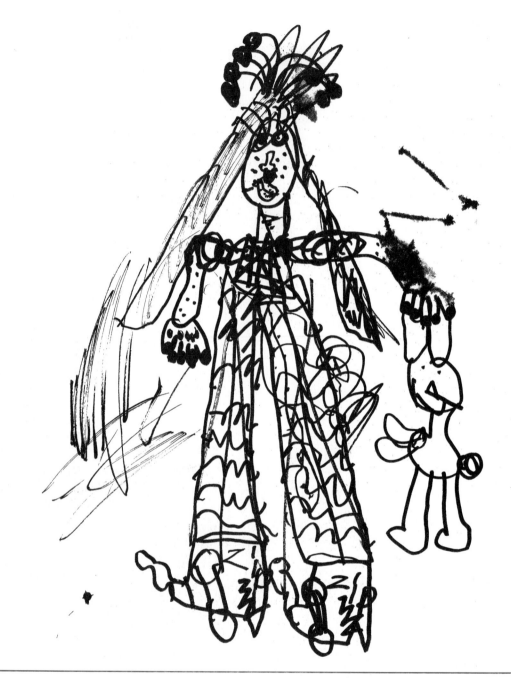

Fig. 26-12 A 10-year-old girl with Asperger's syndrome draws herself in a frantic way, with incredible detail. She can hardly stop adding detail. Her anxious state and obsessive-compulsive characteristiscs are evident in the drawing. She was able to function better and live at home when placed on medication.

TABLE 26-2 ■ Interpretation of Elements in Kinetic Family Drawings

Element	Interpretation
A's	Associated with an emphasis on high academic achievement
Beds	Relatively rare; associated with sexual or depressive themes
Bikes	A common activity of normal children; when overemphasized, may reflect the child's (usually a boy) significant strivings; more common in adolescents when power of the bike and motorbike become particularly important
Brooms	A recurrent symbol; seen particularly in the hands of mothers who put much emphasis on household cleanliness
Butterflies	Associated with the search for elusive love and beauty
Cats	Often symbolic of conflict in identification with mother; *ambivalence, conflict*
Clowns	A preoccupation often seen in a child with significant feelings of inferiority
Cribs	A new baby in the family often produces jealousy in older siblings; because of their "magical thinking," they frequently insist on staying home from school out of fear that something will happen to the baby.
Dirt	Theme of digging or shoveling dirt is associated with negative connotations about dirty thoughts or dirty clothes.
Drums	Displaced anger
Electricity	An extreme need for warmth and love
Fire	An intense need for warmth and love; the fact that love may turn into hate—a destructive force (most fire setters are passive-aggressive personality types)
Flowers	Love of beauty, growth process; in girls, flowers below the waist reflect feminine identification
Garbage	"Taking out the garbage" for many children is equivalent to taking out the unwanted and "dirty" parts of the family existence; frequently found in kinetic family drawings when there is a new baby in the house, or a new foster child; without young infants, garbage may reflect significant guilt about feelings of ambivalence and rivalry toward a younger sibling.
Heat	Need for warmth and love
Horses	A safe comfortable sexual symbolic identification found universally in Western culture among adolescent girls
Ironing board	With an "X" by adolescent boys may reflect conflict and ambivalence toward mother; the iron may reflect the intensity of the feelings
Jump rope	The encapsulation of a rival or protection for the self
Kites/balloons	Attempts to escape from restrictive family environments; escape and freedom

Continued

TABLE 26-2 ■ Interpretation of Elements in Kinetic Family Drawings—cont'd

Element	Interpretation
Ladders	Tension, precarious balance
Lamps	The need for warmth and love
Lawnmower	A cutting symbol that is usually associated with a castrating figure; usually drawn by boys.
Leaves	Dependency; a symbol of that which clings to the source of nurturance.
Light bulbs	Need for warmth and love; also *flashlights*
Logs	Hypermasculinity or masculine strivings
Paint brush	Often an extension of the hand and associated with a punishing figure
Rain	Associated with depressive tendencies
Refrigerator	Associated with deprivation and depressive reactions to deprivation; the refrigerator is a source of nurturance but is still a cold object.
Skin diving	Usually drawn by boys; associated with withdrawal and depressive tendencies
Snakes	An infrequent but well-known phallic symbol
Stars	Associated with deprivation—physical or emotional; stars are usually cold and distant
Stop sign	"Keep out"; attempt at impulse control
Sun	In young children, the sun is stereotyped and has little meaning; a darkened sun drawn by older children may reflect depression; the sun's face may reflect pertinent emotions; if figures are facing the sun—the need for warmth and love; if facing away from the sun—rejection.

REFERENCES

1. Stein MT: Challenging case: the use of family drawings by children in pediatric practice, *J Dev Behav Pediatr* 18(5): 334, 1997.
2. Kellog R: *Analyzing children's art*, Palo Alto, Calif, 1969, National Press.
3. Gardner H: *Artful scribbles: the significance of children's drawings*, New York, 1980, Basic Books.
4. Goodenough FL: *Measurement of intelligence by drawings*, New York, 1926, World Books.
5. Harris DB: *Children's drawings as measures of intellectual maturity*, New York, 1963, Harcourt.
6. Luquet GF: *Les dessins d'un enfants: etude psychologique*, Paris, 1917, Alcain.
7. DiLeo JH: *Young children and their drawings*, New York, 1970, Brunner-Mazel.
8. Gillespie J: *The projective use of mother-and-child drawings: a manual for clinicians*, New York, 1994, Brunner-Mazel.
9. Burns RC, Kaufman SH: *Actions, styles and symbols in kinetic family drawings: an interpretive manual*, New York, 1972, Brunner-Mazel.

10. O'Brien RP, Patton WW: Development of an objective scoring method for kinetic family drawings, *J Pers Assess* 58:156, 1974.
11. DiLeo, JH: *Interpreting children's drawings*, New York, 1983, Brunner-Mazel.
12. Vohr B, Garcia-Coll CT: Neurodevelopmental and school performance of very low birth weight infants: a seven year longitudinal study, *Pediatrics* 76:345, 1985.
13. Spinetta, J et al: The kinetic family drawing in childhood cancer: a revised application of an age-independent measure. In Spinetta J, Deasy-Spinetta P, editors: *Living with childhood cancer*, St. Louis, 1981, Mosby, pp 86-120.
14. Instone SL: *Children with HIV: how they feel about what parents say*, unpublished doctoral dissertation, San Diego, 1996, University of San Diego.
15. Koppitz EM: *Psychological evaluation of children's human figure drawings*, New York, 1968, Grune & Stratton.

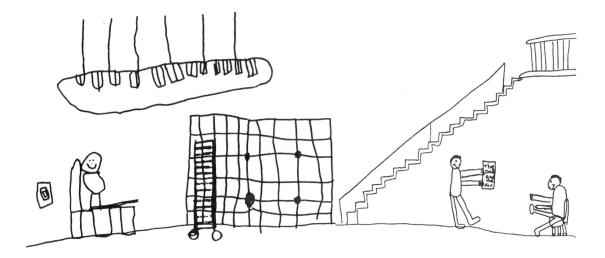

"Reading together." Left illustration by Ben Stein, age 5. Right illustration by Josh Stein, age 8.

CHAPTER 27

BOOKS FOR PARENTS: AN ANNOTATED BIBLIOGRAPHY

- Nancy Mann
- Suzanne D. Dixon
- Martin T. Stein

Pediatric professionals recommend books for parents to read for various reasons. Books often serve as an adjunct to the teaching done in the office. Some parents need or request additional information on topics discussed briefly in the office visit. Books can provide a reinforcing or differing view, as needed. Parents of children with special needs may be especially appreciative of such resources. **Books do not substitute for direct, personal guidance, but are an important adjunct to care.**

Several factors should be considered before recommending a book, such as the following:

- Parents' particular need
- Child's developmental level
- Parents' ability to use written material
- What is affordable and available
- Parental motivation

Clinicians should be clear about the goals to be achieved in recommending books. A pernicious belief exists that parenting can only be done by professionals and that more information automatically ensures better parenting. The clinician can unconsciously support that belief and add to anxiety by wholesale or routine reading suggestions. Giving people confidence is the goal here—not overwhelming them with "professionalism."

Maximal availability of the books will offer the opportunity for ready use. Strategies include keeping copies of selected books in the waiting room or examining room, having books available to purchase at cost in the office, compiling a lending library, and requesting a nearby bookstore to stock selected favorites. A printed reading list can be developed, but should be given out with *specific* notation from the clinician to point parents in a good direction.

A few cautions are in order. First, it is essential for the clinician to read the books. One must be familiar with an author's philosophy and recommendations to determine if the book would be compatible with the clinician's own philosophy and information as imparted to parents in the office.

BOX 27-1	CRITERIA FOR INCLUSION IN LIST

1. Clarity—succinct, easy to comprehend vs. wordy and rambling
2. Organization—well-defined topics, headings, and subheadings
3. Author's attitude—reassuring and supportive vs. condescending and guilt-inducing
4. Author's qualifications
5. Availability—books available in bookstores or libraries
6. Credibility of actual content

Second, the list in this chapter has been selected from the vast and ever-growing literature available for parents. Many books that are no doubt excellent escaped our review. Box 27-1 gives the criteria for inclusion in our list.

The clinician should periodically peruse the child development section at the local bookstore in order to be familiar with the most-current books. A few we have found helpful are listed below by category and then alphabetically by first author.

BIBLIOGRAPHY FOR PARENTS
Child Development

1. Ames LB, Ilg F: *Your One Year Old: The Fun Loving Fussy* (1982); *Your Two Year Old: Terrible or Tender* (1976); *Your Three Year Old: Friend or Enemy* (1976); *Your Four Year Old: Wild and Wonderful* (1976); *Your Five Year Old: Sunny and Serene* (1979); *Your Six Year Old: Loving and Defiant* (1980), New York, Dell Books. Codirectors of the Gesell Institute of Child Development, these authors display their knowledge, experience, and sense of humor in their uncanny skill of depicting accurate portraits of children's behavior. Very practical advice combined with a reassuring style make these books invaluable reading for a frustrated parent. Although they are now more than two decades old, their insights have passed the test of time and are still applicable.

2. Brazelton TB: *Infants and Mothers,* New York, 1969, Dell. In describing the behavior of three normal babies, Dr. Brazelton makes extremely clear how different infants can be. His descriptions of the interactions between average, quiet, and active babies and their families during the first year of life make worthwhile reading for new parents and also for parents who make frequent comparisons between their infant and other babies. This has been updated somewhat. Highlights individuality and temperament. Now a "classic" in infant development.

3. Brazelton TB: *Toddlers and Parents,* New York, 1974, Dell. With empathy and humor, Dr. Brazelton presents a realistic family profile in the turbulent life of a child from the ages of 1 to 2 years. He explores the toddler's developmental work of self-assertion, as well as the issues of toilet training, sibling rivalry, working parents, and single parents.

4. Brazelton TB: *Touchpoints,* Reading, Mass, 1992, Addison-Wesley. An easy-to-read reference book in which parents' questions and concerns about their child's behavior, devel-

opment, and feelings are anticipated and answered in chronological (part I) as well as problem (part II) form.

5. Caplan F, editor: *The First Twelve Months of Life,* ed 2, New York, 1993, Grosset & Dunlap. In this new edition Caplan has continued to use much of the most recent research on infants in an effort to help parents understand why babies behave as they do. Descriptions of a baby's month-by-month development, numerous photographs, and growth charts make the book reader friendly. Like the first edition, this excellent book has a wealth of information that is both fun to discover and helpful to know.

6. Comer JP, Poussaint AF: *Raising Black Children,* New York, 1992, Penguin Books. A revision of *Black Child Care,* this general guide to parenting focuses on special concerns of black families. More ethnic specific than the first edition with main focus still on child development.

7. Fraiberg S: *The Magic Years,* New York, 1959, Charles Scribner's Sons. Now a child development classic—a "must read" for students of early childhood! Child psychoanalyst Fraiberg discusses early psychological development (birth to 6 years) as if the reader were experiencing the child's inner world. More theoretical than most books in this list, it discusses typical developmental problems and their management. Very sensible observations. A big favorite for pediatricians, both in the making and established.

8. Greenspan S, Greenspan NT: *First Feelings,* New York, 1985, Viking. This book chronicles the stages of emotional and cognitive development from birth through age 4. Six stages in the emotional life of the young child are seen as critical to healthy development: the awakening of the infant, the discovery of communication, the deepening of relationships, the developing of a sense of self, the ability to create new ideas, and the development of complex feelings. Descriptions of children and families are strategically used to clarify each stage. Practical advice assists parents as they encounter the range of children's emotions, fears, and struggles. College educated audience.

9. Klaus M, Kennell J, Klaus P: *Bonding,* Reading, Mass, 1995, Addison-Wesley. A readable text for parents and professionals that discusses the formation of the emotional bonds between parent and child from pregnancy through early infancy. Sensitive and insightful coverage of premature births and birth defects. Includes a discussion of the benefits of a doula, a social support person for the laboring mother.

10. Klaus M, Klaus P: *Your Amazing Newborn,* Reading, Mass, 1998, Perseus Books. A photographic journey into the readiness of newborns to engage and be engaged by their environment. The authors make research in early child development available to parents with clear narrative and photographs on nearly every page.

11. Kutner L: *Toddlers and Preschoolers,* New York, 1994, William Morrow & Co. Easy, practical, small book. Short chapters, issues of temperament, choosing a preschool.

Parenting

1. Brown J, Davis J: *No More Monsters in the Closet,* New York, 1995, Crown Publishers. A guide for teaching a child to use imagination to overcome every fear from doctors to nightmares, social situations, school plays, and relatives visiting. The perspective and

writing is reader friendly. Helpful for motivated parents and professionals who are interested in imagery.

2. Clark L: *S.O.S! Help for Parents,* Bowling Green, Kentucky, 1985, Parents Press. A well-organized book that covers a variety of discipline methods (positive reinforcement, parents as models, active ignoring, and time out) in an easy-to-read format. Helpful charts, illustrations, and highlighted points make this book a good source for professionals and parents of all educational levels. Excellent coverage of time out at any age.

3. Coles R: *The Moral Intelligence of Children,* New York, 1997, Plume. This book focuses on the connection between the behaviors of parents and teachers and raising children with a spirit of generosity and empathy. A major contribution to parent guides.

4. Faber A, Mazlish E: *Siblings Without Rivalry,* New York, 1987, Avon Books. This book offers practical guidelines supplemented with the views and experiences of parents in a parenting workshop. Thought-provoking ideas for role playing. Helpful comic strips and reminder strips on how to handle different situations make this book a good source for parents and professionals.

5. Ferber R: *Solve Your Child's Sleep Problems,* New York, 1985, Simon & Schuster. Excellent explanations of the developmental basis of sleep disturbances in a family context. Specific, sensible suggestions for solving problems from sleep rhythm disturbances to enuresis. Highly recommended; for educated parents only.

6. Gordon T: *P.E.T.: Parent Effectiveness Training,* New York, 1975, Plume Books. One of the best books in presenting the basic, essential communication skills needed in families: how to listen, how to communicate your feelings, how to solve conflicts. Recipe format. Gives parents a concrete place to manage issues and sets up an approach to solving problems. May be too prescriptive for some families, just right for others.

7. Greenspan S, Greenspan NT: *The Essential Partnership,* New York, 1989, Penguin. This book builds on the information presented in *First Feelings,* offering guidelines on everyday child-rearing issues from infancy through age 4. The authors discuss relationship building, self-esteem, independence, anger, aggression, tantrums, and peer relationships. Case histories, including ones from single and dual career families, clarify concepts and offer practical advice. Offers an excellent discussion on the use of play time or "floor time" as an opportunity to observe and learn about children.

8. Greenspan S: *The Challenging Child,* New York, 1995, Addison-Wesley. A valuable book for motivated parents of "difficult" children that gives insight to the child while offering child-rearing guidelines. Dr. Greenspan describes five personality patterns and devotes a chapter to each (sensitive child, self-absorbed child, defiant child, inattentive child, and active-aggressive child). A nice neutral chapter of environmental and dietary influences on children's behavior also is included.

9. Hopson DP, Hopson D: *Different and Wonderful: Raising Black Children in a Race Conscious Society,* New York, 1990, Prentice Hall. Black children in America are born into a society with strong racist undercurrents that can damage self-esteem and reduce control over their environment. Black parents are faced with the challenge of raising children with a positive sense of self-worth in a society that judges them as less intelligent, attractive, and trustworthy. This book guides black parents through each phase of child devel-

opment in the context of race issues and self-esteem. Explores tough issues affecting black middle-class families. Provides parents with practical tools for recognizing their own racial attitudes, instilling ethnic pride, and discussing race-related issues. Offers a resource guide to direct parents toward children's books and toys that celebrate African-American culture.

10. Kurcinka MS: *Raising Your Spirited Child: A Guide for Parents Whose Child is More Intense, Sensitive, Perceptive, Persistent and Energetic,* New York, 1991, Harper Collins. An encouraging book for parents that addresses understanding, working, living with, and enjoying "difficult" children. Emphasis is on the positive aspects of these children. Good for frustrated parents who are willing to follow good, solid advice.

11. Phelan T: *1-2-3 Magic,* Glen Ellyn, Ill, 1995, Child Management Inc. A simple, proven method of discipline that uses counting to help parents stop unwanted behavior and start wanted behavior without arguing, yelling, or spanking. Easy-to-follow steps for the very motivated parent.

12. Pipher M: *Raising Ophelia: Saving the Selves of Adolescent Girls,* New York, 1994, Ballantine Books. The theme of this book is that many girls experience a loss of spirit and self-esteem as they enter adolescence. The author points to cultural values and expectations as the source of change. She illustrates her ideas with cases from her practice as a child psychologist. The emphasis is on prevention.

13. Turecki S: *The Difficult Child,* New York, 1989, Bantam Books. Parents have found this book to be useful to help them understand their child with difficult-to-manage behaviors. Practical strategies are described for behavior change in the child and family.

14. Turecki S, Wernick S: *The Emotional Problems of Normal Children,* New York, 1994, Bantam Books. Dr. Turecki describes emotional difficulties that can happen to typical children and offers management strategies for parents to help children overcome these challenges. Best for educated, highly motivated parents.

Parenting Teenagers

1. Greydanus D, editor: *Caring for Your Adolescent,* New York, 1995, Bantam Books (for American Academy of Pediatrics). The third of a three-book series developed by the American Academy of Pediatrics. Well-written and easy-to-use comprehensive guide for parents of 12- to 21-year-olds. Practical advice on everything from typical development to nutrition to school failure to family conflicts. Straightforward coverage of sexuality, signals of substance abuse, sexually transmitted diseases, birth control, and eating disorders. Reader-friendly format and illustrations make it informative for all parents.

2. Kutner L: *Making Sense of Your Teenager,* New York, 1997, William Morrow. Straightforward and easy-to-read book that offers insights and tools to help parents understand their teenagers and find solutions to common problems.

3. Wolf A: *Get Out of My Life—But First Could You Drive Me and Cheryl to the Mall?* New York, 1991, Noonday Press. An accurate description of the behavior of teenagers and the psychological aspects behind these behaviors. The humorous approach makes it easy and enjoyable to read.

Child Health and Physical Care

1. Blocker A: *Baby Basics: A Guide for New Parents,* Minneapolis, 1997, Chronimed Publishing. Straightforward, practical advice for new parents that covers a wide range of topics, such as planning for the arrival of the baby, investing in the future, making wills, nutrition, babyproofing, and clothing. Good checklist and resource list in each chapter. Very easy to use.

2. Eisenberg A, Murkoff HE, Hathaway SE: *What to Expect the First Year,* New York, 1989, Workman. Comprehensive guide to newborn and infant care. Offers up-to-date practical information. Format is easy to read with chapters that identify issues at monthly stages. Useful sections on nutrition, language development, and safety.

3. Leach P: *Your Baby and Child,* ed 2, New York, 1989, Alfred A Knopf. Developmental psychologist Penelope Leach has written an outstanding encyclopedia for parents of children from birth to 5 years. Leach uses an approach to everyday care and common behavioral issues that is based on the development of the child and the family. Subtitles within the chapter, many excellent drawings and pictures, and a superb index with definitions facilitate reading this comprehensive book and make it accessible to most parents.

4. Leach P: *Your Growing Child,* New York, 1989, Alfred A Knopf. An encyclopedia of child care issues, from health to nutrition to development. Solid and clear, although brief sections. Alphabetical format a bit difficult to use. However, it does cover issues through adolescence, with a strong section on teenage issues.

5. Nathanson LW: *The Portable Pediatrician,* New York, 1994, Harper Collins. A practical guide for parents of young children, written in an engaging style by an experienced pediatrician. Drawings and highlighted advice make this an easy and informative read.

6. Pantell R, Fries JF, Vickery DM: *Taking Care of Your Child: A Parent's Guide to Medical Care,* ed 3, Reading, Mass, 1990, Addison-Wesley. Pediatrician Pantell and his colleagues outline many aspects of health promotion, approaches to common symptoms, and home management for parents. Through a series of algorithms designed for parents faced with specific symptoms, the format is especially lucid and practical.

7. Schmitt BD: *Your Child's Health: A Pediatric Guide for Parents,* New York, 1991, Bantam. A revision of the first guidebook on children's common illnesses, on behavior problems, and on health promotion from infancy through adolescence. Offers parents appropriate and safe home remedies and guidelines for seeking emergency and nonemergency medical care. The behavior modification protocols for common developmental problems are readily accessible and practical for most parents. It is especially valuable for parents who will benefit from specific, detailed recommendations.

8. Schiff D, Shelov S, editors: *Guide to Your Child's Symptoms,* New York, 1997, Bantam Books (for American Academy of Pediatrics). A home reference developed by the American Academy of Pediatrics to aid parents in assessing a problem and deciding what action should be taken. Easy to use with alphabetical listing of symptoms accompanied by age-specific charts with questions to consider, possible cause, and actions to take. Illustrated First Aid manual section is practical and comprehensive.

9. Schor E, editor: *Caring for Your School Age Child,* New York, 1995, Bantam Books (for American Academy of Pediatrics). The second in a three-book series developed by the

American Academy of Pediatrics. Well-written and easy-to-use comprehensive guide for parents of 5- to 12-year-olds. Useful information on typical health, and physical, social, and personal development. Extensive coverage of emotional, behavioral, and discipline problems and family and school matters, as well as health problems. Reader-friendly format and illustrations make it informative for all parents.

10. Shelov S, editor: *Caring for Your Baby and Young Child: Birth to Age 5,* New York, 1991, Bantam Books (for American Academy of Pediatrics). Written especially for new parents, this well-written guide was developed by the American Academy of Pediatrics. Details about physical and psychological growth, development, and common problems of early childhood are described in appropriate detail to be of help to all parents. The index and organization of the book provide quick access to questions and concerns.

11. Spock B, Parker S: *Dr. Spock's Baby and Child Care,* New York, 1998, Pocket Books (softcover), EP Dutton (hardcover). This 7th edition of Dr. Spock's classic guide to parenting and child rearing is a compilation of information on child development, principles, parenting skills, and common medical conditions. Dr. Spock's advice on parenting (captured in the book's opening statement, "Trust yourself. You know more than you think.") has engaged parents for three generations. The index is particularly useful for rapid retrieval of information by concerned parents.

12. Tristram C, Tristram L: *Have Kid Will Travel: 101 Survival Strategies for Vacation With Babies and Young Children,* Kansas City, 1997, Andrews McMeel. Practical advice on planning trips and traveling with children. Excellent points on where not to go, how to babyproof a hotel room, and how to fly with small children. Good list of references.

13. US Department of Health and Human Services: *Infant Care,* DHHS Publication No HRS-M-CH-89-2, 1989, 109 pp. A short and easy-to-read manual, it contains helpful basic information for new parents, such as care of the baby, special problems that may develop (e.g., illness or accidents), developmental characteristics of infants, ways to enhance babies' growth through play, and a discussion of temperamental differences among babies. Available in Spanish. A single copy is free from the National Maternal and Child Health Clearinghouse, 38th and R Streets NW, Washington, DC 20057. Additional copies can be purchased for $1.50 each.

14. US Department of Health and Human Services: *Your Child from 1 to 6,* Superintendent of Documents, US Government Printing Office, DHHS Publication No OCD 91-30026, 1991. This 92-page booklet begins where *Infant Care* leaves off. It contains material relating to the emotional and intellectual development of the child, as well as medical information. It makes helpful suggestions for handling special situations, such as going to the hospital, moving, disabilities, illnesses, and accidents. Available in Spanish. A single copy is available free from the National Maternal and Child Health Clearinghouse, 38th and R Streets NW, Washington, DC 20057. Additional copies are $1.00 each.

15. Williams F: *Babycare for Beginners,* New York, 1996, Harper Collins. Large step-by-step photos with captions demonstrate everything from handling the baby to feeding to dressing and grooming. Helpful for inexperienced parents who would like to be reassured that they are doing the basics correctly.

Day Care

1. Cochran E, Cochran M: *Child Care that Works,* New York, 1997, Houghton Mifflin Co. A complete, easy-to-use guide that gives parents the information for finding good child care. The appendices are extremely useful with checklists for the different types of child care, lists of local and national resources, suggested reading, and questions to ask providers. Highly recommended for parents exploring day-care options.
2. Katzev AR, Bragdon NH: *Child Care Solutions,* New York, 1990, Avon Books. Comprehensive guide for the selection of day care from infancy to after-school care. Identifies strategies for parents to use as they search for, evaluate, and choose among various child care environments. Includes practical advice for parents as they manage day-to-day child care issues and strive to work effectively with providers.
3. US Department of Health and Human Services, Office of Human Development Services, Daycare Division: *A Parent's Guide to Daycare,* DHHS Publication No (OHDS) 80-30254, Superintendent of Documents, US Government Printing Office, 1980. A practical, readable, and inexpensive booklet for parents. Part I discusses the components of quality day care and pragmatic considerations to be made before seeking it. Part II details the step-by-step process of finding day care. The checklists are particularly valuable. In addition to noting the age-related needs of children and individual parent preferences, special situations such as nighttime care, single parenting, and children with special needs are considered. Part III covers a multitude of common day-care problems and suggestions for management. Part IV offers resources of organizations and agencies that may be useful when selecting day care for children with disabling conditions. In addition to the manual's reasonable length (75 pages), sections are designed to ease finding the particular information needed by having headlines in the left column and boldface headings in the text. Highly recommended.
4. Woolever E, editor: *Your Child: Selecting Day Care,* Des Moines, Iowa, 1990, Better Homes and Gardens Books. Brief, but thorough review of issues that parents face as they evaluate and select child care. Includes checklists for evaluating the child care providers, identifying quality of programs and safety. Provides excellent information on parent-child care provider relationships.

Families with Special Needs

Prematurity

1. Harrison H: *The Premature Baby Book,* New York, 1983, St. Martin's Press. Parents will appreciate this book as the most complete compilation of information about preemies. Written by the mother of a preemie with extensive consultation from neonatology experts, this is a superb resource. Numerous vignettes of families' responses and adaptation make this a "must" for neonatal staff as well. Some medical issues may be dated, but the essence here is still sound.
2. Ludington-Hoe S, Golant S: *Kangaroo Care,* New York, 1993, Bantam Books. A guide to the Kangaroo Care holding program. The book reviews the program's history, the research supporting its benefits, who can follow the program, and how. This book also has excellent coverage of life in the neonatal intensive care unit for parents and the baby. Rec-

ommended for parents who would like to participate more in the care of their premature infant.

Twins

1. Gromada K, Hulburt M: *Keys to Parenting Twins,* New York, 1992, Barrons. Written by parent educators and mothers of twins who publish a newsletter for parents of twins, this guide touches on baby basics (feeding, sleeping, family adjustment) with emphasis on individuality. Most topics are briefly covered; however, a good resource list for more in-depth coverage is provided.

Disabled

1. Charkins H: *Children with Facial Difference: A Parents' Guide.* Bethesda, Maryland, 1997, Woodbine House. Informative book that covers all aspects of having a child with a facial difference, from basic genetics to emotional challenges. Written by the mother of a child born with Treacher Collins syndrome, in collaboration with professionals. It offers the support and resources that only a parent who has been there can offer. A must for parents of a child born with a facial difference.

2. Freeman RD, Carvin CF, Boese RJ: *Can't Your Child Hear? A Guide for Those who Care for the Deaf,* Baltimore, 1981, University Park Press. Complete, clear guide for a child with any degree of hearing impairment from birth onward. Good resource for professionals, too.

3. Miller N: *Nobody's Perfect: Living and Growing with Children who Have Special Needs,* Baltimore, Maryland, 1994, Paul F. Brooks. Excellent practical, insightful, and supportive book for parents of children with special needs; it addresses the theoretical (model for adapting) to the practical (how to handle parents, friends, going out in public, etc.). Many anecdotes from mothers of children with special needs. A helpful list of readings and resources is included.

4. Schleichkorn J: *Coping with Cerebral Palsy,* Austin, Texas, 1983, ProEd. This paperback book provides concise guidelines toward an understanding of the issues facing children with cerebral palsy, definitions of medical terms, psychosocial issues, and educational concerns. It has a particularly valuable section describing issues that affect the older child and adult and a further list of readings. Appropriate for beginning a discussion with a family after an initial postdiagnosis adjustment period.

5. Thompson CE: *Raising a Handicapped Child,* New York, 1986, William Morrow & Co. Written by a pediatrician and mother, this book addresses issues facing a family with a child who has a major handicapping condition. A significant portion is dedicated to the feelings of parents and helpful approaches to coping. Strategies for working with medical and educational systems are discussed. This book is for parents of a child with an established disability, particularly for those in a "dawn time" of grief, frustration, or hopelessness.

6. The **Woodbine House Special Needs Collection** has books covering many topics, such as visual impairments, Down syndrome, autism, Tourette's, and teaching communication skills to children with special needs, all of which are well written and practical (for information, phone 800-843-7323).

Attention Deficit Hyperactivity Disorder

1. Barkley R: *Taking Charge of ADHD,* New York, 1995, Guilford Press. A well-organized guide of suggestions for helping children with ADHD. Practical lists of suggestions and charts. The text can get a bit technical, but the advice given is excellent. Good for motivated, well-educated parents.
2. Hallowell E, Ratey J: *Driven to Distraction,* New York, 1994, Touchstone. A bestselling book that any parent who thinks they or their children have ADHD probably will have read. The authors use stories from their patients to demonstrate the different forms of ADHD. Despite the media hype, it offers sound advice on how to identify ADHD and what to do about it.
3. Ingersoll B: *Your Hyperactive Child: A Parent's Guide to Coping with ADD,* New York, 1988, Doubleday. One of the best books written on what ADD is and what treatments work and don't work. Supports behavior modification, parent-teacher cooperation, and medication and debunks nutritional remedies. Easy to read, this book should be recommended for any parent of a child with ADHD.
4. Quinn P, Stern J: *Putting on the Brakes: Young People's Guide to Understanding Attention Deficit Hyperactivity Disorder,* New York, 1991, Magination Press. A book written for 8- to 13-year-olds that uses wonderful analogies to explain what ADHD is and how to address the problems that it presents. Practical and straightforward.

Gifted Children

1. Ehrlich VZ: *Gifted Children: A School for Parents and Teachers,* Englewood Cliffs, NJ, 1982, Prentice-Hall. General overview for parents of children who have special educational needs that are not being met by standard or enriched programs. The focus is on schooling issues.
2. Walker SY: *The Survival Guide for Parents of Gifted Kids,* Minneapolis, 1991, Free Spirit Publishing. Although this book does not offer too many recommendations for overcoming problems, it does have a good list of other references at the end of each chapter and a good "when to worry" list. A chapter on educational programs and advocacy is included.

Divorce and Stepfamilies

1. Bernstein AC: *Yours, Mine and Ours,* New York, 1990, Norton. This book explores how families change when remarried parents have a child together. Based on the author's experiences as a stepmother and family therapist and on interviews with "mixed" families, this book explores the psychology and social influences of stepfamilies. Bernstein details the interdependent roles of each member in a stepfamily and analyzes the issues of resentment, competition, and anger.
2. Boyd H: *The Stepparent's Survival Guide,* London, 1998, Ward Lock. Small paperback with all the issues clearly identified. British words a little distracting to the American reader, but no problem with the content.
3. Brown LK, Brown M: *Dinosaurs Divorce,* New York, 1986, Little, Brown. Cartoon dinosaurs explain in a straightforward, easy-to-understand fashion what divorce is, why it happens, and what the child can expect in the future. The familiar illustrations by Marc Brown make it reader friendly for the elementary school–age child.

4. Evans MD: *This is Me and My Single Parent* (1989), *This is Me and My Two Families* (1988), New York, Magination Press. Fill-in-the-blanks workbooks for parent(s) and children to do together to open up discussion on the stress points in these "special families."

5. Ives S, Fassle D, Rash M: *The Divorce Workbook*, Burlington, Vt, 1985, Waterfront Books. A workbook for parents, relatives, or counselors to use with elementary school–age children. Explains marriage, separation, divorce, legal "stuff" and feelings. Encourages creative expression of thoughts and feelings through picture drawing. Good for use in conjunction with therapy.

6. Kalter N: *Growing up with Divorce*, New York, 1990, Free Press. Informative discussion of the impact of divorce on children at specific ages with practical suggestions for parents. Focus is on observing the individual child, respecting the stage of development, and communicating clearly. Case histories provide insight into children's perceptions of the immediate and long-term issues in divorce and the ways families have learned to cope with their children's anger, fears, and maladaptive behaviors.

7. Wallerstein J, Blakeslee S: *Second Chances: Men, Women, and Children a Decade After Divorce*, New York, 1989, Ticknor and Fields. The authors interviewed 60 families with 131 children at the time of their divorce and again at 5- and 10-year intervals. The long-term psychological effects and economic impact of divorce are analyzed. Descriptions of the effects of divorce on children's thoughts and feelings, social relationships, work, family life, and economic stability are candid and comprehensive. The psychological stages of divorce are defined for children and adults. Case vignettes add a valuable personal dimension to the research findings. This is really a scholarly work for families who wish to explore the issue at this depth.

Adoption

1. Cole J: *How I Was Adopted*, New York, 1995, William Morrow & Co. A straightforward story that explains to early school-age children what adoption is and how it happens.

2. Hicks R: *Adopting in America*, Sun City, California, 1995, Wordsing Press. A comprehensive book that covers the technicalities of adoption. It explains different types of adoption, lists resources in every state, reviews laws and procedures, and includes sample letters.

3. Register C: *Are those Kids Yours? American Families with Children Adopted from Other Countries*, New York, 1991, The Free Press. Comprehensive look at the issues for families who are contemplating interracial adoption or for those with multiethnic families. Explores real issues facing such families as they mature together.

4. Schaffer J, Lindstrom C: *How to Raise an Adopted Child*, New York, 1989, Penguin Books. An age-correlated guide that covers the physical and psychological development from birth to adolescence and the special needs of adoptive children. Answers many common questions. Somewhat dense.

Serious Illness and Death

1. Family Living Series: *Children Die Too* and *Why Mine?* Omaha, 1981, Centering Corp. Two simply and sensitively written, brief (20 pages) booklets that can be used at any stage of parental grief. An added dimension of support and insight through quotes from parents.

Recommend purchase in bulk by health care professionals as an adjunct in their support of parents. Free catalogue available from: Centering Corp, PO Box 3367, Omaha, NE 68103.

2. Grollman E, editor: *Bereaved Children and Teens*, Boston, 1995, Beacon Press Books. A comprehensive guide for parents who are helping their children cope with the death of someone they know. Each chapter is written by an authority and covers, in a developmentally appropriate fashion, everything from how to talk about death and dying to how bereavement affects a child to different religious customs about death and how to explain them to children. The last section addresses useful treatments and therapies that can help children cope with death and alerts parents to signs that a child needs professional care. The in-depth style makes it valuable for the highly educated parent and professional.

3. Grollman E: *Talking about Death*, Boston, 1990, Beacon Press Books. A frank guide for parents. The book begins with a straightforward read-along "story" explaining what death is. The rest of the book explains to parents how children view and react to death and how they can help. Excellent list of resources parents can use locally, as well as nationally.

4. Kübler-Ross E: *On Children and Death*, New York, 1983, MacMillan. From the person who gave the classic descriptions of the grieving process, this book explains children's understanding of death and how to assist in the process.

5. Trozzi M: *Talking with Children About Loss: Words, Strategies and Wisdom to Help Children Cope with Death, Divorce, and Other Difficult Times*, New York, Putnam (1999). Intended for parents and professionals, this book gently leads the reader through the most difficult terrain: how to help your child deal with the painful feelings of significant loss in a way that actually enhances healthy psychological development. This easy-to-read book uses lots of examples: facing the death of a family member or a pet, divorce, chronic illness, and welcoming a new sibling born with special needs, as well as the inevitable losses and changes that all children face. Practical suggestions for management and intervention are included. Good for parents who need this perspective and for teachers and other professionals who deal with children facing death of themselves or of family members.

6. The **Good Grief Program:** Books and videos on loss for children and adolescents: An annotated bibliography, Boston, Mass, 1996, Boston Medical Center.

Child Safety Resources

The following organizations and agencies provide pamphlets and leaflets dealing with child safety resources:

1. Action for Child Product Safety, 358 Woburn St, Lexington, MA 02173.

2. Action for Children's Television (ACT), 20 University Road, Cambridge, MA 02138. An advocacy group that continues to be legislatively active, to provide ongoing monitoring of television, and to provide educational materials. A good mailing list to be on.

3. Committee on Accident and Poison Prevention, American Academy of Pediatrics (AAP), 141 Northwest Point Blvd, Elk Grove Village, IL 60009.

4. Parents' Choice, Box 185, Waban, MA 02168. Awards for books, magazines, computer games, television shows, and toys.

5. US Consumer Product Safety Commission (Washington, DC 20207): *Because You Care for Kids* (numerous hazards); *Safety Sampler* (baby equipment and toys); *Super Sitter* (advice to babysitters).

Nutrition

1. Baker S, Henry R: *Boston Children's Hospital Parents' Guide to Nutrition,* Reading, Mass, 1989, Addison-Wesley. Comprehensive, sensible, and usable information on nutritional issues from infancy to adolescence. The authors review the latest research, demystify fad diets, and provide nutritional recommendations. The format is easy to read, and recipes are included.

2. Dietz WH, Stern L, editors: *Guide to Your Child's Nutrition,* New York, 1999, Villard (for the American Academy of Pediatrics). Collaborative effort sponsored by the American Academy of Pediatrics to provide the best nutritional information. Detailed, for newborns to adolescents. Common and uncommon problems. Lots of charts, practical ideas. For the physician or the very interested family.

3. Ikeda J, Naworski P: *Am I Fat? Helping Young Children Accept Differences in Body Size,* Santa Cruz, Calif, 1992, ETR Associates. This perceptive and colorful storybook helps parents and children talk about differences in body sizes and shape. It is easy and fun to read and provides an entry for talking about other kinds of physical differences.

4. Lansky V: *Feed Me: I'm Yours,* Oldhaven, New Jersey, 1996, Simon & Schuster. This long-lasting practical book has an emphasis on feeding toddlers.

5. Piscatella J: *Fat-Proof Your Child,* New York, 1997, Workman Publishing. An in-depth guide for parents that emphasizes parents being the most influential factor on how active and healthy their children will be. Sound advice on diet and exercise. Some parts a bit technical (e.g., figuring out basal metabolic rate).

6. Satter E: *Child of Mine,* Palo Alto, Calif, 1987, Bull. This nutritional guidebook offers information on the developmental and social aspects of feeding from infancy through adolescence. Behaviors that encourage the formation of healthy eating patterns are reviewed, and technical nutrition information is translated into practical and basic concepts.

7. Satter E: *How to Get Your Kid to Eat—But Not Too Much,* Palo Alto, Calif, 1987, Bull. This practical resource shows parents how to help children develop good eating behaviors. It also discusses childhood distortions about eating and feeding that may be precursors to eating disorders in later life.

8. Tamborlane W, editor: *The Yale Guide to Children's Nutrition,* New Haven, 1997, Yale University Press. A comprehensive reference that addresses all aspects of nutrition (e.g., eating disorders, childhood obesity, diabetes, cholesterol, food allergies), using the most current research findings. Reader friendly with charts and tables that provide information on everything from healthy snacks to nutrition for the breast-feeding mother. Good for professionals and parents who like to be well informed.

Sports and Child Development

1. Schreiber LR: *The Parent's Guide to Kids' Sports,* Boston, 1990, Little, Brown & Co. This book provides essential information on the physical, psychological, and social issues in children's sports. Parental involvement, coaching, competition, and girls' participation in sports are emphasized. Exercise, nutrition, and injury prevention are also reviewed. It is a useful guide to the equipment needs, costs, and injuries in common sports. A bibliography and resource list is included.

BOOKS FOR CHILDREN
Developmental and Situational Conflicts

1. Berenstain S, Berenstain J: First Time Books: *The Berenstain Bears: Go to the Doctor; Go to Visit the Dentist; Moving Day; and the Sitter; Get in a Fight; Trouble with Friends; Trouble with Money; and the Messy Room; Learn About Strangers; and Too Much TV; and Too Much Junk Food; Go Out for the Team; and Mama's New Job; Forget their Manners; and the Truth; Get Stage Fright; Trouble at School; in the Dark; and the Bad Habit,* New York, 1981 to 1997, Random House. Inexpensive picture books that highlight some stressful experiences. Written for older toddlers and preschoolers in pleasant and reassuring manner. Available in bookstores and children's stores.

2. Berger T: *I Have Feelings,* New York, 1977, Human Sciences Press. Nice, reflective book for kindergarten through sixth grade. An example of several books that help children to reflect on themselves through another child's eyes.

BOOKS FOR TEENAGERS

1. Edelstein B: *The Women Doctor's Diet for Teenage Girls,* Englewood Cliffs, NJ, 1980, Prentice-Hall. This is a good book for bright parents and their teenage girls from the middle to upper-middle class. The author offers sound guidelines for losing weight tailored to the needs of young women. It is sensitive to issues of body image, junk food, crash diets, and family pressures. Although the book is written for teens, parents (AND CLINICIANS!) may find it helpful.

2. Lindsay JW: *Pregnant Too Soon: Adoption Is an Option,* Buena Park, Calif, 1980, Morning Glory Press. This soft-cover book uses case histories of pregnant teenagers to illustrate the problems of young women who become mothers in their teen years. The author emphasizes the option of adoption, and this book serves as a good resource for pregnant teenagers who want to learn or read more about the process of adoption.

3. Mayle P: *What's Happening to Me?* Secaucus, NJ, 1975, Lyle Stuart. This delightful, slim, inexpensive soft-cover book is described as a guide to puberty and is produced by the same authors who wrote *Where Did I Come From?* With amusing drawings and a brief, compassionate narrative, the authors present various aspects of pubertal development from breasts to erections. This book is probably best suited for those in early adolescence.

4. McCoy K, Wibbelsman C: *The Teenage Body Book,* New York, 1978, Simon & Schuster. This book is based on questions commonly asked by teenagers concerning their bodies and bodily changes. The authors are a former editor of *Teen Magazine* and a physician who specializes in adolescent medicine. The authors cover a wide range of topics, including normal physical development and birth control. Case vignettes and examples of letters from teens are used to illustrate various problems. Detailed line drawings are plentiful and excellent. This book is more appropriate for those in mid to late adolescence; it may be too sophisticated for younger adolescents.

5. Riera M: *Surviving High School,* Berkeley, California, 1997, Celestial Arts Publishing. This book, written for 13- to 20-year-olds, covers all aspects of adolescence—sex, parents, safety, money, and college. The format of teenagers' commentaries intermixed with expla-

nations and questions from a counselor sets a friendly tone. Riera encourages reflections through "think about it" questions at the end of each chapter.

SEX EDUCATION

1. An eight-page annotated **bibliography of books on sex education** (and sibling preparation and rivalry), with age-level recommendations developed by and available from nurse-mother Philothea T Sweet, RN; Obstetrics Clinic, Outpatient Department; University of Minnesota Hospitals; Minneapolis, Minn. A free, annotated resource list of sex-education books is available from the local Planned Parenthood Association. List has separate sections for parents, teens, and children. Free reprints of some articles also available.

2. Gordon S, Gordon J: *Raising a Child Conservatively in a Sexually Permissive World,* New York, 1989, Fireside. This book offers useful guidelines for parents who would like to talk with their children about sexual, social, and moral issues. The author believes that parents have the responsibility to be their children's primary sex educators and that informed children will grow into responsible adults. The format is well organized, and the writing is thoughtful and readable. Sample questions are included in anticipation of a child's curiosity at different developmental stages. This book also provides a comprehensive bibliography with recommendations for parents who want to know more.

3. Harris R: *It's Perfectly Normal: Changing Bodies, Growing up, Sex and Sexual Health,* Cambridge, Mass, 1994, Candlewick Press. A wonderful book for preteens and their parents. Informative, easy to read, accurate, and unbiased. Nice cartoons and illustrations.

4. Maderas L: *What's Happening to My Body? A Book for Girls* (1983) and *What's Happening to My Body? A Book for Boys* (1988); ed 2, New York, New Market Press. Excellent comprehensive books to be read with preadolescents. New edition has information on AIDS and sexually transmitted diseases.

5. Stoppard M: *Sex Ed,* New York, 1997, DK Publishing. In a comic book fashion, Dr. Stoppard debunks myths and encourages safe sex and contraception. A strong emphasis on seeking additional help.

6. Weisman BA, Weisman MH: *What We Told Our Kids About Sex,* San Diego, 1987, Harvest/Harcourt. This concise book offers parents guidelines for sensitive and factual discussion of human sexuality. Recognizing the emotional nature of sexual issues and human values, the authors recommend that parents begin discussing sex and family values before the teenage years. Chapters are designed to be read as background for a discussion or by a preteen.

INTERNET RESOURCES

The Internet offers the opportunity to find information readily and easily. This is a growing avenue to provide parent education, referral, and a lot of valuable information. Caution must be exercised, however, because no overall process for review or oversight exists. Some information may reflect personal or ideological viewpoints that are not mainstream or in line with the goals and values of a family. This must be evaluated for each site. Some services purport to identify legitimate sources of medical information on the Web, but these may not have kept up with the rapid influx of information.

The clinician cannot stop families from getting information from the web. Honest interaction about this issue and joint review of material will help clinicians and parents use the information together. Following are some things to consider that will help the health care provider and a family evaluate Internet advice on a parenting or child care site:

■ **Who is writing the material?** In addition to the name of the author(s), the site should provide the background and credentials of the contributors. These should be highly qualified professionals with specific education and training in the issues on which they write.

■ **The organizational affiliates should all be identified.** These should be mainstream, professional, and official linkages, not just "the author is a member of . . ." Clear distinctions between organizational backing versus individual perspective alone is important.

■ **The site sponsorship should be identified.** Who is paying for site development and oversight? The *.org* address suffix, indicating supposedly non-profit organizational sponsorship, is not a guarantee of legitimacy. Conversely, a *.com* suffix doesn't mean that the material is invalid because of commercial sponsorship. Sometimes these sites have the best material because resources are available to develop and maintain the site at a high level of excellence. For commercially sponsored sites, the commercial components should be explicit ad units, clearly demarcated from the content as one would see in a magazine. The *.edu* designation indicates an educational entity as the base site. These, too, call for scrutiny of content, although commercialization is less likely.

■ **The processes for the development, oversight, and updating of content should be available for review** so that the reader knows how the material is scrutinized before being posted. This gives some assurance that it is not just the views of one individual.

■ **The dating of the material should be stated.** This ensures the timeliness of the information. Archival material can be of great worth, but one should be able to find out how old the material is and how often it is reviewed and updated.

These criteria are similar to those developed for the appraisal of medical information generally as stated in a multidisciplinary conference on the uses of the Web in medical practice.[1-3] Physicians should develop ways to address the use of the Internet in their practices because it probably will have increasing impact on their work.[4]

Families should be encouraged to bring in the material that they get on the Internet for review with the child health care provider. They can look it over together, and sharing of the materials with other families can be facilitated if the material looks good to the clinician. Dismissal of this growing medium as a resource will only result in the hiding of the material from this shared review.

Some sites that offer general parenting and child care advice to parents are listed here:

1. **totalbabycare.com** This site contains an encyclopedia of information about pregnancy to age 3 on development, health and safety, and current news issues; it also has a Q&A section, monthly age-adjusted e-mail newsletters, and a lot of special features. Sponsored by Proctor and Gamble, Pampers division, it brings high level and seasoned professionals and organizations together to provide to provide a wealth of information.

2. **babycenter.com** This site focuses largely on pregnancy and the first year. Many features on this site change daily, including polls, news, games, and the largest baby name reference available. Monitored chat, Q&As, and lots of special features. Well written and reviewed. Webby award winner: "Best on the Web" several years in a row.
3. **parenttime.com** A Time/Warner production, this contains a lot of material from several sources, much of it archived. Under renovation at the time of this review.
4. **parentsoup.com** Lots of good things here from a lot of different perspectives. Needs some wading through. Parent and professional contributions. Quality varies widely.
5. **aap.org** The American Academy of Pediatrics site, contains abstracts from *Pediatrics*, AAP policy statements, and important news that affects children, families, and clinicians who provide care for children and adolescents.

Other sites may be identified through search engines by using *parenting, healthcare, newborn, child health, child development,* and *baby care* in a search. Sites that deal with specialty information can be searched through identification by the term or professional organization.

REFERENCES

1. Silberg W, Lunberg G, Musacchio R: Assessing, controlling and assuring the quality of medical information on the Internet, *JAMA* 277:1244, 1997.
2. Rippen H: Criteria for assessing the quality of health information on the Internet. At: http://www.mitretek.org/hiti/showcase/documents/criteria.html.
3. Lamp JM, Howard PA: Guiding parents' use of the Internet for newborn education, *MCN* 24:33, 1999.
4. Blumenthal D: The future of quality measurement and management in a transforming health care system, *JAMA* 278:1622, 1997.

ADDITIONAL READING ABOUT THE USE OF INTERNET RESOURCES IN MEDICAL PRACTICE

Hancock L: *Physicians' guide to the internet,* Philadelphia, 1996, Lippincott-Raven.
Kiley R: *Medical information on the internet,* New York, 1998, Churchill Livingstone.
Smith RP, Edwards MJA: *The internet for physicians,* New York, 1997, Springer.

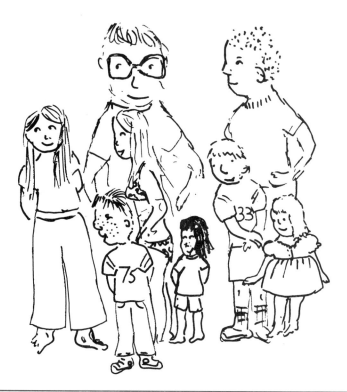

"My family." By a girl, age 13. The profiles, perspectives in arrangement, and lots of detail testify to some sophisticated drawing skills.

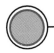

APPENDIX

Section I: Screening Checklists as Aids to Interview

A basic principle of this book is that the acquisition of information about development, behavior, and family function is acquired optimally from interviewing children, youth, and parents. Many clinicians have discovered the benefits of selected screening checklists as a way to supplement or focus the clinical interview. These tests, when administered before seeing a child, can trigger questions, raise issues, and prevent omissions in data collection.

Every assessment is an interaction between the examiner and the child. It is influenced by the state, temperament, and availability of the child, as well as the training, ease, skill, and style of the examiner. The results of screening tests must always be interpreted with these factors in mind. They should never be a substitute for face-to-face clinical encounters in primary care practice. Screening tests serve as an adjunct, a time saver, and a structure on which to focus behavioral and developmental concerns.

REFERENCES

Glascoe FP: Developmental screening. In Wolraich ML: *Disorders of development and learning,* ed 2, St. Louis, 1996, Mosby, pp 89-128.

Blackman JA: Developmental screening: infant, toddler and preschooler. In Levine MD, Carey WB, Crocker AC: *Developmental-behavioral pediatrics,* ed 3, Philadelphia, 1993, WB Saunders, pp 689-695.

TABLE A-1 ■ **Standardized Developmental-Behavioral Screening Instruments**

Tool, Source & Price	Age Range	Description	Scoring	Accuracy	Time Frame
Child Development Inventories (formerly Minnesota Child Development Inventories), 1992. Behavior Science Systems, Bx 580274, Minneapolis, MN 55458 (ph: 612-929-6220) ($41.00 +s/h)	3-72 mo	Three separate instruments, each with 60 yes/no descriptions. Can be mailed to families, completed in waiting rooms, administered by interview or by direct elicitation.	A single cutoff tied to 1.5 standard deviations below the mean	Sensitivity in detecting children with difficulties is greater than 75% (across studies), and specificity in correctly detecting normal development is 70% (across studies).	About 10 min
Parents' Evaluations of Developmental Status (PEDS), 1997. Ellsworth & Vandermeer Press, Ltd. 4405 Scenic Dr., Nashville, TN, 37204 (ph: 615-386-0061/fax: 615-386-0346) http://edge.net/~evpress ($30.00 +s/h)	Birth to 8 years	Ten questions eliciting parents' concerns. Can be administered in waiting rooms or by interview in Spanish and English. Determines when to refer, provide a second screen, counsel, reassure, or carefully monitor development, behavior, and academic progress.	Identifies levels of risk for various kinds of emotional and developmental problems and delays	Sensitivity ranges from 74% to 79%, and specificity ranges from 70% to 80% across age levels.	About 2 min

Ages and Stages Questionnaire (formerly Infant Monitoring System), 1994. Paul H. Brookes Publishers, P.O. Bx 10624, Baltimore, MD 21285 (ph: 800-638-3775) ($130.00 +s/h)	0-60 mo	Clear drawings and simple directions help parents report on children's skills. Separate copyable forms of 30 items for each age range (tied to well-child visit schedule). Can be used in mass mailings for child-find programs.	Single pass/fail score	Sensitivity ranges from 70% to 90% at all ages except the 4-month level, and specificity ranges from 75% to 91%.	About 7 min
Pediatric Symptom Checklist, Jellinek MS, Murphy JM, Robinson J et al: Pediatric Symptom Checklist: Screening school age children for psychosocial dysfunction, *J Pediatr* 112:201, 1988 (Test is included in the article.)	4-16 yrs	Thirty-five short statements of problem behaviors including both externalizing (conduct) and internalizing (depression, anxiety, adjustment, etc). Ratings of never, sometimes, or often are assigned a value of 0, 1, and 2, and scores above cutoffs indicate when referrals are needed.	Single refer/nonrefer score	All but one study showed high sensitivity (80%-95%) but somewhat scattered specificity (68%-100%).	About 7 min
Denver II (1990), Denver Developmental Materials (DDM), PO Box 6169, Denver, CO 80206 (ph: 303-355-4729)	0-6 yr	Administered by trained person, who asks parent questions and assesses child's skills in motor, language, and social domains. A helpful visual aid of a child's development for parents. Helps to clarify concerns. Gives a structure for observation.	Scoring chart with bar graphs that display 25th to 90th percentile for each milestone; produces a single score—normal, suspect and untestable.	It is not meant to predict specific developmental conditions. Rather, the validity is based on its accuracy to detect the normal range of each developmental milestone.	20 min

Modified with permission from Glascoe FP: *Collaborating with parents*, Nashville, Tenn 1998, Ellsworth & Vandermeer.

TEMPERAMENT (see Chapter 2)

Examples of selected questionnaires from Carey scales follow.

Carey Infant Temperament Scale

Using the scale below, please mark the space that tells how often the infant's recent and current behavior has been like the behavior described by each item.

1. almost never
2. rarely
3. variable, usually not
4. variable, usually does
5. frequently
6. almost always

1. The infant is fussy on waking up and going to sleep (frowns, cries). 1 2 3 4 5 6
2. The infant plays with a toy for under a minute and then looks for another toy or activity. 1 2 3 4 5 6
3. The infant plays continuously for more than 10 minutes at a time with a favorite toy. 1 2 3 4 5 6
4. The infant indicates discomfort (fusses or squirms) when diaper is soiled with bowel movement. 1 2 3 4 5 6
5. The infant lies quietly in the bath. 1 2 3 4 5 6
6. The infant objects to being bathed in a different place or by a different person, even after 2 or 3 tries. 1 2 3 4 5 6
7. The infant is pleasant (coos, smiles, etc.) during procedures like hair brushing or face washing. 1 2 3 4 5 6
8. The infant continues to cry in spite of several minutes of soothing. 1 2 3 4 5 6
9. The infant adjusts easily and sleeps well within 1 or 2 days with changes of time or place. 1 2 3 4 5 6
10. The infant cries for less than one minute when given an injection. 1 2 3 4 5 6
11. The infant shows much body movement (kicks, waves arms) when crying. 1 2 3 4 5 6

Middle Childhood Temperament Questionnaire

Using the scale below, please mark the space that tells how often the child's recent and current behavior has been like the behavior described by each item.

1. almost never
2. rarely
3. variable, usually not
4. variable, usually does
5. frequently
6. almost always

1. Runs to get where he/she wants to go.	1 2 3 4 5 6
2. Avoids (stays away from, doesn't talk to) a new sitter on first meeting.	1 2 3 4 5 6
3. Easily excited by praise	1 2 3 4 5 6
4. Frowns or complains when asked by parent to do a chore	1 2 3 4 5 6
5. Notices (looks toward) minor changes in lighting (changes in shadows, turning on lights, etc.)	1 2 3 4 5 6
6. Loses interest in a new toy or game the same day he/she gets it.	1 2 3 4 5 6

From: Behavioral-Developmental Initiatives, 14636 N. 55th Street, Scottsdale, AZ 85254 (ph: 800-405-2313; website www.b-di.com). Temperament scales available for early infancy (EITQ), infancy (RITQ), toddler (TTS), 3-7 years old (BSQ), and middle childhood (MCTQ).

Pervasive Developmental Disorder Screening Test
Stage One—Primary Care Screening

©1994 Bryna Siegel, Ph.D., University of California, San Francisco

Name of child _____ Today's date _____

Age in months _____   Sex   M/F

Directions: Fill in answers to show any difficulty you may have experienced with your child up to now. Answer the questions to show what is most often true about your child, not 'best' or 'worst'.

	Usually true YES	Usually false NO
Did your baby avoid playing with dolls or stuffed animals, or even seem to dislike them?	____	____
Did your baby have a hard time getting used to playing with new toys, or playing new games, even though he might enjoy them once he got used to them?	____	____
Did your baby seem uninterested in learning to talk?	____	____
Did you feel afraid because your baby seemed unafraid or unaware of things that were dangerous?	____	____
At times, did you get upset because your baby didn't seem to care if you were there or not?	____	____
Did your baby's mood sometimes change all of a sudden for no real reason?	____	____
Did your toddler usually enjoy being tickled or being chased, but did not usually enjoy playing patty-cake or peek-a-boo?	____	____
Did people ever say that your toddler seemed more solemn or serious than others of the same age?	____	____
Could your child do some things so well that it surprised you when he couldn't do other things?	____	____

PDDST-Stage One-Primary Care Screening

	Usually true YES	Usually false NO
Did your child prefer things he could play with the same way, over and over, such as a "See 'n'Say" (a pull-the-string toy, or toys with buttons he could push (such as a toy telephone or typewriter)?	——	——
Did your child only seem to understand only part of what was said to him?	——	——
Did it seem that your child could pretty much understand what you said but usually would not follow directions?	——	——
Did your child understand most or all of what was said to him, but did not yet say any, or more than a few words?	——	——
Did your child only try to communicate when there was something he wanted and couldn't get for himself?	——	——
Would your child lead you to a desired object as his way of showing you what he wanted?	——	——
Did your child try to get away with using as few words as possible? (For example, saying "Juice" for anything he wanted to eat?) Write N/A if he did not talk at this age.	——	——
Up to this age, had your child ever gone through a time when he stopped using words he once used?	——	——
Did your child seem like he couldn't keep track of his arms and legs? For example, did he stand or carry himself awkwardly, or bump into things; and you didn't know any reason he should act like this?	——	——
Total for all Stage I questions (co=3)	——	——

Page 2 of 2

Pervasive Developmental Disorder Screening Test
Stage Two-Developmental Disorders Clinic Screening

©1994 Bryna Siegel, Ph.D., University of California, San Francisco

Name of child _____ Today's date _____

Age in months _____ Sex   M/F

Directions: Fill in answers to show any difficulty you may have experienced with your child up to now. Answer the questions to show what is most often true about your child, not 'best' or 'worst'.

	Usually true YES	Usually false NO
Did your baby only sleep for short bouts, or show a great deal of unpredictability in sleep patterns?	____	____
Did your baby sometimes stare or tune out, making it hard to get his attention?	____	____
Did your baby either ignore toys most of the time, or play almost all the time with one or two things?	____	____
Did your baby's mood sometimes change all of a sudden for no real reason?	____	____
Did your baby seem uninterested in learning to talk?	____	____
Did your baby usually enjoy being tickled or being chased, but did not usually enjoy playing patty-cake or peek-a-boo?	____	____
Did your child cry when you left, but seemed not to notice when you returned?	____	____
Did your child often seem to understand only part of what was said to him? (For example, was it hard to tell if he was disobeying, or just not understanding you?)	____	____

Page 1 of 2

PDDST-Stage Two-Developmental Disorders Clinic Screening

	Usually true YES	Usually false NO
Did your child like things he could play with the same way, over and over, such as "See 'n'Say" (a pull-the-string toy) or toys with buttons he could push (such as a toy telephone or typewriter)?	——	——
Did your child seem exceptionally independent, only coming to get you if there was something he wanted and couldn't get for himself?	——	——
Had you worried that your child didn't seem too interested in other children?	——	——
Did your child seem unusually interested in mechanical things, such as light switches, door latches, locks, fans, vacuums, or clocks?	——	——
Was your child mostly uninterested in watching TV, or only liked things a child his age wouldn't watch—like adult music videos, certain game shows, or certain commercials?	——	——
Did your child not yet imagine make-believe people and actions when he played?	——	——
Had you ever worried that your child couldn't see well because he held things very close to his eyes and looked at them closely for a long time?	——	——
Does your child seem very tuned in to order and neatness when he plays? For example, does he like to line things up, or sort things by category over and over, or insist on putting things away when finished?	——	——
When excited, does you child flap his hands or fingers?	——	——
Total for all Stage II questions (co=4).	——	——

Page 2 of 2

Pervasive Developmental Disorder Screening Test
Stage Three-Autistic Spectrum Disorders Screening

©1994 Bryna Siegel, Ph.D., University of California, San Francisco

Name of child _____ Today's date _____

Age in months _____ Sex   M/F

Directions: Fill in answers to show any difficulty you may have experienced with your child up to now. Answer the questions to show what is most often true about your child, not 'best' or 'worst'.

	Usually true YES	Usually false NO
Did your baby sometimes stare or tune out, making it hard to get his attention?	____	____
Did your baby either ignore toys most of the time, or play all of the time with one or two things?	____	____
Did your baby ever seem bored or uninterested in conversations around him?	____	____
Did your baby often stare at his own hands or fingers, perhaps turning them over at times?	____	____
When you were trying to get your baby's attention, did you ever feel that your baby would avoid looking right at you?	____	____
Did your baby's mood sometimes change all of a sudden for no real reason?	____	____
Did your child usually enjoy being tickled or being chased, but did not usually enjoy playing patty-cake or peek-a-boo?	____	____
Did people ever say that your toddler seemed more solemn or serious than others of the same age?	____	____
Did your child often cry when you left, but seem not to notice you much when you returned?	____	____

PDDST-Stage Three-Autistic Spectrum Disorders Screening

	Usually true YES	Usually false NO
Did your child seem particularly fascinated by motion? For example, would he flip pages of a book, sift sand, spin objects, or watch running water just to see the movement?	——	——
Did your child often seem to understand only part of what was said to him? (For example, was it hard to tell if he was disobeying, or just not understanding you?)	——	——
Had you worried that your child didn't seem too interested in other children?	——	——
Was your child mostly uninterested in watching TV, or only liked things a child his age usually wouldn't watch—like adult music videos, certain game shows or even certain TV commercials?	——	——
Did your child seem unable to learn to do things through watching and copying others (like catching a ball or swinging on a swing)?	——	——
Does you child play with toys in ways that aren't really the main way the toy was meant to be used?	——	——
When excited, does you child flap his hands or fingers?	——	——
Total for all Stage III questions (co=6).	——	——

Page 2 of 2

Siegel B: *The world of the autistic child*, New York, 1996, Oxford University Press.

PEDS RESPONSE FORM

Child's Name _Billy Morris_   Parent's Name _Linda Morris_

Child's Birthday _4/17/94_   Child's Age _3_   Today's Date _4/27/97_

1. Please list any concerns about your child's learning, development, and behavior.

As I said, I don't think he talks as well as he should for his age. Otherwise, he's just a great little boy, very loving, watches everything carefully. Figures things out quickly. Very bright!

2. Do you have any concerns about how your child talks and makes speech sounds?

Circle one: No   Yes   (A little)   COMMENTS:

He's kind of quiet and doesn't say very much. Seems to prefer watching to interacting.

3. Do you have any concerns about how your child understands what you say?

Circle one: (No)   Yes   A little   COMMENTS:

4. Do you have any concerns about how your child uses his or her hands and fingers to do things?

Circle one: (No)   Yes   A little   COMMENTS:

5. Do you have any concerns about how your child uses his or her arms and legs?

Circle one: (No)   Yes   A little   COMMENTS:

6. Do you have any concerns about how your child behaves?

Circle one: (No)   Yes   A little   COMMENTS:

7. Do you have any concerns about how your child gets along with others?

Circle one: (No)   Yes   A little   COMMENTS:

8. Do you have any concerns about how your child is learning to do things for himself/herself?

Circle one: (No)   Yes   A little   COMMENTS:

9. Do you have any concerns about how your child is learning preschool or school skills?

Circle one: (No)   Yes   A little   COMMENTS:

10. Please list any other concerns.

None

The PEDS developmental screening instrument is accompanied by a recording page that displays results at different exams throughout childhood. A third page of the test scores the exam and guides the clinician in consideration of retesting, observation, consultation, or referral.

	YES	SOMETIMES	NOT YET

COMMUNICATION   *Be sure to try each activity with your child.*

1. If you call to your baby when you are out of sight, does he look in the direction of your voice? ☐ ☐ ☐ ____

2. When a loud noise occurs, does your baby turn to see where the sound came from? ☐ ☐ ☐ ____

3. If you copy the sounds your baby makes, does your baby repeat the same sounds back to you? ☐ ☐ ☐ ____

4. Does your baby make sounds like "da," "ga," "ka," and "ba"? ☐ ☐ ☐ ____

5. Does your baby respond to the tone of your voice and stop her activity at least briefly when you say "no-no" to her? ☐ ☐ ☐ ____

6. Does your baby make two similar sounds like "ba-ba," "da-da," or "ga-ga"? (He may say these sounds without referring to any particular object or person.) ☐ ☐ ☐ ____

COMMUNICATION TOTAL ____

GROSS MOTOR   *Be sure to try each activity with your child.*

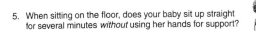

1. When you put her on the floor, does your baby lean on her hands while sitting? (If she already sits up straight without leaning on her hands, check "yes" for this item.) ☐ ☐ ☐ ____

2. Does your baby roll from his back to his tummy, getting both arms out from under him? ☐ ☐ ☐ ____

3. Does your baby get into a crawling position by getting up on her hands and knees? ☐ ☐ ☐ ____

4. If you hold both hands just to balance him, does your baby support his own weight while standing? ☐ ☐ ☐ ____

5. When sitting on the floor, does your baby sit up straight for several minutes *without* using her hands for support? ☐ ☐ ☐ ____ *

6. When you stand him next to furniture or the crib rail, does your baby hold on without leaning his chest against the furniture for support? ☐ ☐ ☐ ____

GROSS MOTOR TOTAL ____

If gross motor item 5 is marked "yes" or "sometimes," mark gross motor item 1 as "yes."

 ASQ   **8 months**

	YES	SOMETIMES	NOT YET

FINE MOTOR   *Be sure to try each activity with your child.*

1. Does your baby reach for a crumb or Cheerio and touch it with her finger or hand? (If she already picks up a small object, check "yes" for this item.)   ❏ ❏ ❏ ___

2. Does your baby pick up a small toy, holding it in the center of his hand with his fingers around it?   ❏ ❏ ❏ ___

3. Does your baby *try* to pick up a crumb or Cheerio by using her thumb and all her fingers in a raking motion, even if she isn't able to pick it up? (If she already picks up a crumb or Cheerio, check "yes" for this item.)   ❏ ❏ ❏ ___

4. Does your baby pick up small toys with only one hand?   ❏ ❏ ❏ ___

5. Does your baby *successfully* pick up a crumb or Cheerio by using his thumb and all his fingers in a raking motion? (If he already picks up a crumb or Cheerio, check "yes" for this item.)   ❏ ❏ ❏ ___

6. Does your baby pick up a small toy with the *tips* of her thumb and fingers? (You should see a space between the toy and her palm.)   ❏ ❏ ❏ ___*

FINE MOTOR TOTAL ___

If fine motor item 6 is marked "yes" or "sometimes," mark fine motor item 2 as "yes."

PROBLEM SOLVING   *Be sure to try each activity with your child.*

1. Does your baby pick up a toy and put it in his mouth?   ❏ ❏ ❏ ___

2. When she is on her back, does your baby try to get a toy she has dropped if she can see it?   ❏ ❏ ❏ ___

3. Does your baby play by banging a toy up and down against the floor or table?   ❏ ❏ ❏ ___

4. Does your baby pass a toy back and forth from one hand to the other?   ❏ ❏ ❏ ___

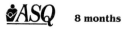 **8 months**

	YES	SOMETIMES	NOT YET

PROBLEM SOLVING *(continued)*

5. Does your baby pick up two small toys, one in each hand, and hold onto them for about 1 minute? ☐ ☐ ☐ ____

6. When holding a toy in his hand, does your baby bang it against another toy on the table? ☐ ☐ ☐ ____

PROBLEM SOLVING TOTAL ____

PERSONAL-SOCIAL   *Be sure to try each activity with your child.*

1. While lying on her back, does your baby play by grabbing her foot? ☐ ☐ ☐ ____

2. When in front of a large mirror, does your baby reach out to pat the mirror? ☐ ☐ ☐ ____

3. Does your baby try to get a toy that is out of reach? (He may roll, pivot on his tummy, or crawl to get it.) ☐ ☐ ☐ ____

4. While on her back, does your baby put her foot in her mouth? ☐ ☐ ☐ ____

5. Does your baby drink water, juice, or formula from a cup while you hold it? ☐ ☐ ☐ ____

6. Does your baby feed himself a cracker or a cookie? ☐ ☐ ☐ ____

PERSONAL-SOCIAL TOTAL ____

OVERALL   *Parents and providers may use the bottom of the next sheet for additional comments.*

1. Do you think your child hears well?   YES ☐   NO ☐

   If no, explain: _____

2. Does your baby use both hands equally well?   YES ☐   NO ☐

   If no, explain: _____

3. When you help your baby stand, are her feet flat on the surface most of the time?   YES ☐   NO ☐

   If no, explain: _____

 ASQ   **8 months**

OVERALL *(continued)*

4. Does either parent have any family history of childhood deafness or hearing impairment? YES ☐ NO ☐

   If yes, explain: _____

5. Has your child had any medical problems in the last several months? YES ☐ NO ☐

   If yes, explain: _____

6. Does anything about your child worry you? YES ☐ NO ☐

   If yes, explain: _____

 8 months

BOX A-1	PEDIATRIC SYMPTOM CHECKLIST: SCREENING FOR PSYCHOSOCIAL PROBLEMS

Mark Under the heading that best fits your child.

	Never (0)	Sometimes (1)	Often (2)
Complains of aches and pains			
Spends more time alone			
Tires easily, little energy			
Fidgety, unable to sit still			
Has trouble with a teacher			
Less interested in school			
Acts as if driven by a motor			
Daydreams too much			
Distracted easily			
Is afraid of new situations			
Feels sad, unhappy			
Is irritable, angry			
Feels hopeless			
Has trouble concentrating			
Less interest in friends			
Fights with other children			
Absent from school			
School grades dropping			

A cumulative score ≥28 suggests the need for evaluation for a significant behavioral problem.
From Jellinek M, Murphy JM: Screening for psychosocial disorders in pediatric practice, *Am J Dis Child*, 142:1153-1157, 1988. Used by permission.

Continued

BOX A-1	PEDIATRIC SYMPTOM CHECKLIST: SCREENING FOR PSYCHOSOCIAL PROBLEMS—cont'd

Mark Under the heading that best fits your child.

	Never (0)	Sometimes (1)	Often (2)
Is down on him or herself			
Visits doctor with doctor finding nothing wrong			
Has trouble with sleeping			
Worries a lot			
Wants to be with you more than before			
Feels he or she is bad			
Takes unnecessary risks			
Gets hurt frequently			
Seems to be having less fun			
Acts younger than children his or her age			
Does not listen to rules			
Does not show feelings			
Does not understand other people's feelings			
Teases others			
Blames others for his or her troubles			
Takes things that do not belong to him/her			
Refuses to share			

A cumulative score ≥28 suggests the need for evaluation for a significant behavioral problem.
From Jellinek M, Murphy JM: Screening for psychosocial disorders in pediatric practice, *Am J Dis Child*, 142:1153-1157, 1988. Used by permission.

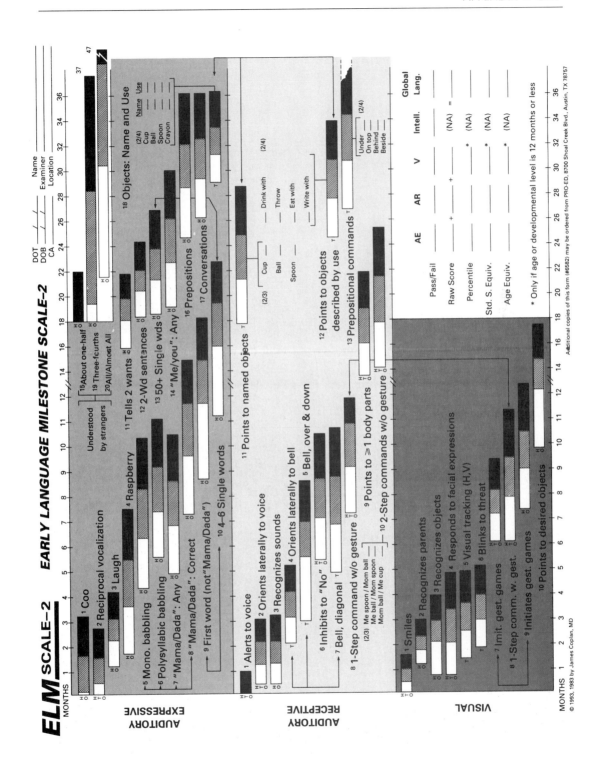

Additional copies of this form (#6582) may be ordered from PRO-ED, 8700 Shoal Creek Blvd., Austin, TX 78757

AR 3. H: Does baby seem to respond in a specific way to certain sounds (becomes excited at hearing parents' voices, etc.)?

AR 4. T: Sit facing baby, with baby in parent's lap. Extend both arms so that your hands are behind baby's field of vision and at the level of baby's waist. Ring a 2"-diameter bell, first with 1 hand, then the other. Repeat 2 or 3 times if necessary. Pass if baby turns head to the side at least once.

AR 5. T: See note for AR 4. Pass if baby turns head first to the side, then down, to localize bell, at least once. (Automatically passes AR 4.)

AR 6. H: Does baby understand the command "no" (even though he may not always obey)? T: Test by commanding "(Baby's name), no!" while baby is playing with any test object. Pass if baby temporarily inhibits his actions.

AR 7. T: See note for AR 4. Pass if baby turns directly down on diagonal to localize bell, at least once. (Automatically passes AR 5 and AR 4.)

AR 8. H: Will your baby follow any verbal commands without you indicating by gestures when it is you want him to do ("Stop" "Come here" "Give me" etc.)? T: Wait until baby is playing with any test object, then say "(Baby's name), give it to me." Pass if baby extends object to you, even if baby seems to change his mind and take the object back. May repeat command 1 or 2 times. If failed, repeat the command but this time hold out your hand for the object. If baby responds, then pass item V 8 (1-step command with gesture).

AR 9. H: Does your child point to at least 1 body part on command? T: Have mother command baby "Show me your..." or "Where's your...." without pointing to the desired part herself.

AR 10. H: "Can child do 2 things in a row if asked? For example 'First go get your shoes, then sit down'? T: Set out ball, cup, and spoon, and say "(Child's name), give me the spoon, then give the ball to mommy." Use slow, steady voice but do not break command into 2 separate sentences. If no response, then give each half of command separately to see if child understands separate components. If child succeeds on at least half of command, then give each of the following:" "(Child's name), give me the ball and give mommy the spoon." May repeat once but do not break into 2 commands. Then "Give mommy the ball, then give me the cup." Pass if at least two 2-step commands executed correctly. (Note: Child is credited even if the order of execution of a command is reversed.)

AR 11. T: Place a cup, ball, and spoon on the table. Command child "Show me/where is/give me.... the cup/ball/spoon." (If command is "Give me," be sure to replace each object before asking about the next object.) Pass = 2 items correctly identified.

AR 12. T: Put cup, ball, spoon, and crayon on table and give command "Show me/where is/give me... the one we drink with/eat with/draw (color, write) with/throw (play with)." If the command "Give me" is used, be sure to replace each object before asking about the next object. Pass = 2 or more objects correctly identified.

AR 13. T: Put out cup (upside down) and a 1" cube. Command the child "Put the block under the cup." Repeat 1 or 2 times if necessary. If no attempt, or if incorrect response, then demonstrate correct response, saying, "See, now the block is under the cup." Remove the block and hand it to the child. Then give command "Put the block on top of the cup." If child makes no response, then repeat command 1 time but do not demonstrate. Then command "Put the block behind the cup," then "Put the block beside the cup." Pass = 2 or more commands correctly executed (prior to demonstration by examiner, if "under" is scored).

IV. Visual

V 1. H: "Does your baby smile—not just a gas bubble or a burp but a real smile?" T: Have parent attempt to elicit smile by any means.

V 2. H: "Does your baby seem to recognize you, reacting differently to you than to the sight of other people? For example, does your baby smile more quickly for you than for other people?"

V 3. H: "Does your baby seem to recognize any common objects by sight? For example, if bottle or spoon fed, what happens when bottle or spoon is brought into view before it touches baby's lips?" Pass if baby gets visibly excited, or opens mouth in anticipation of feeding.

V 4. H: "Does your baby respond to your facial expressions?" T: Engage baby's gaze and attempt to elicit a smile by smiling and talking to baby. Then scowl at baby. Pass if any change in baby's facial expression.

V 5. T: Horizontal (H): Engage child's gaze with yours at a distance of 18". Move slowly back and forth. Pass if child turns head 60° to left and right from midline. Vertical (V): Move slowly up and down. Pass if child elevates eyes 30° from horizontal. Must pass both H & V to pass item.

V 6. T: Flick your fingers rapidly towards child's face, ending with fingertips 1-2" from face. Do not touch face or eyelashes. Pass if child blinks.

V 7. H: Does child play pat-a-cake, peek-a-boo, etc., in response to parents?

V 8. T: See note for AR 8 (always try AR 8 first; if AR 8 is passed, then automatically give credit for V 8).

V 9. H: Does child spontaneously initiate gesture games?

V 10. H: "Does child ever point with index finger to something he/she wants? For example, if child is sitting at the dinner table and wants something that is out of reach, how does child let you know what he/she wants?" Pass only index finger pointing not reaching with whole hand.

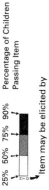

I. General Instructions

25% 50% 75% 90% Percentage of Children Passing Item

Item may be elicited by
H = History
T = Direct Testing
O = Incidental Observation

• Always start with H, where allowed.
• Child passes item if passed by any of the allowable means of elicitation for that item.
• Basal = 3 consecutive items passed (work down from age line).
• Ceiling = 3 consecutive items failed (work up from age line).

II. Auditory Expressive (AE)

A. Content

AE 1. H: Makes prolonged musical vowel sounds in a sing-song fashion (ooo, aaa, etc.), not just grunts or squeaks.

AE 2. H: Does baby watch speaker's face and appear to listen intently, then vocalize when the speaker is quiet? Can you "have a conversation" with your baby?

AE 4. H: Blows bubbles or gives "Bronx cheer"?

AE 5. H: Makes isolated sounds such as "ba," "da," "ga," "goo," etc.

AE 6. H: Makes repetitive string of sounds: "babababa," or "lalalalala," etc.

AE 7. H: Says "mama" or "dada" but uses them at other times besides just labelling parents.

AE 8. H: Child spontaneously, consistently, and correctly uses "mama" or "dada," just to label the appropriate parent.

AE 9, AE 10, AE 13. H: Child spontaneously, consistently, and correctly uses words. Do not count "mama," "dada," or the names of other family members or pets.

AE 11. H: Uses single words to tell you what he/she wants. "Milk!" "Cookie!" "More!" etc. Pass = 2 or more wants. List specific words.

AE 12. H: Spontaneous, novel 2-word combinations ("Want cookie" "No bed" "See daddy" etc.) Not rotely learned phrases that have been specifically taught to the child or combinations that are really single thoughts (e.g., "hot dog").

AE 14. H: Child uses "me" or "you" but may reverse them ("you want cookie" instead of "me want cookie," etc.)

AE 17. H: "Can child put 2 or 3 sentences together to hold brief conversations?"

AE 18. T: Put out cup, ball, crayon, & spoon. Pick up cup & say "What is this? What do we do with it? (What is it for?)" Child must name the object and give its use. Pass = "drink with," etc., not "milk" or "juice." Ball: Pass = "throw," "play with," etc. Spoon: Pass = "Eat" or "Eat with," etc. not "Food," "Lunch." Crayon: Pass = "Write (with)," "Color (with)," etc. Pass item if child gives name and use for 2 objects.

B. Intelligibility

AE 15, AE 19, AE 20. T: "How clear is your child's speech? That is, how much of your child's speech can a stranger understand?"

—Less than one-half
—About one-half (AE 15)
—Three-fourths (AE 19)
—All or Almost All (AE 20)

Pick one (H, O)

To score:
If less than one-half: Fail all 3 items in cluster.
If about one-half: Pass AE 15 only.
If three-fourths: Pass AE 19 and AE 15.
If all or almost all: Pass all 3 items in cluster.

III. Auditory Receptive (AR)

AR 1. H, T: Any behavioral change in response to noise (eye blink, startle, change in movements or respiration, etc.)

AR 2. H, T: What does baby do when parent starts talking while out of sight? Pass if any shift of head or eyes to voice.

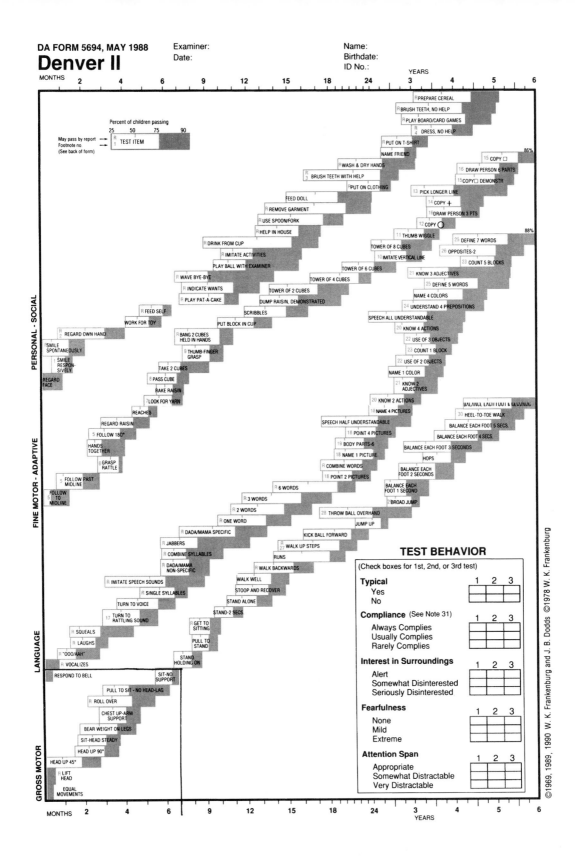

DIRECTIONS FOR ADMINISTRATION

1. Try to get child to smile by smiling, talking or waving. Do not touch him/her.
2. Child must stare at hand several seconds.
3. Parent may help guide toothbrush and put toothpaste on brush.
4. Child does not have to be able to tie shoes or button/zip in the back.
5. Move yarn slowly in an arc from one side to the other, about 8" above child's face.
6. Pass if child grasps rattle when it is touched to the backs or tips of fingers.
7. Pass if child tries to see where yarn went. Yarn should be dropped quickly from sight from tester's hand without arm movement.
8. Child must transfer cube from hand to hand without help of body, mouth, or table.
9. Pass if child picks up raisin with any part of thumb and finger.
10. Line can vary only 30 degrees or less from tester's line.
11. Make a fist with thumb pointing upward and wiggle only the thumb. Pass if child imitates and does not move any fingers other than the thumb.

12. Pass any enclosed form. Fail continuous round motions.

13. Which line is longer? (Not bigger.) Turn paper upside down and repeat. (pass 3 of 3 or 5 of 6)

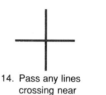

14. Pass any lines crossing near midpoint.

15. Have child copy first. If failed, demonstrate.

    When giving items 12, 14, and 15, do not name the forms. Do not demonstrate 12 and 14.

16. When scoring, each pair (2 arms, 2 legs, etc.) counts as one part.
17. Place one cube in cup and shake gently near child's ear, but out of sight. Repeat for other ear.
18. Point to picture and have child name it. (No credit is given for sounds only.)
    If less than 4 pictures are named correctly, have child point to picture as each is named by tester.

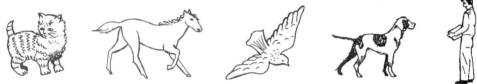

19. Using doll, tell child: Show me the nose, eyes, ears, mouth, hands, feet, tummy, hair. Pass 6 of 8.
20. Using pictures, ask child: Which one flies?... says meow?... talks?... barks?... gallops? Pass 2 of 5, 4 of 5.
21. Ask child: What do you do when you are cold?... tired?... hungry? Pass 2 of 3, 3 of 3.
22. Ask child: What do you do with a cup? What is a chair used for? What is a pencil used for? Action words must be included in answers.
23. Pass if child correctly places and says how many blocks are on paper. (1, 5).
24. Tell child: Put block **on** table; **under** table; **in front of** me, **behind** me. Pass 4 of 4. (Do not help child by pointing, moving head or eyes.)
25. Ask child: What is a ball?... lake?... desk?... house?... banana?... curtain?... fence?... ceiling? Pass if defined in terms of use, shape, what it is made of, or general category (such as banana is fruit, not just yellow). Pass 5 of 8, 7 of 8.
26. Ask child: If a horse is big, a mouse is __? If fire is hot, ice is __? If the sun shines during the day, the moon shines during the __? Pass 2 of 3.
27. Child may use wall or rail only, not person. May not crawl.
28. Child must throw ball overhand 3 feet to within arm's reach of tester.
29. Child must perform standing broad jump over width of test sheet (8 1/2 inches).
30. Tell child to walk forward, ⚯⚯⚯⚯➤ heel within 1 inch of toe. Tester may demonstrate. Child must walk 4 consecutive steps.
31. In the second year, half of normal children are non-compliant.

OBSERVATIONS:

DENVER PRESCREENING DEVELOPMENTAL QUESTIONNAIRE II

(PDQ-II)

0-9 MONTHS

Child's Name _____

Person Completing PDQ-II _____

Relation to Child _____

For Office Use			
Today's Date	___ yr	___ mo	___ day
Child's Birthdate	___ yr	___ mo	___ day
Subtract to get Child's Exact Age	___ yr	___ mo	___ day
PDQII Age:			___ completed wks

CONTINUE ANSWERING UNTIL 3 "NOs" ARE CIRCLED

1. Equal Movements
When your baby is lying on his back, can he move each of his arms as easily as the other and each of his legs as easily as the other? Circle **NO** if your baby makes jerky or uncoordinated movements with one or both of his arms or legs.   **YES   NO**

For Office Use 90% 75%		
0	0	GM

2. Responds to Sounds
Does your baby respond (with eye movements, change in breathing or other change in activity) to a new sound outside his line of vision?   **YES   NO**

0	0	L

3. Regards Face
When your baby is lying on her back, does she look at you and watch your face?   **YES   NO**

0	0	PS

4. Vocalizes
Does your baby make sounds other than crying, such as uh, eh or cooing?   **YES   NO**

0-3	0	L

5. Smiles Responsively
When you smile and talk to your baby, does he smile back at you?   **YES   NO**

1-2	1	PS

6. Head Up 45 Degrees
When your baby is on her stomach on a flat surface, can she lift her head at least as far as this picture?   **YES   NO**

2-3	1-3	GM

7. "Ooo"/"Aaa"
Does your baby make vowel sounds such as "ooo" or "aaa"?   **YES   NO**

2-3	1-2	L

---

8. Head Up 90 Degrees
When your baby is on her stomach on a flat surface, can she lift her head and chest to look straight ahead like this picture?   **YES   NO**

For Office Use 90% 75%		
3-2	2-3	GM

9. Hands Together
Does your baby play with his hands by touching them together?   **YES   NO**

4	2-3	FMA

10. Regards Own Hand
Have you seen your baby stare at his own hand for at least 5 seconds?   **YES   NO**

4	3	PS

11. Squeals
Does your baby make happy, excited, high-pitched squealing sounds which are not crying?   **YES   NO**

4-1	2-3	L

12. Bears Weight on Legs
When you stand your baby up, holding her under the arms, does she try to stand on her feet and support some of her own weight?   **YES   NO**

4-1	3-2	GM

13. Follows 180 Degrees
While your baby is on his back, move your hand from one side to the other above his face. Did your baby watch your hand by turning his head from one side *all the way* to the other side like this picture?   **YES   NO**

4-2	3-3	FMA

(Please turn page)   ©Wm. K. Frankenburg, M.D., 1975, 1986, 1998

SECTION II: SECOND STAGE SCREENING AND COMMON TESTS

Some pediatricians will want to have available developmental screening and assessment tools that are more expansive, detailed, or specific. Many others will see the results of such tests in reports on patients they send for referral and would like to know about these tools. Research in this area may use some of these as outcome measures or predictor variables.

Some of these tools are described below along with the amount of training generally needed.

- **MacArthur Communicative Developmental Inventories (CDI):** Detailed parent questionnaire of language competencies, including gestures, comprehension, production, complexity, and semantics. Two forms: infant—3 to 16 months; toddler—17 to 30 months. Spanish and Italian forms normed in these populations. Gives percentiles on dimensions based on large norming sample. Age equivalent may be reported for delayed language. (Development Psychology Lab, Department of Psychology, San Diego State University, San Diego, CA 92182)
- **Achenbach Child Behavior Check List (CBCL):** Parent questionnaire of behavioral concerns. Ages 2 to 3 and 4 to 18. Deviant scores for internalizing and externalizing scores. Teacher forms also available. (Center for Children, Youth and Families, University of Vermont, 1 South Prospect Street, Burlington, VT 05401)
- **ANSER:** Very detailed parent and teacher questionnaires used to characterize behavior and attentional and learning concerns. Formal scoring in research settings. Often used clinically as an inventory of concerns.
- **Bayley Scales of Infant Development (BSID)** editions 1 and 2: Developmental test of children ages birth to 36 months on mental and motor scales. Yields quotient scores for age, the MDI (Mental Development Index), and PDI (Performance Development Index). Behavioral record component yields good observations collected during the assessment. Training required. An abbreviated form using a subset of items is now available. (The Psychological Corporation, Harcourt Brace Jovanovich)
- **Beery Developmental Test of Visual-Motor Integration (VMI):** Hand-eye coordination in figure drawing. An expansion of the simple figure copying presented in Chapter 24. Gives an age equivalent. Minimal training and familiarization. Ages 3 to 18 (adult). (Modern Curriculum Press, 13900 Prospect Road, Cleveland, OH 44136)
- **Peabody Picture Vocabulary Test–Revised (PPVT-R):** A series of pictures of increasing difficulty shown to child to establish language age level. Ages 22 months to adult (33+ years). Yields a language score. Familiarization and cultural issues may alter the results somewhat. Some training required. (American Guidance Service, Circle Pines, MN 55041-1796)
- **Revised Developmental Screening Inventory (Knobloch):** An adaptation of the Gesell schedules, designed for use in risk populations ages 4 weeks to 36 months. Yields a performance level in each of five areas. A Developmental Quotient is reported by area and an overall classification of normal, questionable, or abnormal is presented, weighted to motor performance. Some training required. (Developmental Evaluation Materials, Inc., Department of Pediatrics, Albany Medical College, Albany, NY 12208)
- **Hawaii Early Learning Profile (HELP):** Developmental screening for early childhood, curriculum based. Divided by area, showing progression. Good to use as a base for indi-

vidual intervention. Ages birth to 3 years. Less useful in population studies. Form itself is seen as an intervention. Familiarization and some training required. (VORT Corporation, PO Box 60132, Palo Alto, CA 94306)
- **Battelle Developmental Inventory Screening Test:** Measures developmental competency for ages 6 months to 8 years in five areas. Yields age competency in each area assessed. Moderate training required. Takes 30 to 45 minutes; really a lot more than a screening.
- **Einstein Assessment of School-Related Skills (EASRS):** Grade level brief achievement screenings. Examiner forms script the directions, so little training is needed. (Modern Curriculum Press, 13900 Prospect Road, Cleveland, OH 44136)

For psychologists or those with special training to administer:
- **Wechsler Intelligence Scale for Children (WISC):** Standard intelligence test. Yields verbal, performance, and full scale or overall IQ measurement with 100 as the norm for age. Subscale scores are also reported to identify any existing discrepancies. Fully trained psychologist required. Ages 6 to 16.
- **Wechsler Preschool Primary Scale of Intelligence–Revised (WPPSI-R):** Ages 3 to 7. Yields IQ measures, full, performance, and verbal.
- **Leiter Test of Nonverbal Intelligence:** Individual test to evaluate nonverbally mediated skills. Useful when there is a known language impairment. Fully trained psychologist required.
- **Wide Range Achievement Test (WRAT):** A measure of what a child knows in several academic areas. A reflection of learning, not necessarily ability. Discrepancy between ability and achievement defines learning difficulties in many school jurisdictions.
- **Woodcock Johnson Psychoeducational Battery–Revised:** Gives performance levels in basic academic areas. Ages 2 to adult.
- **Neonatal Behavioral Assessment Scale (NBAS):** A measure of neonatal behavior on 27 dimensions with a 9-point scale for each. Scores are reported by item and are clustered into three to four dimensions from worrisome to optimal. Valid from birth to 30 days old. Adaptations available for preterm infants. Strict training required for research use. Clinical adaptations of parts of the assessment are useful.
- **School Based Achievement Tests.** Group-administered measure of what a child has learned and can put down in the timed test situation. Multiple tests:
  —California Achievement Tests
  —Iowa Test of Basic Skills
  —Stanford Achievement Test
  —ACT Proficiency Examination
  —Comprehensive Test of Basic Skills

SECTION III: A PEDIATRICIAN'S BOOK SHELF

Recommended Readings for pediatricians and other primary care clinicians who care for children and adolescents.

The authors/editors have found the following books to be insightful and clinically useful in their own development as pediatricians; they are part of the "classics" in this field. They are recommended for those who choose to explore the wide range of behaviors and developmental issues in children that are beyond the scope of this book.

Brazelton TB: *Infants and mothers: individual differences in development*, New York, 1969, Delacourt.

Bronfenbrenner U: *The ecology of human development: experiments by nature and design*, Cambridge, Mass, 1979, Harvard University Press.

Erikson EH: *Childhood and society*, ed 2, New York, 1963, WW Norton & Co.

Fraiberg S: *The magic years: understanding and handling the problems of early childhood*, New York, 1959, Scribner.

Freud A: *Normality and pathology in childhood: assessments of development*, New York, 1965, International Universities Press.

Illingsworth RS: *The development of the infant and young child: normal and abnormal*, London, 1960, Livingstone.

Kagan J: *The nature of the child*, New York, 1984, McGraw-Hill.

Spock B, Parker S: *Dr. Spock's baby and child care*, ed 7, New York, 1998, Pocket Books.

Thomas A, Chess S: *Temperament and development*, New York, 1977, Brunner Mazel.

Werner EE: *Cross-cultural child development: a view from planet earth*, Monterey, Calif, 1979, Brooks-Cole Publishing.

Whiting B, Whiting JWM: *Children of six cultures: a psychocultural analysis*, Cambridge, Mass, 1975, Harvard University Press.

Winnicott DW: *The child, the family and the outside world*, Reading, Mass, 1987, Perseus Books.

SECTION IV: PARENT AND CHILD GUIDES FOR PEDIATRIC VISITS

The Parent and Child Guides to Pediatric Visits can be filled out by parents and older children and adolescents before a health supervision visit. They are intended to inform parents and kids about normal aspects of development, as well as provide a checklist for concerns about behavior, development, and other areas of health care. The guides were developed by the American Academy of Pediatrics and are published in the appendix of *Guidelines for Health Supervision III*. They are available from the American Academy of Pediatrics, Publications Department, 141 Northwest Point Blvd., PO Box 927, Elk Grove Village, IL 60009-0927 (phone: 888-227-1770; fax: 847-228-1281).

Children 6 TO 11 YEARS OLD

In the past year or two you have learned a lot of new information and skills, both at home and at school. You can now do more on your own and you probably are involved in a lot of activities. You may have discovered new people and new experiences that are important to you.

You are also becoming able to make good decisions about your health and safety. For example, you can remember to *wear your helmet* when you are riding your bike, *buckle up your seat* belts anytime you ride in a car, *brush your teeth, eat nutritious foods, and avoid alcohol and tobacco use.* You can also let your doctor know how you are feeling, and ask any questions you have about your health, your friends, school, your family, or experiences you have had.

It would be helpful if you could take a few minutes now to think about what things you would like to discuss during your visit with your doctor today. The following list is intended to give you a few suggestions.

What is one thing you are proud of about yourself?

Please put a check (✔) by all areas you would like to discuss:

_____ 1. Your general health, or particular symptoms or concerns

_____ 2. Your physical growth

_____ 3. Questions about any aspect of your medical care or what will happen at today's visit

_____ 4. Your school work

_____ 5. Sports and other activities

_____ 6. Urinating or having bowel movements

_____ 7. Your appetite or diet

_____ 8. Your sleeping

_____ 9. Your energy or activity level

_____ 10. How you get along with other children

_____ 11. How you get along with your brothers and sisters

_____ 12. How you get along with your mother and father

_____ 13. Any aches and pains you have frequently

_____ 14. Any things you have been worrying about

_____ 15. Any injuries you have had

_____ 16. The effects of tobacco, alcohol, and other drugs of abuse

Are there any *other* concerns you would like to be able to talk about with the doctor or nurse?

Your name:

Today's date:

Date of birth:

Parent(s)' name(s):

Other people in the household:

Guide to Pediatric Visits

Younger Adolescents 11 TO 15 YEARS OLD

As an adolescent, during your visits to the pediatrician, you will have the opportunity to meet with the doctor or nurse to talk confidentially about issues that concern you.

It is common for young adolescents to have concerns about their rapid physical growth and sexual development (puberty). It is important to feel accepted among your peers over standards for dress, recreation, behavior, and values. Adolescents experiment with many risk-taking behaviors. Conflicts with parents over issues of independence are common.

During these visits, you may bring up for discussion anything that concerns you. Some issues that commonly worry children and teenagers are listed below. Be assured that confidentiality will be maintained unless the doctor or nurse is concerned that you are going to hurt yourself or someone else.

What are some of the things that make you feel proud of yourself?

Please put a check (✔) by all areas you would like to discuss:

_____ 1. Any health issue, specific symptom or concern

_____ 2. Your eating or weight

_____ 3. Sleeping pattern and routines

_____ 4. Bowel and urine elimination

_____ 5. For girls — menstrual history (regularity/length of period/pain) For boys — "nocturnal emissions" (wet dreams)

_____ 6. School grades

_____ 7. Any problems with school

_____ 8. Sports, hobbies, or other activities

_____ 9. Your friends

_____ 10. Interactions with your brothers and sisters

_____ 11. Interactions with your parent(s)

_____ 12. Responsibilities at home, chores, household rules

_____ 13. Feelings of sadness, mood changes

_____ 14. Worrying a lot

_____ 15. Trouble concentrating

_____ 16. Frequent aches and pains

_____ 17. Feeling angry or hopeless

_____ 18. Taking unnecessary risks

_____ 19. Use of tobacco or alcohol

_____ 20. Other drugs

_____ 21. Sexual activity, contraceptives, sexually transmitted diseases

_____ 22. Your sexual orientation

_____ 23. Fears

_____ 24. Family problems, such as money problems, violence, alcohol or other drug abuse, conflicts between parents or separation

_____ 25. Death or illness of a family member

_____ 26. Any trauma or abuse you have experienced

Are there any *other* concerns you would like to be able to talk about with the doctor or nurse?

Your name: _____   Today's date: _____

Date of birth: _____

Parent(s)' name(s): _____

Other people in the household: _____

Older Adolescents 16 TO 21 YEARS OLD

As an older adolescent, we would like to acknowledge your individuality by examining you without your parents present. We promise you confidentiality. We will inform your parents about our discussions only if you are doing or thinking things that pose a serious risk to yourself or to others. We may encourage you to discuss some issues openly with your family. We can brainstorm with you about how to do this.

During these years, teens typically show increasing intellectual, moral, social, and emotional independence. You may have substituted your own or your friends' standards for your family's value system. You may be experimenting with behaviors that put you at physical, psychological, or social risk. Many teens develop intimate relationships during this age and begin thinking about sexual activity. The possibility of conflict within the family increases in this period.

It would be helpful if you could take a few minutes to think about what things you would like to discuss during your visit today; the following list is intended to offer a few suggestions.

What are you happy about or proud of in yourself?

Please put a check (✔) by all areas you would like to discuss:

_____ 1. Your overall health, or specific symptoms or concerns

_____ 2. Your physical development or stage of puberty

_____ 3. Menstrual patterns or problems

_____ 4. Your social and emotional needs

_____ 5. Appetite, eating patterns, or nutrition

_____ 6. Your sleeping patterns

_____ 7. Emotional problems, such as depression or anxiety

_____ 8. Family problems, such as money problems, violence, alcohol or other drug use, separation or divorce

_____ 9. Communication patterns in your family

_____ 10. Problems with your parents

_____ 11. Any problems at school

_____ 12. Your school performance

_____ 13. Preparation for future education or job

_____ 14. Sports participation

_____ 15. Your friends and peer group

_____ 16. Angry or irritable moods

_____ 17. Smoking

_____ 18. Fears or anxiety you may have

19. Alcohol use

_____ 20. Use of other drugs

_____ 21. Your sexual orientation

_____ 22. Your sexual activity

_____ 23. Unsafe, high-risk activities or practices

_____ 24. Immunizations required at this age

_____ 25. Special screening tests

_____ 26. Any abuse or trauma you have experienced

_____ 27. Planning for job or further education

Are there any *other* concerns you would like to be able to talk about with the doctor or nurse?

Your name: _____ Today's date: _____

Date of birth: _____

Parent(s)' name(s): _____

Other people in the household: _____

Infants BIRTH TO 12 MONTHS

Children do best when their parent(s) and their doctors and nurses *work together* to observe them, listen to them, and understand them.

Your first year with your baby is one of the most exciting and important times you will have. It can also be one of the hardest. All babies are different. Perfectly healthy babies have different styles and schedules for eating, sleeping, reacting to noise and touch, and calming themselves when they get upset. Some babies will be very active, and some will seem more calm. Most will enjoy being cuddled, but some will feel more comfortable when they are not held so much. As you watch your baby, you will become the expert on what he or she does more easily, and what your baby needs more help with. Your doctor and nurse can help you with ways to make feeding, sleeping, and discovering the world go well. However, they will need to rely on your report of how your baby does things and what will work best in your household.

As babies grow, they become more regular about when and how long they sleep, when and how they eat, and how they react to you and other important people in their world. You should see signs that your baby hears even soft sounds and sees light and faces. Your baby may turn toward them, watch them, smile at them, and even imitate them. As your baby grows, you will see him or her lifting his/her head, pushing his/her upper body up, and even holding himself/ herself up to sit — all so she/he can do even more to see you and the sights and sounds around him/ her. If you have a "gut feeling" that there is something wrong or unusual about the way your baby does these things, be sure to talk to your pediatrician about it. Any observation or concern you have is important, and discussing it may help you do even more to help your baby.

It would be helpful if you could take a few minutes to think about what things you would like to discuss during your visit today; the following list is intended to offer a few suggestions.

What are you enjoying most about your baby?

Please put a check (✔) by all areas you would like to discuss:

_____ 1. The baby's health, specific symptoms or concerns

_____ 2. Questions about shots (immunizations) the baby needs

_____ 3. Vision, and how the baby reacts to things she/he sees

_____ 4. Hearing, and how the baby reacts to things she/he hears

_____ 5. How it feels to hold the baby — does she/he feel "tense" or "floppy" or in any way uncomfortable?

_____ 6. When the baby sleeps and for how long

_____ 7. What the baby eats and how often

_____ 8. How active and alert the baby seems to be

_____ 9. Concerns about spoiling the baby

_____ 10. Questions about when the baby might do new things, like sitting or talking

_____ 11. The baby's moods

_____ 12. Questions about bathing or diapering the baby

_____ 13. Questions about child care

_____ 14. Questions about how brothers or sisters interact with the baby

_____ 15. Recovery from pregnancy; questions about family planning or avoiding another pregnancy

_____ 16. Death or illness of a family member

_____ 17. Depression or other psychological problems in a family member

_____ 18. Any accidental injury, trauma, or abuse the child or a parent may have experienced

_____ 19. Other family problems, such as money problems, violence, alcohol, or other drug abuse, conflict between parents, or separation

Are there any *other* concerns you would like to be able to talk about with the doctor or nurse?

Child's name: _____   Today's date: _____

Date of birth: _____

Your name: _____

Your relationship to child: _____

Other people in the household: _____

HE0221

Toddlers 12 TO 36 MONTHS

Children do best when their parent(s) and their doctors and nurses *work together* to observe them, listen to them, and understand them.

The toddler years are fascinating, exciting, and challenging for parents and children alike. Children are learning to do so many new things so quickly — to walk, to talk, to use the toilet, and to play with other children! They are learning to be more independent and to "have a mind of their own." Children are more and more interested in looking at books and having stories read to them as they advance through the toddler period.

Most parents of toddlers have seen a tantrum, and have had experience with a child who refused to cooperate. Some parents are surprised at how angry they feel under these circumstances. Discussing these issues with family members, friends, or physicians may help parents to think about their preferred approach to discipline.

It would be helpful if you could take a few minutes to think about what things you would like to discuss during your visit today; the following list is intended to offer a few suggestions.

What are you enjoying most about your child at this age?

Please put a check (✔) by all areas you would like to discuss:

_____ 1. The child's health, specific symptoms or concerns

_____ 2. Questions about necessary screening tests or immunizations

_____ 3. Vision or hearing

_____ 4. Appetite or eating patterns

_____ 5. Sleeping patterns and routines, naps

_____ 6. The child's energy or activity level

_____ 7. The child's overall development

_____ 8. The child's ability to speak and be understood

_____ 9. The child's ability to walk, run, climb

_____ 10. Toilet training

_____ 11. Good ways to discipline

_____ 12. Temper tantrums

_____ 13. Fears

_____ 14. How the child behaves with adults

_____ 15. How the child behaves with other children

_____ 16. How the child plays; good ideas for toys and activities

_____ 17. Child care or preschool

_____ 18. The child's relationship with brothers or sisters

_____ 19. Death or illness of a family member

_____ 20. Depression or other psychological problems in a family member

_____ 21. Other family problems, such as money problems, violence, alcohol or other drug abuse, conflicts between parents, or separation

_____ 22. Any trauma or abuse the child may have experienced

_____ 23. Any issues about your own childhood that you think may affect your parenting

Are there any *other* concerns you would like to be able to talk about with the doctor or nurse?

Child's name:

Date of birth:

Your name:

Your relationship to child:

Other people in the household:

Today's date:

HE0222

Preschool Children 3 TO 5 YEARS OLD

Children do best when their parent(s) and their doctors and nurses *work together* to observe them, listen to them, and understand them.

The preschool years are busy and exciting times for both parents and children. Children now want to do more and more things for themselves and need help to learn the best ways to dress and feed themselves, take care of bathing and toileting needs, and to explore and play safely. Often they feel "big" enough to try things on their own, but they still need a lot of teaching, supervision, and limits. They are beginning to understand some important learning concepts — numbers, letters, sounds, colors, and shapes. They also are beginning to consider concepts of how to get along — waiting, politeness, sharing, helping, resting. They may be having important experiences of "leaving home" for preschool or recreation activities. There are many differences in how quickly children learn at this age, and their attitudes and interests may be different from those of their brothers, sisters, and friends. They and their parents are learning together about their special skills, interests, and personalities.

It would be helpful if you could take a few minutes to think about what things you would like to discuss during your visit today; the following list is intended to offer a few suggestions.

What are you enjoying most about your child at this age?

Please put a check (✔) by all areas you would like to discuss:

_____ 1. The child's health, specific symptoms or concerns

_____ 2. Questions about necessary screening tests or immunizations

_____ 3. Vision or hearing

_____ 4. Appetite or eating patterns

_____ 5. Sleeping patterns and routines, naps

_____ 6. The child's overall development

_____ 7. The child's ability to speak and be understood

_____ 8. The child's ability to walk, run, and climb

_____ 9. The child's ability to draw, play with blocks and puzzles

_____ 10. The child's energy or activity level

_____ 11. Fears

_____ 12. The child's ability to pay attention to directions or tasks

_____ 13. Toilet training

_____ 14. Sexual behavior or masturbation

_____ 15. Temper tantrums

_____ 16. Good ways to discipline

_____ 17. Child care or preschool arrangements, plans for kindergarten

_____ 18. How the child plays; good ideas for toys and activities

_____ 19. How the child behaves with adults

_____ 20. How the child behaves with other children

_____ 21. The child's relationship with brothers or sisters

_____ 22. Death or illness of a family member

_____ 23. Depression or other psychological problems in a family member

_____ 24. Other family problems, such as money problems, violence, alcohol or other drug abuse, conflicts between parents, or separation

_____ 25. Any trauma or abuse the child may have experienced

_____ 26. Any issues from your childhood that you think may affect your parenting

Are there any *other* concerns you would like to be able to talk about with the doctor or nurse?

Child's name:

Today's date:

Date of birth:

Your name:

Your relationship to child:

Other people in the household:

HE0223

Parents' Guide to Pediatric Visits

School-age Children 6 TO 11 YEARS OLD

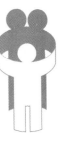

Throughout the school years, children are becoming increasingly independent individuals. They are rapidly obtaining new skills, knowledge, and interests. Experiences outside of the home contribute increasingly to their psychological and social growth. During this period, children become increasingly able to make important decisions that influence their health.

The health supervision of school-age children includes attention to their physical, psychological, and social well-being. Health supervision visits provide opportunities to help children gain knowledge about their health and bodies and feel growing responsibility for making healthy decisions. For this reason, it is often helpful for children to be involved directly in discussions during these visits.

It would be helpful if you could take a few minutes to think about what things you would like to discuss during your visit today; the following list is intended to offer a few suggestions.

What are you enjoying most about your child at this age?

Please put a check (✔) by all areas you would like to discuss:

_____ 1. The child's general health, including specific symptoms or concerns

_____ 2. Physical growth and development

_____ 3. Questions about necessary screening tests, immunizations, or the physical examination

_____ 4. Gross- or fine-motor skills

_____ 5. The child's ability to communicate

_____ 6. Bowel and bladder function

_____ 7. Appetite or diet

_____ 8. Sleeping patterns and difficulties

_____ 9. Energy or activity level

_____ 10. Mood (sad, angry, hopeless)

_____ 11. Discipline strategies

_____ 12. School performance or adjustment

_____ 13. School absences

_____ 14. Fears

_____ 15. How the child gets along with other children

_____ 16. How the child interacts with adults

_____ 17. The child's interests and activities

_____ 18. Frequent aches and pains

_____ 19. Questions about sexuality

_____ 20. Annoying habits (like biting nails, sucking thumb)

_____ 21. The child's ability to deal with frustrations

_____ 22. The child's ability to be independent

_____ 23. Attention span

_____ 24. Child care or after-school arrangements

_____ 25. Relationship among family members

_____ 26. Death or illness of a family member

_____ 27. Depression or other psychological difficulties in a family member

_____ 28. Other family stresses (like employment issues, money problems, violence, alcohol or other drug use, conflicts between parents, separation)

_____ 29. Any trauma or abuse the child may have experienced

_____ 30. Any issues from your own childhood that you think might affect your parenting

Are there any *other* concerns you would like to be able to talk about with the doctor or nurse?

Child's name:	Today's date:
Date of birth:	
Your name:	
Your relationship to child:	
Other people in the household:	

HE0224

Parents' Guide to Pediatric Visits

Younger Adolescents 11 TO 15 YEARS OLD

As children mature, they become much more interested in and capable of assuming responsibility for their own health needs. They show increased concern with their developing body and compare themselves with peers to reassure themselves that they are "normal." Psychological and social independence is increasing, and often teenagers begin to show unwillingness to participate in some family activities. They concentrate instead on peer relationships and social activities. Their social and emotional life can greatly influence their physical health. Risk-taking behaviors are more commonly observed during these years. Early adolescence may be a particularly trying time for both parents and adolescents.

During these years, it becomes appropriate to emphasize the opportunity for adolescent-initiated visits and confidential discussion/examination without a parent present. It is also important for the parent(s) to speak with the pediatrician alone to communicate your observations and concerns.

What are some of the things that make you especially proud of your adolescent?

Please put a check (✔) by all areas you would like to discuss:

_____ 1. Health, specific symptoms or concerns

_____ 2. Appetite, eating habits, nutrition

_____ 3. Physical growth and development

_____ 4. Sexual development, sexual behavior, or sexual orientation

_____ 5. Sleeping patterns and routines

_____ 6. School performance this year (grades, frequency of absences)

_____ 7. Participation in sports

_____ 8. Friendships/response to peer pressures

_____ 9. Relationships with brothers and sisters

_____ 10. Interactions with parent(s)

_____ 11. Disciplinary methods, privileges, chores

_____ 12. Communicating feelings and concerns

_____ 13. Sadness, depression

_____ 14. Use of tobacco, alcohol, or illicit drugs

_____ 15. Family problems, such as money problems, violence, alcohol or other drug abuse, conflicts between parents or separation

_____ 16. Death or illness of a family member

_____ 17. Any trauma or abuse the adolescent may have experienced

_____ 18. Any particular fears

_____ 19. Your experience as a teenager and the impact it has on your parenting

Are there any *other* concerns you would like to be able to talk about with the doctor or nurse?

Adolescent's name:

Date of birth:

Your name:

Your relationship to adolescent:

Other people in the household:

Today's date:

Older Adolescents 16 TO 21 YEARS OLD

Adolescents 16 to 21 years of age typically show increasing intellectual, moral, social, and emotional independence. Many teenagers substitute their own or their friends' standards for their family's value system. They may experiment with behaviors that put them at physical, psychological, or social risk. They enter into intimate relationships. Parents are excited and challenged by these developments. Conflicts within the family may occur during this period.

Adolescents do best when their parents and their doctors and nurses respect their autonomy and offer nonjudgmental support and advice. We demonstrate our respect for teenagers by examining them without their parents present and by promising them confidentiality. We want to assure you we will inform you if your adolescent poses a serious risk to himself or herself or to others. We will answer your questions as completely as possible without violating confidentiality. We usually encourage adolescents to discuss issues openly with their families.

It would be helpful if you could take a few minutes to think about what things you would like to discuss during your visit today; the following list is intended to offer a few suggestions.

What are you enjoying most about your adolescent at this age?

Please put a check (✔) by all areas you would like to discuss:

_____ 1. Your adolescent's overall health, or specific symptoms or concerns

_____ 2. Physical growth, development, or stage of puberty

_____ 3. Menstrual patterns or problems

_____ 4. Psychological and social development

_____ 5. Appetite, eating patterns, or nutrition

_____ 6. Sleeping patterns

_____ 7. Emotional outbursts or withdrawal

_____ 8. Evidence of depression or anxiety

_____ 9. Conflicts in the family

_____ 10. Family problems, such as money problems, violence, alcohol or other drug use, separation or divorce

_____ 11. School attendance or performance

_____ 12. Stealing or taking things that do not belong to him/her

_____ 13. Sports participation

_____ 14. Fears

_____ 15. Friends and peer group

_____ 16. Angry or irritable moods

_____ 17. Smoking

_____ 18. Alcohol use

_____ 19. Use of other drugs

_____ 20. Sexual orientation

_____ 21. Sexual activity

_____ 22. Unsafe activities or practices

_____ 23. Immunizations required at this age

_____ 24. Special screening tests

_____ 25. Any trauma or abuse

_____ 26. Planning for job or further education

Are there any *other* concerns you would like to be able to talk about with the doctor or nurse?

Adolescent's name:

Date of birth:

Your name:

Your relationship to adolescent:

Other people in the household:

Today's date:

HE0226

INDEX

---

* References with "t" denote tables; "f" denote
figures; "b" denote boxes

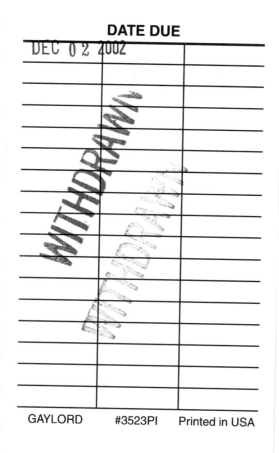